Drugs and Society

Fifth Edition

Glen Hanson

Department of Pharmacology and Toxicology
University of Utah
Salt Lake City, Utah

Peter J. Venturelli

Department of Sociology
Valparaiso University
Valparaiso, Indiana

JONES AND BARTLETT PUBLISHERS

Sudbury, Massachusetts

Boston   London   Singapore

Editorial, Sales, and Customer Service Offices
Jones and Bartlett Publishers
40 Tall Pine Drive
Sudbury, MA 01776
978-443-5000
info@jbpub.com
http://www.jbpub.com

Jones and Bartlett Publishers International
Barb House, Barb Mews
London W6 7PA
UK

Library of Congress Cataloging-in-Publication Data
Hanson, Glen, (Glen R.)
    Drugs and Society/Glen Hanson, Peter J. Venturelli,
    Peter L. Myers. — 5th ed.
    p. cm.
    Includes bibliographical references and index.
    ISBN 0-7637-0291-9
    1. Drugs. 2. Drugs—Toxicology. 3. Drug abuse.
        I. Venturelli, Peter J. II. Myers, Peter L. III. Title.
    RM301.W58 1997
615'.1—DC21   97-19862
                                                                      CIP

Acquisitions Editor: Joseph E. Burns
Developmental Editor: Maxine Effenson Chuck
Production Editor: Nindy LeRoy
Design, Art, Editorial and Electronic Production Service:
    Thompson Steele Production Services
Cover Design: Marshall Hendrichs
Cover Photographs: *(top)* © John Lei, Stock Boston / PNI;
    (lower left) © Jim Leavitt, Impact Visuals / PNI; *(lower
    right)* © Bob Daemmrich, Stock Boston / PNI;
    (middle) © Dan Habib, Impact Visuals / PNI
Cover Printer: Coral Graphics
Printer and Binder: World Color

Printed in the United States of America
01 00 99 98 97   10 9 8 7 6 5 4 3 2 1

Brief Contents

Detailed Contents

Chapter 5
How and Why Drugs Work   110

Chapter 6
Homeostatic Systems and Drugs 136

Chapter 7
CNS Depressants:
Sedative-Hypnotics   158

Preface

Drugs and Society is intended to convey to students the impact of drug use and/or abuse on the lives of ordinary people. The authors have combined their expertise in the fields of drug abuse, pharmacology and sociology with their extensive experiences in research, teaching, and drug-policy implementation to improve this fifth edition over the previous four versions of this book. To make the fifth edition of *Drugs and Society* an exceptional text on drug-related problems, this book is written at a more personal level and directly addresses college students by incorporating personal experiences and attitudes throughout the chapters. This significant improvement makes *Drugs and Society* truly unique. The approach was implemented in response to suggestions from readers and instructors to further stimulate students' comprehension and assimilation of this information.

Drugs and Society was written to assist university students from a wide range of disciplines to gain a realistic perspective of drug-related problems in our society. Students in nursing, physical education and other health sciences, psychology, social work, and sociology will find that our text provides useful current information and perspectives to help them understand:

1. why and how drug abuse occurs;

2. the results of drug abuse;

3. how to prevent drug abuse;

4. how drugs can be used effectively for therapeutic purposes.

To achieve this goal, we have presented the most current and authoritative views on drug abuse in an objective and easily understood manner. To help students appreciate the multifaceted nature of drug-related problems, this edition exposes readers to drug abuse issues from pharmacological, psychological and sociological perspectives. Besides including the most current information concerning drug abuse topics, each chapter also includes helpful learning aids for students. These include:

▲ *Fighting the Drug War* Vignettes intended to help the readers assess governmental efforts to deal with drug-related problems.

▲ *Finding a Balance* These short essays by Brian Luke Seaward present creative ways of dealing with personal problems that help students see that there are effective alternatives to drugs.

▲ *Case in Point* Examples of relevant clinical issues that arise from the use of each major group of drugs discussed.

▲ *Exercises for the Web* Questions based on information available in identified web sites. These exercises guide students' access to constantly updated web material on drug use and abuse, and encourage students to research organizations or groups which have relevance to the topics of the associated chapter.

▲ *Here and Now* Current events that illustrate the personal and social consequences of drug abuse issues.

▲ *Highlighted definitions* Definitions of new terminology. These are conveniently located adjacent to their discussion in the text throughout the chapters.

▲ *Learning objectives* Goals for learning identified at the beginning of each chapter to help students identify the principal concepts being taught.

▲ *Summary statements* Concise summaries found at the end of each chapter which correlate with the learning objectives mentioned above.

▲ *Chapter questions* Provocative questions at the end of each chapter. These encourage

students to discuss, ponder, and critically analyze their own feelings and biases about the information presented in the book.

▲ *Concise and well-organized tables and figures*
Updated features found throughout the book
present the latest information to students in an
easily understood format.

▲ *New color photographs and drawings* These
additions graphically illustrate important concepts and facilitate comprehension as well as
retention of information.

Because of these new and updated features, we
believe that this edition of *Drugs and Society* is
much more "user friendly" than the previous editions and will encourage student learning and motivation.

The new topical coverage in the fifth edition of
Drugs and Society includes:

▲ Extensive, updated material and references
with many citations from studies published
between 1994 and 1997

▲ New material on drug use and abuse within
college student and the entertainment subcultures, including an example of how a new
media subculture promotes drug use.

▲ New and updated information on positive
wellness and the holistic health approach to
drug use.

The material in the text encompasses biomed-
ical, sociological and social-psychological views.

Beginning with Chapter 1, *Drugs and Society*
introduces an overview: the current dimensions of
drug use (statistics and trends) and the most commonly abused drugs at the turn of the century.
Chapter 2 comprehensively explains drug use and
abuse from a theoretical standpoint. The latest biological, psychological, social-psychological and
sociological perspectives are explained. Chapter 3
discusses how the law deals with drug use and/or
abuse of both licit (alcohol, OTC and prescription) and illicit (marijuana, hallucinogens and cocaine) drugs. Chapter 4 focuses on addictive
behavior and treating drug dependence. Chapter 5
instructs students about the factors that determine
how drugs affect the body. This chapter details the

physiological and psychological variables that determine how and why people respond to drugs
used for therapeutic and recreational purposes.
Because the addicting properties of most, if not
all, substances of abuse are due to the effects of
drugs on the reward centers of the brain, chapter 6
helps the student understand the basic biochemical operations of the nervous and endocrine systems and explains how psychoactive drugs and
anabolic steroids alter such functions.

Chapters 7 through 14 deal with specific drug
groups that are commonly abused in this country.
Those drugs which depress brain activity are discussed in chapters 7 (sedative/hypnotic agents), 8
and 9 (alcohol), and 11 (opioid narcotics). The
drugs which stimulate brain activity are covered in
chapters 10 (amphetamines, cocaine, and caffeine)
and 12 (tobacco and nicotine). The last main category of substances of abuse is the hallucinogens.
Such drugs alter the senses and create dreamlike
and/or distorted experiences. These substances are
discussed in chapters 13 (hallucinogens such as
LSD, mescaline, and PCP) and 14 (marijuana). Although most drugs that are abused cause more
than one effect (for example, cocaine can be a
stimulant and a hallucinogen), the classification
we have chosen for this text is frequently used by
experts and pharmacologists in the drug abuse
field and is based on the drug effect that is most
likely to predominate following abuse. All of the
chapters in this section are similarly organized.
They discuss the historical origins and evolution
of the agents so students can better understand society's attitudes toward, and regulation of, these
drugs. Previous and current clinical uses of these
drugs are discussed to help students appreciate
distinctions between therapeutic use and abuse.
Next, the patterns of abuse of these substances and
special features which contribute to their abuse
potential are discussed. Finally, non-medicinal
and medicinal therapies for drug-related dependence, withdrawal, and abstinence are presented.

Chapter 15 explores the topic of drugs and
therapy. As with illicit drugs of abuse, nonprescription and prescription drugs can be misused if
not understood. This chapter helps the student to
appreciate the uses and benefits of proper drug use
as well as appreciate that legal drugs can also be
problematic.

Chapter 16 explores drug use in five major subcultures: sport/athletic, women, adolescent, college student, HIV-positive and entertainment. Included in this chapter is a discussion of a new media drug subculture that has just recently arisen.

Chapter 17 of *Drugs and Society* acquaints students with the treatment, rehabilitation, and prevention of the major drugs of abuse. This final chapter describes the principal sociological, psychological and pharmacological strategies used to treat and prevent substance abuse and details their advantages and disadvantages. The discussion in this chapter helps students to better understand why drug abuse occurs, how society currently deals with this problem on an individual and group basis, and the likelihood of rehabilitation of persons dependent on these substances.

The Appendix of the fifth edition includes an explanation of federal agencies with drug abuse missions, and elucidates details of important legislative actions which regulate drug availability and proper use. In addition, a detailed description of schedules for drugs of abuse and the penalties for their illicit manufacturing, selling, or administration is presented.

Instructor's Aids

The ancillary package for the fifth edition has been updated to include the most contemporary technology. For instructors who adopt the fifth edition for classroom use, an instructor's CD-ROM is available. Designed for classroom use, this CD contains lecture outlines in PowerPoint format, as well as web simulations. In addition, a revised instructor's manual written by Peter Venturelli is also available. Please call the sales department at Jones and Bartlett for further details.

Acknowledgments

The many improvements that have made this the best edition yet of the *Drugs and Society* series could not have occurred without the hard work and dedication of numerous people.

Peter L. Myers, Ph.D. rewrote several chapters for this edition. He extensively revised the chapters on Alcohol and Social Behavior and on Marijuana, and added many new pages of updated text. He wrote a new Addiction and Treatment chapter for this edition and collaborated on the new chapter on Prevention. Dr. Myers is Professor and Director of the Addiction Counselor Training Program at Essex County College in Newark, NJ and President of the International Coalition of Addiction Studies Educators.

Brian Luke Seaward, Ph.D., of the Center for Human Caring at the University of Colorado, wrote the Finding a Balance boxes. This important feature of the book benefits from his long experience and deep study of coping strategies and holistic approaches to stress management.

Maxine Effenson Chuck provided invaluable suggestions and encouragement with a constant flow of questions and rewrites and kept the project on track throughout its development. Allan K Workman provided valuable pedagogical material and suggestions, and Andrea Pyenson is also gratefully acknowledged for her contributions.

Lianne Ames shepherded the project through its final production stages and made it all come together into a book.

We are indebted to the many reviewers who evaluated the manuscript at different stages of development. Much of the manuscript was reviewed and greatly improved by comments from:

Steven R. Hawks
Utah State University

Larry Reid
Rensselaer Polytechnic Institute

David M. White
East Carolina University

Dan Denson
McNeese State University

Denise Jackson
Northeastern University

John Janowiak
Appalachian State University

Thomas Shapiro
Northeastern University

Linda Evinger
University of Southern Indiana

Joy Himmel
Pennsylvania State University

Patricia B. Baasel
Ohio University

Frederick A. Newton
California State University—San Bernardino

Stephanie Dorgan
Ohio University

Ann Marie Ellis
South West Texas State University

David Mason
Northern Illinois University

James Orcutt
Florida State University

The authors would like to express, once again, their gratitude for the comments and suggestions of users and reviewers of previous editions of *Drugs and Society.*

At Valparaiso University, Professor Venturelli is grateful to students Jaron Theye, Kirsten Smith, George Corsianos, and Shane Blackstone for their tireless assistance and involvement with this fifth edition. Also gratefully acknowledged are the countless other students and working people who were interviewed regarding their views and/or use of drugs. Finally, noteworthy appreciation also goes to Ellen B. Meyer and Alice M. Koby, reference librarians at Valparaiso University's Moellering Library, especially when references were incomplete and deadlines loomed.

At our respective institutions, the authors would like to thank a multitude of people too numerous to list individually but who have given us invaluable assistance.

Dr. Hanson is particularly indebted to his wife, Margaret, for her loving encouragement. Without her patience and support this endeavor would not have been possible.

Drugs and Society

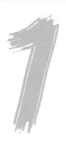

1

Introduction

Drugs and Society

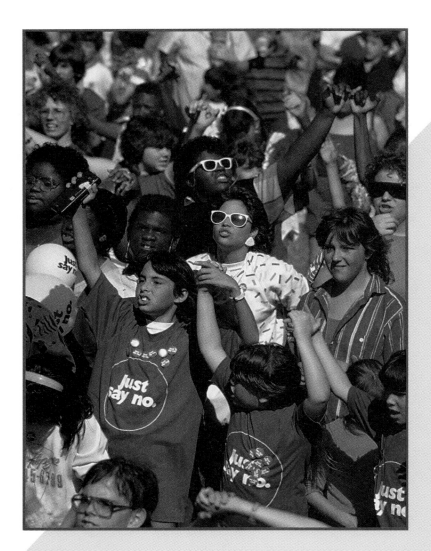

**On completing this chapter
you will be able to:** ▶

- The popular use of legal drugs, particularly alcohol and tobacco, has caused far more deaths, sickness, violent crimes, economic loss, and other social problems than the use of illegal drugs.
- Designer drugs are created for profit and are used as a method for circumventing the laws that make certain substances illegal.
- Attempts to regulate drug use were made as long ago as 2240 B.C.
- Drug use is an "equal-opportunity affliction," meaning that both legal and illegal drugs are consumed in all income, social class, and age groups.
- Approximately 1.5 billion prescriptions for psychoactive drugs are written each year.
- More varieties of drugs are available today. Approximately 80% of all drugs that are currently marketed were either unknown or unavailable 20 years ago.
- The majority of young drug abusers come from homes in which drugs are used extensively.
- In 1995, an estimated 12.8 million Americans were current illicit drug users—that is, they had used an illicit drug in the month prior to their interview. This figure represents 6.1% of the population 12 years old and older.
- The alcohol industry alone spends more than $1 billion annually on advertising.
- Addiction involves five phases that are often independent of one another.
- The majority of illicit drug users are employed. Approximately 70% to 75% of drug users in the United States are employed either full- or part-time; this number represents more than 10 million workers.

Learning Objectives

- Explain how drug use is affected by pharmacological, cultural, social, and contextual factors.
- Recognize the key terms for initially understanding drug use.
- Explain when drugs were first used and under what circumstances.
- Indicate how widespread drug use is and who the potential drug abusers are.
- List four different reasons why drugs are used.
- Rank in descending order, from highest to lowest, the most commonly used licit and illicit drugs.
- Name three types of drug users, and explain how they differ.
- Describe how the mass media promotes drug use.
- Explain when drug use leads to drug abuse.
- List and explain the phases of drug addiction.
- Define employee assistance programs (EAPs) and explain their role in resolving productivity problems.
- Describe the holistic health approach.

Each year the world undergoes a transformation—a form of technological evolution. Technology is driving social change more than ever before. The way people function and interact is constantly in a state of flux. Life is changing so rapidly that a constant pressure is exerted to keep up, stay current, and keep pace with rapid change. To handle this pressure, many people turn to using or abusing drugs. Despite all of our knowledge about the dangers of drug use and abuse, and despite the laws prohibiting such consumption, numerous people use both legal and illegal types of drugs.

Abuse and addiction to any type of drug can happen to anyone. The use of drugs before the onset of potential addiction is easily as seductive and nondiscriminating as its users. Many reasons explain this attraction, as drugs alter body chemistry by interfering with its proper functioning and by altering the reception and transmission of reality. Many would argue that our "reality" would become perilous and unpredictable if people were legally free to dabble in many drugs. Many do not realize, however, that if abused, even legal drugs can alter our perception of reality and become addictive.

In this introductory chapter, we answer some key questions related to drug use:

1. What constitutes a drug?
2. What are the most commonly abused drugs?
3. What are designer drugs?
4. How widespread is drug abuse?
5. What is the extent and frequency of drug use in our society?
6. What are the current statistics on and trends in drug use?
7. What types of drug users exist?
8. How do the mass media influence drug use?
9. What attracts people to drug use?
10. When does drug use lead to drug dependence?
11. When does drug addiction occur?
12. What are the costs of drug addiction to society?
13. What can be gained by learning about the complexity of drug use and abuse?

◢ The Dimensions of Drug Use

To determine the perception of drug use in our country, we asked several interviewees, "What do you think of drug use in our society?" The following are two responses:

> I think it is a big problem, especially when there are so many people doing drugs. Just think how many people are on drugs right now, this very minute, throughout the United States. How many drug users are in the workplace, driving trucks, making investment transactions, and even performing surgery? It's downright horrifying when you think about it. How many kids are not learning much, if anything, in classrooms across the nation because they are flying high while the teacher is talking?
>
> *From Venturelli's research files, 28-year-old female newspaper reporter in a Midwestern city, October 8, 1996*

[Another respondent answering the same question]

> Every effort by the government to stop illegal drug use has failed miserably. Even legal drug use, like alcohol and cigarettes, continues despite what the governmental public health media say. People should be left alone about their drug use unless such drug use is potentially harmful to others. I know that if I ever quit using both legal and illegal drugs it will be my own decision, not because the law can punish me. Yes, drug use is a problem for the addicted, but all throughout our history, drug use has been there. So why worry about it now?
>
> *From Venturelli's research files, 24-year-old male graduate student, October 3, 1996*

These two interviews reflect contrasting attitudes with regard to drug use. The greatest differences of opinion often result from prior socialization experiences, such as family upbringing, peer group relationships, exposure to drug use or drug users, age, and so on.

In its entirety, this book views pharmacological, cultural, social, and contextual issues as the four principal factors responsible for determining how a drug user experiences drug use. These factors are defined as follows:

Pharmacological factors: How the ingredients of a particular drug affect the functions of the body and how the nervous system reacts to the drugs by affecting social behavior.

Cultural factors: How society's views of drug use, as determined by custom and tradition, affect consumption of a particular drug.

Social factors: How the motivation for taking a particular drug is affected by such needs as diminishing physical pain, curing an illness, providing relaxation, relieving stress or anxiety, trying to escape reality, heightening awareness, providing visual, auditory, or sensory distortion, or bolstering confidence. Included in this issue is the belief that drug use develops through the values and attitudes of drug-using communities, subcultures, peer groups, and families, as well as through the extent and quality of users' experiences with personal and social use of drugs.

Contextual factors: How specific contexts define and determine personal dispositions toward drug use, as demonstrated by moods and attitudes about such activity. Specifically, the factors involve the drug-taking social behavior that develops from the physical surroundings where the drug is used. For example, are the drugs taken out-of-doors, in private homes, or at rock concert settings?

Examining the cultural, social, and contextual factors of drug use leads us to explore the sociology and psychology of drug use, while examining the pharmacological factors allows us to explore how drugs affect the body (primarily the central nervous system).

Although the common term for substances that affect both mind and body functioning is popularly called a **drug,** researchers use the term **psychoactive drugs** or **psychoactive substances** because it is more precise in explaining how drugs affect the body. The term *psychoactive drugs* specifically refers to the effect these substances have on the central nervous system and how they alter consciousness and/or perceptions. Because of their effects on the brain, these drugs can be used to treat

> **drug**
> any substance that modifies body functions, such as the nervous system

> **psychoactive drugs or psychoactive substances**
> substances that affect the central nervous system and alter consciousness and/or perceptions

physical or mental illness. Because the body can tolerate increasingly large doses, however, many psychoactive drugs may be used in progressively greater and more uncontrollable amounts. For many substances, a user is at risk of moving from occasional to more regular use, or from moderate use to heavy and chronic use. A chronic user may then risk addiction and withdrawal symptoms whenever the drug is not supplied to the body.

Generally speaking, any substance that modifies the nervous system and states of consciousness is a *drug.* Such modification can enhance, inhibit, or distort the functioning of the body, thus also affecting patterns of behavior and social functioning.

Psychoactive drugs are classified as either **licit** (legal) or **illicit** (illegal). Coffee, tea, cocoa, alcohol, tobacco, and **over-the-counter (OTC)** drugs are licit, or legal substances and, when used in moderation, are usually socially acceptable. Marijuana, cocaine, and LSD are examples of illicit drugs.

> **licit drugs**
> legal drugs, such as coffee, alcohol, and tobacco
>
> **illicit drugs**
> illegal drugs, such as marijuana, cocaine, and LSD. Other commonly used terminology for drug use is highlighted in Table 1.1
>
> **(OTC)**
> over-the-counter drugs

Researchers have made some interesting findings about legal and illegal drug use:

1. The use of such legal substances as alcoholic beverages and tobacco is considerably more common than is the use of illegal drugs such as marijuana, heroin, and LSD. Other legal drugs, such as depressants and stimulants, though less popular than alcohol and tobacco, are still more widely used than heroin and LSD.

2. The popular use of legal drugs, particularly alcohol and tobacco, has caused far more deaths, sickness, violent crimes, economic

loss, and other social problems than the use of illegal drugs.

3. Societal reaction to various drugs changes with time and place. Opium is today an illegal drug and widely condemned as a *pano-pathogen* (a cause of all ills), but in the last two centuries it was a legal drug and was popularly praised as a *panacea* (a cure of all ills). Alcohol use was widespread in the United States in the early 1800s, became illegal during the 1920s, and then was relegalized and has been widely used since the 1930s. In contrast, cigarette smoking is legal in all countries today, but in the seventeenth century it was illegal in most countries and the smoker was harshly punished in some. For example, the penalty for cigarette smoking was having the nose cut off in Russia, lips sliced off in Hindustan (India), and head chopped off in China (Thio 1983, 332–333; Thio 1995).

Marijuana can be grown almost anywhere.

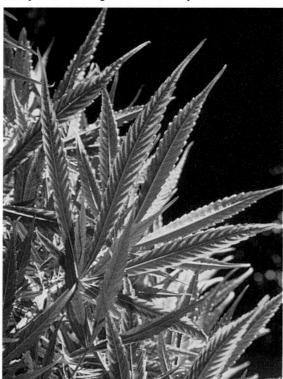

Today, new emphasis in the United States on public health hazards from cigarettes again is leading some people to consider new measures to restrict or even outlaw tobacco smoking.

Table 1.1 introduces some of the terminology that you will encounter throughout this text. It is important that you understand some of the distinctions drawn between the types of drug use and abuse.

Most Commonly Abused Drugs

This book examines the drugs most subject to abuse—those that are taken for pleasure or relief from boredom or stress. The categories that are examined include marijuana, stimulants, hallucinogens, narcotics, depressants, and organic solvents. A brief overview is provided here, and the categories will be discussed in detail throughout this book.

Cannabis, or marijuana and hashish A plant that readily grows in many parts of the world. Marijuana consists of the dried and crushed leaves, flowers, stems, and seeds of the *cannabis sativa* plant. THC (delta 9-tetrahydrocannabinol) is the primary *psychoactive*, mind-altering ingredient in marijuana that produces the euphoria (expressed by those under the influence of this drug as being "high.") Plant parts are usually dried, crushed, and smoked much like tobacco products. Other ways of ingesting marijuana include crushing the leaves into cookie or brownie batter and baking the batter. Hashish is another cannabis derivative that contains the purest form of resin and the highest amount of THC.

Stimulants These substances act on the *central nervous system (CNS)* by increasing alertness, excitation, euphoria, and increased pulse rate and blood pressure. Insomnia and loss of appetite are common outcomes. The user experiences initially pleasant effects, such as a sense of increased energy and a state of euphoria, or "high." Also, users feel restless and talkative and have trouble sleeping. High doses used over the long term can produce personality changes. Stimulants include cocaine (and crack), amphetamines, and caffeine as well as coffee, tea, and tobacco.

Table 1.1	**Commonly Used Terms** Here are some of the most important definitions used for understanding drug use and/or abuse.	

Term	Description
Gateway drugs	The word gateway suggests a path leading to something else. Alcohol, tobacco, and marijuana are the most commonly used drugs. Almost all abusers of more powerfully addictive drugs have first experimented with these three substances.
Medicines	Medicines are used to prevent or treat the symptoms of an illness. They are drugs prescribed by a physician.
Prescription medicines	These drugs are prescribed by a physician. Common examples include drugs prescribed to eliminate drowsiness, stimulation, or relaxation.
Over-the-counter (OTC) drugs	These drugs are sold without a prescription. Recently OTC drugs accounted for "$12 billion a year in retail sales" (Goode 1993, 36). OTC drugs can be purchased at will, without first seeking medical advice. Often these drugs are misused or abused.
Drug misuse	The unintentional or inappropriate use of prescribed or OTC drugs. Misuse includes, but is not limited to, (1) taking more drugs than prescribed, (2) using OTC or psychoactive drugs in excess without medical supervision, (3) mixing drugs with alcohol, (4) using old medicines for self-treating new symptoms of an illness or ailment, (5) discontinuing certain prescribed drugs at will or against a physician's recommendation, and (6) administering prescription drugs to family members without medical consultation and supervision.
Drug abuse	Also known as *chemical* or *substance* abuse. The willful misuse of either licit or illicit drugs for recreation, perceived necessity, or convenience. Drug abuse differs from drug use in that drug *use* is taking or using drugs, while *abuse* is a more intense misuse of drugs, often to the point of addiction.
Drug addiction	Drug addiction involves noncasual or nonrecreational drug use. A frequent symptom includes intense psychological preoccupation with obtaining and consuming drugs. Both physiological and psychological symptoms of withdrawal are often manifested when the craving for the drug is not satisfied. Recently more emphasis has been placed on defining the psychological craving for a drug than on the more biologically based determinants of addiction. (See Chapter 4 for more precise information regarding addiction and the addiction process.)

Hallucinogens These drugs strongly alter perception, thought, and feeling. They most certainly influence the complex inner working of the human mind, causing users to refer to these drugs as psychedelics. Hallucinogens include LSD (lysergic acid diethylamide), mescaline, and peyote.

Depressants These sedative drugs are used to relieve stress and anxiety and, in some cases, to induce sleep. The effects of depressants appeal to many people who are struggling with emotional problems and looking for physical and emotional relief. Because some people turn to these drugs for help in coping with problems, CNS depressants can also cause a host of serious side effects, including problems with tolerance and dependence. Depressants include barbiturates, benzodiazepines (such as Valium), methaqualone (Quaalude), and alcohol (ethanol).

Narcotics   These drugs also depress the CNS. If taken in a high enough quantity, they produce insensibility or stupor. Narcotics include opium, morphine, codeine, and heroin.

Inhalants/organic Solvents   This category of drugs is most often used by younger teenagers. Inhalants include gasoline, airplane glue, and paint thinner. When inhaled, the vapors from these solvents can produce euphoric effects. Organic solvents can also refer to certain foods, herbs, and vitamins, such as "herbal ecstasy."

Appendix D, page 500, lists the most commonly abused drugs in society, outlining their medical uses, trade names, slang terms, physical or psychological dependence, tolerance, duration, usual methods of administration, possible effects, effects of overdose, and withdrawal syndromes. Table 1.2 shows some current "street names" for the substances and processes involved in illicit use of these drugs.

Designer Drugs

In addition to the most commonly abused illicit drug categories described above, innovations in technology have produced new categories known as **"designer" drugs.** These relatively new types are created as **structural analogs** of substances already scheduled as forbidden under the Controlled Substances Act (CSA). The term *structural analogs* refers to drugs that result from altered chemical structures of already existing illicit drugs. Generally, these drugs are prepared by underground chemists, whose goal is to make a profit by creating compounds that mimic the

> **"designer drugs"**
> new categories of hybrid drugs

> **structural analogs**
> drugs that result from altered chemical structures of already illicit drugs. These drugs are produced for profit and mimic effects of controlled substances.

Inhalants. These volatile chemicals, which include many common household substances, are often the most dangerous drug, per dose, a person can take. In addition, inhalants are most often used by young children.

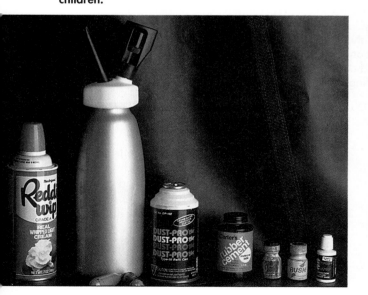

Designer pills made from the illicit drug ecstasy. This drug has some stimulant properties like amphetamines as well as hallucinogenic properties like LSD.

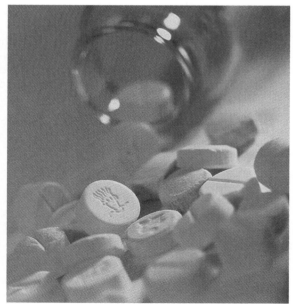

Table 1.2 **Street Terms Relating to Drugs and Drug Use** What slang drug terms do users employ for their drug use in the late 1990s? Below is a sampling of the many different terms used.

Slang Term	What It Means	Slang Term	What It Means
Acapulco gold	A very potent strain of marijuana from Acapulco, Mexico	Lemonade	Poor-quality drugs
Airhead	Under the influence of marijuana	Lid	One ounce or less of marijuana
Alley juice	Very cheap wine, "grapes"	Locker room	Butyl nitrate (inhalant)
Artillery	Equipment for shooting drugs	LSD	Acid, microdots, purple haze, blotters, fry, blaze, tab, dose, gel, pyramid, trips
Bang	To inject narcotics		
Big C	Cocaine		
Big man	Supplier of drugs	Mainliner	A person who injects drugs directly into the vein
Black beauties	Amphetamines		
Black hollies	Amphetamines	Man	Police
Blasted	High on drugs	Manicure	Remove seeds from marijuana
Blotters	LSD	Microdot	A tablet containing LSD
Blunts	A cigar slit open and filled with marijuana	Mule	A carrier of drugs
Bong	A cylindrical water pipe for smoking narcotics, especially marijuana	Papers	Rolling papers that are used to make marijuana or tobacco cigarettes
Brick	One kilogram (2.2 pounds) of tightly compacted marijuana or sometimes hashish; hashish remains rare in the United States but much more prevalent in Europe and in the Middle East	Party	To have a good time using alcohol and other drugs
		Poppers	Amyl nitrate capsules (an inhalant)
		Red devils	Seconal (a barbiturate)
		Reefer	Marijuana
		Roach	The stub of a marijuana cigarette
Buds	Marijuana	Roach clip	Any tweezers-like device used to completely finish smoking a marijuana cigarette stub that is too short to hold in the fingers
Burn	Cheated by a pusher		
Burnout	Heavy user of drugs		
Busted	Arrested on a drug-related charge		
Buttons	Peyote or mushrooms	Rush	An intense surge of pleasure; butyl nitrate inhalant
Candyman	Drug supplier		
Chasing the dragon	A particular way of inhaling heroin	Score	To locate and purchase a quantity of drugs
China white	A very pure white heroin		
Chipping	Occasional use of drugs	Script writer	A doctor willing to write a prescription for faked symptoms
Chippy	A person who uses drugs infrequently		
Coke broke	Financially incapacitated from supporting a cocaine habit	Shotgun	A way of sharing marijuana, by blowing smoke back from someone's lungs into the mouth of another participant so that the exhaled smoke is not "wasted"
Colombo	Marijuana grown in Colombia		
Connect	To purchase drugs		
Crystals	Methamphetamine		
Dexies	Dexadrine, or "dex"	Snow	Cocaine
Dime bag	$10 worth of a narcotic	Snowbird	Dependent on cocaine
Dusting	Sprinkling a narcotic powder on another drug, such as PCP sprinkled on marijuana	Spaced out	Under the influence of drugs
		Speedball	A mixture of cocaine and heroin; "bombita"
Flea powder	Poor-quality drugs		
Freebase	Smoking cocaine from a special water pipe	Spoons	Paraphernalia associated with cocaine, often worn as jewelry
Gluey	A glue sniffer		
Gold	Marijuana, also called Acapulco	Stardust	Cocaine
Goofballs	Barbiturates	Stash	A place where drugs are hidden
Gun	Equipment for injecting drugs	Strung out	Heavily addicted to drugs
Head shop	Store specializing in the sale of drug paraphernalia	Stuff	Drugs
		Superman	LSD blotter with a "Superman" imprint
Heavy burner	A person who smokes a lot of dope; a burnout	Thai sticks	Marijuana laced with opium
		Toot	To sniff cocaine
Hit	A single dose of drugs	Tooter	A small, hollow tube (straw-like) used to sniff cocaine
Home grown	Locally grown marijuana; local weed; ditch weed		
Joint	A marijuana cigarette	Tweezes	A wild variety of psilocybin mushrooms (hallucinogen)
Joy popping	Occasional use of drugs		
Juice	Alcohol		
Junk	Heroin, so named because it's never pure when sold on the street	Uncle	Federal agent
		Wacky tobaccky	Marijuana
Kiddie dope	Usually prescription drugs	Wasted	Intoxicated, strung out
Killer	Strong drug	White lightning	LSD
Killer weed	Strong marijuana, or marijuana sprinkled with PCP	Wired	Addicted to amphetamines or heroin
		Zigzag	A brand of rolling papers used to make marijuana cigarettes
Laughing gas	Nitrous oxide (an inhalant)		

Source: Available at http://www.lec.org/drug search/documents/slangterms.html

psychoactive effects of controlled substances. The number of designer drugs that are created and sold illegally is very large. Anyone with knowledge of college-level chemistry can alter the chemical ingredients and produce new designer drugs, although it may be nearly impossible to predict their properties or effects except by trial and error. Currently, three major types of synthetic analog drugs are available through the illicit drug market: analogs of phencyclidine (PCP), analogs of fentanyl and meperidine (both synthetic narcotic analgesics) such as Demerol, MPPP, (called MPTP), PEPAP, and analogs of amphetamine and methamphetamine (which have stimulant and hal-

MDMA

a type of illicit drug known as "Ecstasy" or "Adam" having stimulant and hallucinogenic properties

lucinogenic properties) such as **MDMA,** known as "Ecstasy" or "Adam," which is widely used on college campuses as a euphoriant and, to some extent, by clinicians as an adjunct to psychotherapy (NIDA 1986). The arrival of these high-technology psychoactive substances is a sign of the new high levels of risk and unpredictable outcome faced by drug users in the 1990s and beyond. As the pace of such risks in substance use increases, the need for a broader, more well-informed view of drug use becomes even more important than in the past.

◢ An Overview of Drugs in Society

Many people think that problems with drugs are unique to this era. Drug use and abuse have always been part of human society, however. For example, the Grecian oracles of Delphi used drugs, Homer's Cup of Helen induced sleep and provided freedom from care, and the mandrake root mentioned in Genesis supplied a hallucinogenic belladonna compound. In Genesis 30:14–16, the mandrake is mentioned in association with lovemaking:

> In the time of wheat harvest Reuben went out and found some mandrakes in the open country and brought them to his mother Leah. Then Rachel asked Leah for some of her son's mandrakes, but Leah said, "Is it so small a thing to have taken away my husband, that you should

take my son's mandrakes as well?" But Rachel said, "Very well, let him sleep with you tonight in exchange for your son's mandrakes." So when Jacob came in from the country in the evening, Leah went out to meet him and said, "You are to sleep with me tonight; I have hired you with my son's mandrakes." That night he slept with her.

Ancient literature is filled with references to the use of mushrooms, datura, hemp, marijuana, opium poppies, and so on. Under the influence of some of these drugs, many people experienced extreme ecstasy or sheer terror. Some old pictures of demons and devils look very much like those described by modern drug users during so-called bummers, or bad trips. The belief that witches could fly may also have been drug-induced because many natural preparations used in so-called witches' brews induced the sensation of disassociation from the body, as in flying or floating.

As far back as 2240 B.C., attempts were made to regulate drug use. For instance, in that year, problem drinking was addressed in the Code of Hammurabi, where it was described as "a problem of men with too much leisure time and lazy dispositions." Nearly every culture has, as part of its historical record, laws controlling the use of a wide range of drugs.

How Widespread Is Drug Abuse?

As mentioned earlier, drug abuse today is more acute and widespread than in any previous age. The evidence for this development is that drug busts are an everyday occurrence in the United States. On any given day, you can scan most major national and international newspapers and undoubtedly run across stories about illegal drug manufacturing, distribution or use.

Drug use is an **"equal-opportunity affliction"** in that no one is immune from it. Research shows that drug consumption cuts across income, social class, and age groups. Drugs are as seductive to the poor as they are to the wealthy, to the

equal-opportunity affliction

drug use, in that it cuts across all members of society regardless of income, social class, and age category

highly educated and the school dropout, and to the young and the old.

Many of us, for example, are a little dismayed when we discover that certain individuals we admire—such as celebrities, politicians, athletes, clergy, and academics—admit to or are apprehended for abusing illicit drugs. We are also taken aback when we hear that cigarettes, alcohol, and marijuana abuse are commonplace in some junior high and even grade schools. Further, most of us know of at least one close friend or family member who abuses drugs.

Extent and Frequency of Drug Use in Society

Erich Goode (1994), a much-respected sociologist, lists four types of drug use:

1. *Medical use*—prescription drugs and OTC drugs used to relieve or treat mental or physical symptoms

2. *Legal recreational use*—use of such licit drugs as tobacco, alcohol, and caffeine to achieve a certain mental or psychic state by the user

3. *Illegal instrumental use*—taking drugs without a prescription to accomplish a task or goal, such as taking nonprescription amphetamines to drive through the night, or relying excessively on barbiturates to get through the day

4. *Illegal recreational use*—taking illicit drugs for fun or pleasure to experience euphoria

Why has the prevalence of licit and illicit drug use remained fairly consistent since 1988? Recent data also indicate that drug use increased from 1994 to 1995 (see Table 1.3). Why has this trend

Table 1.3   Trend Data on the Prevalence of Illicit Drug Use, 1988–1995

	1988	1991[a]	1992[b]	1994[c]	1995[c]
Use in Past Month					
All ages 12+	7.3%	6.3%	5.5%	6.0%	6.1%
12–17	9.2	6.8	6.1	8.2	10.9
18–25	17.8	15.4	13.0	13.3	14.2
26–34	13.0	9.0	10.1	8.5	8.3
35+	2.1	3.1	2.2	3.2	2.8
Use in Past Year					
All ages 12+	14.1	12.7	11.1	10.8	10.7
12–17	16.8	14.8	11.7	15.5	18.0
18–25	32.0	29.1	26.4	24.6	25.5
26–34	22.6	18.4	18.3	14.8	14.6
35+	5.8	6.4	5.1	5.7	5.0
Use in Lifetime (ever used)					
All ages 12+	36.6	37.0	36.2	34.4	34.2
12–17	24.7	20.1	16.5	20.3	22.2
18–25	58.9	54.7	51.7	46.3	45.8
26–34	64.2	61.8	60.8	56.1	54.8
35+	23.0	27.3	28.0	27.7	27.9

Note that this table shows a gradual yearly decline in drug use across all age groups only through 1992.
Note: These figures include use of marijuana, cocaine, hallucinogens, inhalants (except in 1982), heroin, and nonmedical use of sedatives, tranquilizers, stimulants, and analgesics. Data on inhalant use were not collected in 1982, which may lower overall prevalence figures for that year, especially for 12- to 17-year-olds.
(a) Source for all figures in this column: National Institute on Drug Abuse, *National Household Survey on Drug Abuse* (Rockville, MD: NIDA, 1992).
(b) All figures in this column: National Institute on Drug Abuse, *National Household Survey on Drug Abuse* (Rockville, MD: NIDA, 1993).
(c) All figures in this column: Substance Abuse and Mental Health Services Administration (SAMHSA), Office of Applied Studies. *Preliminary Estimates from the 1995 National Household Survey on Drug Abuse.* (Rockville, MD: U.S. Department of Health and Human Services, August 1996).
Sources: National Institute of Drug Abuse. NIDA Notes 5, no. 1 (Winter 1989–1990): 4.

In the 1990s, a variety of factors came together in the United States to extend drug abuse beyond just the very rich or the urban poor. The ease of brewing cheaper, more potent strains of speed (methamphetamine, or "meth") and heroin, coupled with the fact that enforcement officials tended to focus on drug abuse and traffic in urban areas on the East and West Coasts, left middle class and rural populations throughout the country largely overlooked. Suddenly the illicit drug market was booming where no one had been looking.

By the late 1990s, speed—which had gained popularity in the 1970s among outlaw bikers, college students facing exams, all-night party-goers, and long-haul truckers—was more sought after than ever. Teenagers, middle-class workers, and suburbanites joined the ranks of methamphetamine users. "We've been fighting it really strongly for nearly seven years," Edward Synicky, a special agent with California's Bureau of Narcotics Enforcement, told *Time* magazine in early 1996. "But cocaine gets all the publicity because it's glamorous. And law enforcement in general doesn't put the resources into meth that it should."

Increasingly, the illegal substance was produced in clandestine labs set up by both major drug dealers and individual users. By January 1996, John Coonce, head of the U.S. Drug Enforcement Administration's (DEA) meth-lab task force, said meth use was "absolutely epidemic." The surge was attributed largely to powerful Mexican drug syndicates and motorcycle gangs that sold their goods on street corners. Speed acquired the nickname "crank" because it was frequently concealed in motorcycle crankcases.

Clandestine manufacture and use of speed were especially high in the West and Southwest. Speed kitchens flourished in California because it was relatively easy for the Mexican syndicates to smuggle in ephedrine, a key ingredient that is tightly controlled in the United States. From the mid-1980s to the mid-1990s, meth-related hospitalizations in California rose approximately 366%. In Arizona's Maricopa County, methamphetamine-linked crimes jumped nearly 400% over a three-year period in the early 1990s.

Soon this easy-access drug began spreading across the United States. In 1994, DEA field offices in Houston, Denver, Los Angeles, New Orleans, Phoenix, St. Louis, San Diego, and San Francisco were responsible for approximately 86% of the meth laboratory seizures in the country. By 1996, however, officials were seizing huge shipments of methamphetamine that originated in Mississippi and Tennessee.

But speed was not the only drug barreling its way across the country. Use of heroin ran rampant as well. In a Southeastern Massachusetts fishing community, at least 50 fishermen died of AIDS or other drug-related causes between 1991 and 1996. The captain of one scalloper told a local newspaper, "As a wild guess, I would say that if the fishing industry were to run a blood test and eliminate the people that had drug problems, there would be very few boats sailing with a full crew." Many skippers cited the ease with which drug users and dealers could find jobs on board ships as one reason for the alarming rise in drug abuse among their ranks.

Even crack cocaine, which was first seen primarily in New York and Los Angeles, infiltrated rural areas. According to the DEA, a combination of factors forced some crack distributors to develop new markets in smaller towns and rural areas. Pike County, Mississippi, was hit especially hard. Enforcement officials believed most of the crack in Mississippi came from New Orleans; but some drug shipments originating in South America were flown to remote landing strips in the middle of Mississippi farmland.

Whatever people's reasons for using these dangerous substances, it is clear that an important step toward stemming abuse is drying up the supply lines to middle America. To accomplish that goal, the law enforcement community must look beyond traditional hotbeds of activity among the urban poor. ∎

Sources Associated Press. "Survey: Drug Use Pervading New Bedford Fleet." *Maine Sunday Telegram* (July 21, 1996).
National Narcotics Intelligence Consumers Committee. *The NNICC Report, 1994.* Washington, DC: U.S. Drug Enforcement Agency, (1994) 70.
NPR. "All Things Considered." *PM News* (Sept. 18, 1996).
Toufonio, A., et al. "There Is No Safe Speed." *Time* (Jan. 8, 1990).
Wilkie, C. "Crack Cocaine Moves South." *Boston Globe* (June 23, 1996).

occurred, when expenditures for fighting the drug war by the federal, state, and local governments have been increasing in the past five years?

There are several possible answers, none of which by itself offers a satisfactory solution. One perspective notes that practically all of us use drugs in some form, with what constitutes "drug use" being merely a matter of degree. A second explanation is that more varieties of both licit and illicit drugs are available today. One source estimates that approximately 80% of all currently marketed drugs were either unknown or unavailable 20 years ago (Critser 1996). "Roughly 1.5 billion prescriptions are written for drugs in the United States each year, about half of which are new prescriptions and the other half are refills" (Goode 1994, 172). A third explanation is that " . . . in the modern age, increased sophistication has brought with it techniques of drug production and distribution that have resulted in a worldwide epidemic of drug use" (Kusinitz 1988, 149).

In the last decade, for example, illicit drug cartels have proliferated, and varieties of marijuana with ever-increasing potency have infiltrated all metropolitan areas. Many of these varieties are cross-bred with ultra-sophisticated techniques and equipment available everywhere. Finally, even coffee with high caffeine content (a stimulant-type drug) has become available worldwide. This trend has led to the explosion in cappucino-type coffees, the sale of espresso coffee makers for home use, and the unprecedented growth of companies such as Starbucks and Three Brothers Coffee. Twenty years ago, it was difficult to purchase a cup of espresso or cappucino in a typical restaurant; today such types of coffee are commonplace. Even at airports, shopping malls, pool halls, and small town restaurants, it is not unusual to hear an espresso maker hissing away, producing cup after cup for customers ordering fast food.

Drug Use: Statistics and Trends An incredible amount of money is spent each year for legal chemicals that alter consciousness, awareness, or mood. Four classes of these legal chemicals exist:

1. *Social drugs*—$60 billion for alcohol; $25 billion for cigarettes (add another $1.4 billion for cigars, chewing, pipe, and roll-your-own to-bacco, as well as snuff tobacco); $5.7 billion for coffee, tea, and cocoa

2. *Prescription (ethical) drugs*—$700 billion worldwide sales (Critser 1996, 40)

3. *Over-the-counter (patent) drugs*—$14 billion in sales, including cough and cold items, external and internal analgesics, antacids, laxatives, antidiarrheal products, and sleep aids and sedatives

4. *Miscellaneous drugs (such as aerosols, nutmeg, morning glory seeds, and others)*—amount unknown

Studies carried out by the Social Research Group of George Washington University, the Institute for Research in Social Behavior in Berkeley, California, and others provide detailed, in-depth data showing that drug use is universal. A major purpose of their studies was to determine the level of psychoactive drug use among people aged 18 through 74, excluding those people hospitalized or in the armed forces. Data were collected to identify people using specific categories of drugs (that is, caffeine, sleeping pills, nicotine, alcohol, and other psychoactive drugs). Other studies have shown that people in the 18- to 25-year-old age groups are by far the heaviest users and experimenters in terms of past-month and past-year usage (see Table 1.3).

More than 80% of respondents in the studies reported that they drank coffee during the previous year, and over 50% said that they drank tea. In addition, nearly one-third of the population reported consuming more than five cups of caffeine-containing beverages each day.

In 1995, 395 billion doses of caffeine were consumed in the United States. Other research data support the findings of the Social Research Group of George Washington University. For example, an estimated 61 million Americans smoked tobacco in 1995, or 29% of the total U.S. population (SAMHSA 1996a). Statistics also reveal that, in 1995, 111 million Americans age 12 and older had used alcohol in the past month (52% of the population) (SAMHSA 1996a). Illicit drug use was also determined to represent an ongoing problem. For example, marijuana remained the most commonly used illicit drug (as of 1994), with approximately

81% of current illicit drug users being marijuana or hashish users. Also in 1994, about 65 million individuals, out of the 290 million person total, or 31%, reported marijuana use in their lifetime, 18 million (9%) reported use in the past year, and 10 million (5%) reported current use (in the past month) (SAMHSA 1996c).

Finally, other reliable estimates report that in 1995, 34.2% of the U.S. population aged 12 and older reported using illicit drugs, alcohol, and tobacco at some point in their lives. Leading illicit drugs, from highest to lower percentages, were marijuana and hashish (31%), cocaine (10.3%), hallucinogens or PCP (2%), and LSD (7.5%).

The average household owns about 35 drugs, of which one out of five is a prescription drug and the other four are OTC drugs (NIDA 1993). Of the many prescriptions written by physicians, approximately one-fourth modify moods and behaviors in one way or another. Surveys report that over 50% of adults in the United States have, at some time in their lives, taken a psychoactive drug (one that affects mood or consciousness). Over one-third of adults have used or are using depressants or sedatives.

A NIDA study and other research (Horton 1992, 79) indicate drug use trends based on gender. Men are most likely to use stimulants in their thirties, depressants in their forties and fifties, and sedatives from age 60 on. Women however, are most likely to use stimulants from age 21 through age 39 and depressants more frequently in their thirties. Women's use of sedatives shows a pattern similar to use by men, with the frequency of use increasing with age. Women tend to use pills to cope with problems, whereas men tend to use alcohol for this purpose. In addition, people over 35 are more likely to take pills, whereas younger people prefer alcohol. Among those using pills, younger people and men are more likely to use stimulants than older people and women, who take sedatives (Chambers and Griffey 1975; Horton 1992, 78–81).

The actual figures for use of all psychoactive drugs are probably 35% higher than reported. This discrepancy exists partly because a large number of people obtain psychoactive drugs on the "black market" and from friends and relatives who have legitimate prescriptions. An estimated 70% of all psychoactive prescription drugs used by people under 30 are obtained without the user having a prescription. Pharmacists' records show that about $60.7 billion is spent on psychoactive drug prescriptions (U.S. Bureau of the Census 1993, 108), with the rate of increase estimated at about 9% per year. Such figures indicate that it may be more difficult to find people who do not use psychoactive drugs than individuals who do.

Types of Drug Users/Abusers

Just as a diversity set of personality traits (for example, introverts, extraverts, type A, obsessive-compulsive, and so on) exists, drug users vary according to their general approach or orientation, frequency of use, and the amount of the drugs they consume. Some are occasional or moderate users, while others display much stronger attachment to drug use. In fact, some display such obsessive-compulsive behavior that they cannot let a morning, afternoon, and evening pass without using drugs. Such variability in the frequency and extent of usage has been classified by some researchers as fitting into three basic patterns: experimenters, compulsive users, and floaters or "chippers" (members of the last category drift between experimentation and compulsive users).

Experimenters begin using drugs largely because of peer pressure and curiosity, and confine their use to recreational settings. Tobacco, marijuana, and alcohol are the usual limits of their drug-taking behavior, and they are more likely to know the difference between light, moderate, and chronic use.

experimenters
type of drug user: experimenters are novel users

Compulsive users, in contrast, "... devote considerable time and energy to getting high, talk incessantly (sometimes exclusively) about drug use, and become connoisseurs of street drugs" (Beschner 1986, 7). For compulsive users, recreational fun is impossible without getting "high." Other charac-

compulsive users
type of drug user: compulsive users are often addicted users

Table1.4   **National Household Survey on Drug Abuse, 1994** Percentage of population and estimated number of alcohol, tobacco, and illicit drug users in the United States

	Lifetime*		Past Month	
	Percent	Number of Users	Percent	Number of Users
Alcohol	85.3	178,551,000	52.6	110,249,000
Cigarettes	71.2	149,161,000	23.4	48,939,000
Marijuana/hashish	34.1	71,454,000	4.7	9,764,000
Smokeless tobacco	15.0	31,510,000	3.0	6,351,000
Nonmedical use of any psychotherapeutic[†]	10.1	21,047,000	0.8	1,609,000
Cocaine	9.7	20,314,000	0.6	1,265,000
Hallucinogens	8.1	16,964,000	0.3	686,000
Stimulants	5.5	11,583,000	0.1	276,000
Inhalants	5.1	10,734,000	0.7	1,503,000
Analgesics	5.0	10,475,000	0.6	1,183,000
PCP	4.3	9,023,000	0.1	201,000
Tranquilizers	4.1	8,617,000	0.2	332,000
Sedatives	3.5	7,412,000	0.1	217,000
Crack	1.8	3,768,000	0.2	331,000
Any illicit drug	37.6	78,660,000	5.8	12,216,000

Notes: Total population = 209 million.   * Lifetime refers to ever used.   † Nonmedical use of any prescription stimulant, sedative, tranquilizer, or analgesic; does not include over-the-counter drugs.

Source: Substance Abuse and Mental Health Services Administration (SAMHSA), Office of Applied Studies (OAS) *National Household Survey on Drug Abuse: Main Findings 1994.* Rockville, MD: NIDA, 1996.

teristics of these users include the need to escape or postpone personal problems, to avoid stress and anxiety, and to enjoy the sensation of the drugs' euphoric effects. Often, they have difficulty in assuming personal responsibility and suffer from low self-esteem. Many compulsive users are from dysfunctional families, and often serious psychological problems underlie their drug-taking behavior. Problems of personal identity, sexual orientation, boredom, family discord, academic pressure, and chronic depression all contribute to the inability to cope with issues without drugs (Carroll 1996, 45).

Floaters or **"chippers"** focus more on using other people's drugs without maintaining a personal supply. Nonetheless, "chippers," like exper-

floaters or "chippers"

type of drug user: floaters or "chippers" are users who vacillate between the need to seek pleasure and the need to relieve serious psychological problems

imenters, are generally light to moderate consumers of drugs. "Chippers" vacillate between the need for pleasure seeking and the desire to relieve moderately serious problems. As a result, they drift between experimental drug-taking peers to chronic drug-using peers. In a sense, these drug users are marginal individuals who do not strongly identify with experimenters or compulsive users. (An example of how the various types of drug users are often adversely affected by peers is discussed in more detail in Chapters 2 and 4.)

Mass Media Influences on Drug Use in Everyday Life

Studies have shown that the majority of young drug users comes from homes in which drugs are liberally used (Goode 1993, 1994; Coombs 1988; SAMHSA 1996b). These children frequently witness drug use at home. For instance, in the morning, parents may consume large quantities of coffee to wake up and other forms of medication throughout the day: tablets for an upset stomach, vitamins for stress, or aspirin for a headache. Finally, before retiring, the grown-ups may take a "little night cap" or a sleeping pill to relax. Pills alone are taken in almost unbelievable volume. Such everyday consumption of legal drugs—caffeine, prescription or OTC drugs and alcohol—is fueled by the pace of modern lifestyles and greatly accelerated by the influence of today's increasingly sophisticated mass media.

If you look around your classroom building, the dormitories at your college, or the surroundings of your own homes, evidence of mass media and electronic equipment can be found everywhere. Cultural knowledge and information is transmitted via media and electronic gadgets we simply "can't live without," to the point where these surroundings help us define *and* shape our everyday reality.

Although over 70% of the adult population are regular newspaper readers, television remains the most influential medium. Almost 93 million American homes have television sets; 59% have more than one set, and 96% have color sets. In the United States, the number of hours spent watching television is staggering. Statistics indicate that the average household spends 49 hours and 49 minutes per week watching television (Nielsen, 1995). This total represents over 7 hours per day!

Advertisers invest huge amounts of money in television commercials because of the popularity of the medium. For example, the alcohol industry spends more than $1 billion on yearly advertising (Kilbourne 1989; Critser 1996). "The advertising budget for one beer—Budweiser—is more than the entire budget for research on alcoholism and alcohol abusers" (Kilbourne 1989, 13). In 1995, this advertising resulted in spirits, wine, and beer sales totaling $103.9 billion with the largest sales—those of beer—reaching $62.6 billion (Critser 1996). Such sales figures clearly indicate that advertising is both highly effective and very lucrative in promoting drinking.

Radio, newspapers, and magazines are also saturated with advertisements for OTC drugs, constantly offering relief from whatever illness you may have. There are pills for inducing sleep and staying awake, as well as for treating indigestion,

headache, backache, tension, constipation, and the like. Mood, level of consciousness, and physical discomfort can be significantly altered by using these medicinal compounds. Experts warn that such drug advertising is likely to increase geometrically. In the early 1990s, the FDA lifted a two-year ban on consumer advertising of prescription drugs that is expected to bring an onslaught of new sales pitches.

In their attempts to sell drugs, product advertisers use the authority of a physician or health expert or the seemingly sincere testimony of a mesmerized product user. Adults are strongly affected by testimonial advertising because these drug commercials can appear authentic and convincing to large numbers of viewers, listeners, or readers.

The constant barrage of commercials, including many for OTC drugs, relay the message that, if you are experiencing restlessness or uncomfortable symptoms, taking drugs is acceptable (or normative). As a result, adults and eventually children are led to believe that drugs are necessary to maintain well-being.

◢ The Attraction of Drug Use and Some Patterns of Drug Abuse

Why are people so attracted to drugs? Like the ancient Assyrians, who sucked on opium lozenges, and the Romans, who ate hashish sweets some 2000 years ago, many users claim to be bored, in pain, frustrated, unable to enjoy life, or alienated. They turn to drugs in the hope of finding oblivion, peace, "togetherness," or euphoria. The fact that few drugs cause all the effects for which they are taken doesn't seem to be a deterrent. People continue to take drugs for a number of reasons:

1. They may be searching for pleasure, and drugs may make them feel good.

2. Drugs may relieve stress or tension or provide a temporary escape for people with anxiety.

3. Peer pressure is strong, especially for young people. The use of drugs has become a rite of passage in some subcultures of society.

4. In some cases, drugs may enhance religious or mystical experiences. A few cultures teach children how to use specific drugs for this purpose.

5. Drugs can relieve pain and some symptoms of illness.

Since historically many people have been unsuccessful in eliminating the fascination with drugs, it is important that we come to understand it. To reach such an understanding, we will address why people are attracted to drugs, how different types of drugs affect the body and the mind, and what forms of treatment are available for eliminating abuse. These questions are addressed at a general level in Chapter 2, and at the level of specific substances in each chapter from 7 through 15.

When Does Use Lead to Abuse?

Views on the use of drugs depend on one's perspective. For example, from a pharmacological perspective, if a patient is suffering severe pain because of car collision injuries, high doses of a narcotic such as morphine or Demerol should be given to control discomfort. While someone is in pain, no reason exists not to take the drug. From a medical standpoint, once healing has occurred and pain has been relieved, drug use should cease. If the patient continues using the narcotic because it provides a sense of well-being or has become a habit, the pattern of drug intake would then be considered abuse. Thus, the amount of drug taken or the frequency of dosing does not necessarily determine abuse (although individuals who abuse drugs usually consume frequent high doses). Rather, the *motive* for taking the drug is the principal factor in determining the presence of abuse.

Initial drug abuse symptoms include excessive use, constant preoccupation over the availability and supply of the drug, refusal to admit excessive use, early symptoms of withdrawal whenever the user attempts to stop taking the drug, and neglect of important goals or ambitions in favor of using the drug. Even the legitimate use of a drug can be controversial. Often physicians cannot decide even among themselves what constitutes legitimate use of a drug. For example, MDMA ("Ecstasy") is cur-

rently prohibited for therapeutic use, but in 1985, when the Drug Enforcement Administration (DEA) was deciding MDMA's status, some 35 to 200 physicians (mostly psychiatrists) were using the drug in their practice. These clinicians claimed that MDMA relaxed inhibitions and enhanced communications and was useful as a psychotherapeutic adjunct to assist in dealing with psychiatric patients (Shecter 1989; Levinthal 1996). From the perspective of these physicians, Ecstasy was a useful medicinal tool. However, the DEA did not agree and made Ecstasy a Schedule I drug (see Chapter 3). This classification excludes any legitimate use of the drug in therapeutics; consequently, according to this ruling, anyone taking Ecstasy is guilty of drug abuse (Goode 1994).

Other special-interest groups take a more liberal view. They consider drug abuse a statutory problem and describe it as "the use of drugs in an illegal manner." According to such a limited definition, excessive use of alcohol by anyone over 21 years of age would not be considered a form of drug abuse, in spite of the consequences. Obviously, such a narrow view of drug abuse is not very useful in trying to deal with the consequences of extreme or inappropriate drug use, such as alcoholism.

If the problem of drug abuse is to be understood and solutions are to be found, identifying what causes the abuse is most important. When a drug is being abused, it is not legitimately therapeutic; that is, it does not improve the user's physical or mental health. If such drug use is not for therapeutic purposes, what is the motive for using it?

There are many possible answers to this question. Most drug abusers perceive some psychological advantage when using these compounds (at least initially). For many, the psychological lift is significant enough that they are willing to risk social exclusion, arrest, incarceration, and fines to have their drug. The psychological effects that these drugs cause may entail an array of diverse feelings. Different types of drugs have different psychological effects. The type of drug an individual selects to abuse may ultimately reflect his or her own mental state.

For example, people who experience chronic depression, feel intense job pressures, an inability to focus on accomplishing goals, or develop a sense of inferiority may find that a stimulant such as cocaine or amphetamines appears to provide a solution to such dilemmas; these drugs cause a spurt of energy, euphoria, a sense of superiority, and imagined confidence. In contrast, people who experience nervousness and anxiety and want instant relief from the pressures of life may choose a depressant such as alcohol or barbiturates; these agents sedate, relax, and provide relief, and even have some amnesiac properties, allowing users to suspend or forget their problems. People who perceive themselves as creative or who have artistic talents may select hallucinogenic types of drugs to "expand" their minds, heighten their senses, and distort the confining nature of reality. As individuals come to rely more on drugs to inhibit, deny, accelerate, or distort their realities, they run the risk of becoming psychologically dependent on drugs—a process described in detail in Chapter 6.

Drug Dependence

Although Chapters 2 and 4 discuss addiction and drug dependence in detail, we will introduce some underlying factors that lead to drug dependence here. Our discussion emphasizes "drug dependence" instead of "addiction" because the term is both controversial and relative (an issue that came to the forefront during the 1996 Presidential election, for example). *When* drug dependence becomes full-fledged, addiction remains debatable, with many experts unable to agree on the criteria involved. Further, "addiction" is also viewed by some a pejorative label (see Chapter 2, labeling theory).

The main characteristics necessary for addiction are as follows:

1. Both physical and psychological factors precipitate drug dependence. Recently, closer attention has been focused on psychological attachments to drug use as principally indicative of addiction.

2. There is a tendency to eventually become addicted with repeated use of most psychoactive drugs.

3. *Psychological dependence* refers to the need that a user may feel for continued use of a drug so as to experience its effects. *Physical dependence* refers to the need to continue taking the drug to avoid withdrawal symptoms, which often include feelings of discomfort and illness.

4. Generally, addiction refers to mind and body dependence. The process of addiction can be viewed as involving five phases: relief, increased use, preoccupation, dependency, and withdrawal. Initially, relief from using a drug can allow a potential addict to escape one or more of the following feelings: boredom, loneliness, tension, fatigue, anger, and anxiety. Increased use involves taking greater quantities of the drug. Preoccupation consists of a constant concern with the substance—that is, taking the drug becomes "normal" behavior. The dependency phase is synonymous with addiction. More of the drug is sought despite the presence of physical symptoms, such as coughing in cases of cigarette and marijuana addiction or blackouts from advanced alcohol addiction. Withdrawal involves such symptoms as itching, chills, feeling tense, stomach pain, or depression from the nonuse of the addictive drug (Monroe 1996).

◢ The Costs of Drug Use to Society

Society pays a high price for drug addiction. Many of the costs are immeasurable—for example, broken homes, illness, shortened lives, and loss of good minds to industry and professions. The dollar costs are also great. The **National Institute on Drug Abuse (NIDA)** has estimated that the typical narcotic habit costs the user $100 a day or more to maintain, depending on location, availability of narcotics, and other factors. Assuming that a heroin addict has a $100-a-day habit, this addict would need about $36,000 a year just to maintain the drug supply. It is impossible for most addicts to get this amount

NIDA

the National Institute on Drug Abuse, the principal federal agency responsible for directing drug abuse-related research

of money legally, so many resort to criminal activity to support their habits.

Most crimes related to drugs involve theft of personal property—primarily burglary and shoplifting—and less commonly, assault and robbery (mugging). It is estimated that a heroin addict must steal three to five times the actual cost of the drugs to maintain the habit, or roughly $100,000 a year. A number of addicts resort to pimping and prostitution. No accurate figures are available on the cost of drug-related prostitution, although some law enforcement officials have estimated that prostitutes take in a total of $10 to $20 billion per year. It has also been estimated that nearly one out of every three or four prostitutes in major cities has a serious drug dependency.

Another significant concern arises from the recent increases in clandestine laboratories throughout the country that are involved in synthesizing or processing illicit drugs. Such laboratories produce amphetaminelike drugs, heroinlike drugs, "designer" drugs, and LSD and process other drugs of abuse such as cocaine. The **Drug Enforcement Administration (DEA)** reported 390 laboratories seized in 1993, a figure that increased to 967 in 1995. The reasons for such dramatic increases relate to the enormous profits and relatively low risk associated with these operations. As a rule, clandestine laboratories are fairly mobile, relatively crude (often operating in a kitchen, basement, or garage), and operated by individuals with only elementary chemical skills. Because of a lack of training, the chemical procedures are performed crudely, resulting in adulterants and impure products. Such contaminants can be very toxic, causing severe harm or even death to the unsuspecting user (Drug Strategies 1995).

Society continues paying a large sum even after addicts are caught because it takes from $50 to $100 per day to incarcerate each of them. Supporting programs like methadone maintenance costs much less. New York officials estimate that methadone maintenance cost about $2000 per

DEA

the Drug Enforcement Administration, the principal federal agency responsible for enforcing drug abuse regulations

year per patient. Some outpatient programs, such as those in Washington, D.C., claim a cost as low as $5 to $10 per day (not counting cost of staff and facilities), which is much less than the cost of incarceration.

A more long-term effect of drug abuse that has substantial impact on society is the medical and psychological care often required by addicts as a consequence of disease resulting from their drug habit. Particularly noteworthy are the communicable diseases spread because of needle sharing within the drug-abusing population, such as HIV and AIDS (acquired immune deficiency syndrome) and hepatitis. AIDS is the most publicized of these diseases. "An estimated 1 million Americans today are infected with HIV, the immunodeficiency virus, which causes AIDS; as many as 17 million people are infected worldwide" (*NIDA Notes* May/June 1995, 1).

While the transmission of the AIDS virus is primarily associated with male homosexual and/or bisexual contact (43.3% of all cases), the second leading transmission route (31.8% of all cases) is via drug-injecting users who have been exposed to the HIV virus; see Chapter 17). The HIV virus in this population appears to be transmitted in small amounts of contaminated blood left on shared needles. The likelihood of contracting HIV in the drug-abusing population correlates with the frequency of injection and the amount of needle sharing (NIDA May/June 1995; NIDA July 1990). Care for these AIDS patients lasts from months to years in intensive care units at a cost of billions of dollars to the public. Some social workers have advocated that new, uncontaminated needles be made available to drug addicts free of charge to prevent the spread of HIV by contaminated needles. Others argue against this approach, complaining that such a policy encourages abuse of drugs through the more dangerous intravenous route (Goldstein 1994).

Also of great concern is drug abuse by women during pregnancy. Some psychoactive drugs can have profound, permanent effects on a developing fetus. The best documented is fetal alcohol syndrome (FAS), which can affect the offspring of alcoholic mothers (see Chapter 8). Cocaine and amphetamine-related drugs can also cause irreversible congenital changes when used during pregnancy (see Chapter 8). All too often, the affected offspring of addicted mothers become the responsibility of welfare organizations.

Drugs and Crime

There is a long-established close association between drug abuse and criminality. The hypotheses for this association range between the concepts that (1) criminal behavior develops as a means to support addiction, and (2) criminality is inherently linked to the user's personality and occurs independently of drug use (Kokkevi et al. 1993, Drug Strategies 1995). Part of the reason for the controversy about the relationship between criminal activity and drug abuse is that conflicting studies have been conducted in different cultures, employing different methods, focusing on different addictive drugs, and examining recruit samples from different settings (that is, treatment versus criminal justice systems).

Drug-related crimes are undoubtedly overwhelming our judicial system: According to the U.S. Department of Justice, alcohol consumption is associated with 27% of all murders, almost 33% of all property offenses, and more than 37% of robberies committed by young people. In fact, nearly 40% of the young people in adult correctional facilities reported drinking before committing a crime. "In 1993, the DUF (Drug Use Forecasting) program found that the percentage of male arrestees testing positive for an illicit drug at the time of the arrest ranged from 54% in Omaha and San Jose to 81% in Chicago. Female arrestees testing positive ranged from 42% in San Antonio to 83% in Manhattan" (ONDCP June 1995, 6).

It is clear that production, merchandising, and distribution of illicit drugs have developed into a worldwide operation worth hundreds of billions of dollars (Goldstein 1994). These enormous profits have attracted organized crime, both in the United States and abroad, and all too frequently even corrupted law enforcement agencies (McShane 1994). For the participants in such operations, drugs can mean incredible wealth and power. For example, in 1992 Pablo Escobar was recognized as a drug kingpin and leader of the cocaine cartel in Colombia, and acknowledged as one of the world's richest men and Colombia's most powerful man (Wire Services 1992). With his drug-related wealth, Escobar literally financed a private army to conduct a personal war against the government of Colombia (Associated Press 1992); until his death in 1993, he was a serious threat to his country's stability. Such power can be very dangerous and destructive to individuals and even to entire societies.

Violence takes its toll at all levels, as rival gangs fight to control their "turf" and associated drug operations. Innocent bystanders often become unsuspecting victims of the indiscriminate violence. For example, a Roman Catholic cardinal was killed on May 24, 1993, when a car in which he was riding inadvertently drove into the middle of a drug-related shootout between traffickers at the international airport in Guadalajara, Mexico. Five other innocent bystanders were fatally wounded in the incident (Associated Press 1993). Others are injured or killed by drug users who, while under the influence of drugs, commit violent criminal acts.

In addition to the costs to society mentioned above, other costs of drug abuse include drug-related deaths and emergency room visits, newborn health problems, and auto fatalities.

Drugs in the Workplace: A Costly Affliction

Can you make a reservation on American Airlines? Recently the answer to that question was no, you cannot. An employee who had been smoking marijuana at work forgot to load a crucial computer tape into the airline's central reservation system, erasing important information and causing the entire system to crash for eight hours. Cost to the airlines: $19 million. (Woods 1993, 19)

Most adults spend the greatest number of hours per day in some type of family environment (see cartoon on page 21). For most full-time employed adults, the second greatest number of hours is spent in the workplace. Generally, whenever drug use becomes habitual, such behavior does not cease when leaving the family environment. The National Household Surveys, for example, found evidence of significant drug use in the workplace.

In the surveys, the 65.6% of full-time workers reported alcohol use within the past month. Some 9.7% of full-time workers reported marijuana use within the past year. Part-time employees did not differ much in their use of alcohol and marijuana (SAMHSA 1996a).

Approximately 70% to 75% of drug users in the United States are employed (see Figure 1.1) (SAMHSA 1996a), costing American businesses billion of dollars annually in lost productivity and increased health care costs. Over the past several years, many large businesses have instituted substance abuse programs to respond to the problems created by alcohol and other drugs in the workplace.

Other highlights from the National Household Survey on Drug abuse (SAMHSA 1996a) include the following:

1. Heavy alcohol use rates were highest among construction workers, auto mechanics, food preparation workers, light truck drivers, and laborers. The lowest rates of heavy alcohol use were reported by data clerks, personnel specialists, and secretaries.

2. The highest rates of illicit drug use were reported by workers in the following occupations: construction, food preparation, and waiters and waitresses.

3. Workers in occupations that require a considerable amount of public trust, such as police

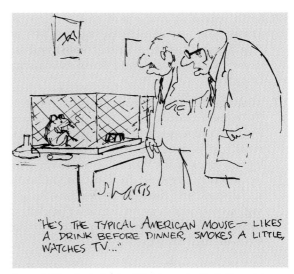

"HE'S THE TYPICAL AMERICAN MOUSE— LIKES A DRINK BEFORE DINNER, SMOKES A LITTLE, WATCHES TV…"

Source: ® Sidney Harris, *American Scientist* magazine. Used with permission.

officers, teachers, and child care workers, report the lowest rates of illicit drug use.

4. Significant differences were found among occupational categories in marijuana use; no differences found in current cocaine use.

5. Age was the most significant predictor of marijuana and cocaine use. Younger employees (18–24 years old) were more likely to report drug use than older employees (25 years or older).

Figure 1.1

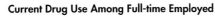

Source: National Institute on Drug Abuse (NIDA). "Research on Drugs and the Workplace." *Capsules (CAP)* Rockville, MD: U.S. Department of Health and Human Services, June 1995.

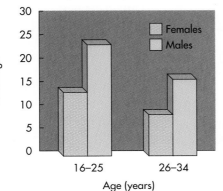

Current Drug Use Among Full-time Employed

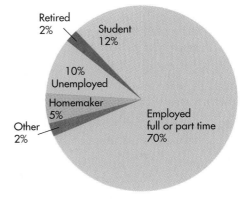

Current Users of Illicit Drugs

6. With regard to marijuana and cocaine use among younger employees (age 18–34), no significant differences in marijuana and cocaine use rates were found across educational categories.

7. *Males* in the following occupations reported the highest rates of illicit drug use: entertainers, food preparation and service, cleaning services, and construction. Among *females,* the highest rates of illicit drug use were reported by workers involved in food preparation, social work, and the legal professions, including lawyers and legal assistants. (In each of these occupations, males reported similar levels of illicit drug use.)

8. In general, unmarried workers reported roughly twice as much illicit drug and heavy alcohol use as married workers. In occupations such as food preparation, transportation drivers, and mechanics, and in industries such as construction and machinery (not electrical), the discrepancy between married and unmarried workers was especially notable.

9. Workers who reported having three or more jobs in the previous five years were twice as likely to be current or past-year illicit drug users as those who held two or fewer jobs over the same period.

10. Approximately 13% of full-time workers, aged 18–49, reported past-year involvement in a mandatory drug test at work.

11. Workers in occupations that impact public safety, including truck drivers, fire fighters, and police, report the highest rate of participation in drug testing.

12. Most youths do not cease drug use when they begin working.

Other findings regarding the topic of drugs and the workplace include additional statistics that negatively impact on job performance:

▲ Drug users are 1.6 times as likely as nonusers to have quit their jobs or have been fired.

▲ They are 1.5 times as likely to have been disciplined by a supervisor.

▲ Approximately 1% of full-time employees reported current cocaine use. In total, 7 million workers reported marijuana and cocaine use.

In summarizing this research on employees who abuse alcohol or other drugs, five major findings emerge: (1) they are three times more likely than the average employee to be late to work; (2) they are three times more likely to receive sickness benefits; (3) they are 16 times more likely to be absent from work; (4) they are four times more likely to be involved in on-the-job accidents; and (5) they are five times more likely to file compensation claims.

Employee Assistance Programs (EAPs) Research data show that more than 10 million employed people currently use illicit drugs. Among full-time employees, 9.2% report current use of any illicit drugs, although certain demographic groups are associated with significantly higher rates of use. For example, 24% of males aged 18–25 years and 15% of males aged 26–34 years are current users. Marijuana and cocaine are the most commonly used illicit drugs.

Many industries have responded to drugs in the workplace by creating **drug testing** and **employee assistance programs (EAPs).** Drug testing generally involves urine screening undertaken to identify employees who are using drugs and who may have current or potential drug problems. EAPs are employer-financed programs administered by a company or through an outside contractor. More than 300,000 EAPs have been established in the United States. The programs are designed to aid in identifying and resolving productivity problems associated with employees' emotional or physical concerns, such as those related to health, marital, family, financial, and substance abuse. Recently, EAPs have expanded their focus to combat employee abuse of OTC and prescription drugs in addition to illicit psychoactive substances. Overall, the programs attempt to formally reduce problems associated with impaired job performance.

drug testing
urine screening to identify employees who may be using drugs

EAPs
employee assistance programs

◢ Venturing Beyond: A Holistic Approach to Drug Use

Throughout this book, we continually emphasize the pharmacological, psychological, and sociological ramifications of most commonly used licit and illicit drugs. Most chapters study and analyze the major drugs and their usage patterns, and emphasize unified approaches for understanding how drugs affect both the mind and the body.

As the reader proceeds through this book, it will become apparent that whenever drug use leads to abuse, it rarely results from single, isolated causes. Instead, it is often caused or preceded by multiple factors, which may include the following:

▲ A combination of genetic factors

▲ Psychological conditioning

▲ Peer group formations

▲ The ability to cope with stress and anxiety of daily living

▲ The quality of role models

▲ The degree of cohesion within the family structure

▲ The level of security with gender identity and sexual orientation

▲ Personality traits

▲ Perceived ethnic and racial compatibility with larger society and socioeconomic status (social class).

The decline in illicit drug use from 1976 to 1994, shown in Figure 1.2, reflects our current view of health as being interrelated with **positive wellness.** Positive wellness—as opposed to wellness—emphasizes the interrelatedness of physical, psychological, emotional, social, spiritual, and environmental factors. No longer are these domains of existence viewed as separate entities. Thus, "no part of the mind, body, or environment is truly separate and independent" (Edlin and Golanty 1992, 5).

positive wellness
an approach that advocates the maintenance of health and wellness as a way of life

Gaining knowledge of how and why drugs work—the subject of these chapters—supports the current holistic approach to health and wellness. As mentioned earlier, understanding drug

---

◖ Figure 1.2 ◗

Use of any illicit drug: trends in annual prevalence among young adults by age group.

Source: Johnston, L. P., P. M. O'Malley, and J. G. Bachman. *National Survey Results from the Monitoring the Future Study, 1975–1994.* Vol. II. Rockville, MD: National Institute on Drug Abuse, 1996, p. 87.

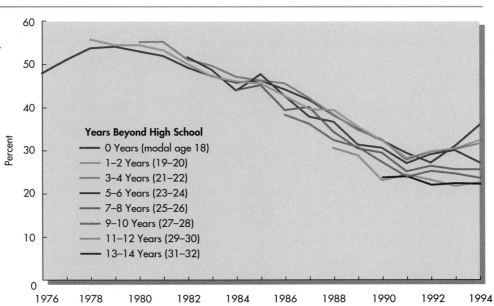

Years Beyond High School
— 0 Years (modal age 18)
— 1–2 Years (19–20)
— 3–4 Years (21–22)
— 5–6 Years (23–24)
— 7–8 Years (25–26)
— 9–10 Years (27–28)
— 11–12 Years (29–30)
— 13–14 Years (31–32)

use is not only important for comprehending our own health, but also for understanding (1) why others are attracted to drugs; (2) what to do (remedies and solutions) when friends or family members abuse drugs; (3) how to help and advise drug abusers about the pitfalls of substance use; (4) the best educational, preventive, and treatment options available for victims of drug abuse; and (5) the danger signals that arise in yourself and others you care about when drug use exceeds normal and necessary use.

Achieving **holistic health** requires self-awareness; it involves the ability to recognize your own drug-use practices. Understanding your own habits and motivations promotes your own self-maintenance. Once you are able to help yourself, you also increase your ability to help others by promoting prevention, education, and treatment of unhealthy drug use.

> **holistic health**
>
> a perspective on health that advocates knowledge about drug use to increase self-awareness and help others

6. Because many experimental drug users do not gravitate to excessive drug use, should experimenters be left alone, or perhaps just given legal warnings or fines?

7. Do the mass media really promote drug use, or do they merely reflect our extensive use of drugs? Provide some evidence for your position.

8. When do you think drug use leads to abuse? When do you think drug use does not lead to abuse?

9. When is drug dependence not considered addiction? When does drug dependence progress to drug addiction?

10. What principal factors are involved in the relationship between drugs and crime?

11. Should all employees be randomly tested for drug use?

12. What is the holistic approach to drug use? Why does this approach stress positive wellness? What is positive wellness?

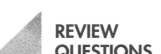 ## REVIEW QUESTIONS

1. Give an example of a drug-using friend and describe how he or she is affected by pharmacological, cultural, social, and contextual factors.

2. Why do you think marijuana is the most commonly used illicit drug?

3. Briefly review the historical uses of drugs. Do you think drug use is innate in our society?

4. Why do Americans use so many legal drugs (for example, alcohol, tobacco, and OTC drugs)? What aspects of our society promote extensive drug use?

5. Why do you think that the use of illicit drugs by young adults who are seniors in high school has increased since 1992 (see Figure 1.2)?

 ## KEY TERMS

drug
psychoactive drugs or psychoactive substances
licit drugs
illicit drugs
over-the-counter (OTC)
gateway drugs
"designer" drugs
structural analogs
MDMA
equal-opportunity affliction
experimenters, compulsive users, and floaters or "chippers"
National Institute on Drug Abuse (NIDA)
Drug Enforcement Administration (DEA)
drug testing
positive wellness
employee assistance programs (EAPs)
holistic health

EXERCISES FOR THE WEB

Exercise 1:
National Institutes of Drug Abuse

NIDA's mission is to lead the nation in bringing the power of science to bear on drug abuse and addiction. This charge has two critical components. The first is to strategically support and conduct research across a broad range of disciplines. The second is to ensure the rapid and effective dissemination and use of the research to significantly improve drug abuse and addiction prevention, treatment, and policy. The National Institutes of Drug Abuse was established in 1974 and, in October 1992, became part of the National Institutes of Health of the Department of Health and Human Services.

Exercise 2:
Beer Advertising

Providing an array of services to non-profit, private, and public sector organizations and educators throughout Wisconsin, the Prevention Resource Center is a statewide program sponsored by the Wisconsin Clearinghouse.   These services include disseminating prevention-related materials, lending curricula, videos, and books, and providing technical assistance in such areas as grant writing and program evaluation. The staff also presents ideas and information at conferences and workshops. The Clearinghouse mails the "Prevention Package" to more than 500 sites, providing information on new publications, successful programs, and a calendar of upcoming conferences and training events.

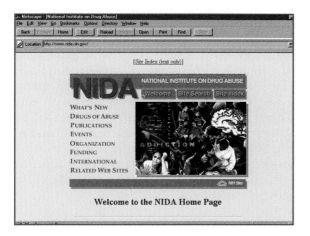

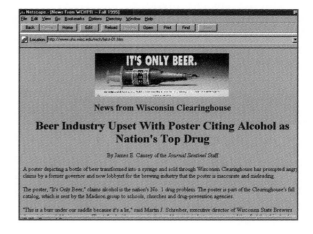

SUMMARY

1. Pharmacological, cultural, social, and contextual issues are the four principal factors responsible for determining how a drug user experiences drug use. Pharmacological factors take into account how a particular drug affects the body. Cultural factors examine how society's views, as determined by custom and tradition, affect use of a particular drug. Social factors include the specific reasons why a drug is taken and how drug use develops from social factors, such as family upbringing, peer group alliances, subcultures, and communities. Contextual factors account for how drug use behavior develops from the physical surroundings where the drug is taken.

2. Initial understanding of drug use includes the following key terms: drug, gateway drugs, medicines and prescription medicines, over-the-counter (OTC) drugs, drug abuse, and drug addiction.

3. Mentions of drug use date back to the Bible, including ancient literature dated 2240 B.C. Under the influence of drugs, many people experienced feelings ranging from extreme ecstasy to sheer terror. At times drugs were used to induce sleep and provide freedom from care.

4. Drug users are found in all occupations and professions, income and social class levels, and all age groups. No one is immune to drug use. Thus, drug use is an "equal-opportunity affliction."

5. According to sociologist Erich Goode, drugs are used for four reasons: (a) legal instrumental use or medical use, (b) legal recreational use, (c) illegal instrumental use, and (d) illegal recreational use.

6. The most commonly used licit and illicit drugs, rated from highest to lowest frequency of use are alcohol, cigarettes, marijuana, smokeless tobacco, nonmedical use of any psychotherapeutic (prescription stimulant, sedative, tranquilizer, or analgesic), cocaine, hallucinogens, stimulants, inhalants, and analgesics. The most commonly abused illicit drugs are cannabis (marijuana), stimulants, hallucinogens, narcotics, depressants, and organic solvents.

7. The three types of drug users are experimenters, compulsive users, and floaters. Experimenters try drugs because of curiosity and peer pressure. Compulsive users use drugs on a full-time basis and seriously desire to escape from or alter reality. Floaters or "chippers" vacillate between experimental drug use and chronic drug use.

8. The mass media tend to promote drug use through advertising. The constant barrage of OTC drug commercials relays the message that, if you are experiencing some symptom, taking drugs is an acceptable option.

9. From a pharmacological perspective, drug use becomes excessive when psychoactive drugs are taken without medical reasons. Initial drug abuse symptoms include excessive use, over-preoccupation with the availability and supply of drugs, denial of excessive use, symptoms of withdrawal whenever the user attempts to stop taking the drug, and neglect of personal goals in favor of using the drug.

10. The five phases of drug addiction are relief, increased use, preoccupation, dependency, and withdrawal.

11. Employee assistance programs (EAPs) are employer-financed programs administered by a company or through an outside contractor. They are designed to aid in identifying and resolving productivity problems associated with employees' emotional or physical concerns, such as those related to health, marital, family, financial, and substance abuse. Recently, EAPs have expanded their focus to combat employee abuse of OTC and prescription drugs as well as illicit psychoactive substances.

REFERENCES

Associated Press. "Program to Fight Drug Smuggling Costs U.S. a Lot, Produces Little." *Salt Lake Tribune* 244 (17 August 1992): A-1.

Associated Press. "Mexican Cardinal, Six Others Killed in Cross-Fire as Drug Battles Erupt in Guadalajara." *Salt Lake Tribune* 246 (25 May 1993): A-1.

Beschner, G. "Understanding Teenage Drug Use." In *Teen Drug Use,* edited by G. Beschner and A. Friedman. Lexington, MA: D. C. Heath 1986: 1–18.

Carroll, C. R. *Drugs in Modern Society,* 4th ed. Madison, WI: Brown & Benchmark, 1996.

Chambers, C. C., and M. S. Griffey. "Use of Legal Substances Within the General Population: The Sex and Age Variables." *Addictive Diseases* 2 (1975): 7–19.

Coombs, R. H., ed. *The Family Context of Adolescent Drug Use.* New York: Harworth, 1988.

Critser, G. "Oh, How Happy We Will Be: Pills, Paradise, and the Profits of the Drug Companies." *Harper's Magazine* (June 1996) 39–48.

Drug Strategies. *Keeping Score: What We Are Getting for Our Federal Drug Control Dollars 1995.* Washington, DC: 1995. Available 080/edres/colleges/boss/depts/cesar/drugs/ks1995.

Edlin, G., and E. Golanty. *Health and Wellness: A Holistic Approach,* 4th ed. Boston, MA: Jones and Bartlett, 1992.

Goldstein, A. "Lessons from the Street." In *Addiction from Biology to Drug Policy.* New York: Freeman, 1994.

Goode, E. *Deviant Behavior,* 3rd ed. Englewood Cliffs, NJ: Prentice-Hall, 1990.

Goode, E. *Deviant Behavior,* 4th ed. Englewood Cliffs, NJ: Prentice-Hall, 1994.

Goode, E. *Drugs in American Society,* 4th ed. New York: McGraw-Hill, 1993.

Horton, J. "Addictive Behaviors." In *The Women's Health Book,* edited by J. Horton. Washington, DC: Jacobs Institute of Women's Health and Elsevier, 1992: 79.

Johnston, C. D., P. M. O'Malley, and J. G. Bachman. *National Survey Results from the Monitoring the Future Study, 1975–1994.* Rockville, MD: National Institute on Drug Abuse, 1996.

Kilbourne, J. "Advertising Addiction: The Alcohol Industry's Hard Sell." *Multinational Monitor* (June 1989): 13–16.

Kokkevi, A., J. Liappas, V. Boukouvala, V. Alevizou, E. Anastassopoulou, and C. Stefanis. "Criminality in a Sample of Drug Abusers in Greece." *Drug and Alcohol Dependence* 31 (1993): 111–21.

Kusinitz, M. "Drug Use Around the World." in *Encyclopedia of Psychoactive Drugs,* edited by S. Snyder. Series 2. New York: Chelsea House, 1988.

"Let's All Work to Fight Drug Abuse." Dallas, TX: L.A.W. Publications, 1991.

Levinthal, C. F. *Drugs, Behavior, and Modern Society.* Boston, MA: Allyn and Bacon, 1996.

McShane, L. "Cops Are Crooks in N.Y.'s 30th Precinct." *Salt Lake Tribune* 238 (18 April 1994): A-5.

Monroe, J. What Is Addiction? *Current Health,* 2 (January 1996): 16–19.

National Institute on Drug Abuse (NIDA). "Designer Drugs." *Capsules (CAPS).* Rockville, MD: NIDA, June 1986.

National Institute on Drug Abuse (NIDA). *NIDA Notes* 5, no. 1 (Winter 1989–1990): 4.

National Institute on Drug Abuse (NIDA). "Drug Abuse and AIDS." *Capsules (CAP 04)* Rockville, MD: NIDA, July 1990.

National Institute on Drug Abuse (NIDA). "Research on Drugs and the Workplace." *Capsules (CAPS).* Rockville, MD: NIDA, 1990a.

National Institute on Drug Abuse (NIDA). *National Household Survey on Drug Abuse.* Rockville, MD: NIDA, 1992.

National Institute on Drug Abuse (NIDA). *National Household Survey on Drug Abuse: Highlights 1993.* Rockville, MD: NIDA, 1993: 7.

National Institute on Drug Abuse (NIDA). "NIDA Plays Key Role in Studying Links Between AIDS and Drug Abuse." *NIDA Notes* 10, no. 3 (May/June 1995): 1.

Nielsen Company. *Television: 1995 Nielsen Report.* Northbrook, IL: Nielsen, 1995.

Office of National Drug Control Policy (ONDCP). *Fact Sheet: Drug Use Trends.* Washington, DC: Drugs and Crime Clearinghouse, NCJ-153518, June 1995.

Schecter, M. "Serotonergic-Dopaminergic Mediation of 3, 4-Methytenedioxy-Methamphetamine (MDMA, Ecstasy)." *Pharmacology, Biochemistry and Behavior* 31 (1989): 817–24.

Substance Abuse and Mental Health Services Administration (SAMHSA), Office of Applied Studies (OAS). *National Household Survey on Drug Abuse: Main Findings 1994.* Rockville, MD: NIDA, 1996a.

Substance Abuse and Mental Health Services Administration (SAMHSA), Office of Applied Studies (OAS). *The Relationship Between Family Structure and Adolescent Substance Use.* Rockville, MD: U.S. Department of Health and Human Services, July 1996b.

Substance Abuse and Mental Health Services Administration (SAMHSA), Office of Applied Studies (OAS). *Preliminary Estimates from the 1995 National Household Survey on Drug Abuse.* Rockville, MD: U.S. Department of Health and Human Services, August 1996c.

Thio, A. *Deviant Behavior,* 4th ed. New York: Harper-Collins College, 1995.

U.S. Bureau of the Census. *Statistical Abstract of the United States, 1993,* 113th ed. Washington, DC: U.S. Government Printing Office, 1993: 108.

Wang, P. "A New Way to Drugs." *Time* (30 December 1985): 33–4.

Wire Services. "Cocaine Kingpin Escapes After Bloody Shootout." *Salt Lake Tribune* 244 (23 July 1992): A-1.

Woods, G. *Drug Abuse in Society: A Reference Handbook.* Santa Barbara, CA: ABC-CLIO, 1993.

2 Explaining Drug Use and Abuse

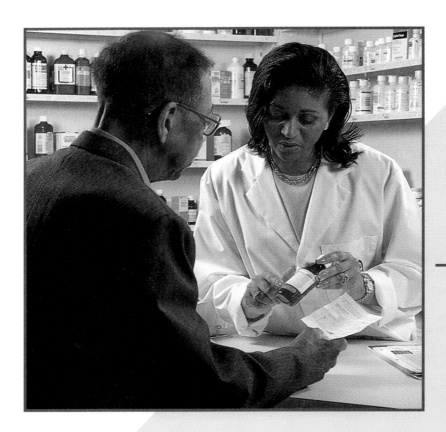

On completing this chapter
you will be able to:

- Drug use and drug dealing are major factors in the growth of crime and violence among the young.
- Biological explanations of drugs trace the desire for drug use to innate physical beginnings and suggest that the tendency to abuse drugs may be an inherited predisposition.
- A strong relationship exists between severe drug addiction and mental illness.
- Sigmund Freud believed that addiction to drugs was an outgrowth of habitual (compulsive) masturbatory activity.
- Such personality traits as extreme forms of introversion and extraversion may explain why many people abuse drugs.
- Drug use is mostly learned from others.
- When drug use becomes consistent and habitual, it usually occurs in the peer group setting, with people we like.
- Drugs are sometimes used to compensate for a lack of self-confidence.
- No single theory can explain why most people use drugs.
- Some theories advocate that an individual's alliance with drug-using peers largely results from an inability to cope with rapid societal change.
- People who perceive themselves as drug users are more likely to develop serious drug abuse problems.

Learning Objectives

- List six reasons why drug use or abuse is a more serious problem today than it was in the past.
- List and briefly describe the following biological theories as they relate to drug use and abuse: genetic pursuit of pleasure, self-medication, and genetic influence.
- Explain the relationships between some mental disorders and possible effects of certain drugs.
- Explain the relationship between introverted or extraverted personality patterns and possible effects of stimulants or depressants.
- Briefly define and explain reinforcement or learning theory and some of its applications to drug use and abuse.
- List and briefly describe the four sociological theories broadly known as *social influence theories*.
- Describe symptoms and indicators of possible drug use or abuse in childhood behavior patterns.
- List and describe three factors in the learning process that Howard Becker believes first-time users go through before they become attached to using illicit psychoactive drugs.
- Define the following concepts as they relate to drug use: primary and secondary deviance, master status, and retrospective interpretation.
- Explain why both internal and external controls against drug use are insufficient to block the allure of drugs (Reckless's containment theory).
- Understand what is meant by making low-risk choices regarding drug use.

In a general sense, Chapter 1 introduced many ramifications of drug use. In this chapter, the perplexing question we will explore is, Why would anyone *voluntarily* consume drugs when they are not medically needed or required? Why subject your body and mind to the harmful effects of repetitive drug use, eventual addiction, and relapse into drug use? What logical reasons could explain such apparently irrational behavior? Following are three perspectives regarding drug use:

> Why do I use weed (marijuana), "booze" (liquor), cigarettes, and occasional "shrooms" (psilocybin mushrooms), and acid (LSD)? Well, why not? I get bored very easily and I am at a time in my life when except studying, there is nothing to do except to party.
>
> *From Venturelli's research files, undergraduate male college student, age 22, May 18, 1996*

[A second interview]

> You are asking the wrong person about drug use. I am against such drugs as marijuana, cocaine, tobacco, and LSD. My friends feel the same. I occasionally drink when I am with friends or at a party, but even one or two drinks make me feel out of it. I just don't like to feel as if I am losing control of reality, I like reality too much. . . . I think people who use drugs liberally are in some way addicted to the feeling of being high. They are not aware of how great it is to be in control of their thinking.
>
> *From Venturelli's research files, male graduate university student, age 28, March 6, 1996*

[A third interview]

> Yes, I have friends who try to tell me to slow down when we are smoking weed and drinking. I just like to get high until I am about to pass out. If I could, I would be high all day without any time out. Never think about quitting or slowing down when it comes to drugs. The only time I am happy is when I am completely zonked out. I guess I am a little attached to these drugs—I am addicted to them!
>
> *From Venturelli's research files, public high school student in a small Midwestern city, age 15, September 9, 1996*

The excerpts above show three variations in the values and attitudes regarding drug use. The first interviewee represents recreational drug users who believe they can potentially control their drug use. The second interviewee represents cautious drug users who shun illicit drug use. The third interviewee represents a type of drug user who is unaware of the "pitfalls" of drug addiction and the problems associated with drug abuse. Beyond these three types of users, other types exist who rarely use licit or illicit drugs. In this chapter we will examine what motivates these different types of users and address issues such as why drugs attract some people but repel others. By learning about these differences, we will develop a better understanding of drug use and abuse.

In this chapter, the different explanations are framed within major theoretical perspectives. Like the United States, nearly all other countries are experiencing increasing amounts of drug use within certain subcultures of people who use or abuse drugs. Moreover, as we attempt to offer major theoretical and scientific explanations for drug use, we will be able to develop an understanding of why drugs are so seductive not only in our society, but also on a global scale.

Drug Use: A Timeless Affliction

Historical records document drug use as far back as 2240 B.C., when Hammurabi, the Babylonian king and lawgiver, addressed the problems associated with drinking alcohol. Even before then, "the Sumerian people of Asia Minor, who created the cuneiform alphabet, included references to a 'joy plant' . . . , which date from about 5000 B.C." (O'Brien 1992, ix). Experts indicate that the plant was an opium poppy used as a sedative.

As noted in Chapter 1, virtually every culture has experienced problems with drug use or abuse. Based on this information, we can verify that today's drug use problems are part of a very rich tradition stemming from long ago.

The quest for explanations and information is more important than ever as the problem continues evolving. We offer six reasons why drug use and abuse are an even more serious issue than they were in the past and thus worthy of study:

1. From 1960 to the present, drug use has become a widespread phenomenon. Before the 1960s, drug use was a serious problem only within certain isolated populations. Today, however, it affects nearly every social group.

2. Today, drugs are much more potent than they were years ago. For example, in 1960, the average THC content of marijuana was 1% to 2%. (THC is the ingredient responsible for making a person "high.") Today, the amount of THC in marijuana varies between 4% and 6%. THC content of marijuana from Colombia ranges between 4% and 6%. Other more refined varieties usually grown without seeds, such as **sinsemilla, northern lights,** and **Geneva sativa** varies between 6% and 8% (Francis 1996, 44–56). To a large extent, the increase of THC content is due to improved cultivation techniques (Mijuriya and Aldrich 1988; Francis 1996, 44). Crack and other manufactured drugs offer potent effects at low cost, vastly multiplying the damage potential of drug abuse.

> **sinsemilla, northern lights, and Geneva sativa**
> a more potent type of marijuana, meaning "without seeds"

3. Whether they are legal or not, drugs have become commonplace, and their sale is a multibillion-dollar-a-year business, with a major influence on many national economies.

4. Drug use endangers the future of a society by physically harming its youth and potentially destroying the lives of many young men and women. When "gateway" drugs such as alcohol and tobacco are used at an early age, a strong possibility exists that the use will progress to other drugs, such as marijuana, cocaine, and amphetamines. Early drug use will likely lead to a lifelong habit, which has serious implications for the future.

5. Drug use and especially drug dealing is becoming a major factor in the growth of crime among the young. Violent delinquent gangs are increasing at an alarming rate (Hutchinson and Kyle 1993; Moore 1993; Chaiken 1996, 1). Violent gun shootings, drive-by killings, car jacking, and "wilding" (Cummings 1993, 49; ONDCP September 1994; Sanders 1994, 85–107) are common in cities (and increasing in small towns), such that the public has reacted with dismay, outrage, and fear (Moore 1993; Kunen 1989; Will 1990, 64).

6. The possibility of near or serious accidents caused by drug users grows as people become more dependent on technology. For instance, the operation of sophisticated machines and electronic equipment requires that workers and professionals be free of the effect of mind-altering drugs. Just imagine if several computer programmers responsible for supervising air traffic control were cocaine users, or if technicians at a major X-ray diagnostic and cancer treatment center smoked marijuana during their lunch breaks. The consequences could be deadly in both cases.

Why does a nation such as ours have a severe drug problem? With remarkable and unsurpassed excellence in scientific, technological, and electronic accomplishments, one might think that in the United States drug use and abuse would appear to be irrational behavior and would begin to diminish. One might also think that the allure of drugs would further diminish when we look at the statistically high proportions of accidents, crimes, marital strife and divorce, addiction, and death rates from the use and abuse of licit and illicit drugs. Yet such social, psychological, economic, and medical costs have not served as a deterrent to drug use.

Considering these costs, what explains the continuing use and abuse of drugs? What could possibly sustain and feed the allure of drugs? Why are drugs used when the consequences are so well documented?

In answering these questions, we need to recall from Chapter 1 some basic reasons why people take drugs:

1. People may be searching for pleasure, and drugs may make them feel good.

2. Drugs may relieve stress or tension or provide a temporary escape for people with anxieties.

3. Peer pressure is a strong influence, especially for young people. The use of drugs has become a rite of passage in some levels of society.

4. In some cases, drugs may enhance religious or mystical experiences. A few cultures teach children how to use specific drugs for this purpose.

5. Drugs can relieve pain and symptoms of illness.

Although these reasons may outline some underlying causes for excessive or abusive drug use, they also suggest that the variety and complexity of explanations and motivations are almost infinite. For any one individual, it is seldom clear when nondestructive use becomes abuse. When we consider the wide use of such licit drugs as alcohol, nicotine, and caffeine, we find that over 88% (U.S. Bureau of the Census 1990, 122; Drug Strategies 1995, 3) of the U.S. population are daily drug users in some form. Further, as we will see in later chapters, almost any of the hundreds of moods humans can experience can be mimicked by some drug.

We can therefore begin to understand why the explanation for drug use and abuse is complicated and cannot be forced into one or two theories. In attempting to answer the question of why people use drugs, researchers have tackled the question from three major theoretical positions—namely, biological, psychological, and sociological perspectives. The remainder of this chapter discusses these three major explanations.

◢ Biological Explanations

As noted in Chapter 1, biological explanations have tended to use genetic theories or the disease model for explaining drug addiction. The view that alcoholism is a sickness dates back approximately 200 years (Conrad and Schneider 1980; Heitzeg 1996). This specific disease perspective is based on E. M. Jellinek's (1960) view that alco-

holism largely involves a loss of control over drinking and that the drinker experiences clearly distinguishable phases in his or her drinking patterns. Thus, the disease model views drug abuse as an illness in need of treatment or therapy. For example, concerning alcoholism, the illness affects the abuser to the point of loss of control.

According to biological theories, drug abuse has an innate physical beginning stemming from constitutional physical characteristics that cause certain individuals either to experiment or to crave the drugs to the point of abusive use. **Genetic and biophysiological theories** explain addiction in terms of genetics, brain dysfunction, and biochemical patterns.

genetic and biophysiological theories
explanations of addiction in terms of genetic brain dysfunction and biochemical patterns

Biological explanations emphasize that the **central nervous system (CNS)** reward sensors are more sensitive to drugs that are abused in some people, making the drug experience more pleasant and more alluring for these individuals (Jarvik 1990; Mathias 1995, 2). (The CNS is defined as one of the major divisions of the nervous system, composed of the brain and spinal cord.) In contrast, others find the effects of drugs of abuse very unpleasant; such people are not likely to be attracted to these drugs (Farrar and Kearns 1989).

CNS
central nervous system (CNS) one of the major divisions of the nervous system, composed of the brain and the spinal cord

Most experts acknowledge that biological factors play an essential role in drug abuse. These factors likely determine how the brain responds to these drugs and why such substances prove addictive. It is thought that by identifying the nature of the biological systems that contribute to drug abuse problems that improved therapy can be developed (Halloway 1991).

All the major biological explanations related to drug abuse assume that these substances exert their **psychoactive effects** (effects on the brain's mental functions) by altering brain chemistry. Specifically, the drugs of abuse interfere with the functioning of **neurotransmitters,** chemical messengers used for communication between brain regions

> **psychoactive effects**
> how drug substances alter and affect the brain's mental functions

(see Chapter 6 for details). The following are three principal biological theories that help explain why some drugs are abused and why certain people are more likely to become addicted when using these substances.

> **neurotransmitters**
> chemical messengers released by neurons (nerve cells) for communication with other cells

Are Abused Drugs Positive Reinforcers?

Biological research has shown that stimulating some brain regions with an electrode causes very pleasurable sensations. In fact, laboratory animals would rather self-administer stimulation to these brain areas than eat or engage in sex. It has been demonstrated that drugs of abuse also activate these same pleasure centers of the brain. Because of this positive reinforcing property, these drugs are repeatedly self-administered by animals and drug addicts (Koob 1992).

It is generally believed that most drugs with abuse potential enhance the pleasure centers by causing the release of a specific brain neurotransmitter called **dopamine** (Izenwasser and Kornetsky 1992): release of dopamine by the functional cells of the brain (neurons) leads to the drug-seeking behavior that is common to all drug addictions (Stolerman 1992; Doweiko 1996, 217–218). In addition, it has been proposed that overstimulation of these brain regions by

> **dopamine**
> the brain transmitter believed to mediate the rewarding aspects of most drugs of abuse

continual drug use "exhausts" these dopamine systems and leads to depression and an inability to ex-

perience normal pleasure. It has been proposed that such a mechanism accounts for the craving and some of the other unpleasant effects experienced during withdrawal from these drugs (Imperato et al. 1992).

Drug Abuse and Psychiatric Disorders

Biological explanations are thought to be responsible for the substantial overlap that exists between drug addiction and mental illness. Because of the similarities, severe drug dependence itself is classified as a form of psychiatric disorder by the American Psychiatric Association (see the discussion of *DSM-IV* classifications later in this chapter). For example, abuse of drugs can in and of itself cause mental conditions that mimic major psychiatric illness, such as schizophrenia, severe anxiety disorders, and suicidal depression (Halloway 1991; American Psychiatric Association 1994). It is believed that these similarities reflect the fact that common chemical factors (changes in neurotransmitter systems in the brain) are altered both by drugs of abuse and during episodes of psychiatric illness (Halloway 1991; NIDA 1993, 20). Several important potential consequences of this relationship may help us understand the nature of drug abuse problems.

1. *Psychiatric disorders and drug addiction often occur simultaneously.* This conclusion is supported by the fact that the incidence of mental illness is higher in the drug-abusing population than among individuals who do not abuse drugs. Thus, psychiatric illness is present in 37% of those with a severe alcoholic disorder and present in 53% of those with a severe nonalcohol drug disorder (Brady and Lydiard 1992). The issue of co-occurrence between drug abuse and mental illness is very important and research to study its prevalence is being encouraged by federal mental health and drug abuse programs ("Epidemiological and Services Research" 1994). Because of the common mechanisms, drug abuse is likely to expose or worsen psychiatric disorders.

2. *Therapies that are successful in treating psychiatric disorders may be useful in treating mental*

problems caused by the drugs of abuse. It is likely that many of the therapeutic lessons we learn about dealing with psychiatric illnesses can be useful in drug abuse treatment, and vice versa.

3. *Abuse of drugs by some people may represent an attempt to relieve underlying psychiatric disorders.* Such people commonly use CNS depressants such as alcohol to relieve anxiety, while CNS stimulants such as cocaine are frequently used by patients with depression disorders (Grinspoon 1993). In such cases, if the underlying psychiatric problem is relieved, the likelihood of successfully treating the drug abuse disorder improves substantially.

Genetic Explanations

One biological theory receiving close scrutiny suggests that inherited traits can predispose some individuals to drug addiction. Such theories have been supported by the observation that increased frequency of alcoholism and drug abuse exists among children of alcoholics and drug abusers (Uhl et al. 1993). Using adoption records of some 3000 individuals from Sweden, Cloninger, Gohman, and Sigvardsson conducted one of the most extensive research studies examining the genetics of alcoholism. They found that " . . . children of alcoholic parents were likely to grow up to be alcoholics themselves, even in cases where the children were reared by nonalcoholic adoptive parents almost from birth" (Doweiko 1996, 217). Such studies estimate that drug vulnerability due to genetic influences accounts for approximately 38% of all cases, while environmental and social factors account for the balance (Uhl et al. 1993).

Other studies attempting to identify the specific genes that may predispose the carrier to drug abuse problems have suggested that a brain target site (called a *receptor*—see Chapter 6 for details) for dopamine is altered in a manner that increases the drug abuse vulnerability (Uhl et al. 1992). Although several genetic studies have confirmed these findings, others have not (Uhl et al. 1992). Studies that test for genetic factors in complex behaviors such as drug abuse are very difficult to conduct and interpret. It is sometimes impossible to design experiments that distinguish among genetic, social, environmental, and psychological influences in human populations. For example, inherited traits are known to be major contributors to psychiatric disorders, such as schizophrenia and depression (Gershon and Rieder 1992). It is also established that substance abuse disorders occur in approximately half of those with severe mental illness (Bartels et al. 1993). Thus, patients who abuse stimulants, such as cocaine, have a high incidence of depression (Grinspoon 1993). Because of this co-occurrence, a high incidence of an abnormal gene in a cocaine-abusing population may not be directly linked to drug abuse behavior, but may be associated with depression, which has a high representation among cocaine abusers (Uhl et al. 1992).

Theoretically, genetic factors can directly or indirectly contribute to drug abuse vulnerability in several ways; for example,

1. Psychiatric disorders that are genetically determined may be relieved by drugs of abuse, thus encouraging their use.

2. In some people, reward centers of the brain may be genetically determined to be especially sensitive to addicting drugs; thus, use of drugs of abuse by these people would be particularly pleasurable and would lead to a high rate of addiction.

3. Character traits, such as insecurity and vulnerability, that often lead to drug abuse behavior may be genetically determined, causing a high rate of addiction in these people.

4. Factors that determine how difficult it will be to break a drug addiction may be genetically determined, causing severe craving or very unpleasant withdrawal effects; such people are less likely to abandon their drug of abuse.

The appeal of the genetic theories for drug abuse is that, once discovered, they may help us to understand the reasons that drug addiction occurs in some individuals but not in others. In addition, if genetic factors play a major role in drug abuse, it might be possible to use genetic screening to identify people who are especially vulnerable to drug abuse problems and to help such individuals avoid exposure to these substances.

◢ Psychological Explanations

Psychological theories mostly deal with internal mental or emotional states, often associated with or exacerbated by social and environmental factors. Primary internal psychological states of existence include one or more of the following: escape from reality, inability to cope with anxiety, destructive self-indulgence to the point of constantly desiring intoxicants, blind compliance with drug-abusing peers, self-destructiveness, and conscious and unconscious ignorance regarding the harmful effects of abusing drugs. Early psychological theories were espoused by Freud, who linked "primal addictions" with masturbation, and postulated that all later addictions, including alcohol and other drugs, were caused by ego impairments. Freud felt that drugs fulfilled insecurities that stem from parental inadequacies, causing difficulty in adequately forming bonds of friendships. He claimed that alcoholism (see Chapter 9) is an expression of the death instinct, as are self-destruction, narcissism, and oral fixations. Although Freud's views present interesting insights often not depicted in other theories, his theoretical concerns are difficult to see in action, test, and provide data for verification.

Distinguishing Between Substance Abuse and Mental Disorders

Widely accepted categories of diagnosis for behavioral disorders, including substance abuse, have been established by the American Psychiatric Association. As standardized diagnostic categories, the characteristics of mental disorders have been analyzed by professional committees over many years and today are summarized in their fourth generation of development in a widely accepted book called the *DSM-IV,* or *Diagnostic and Statistical Manual,* 4th edition (American Psychiatric Association 1994). In addition to categories for severe psychotic disorders and more common neurotic disorders, experts in the field of psychiatry have established specific diagnostic criteria for various forms of substance abuse. All patterns of drug abuse that are described in this text have a counterpart description in the *DSM-IV* manual

for medical professionals. For example, the *DSM-IV* discusses the mental disorders resulting from the use or abuse of sedatives, hypnotics, or antianxiety drugs; alcohol; narcotics; amphetamine-like drugs; cocaine; caffeine; nicotine (tobacco); hallucinogens; phencyclidine (PCP); inhalants; and cannabis (marijuana). This manual of psychiatric diagnoses discusses in detail the mental disorders related to the taking of drugs of abuse, the side effects of medications, and the consequence of toxic exposure to these substances (American Psychiatric Association 1994).

Because of the similarities between, and coexistence of, substance-related mental disorders and naturally occurring (referred to as *primary*) psychiatric disorders, it is sometimes difficult to distinguish between the two problems; however, in order for proper treatment to be rendered, the cause of the psychological symptoms must be determined. According to *DSM-IV* criteria, substance use (or abuse) disorders can be identified by the occurrence and consequence of dependence, abuse, intoxication, and withdrawal. These important distinguishing features of substance abuse disorders are discussed in greater detail in Chapter 5 and in conjunction with each drug group.

According to the *DSM-IV,* the following information can also help distinguish between substance-induced and primary mental disorders: (1) personal and family medical, psychiatric, and drug histories; (2) physical examinations; and (3) laboratory tests to assess physiological functions and determine the presence or absence of drugs. However, the possibility of primary mental disorder should not be excluded just because the patient is using drugs—remember, many drug users are self-medicating primary psychiatric problems with substances of abuse. The coexistence of underlying psychiatric problems in a drug user is suggested by the following circumstances: (1) the psychiatric problems do not match the usual drug effects (for example, use of marijuana usually does not cause severe psychotic behavior); (2) the psychiatric disorder was present before the patient began abusing substances; and (3) the mental disorder persists for more than four weeks after substance use ends. The *DSM-IV* makes it clear that the relationship between mental disorders and substances of abuse is important for proper diagnosis, treatment, and understanding. (See "Psychological and Psychotherapeutic Approaches" in Chapter 4.)

The Relationship Between Personality and Drug Use

Since medieval times, personality theories of increasing sophistication have been used to classify long-term behavioral tendencies or traits that appear in individuals, and these traits have long been considered as influenced by biological or chemical factors. Although such classification systems have varied widely, nearly all have shared two commonly observed dimensions of personality: introversion and extraversion. Individuals who show a predominant tendency to turn their thoughts and feelings inward rather than to direct attention outward have been considered to show the trait of *introversion*. At the opposite extreme, a tendency to seek outward activity and sharing feelings with others has been called *extraversion*. Of course, every individual shows a mix of such traits in varying degrees and circumstances.

In some research studies, introversion and extraversion patterns have been associated with levels of neural arousal in brain-stem circuits (Carlson 1990; J. A. Gray 1987; Apostolides 1996), and these forms of arousal are similar and closely associated with effects caused by drug stimulants or depressants. Such research hypothesizes that people whose systems produce high levels of sensitivity to neural arousal may find high-intensity external stimuli to be painful, and may react by turning inward. With these extremely high levels of sensitivity, such people may experience neurotic levels of anxiety or panic disorders. At the other extreme, individuals whose systems provide them with very low levels of sensitivity to neural arousal may find that moderate stimuli are inadequate to produce responses. To reach moderate levels of arousal, they may turn outward to seek high-intensity external sources of stimulation (Eysenck and Eysenck 1985; Gray 1987; Rousar, Brooner, Regier, et al. 1994).

Since high- and low-arousal symptoms are easy to create by using stimulants, depressants, or hallucinogens, it is possible that these personality patterns of introversion or extraversion may affect how a person reacts to substances. For people whose experience is predominantly introverted or extraverted, extremes of high or low sensitivity may lead them to seek counteracting substances that become important methods of bringing experience to a level that seems bearable.

Theories Based on Learning Processes

How are abuse patterns learned? Research on learning or conditioning explains how humans acquire new patterns of behavior by the close association or pairing of one significant reinforcing stimulus with another less significant or neutral stimulus. In learning by this method, people get used to certain behavior patterns. This process, known as *conditioning,* explains why pleasurable activities may become intimately connected with other activities that are also pleasurable, neutral, or even unpleasant. In addition, people can turn any new behavior into a recurrent and permanent one by the process of **habituation**—repeating certain patterns of behavior until they become established or habitual.

habituation
repeating certain patterns of behavior until they become established or habitual

The basic process by which learning mechanisms can lead a person into drug use is described in Bejerot's **"addiction to pleasure" theory** (Bejerot 1965, 1972, 1975). The theory assumes that it is biologically normal to continue a pleasure stimulus when once begun. Even recent research supports this theory, showing that "a strong, biologically based need for stimulation appears to make sensation-seeking young adults more vulnerable to drug abuse" (Mathias 1995, 1). Sensation-seeking individuals are defined as types of people who characteristically seek new or novel

"addiction to pleasure" theory
theory that assumes that it is biologically normal to continue a pleasure stimulus when once begun

thrills in their experiences. They maintain a constant preoccupation with getting high or are known to have a relentless desire to pursue physical stimulation or dangerous behaviors. The pleasure derived from stimulation may become habitual when new and shorter nerve courses come into function and higher centers are disconnected. For example, the pleasure associated with getting high may become a learned conditioned response if opiate users discover that the drug and sexual stimulation are mutually reinforcing. Opiate use becomes addictive when the two stimuli become mutually reinforcing. At this point, drug use and sexual stimulation are mutually reinforced through paired associative learning.

Another example is when drug use is associated with receiving affection or approval in a social setting, such as within a peer group relationship. Initially, the use of particular drugs may not, in themselves, be very important or pleasurable to the individual. However, the affection experienced during intimate interaction when drugs are used becomes paired with the drug. The pleasure derived from peer approval, and the intimacy often associated with such interaction coupled with drug use can become paired and associated. In this example, drug use and intimacy may become perceived as very worthwhile.

By the conditioning process, a pleasurable experience such as drug taking may become associated with a comforting or soothing environment. When this happens, two different outcomes may result. First, the user may feel uncomfortable taking the drug in any other environment (as marijuana or even a psychedelic drug, taken in another environment, may actually produce tension, insecurity, panic reactions), or—in the case of LSD, for example—a bad trip. Second, the user may become very accustomed or habituated to the familiar environment as part of the drug experience. The likely result is that through the process of developing drug tolerance (see Chapter 5), a comforting or familiar environment may evolve as the body begins to react less severely to the drug. Likewise, taking the drug in a different setting may cause a more severe or "fresh" reaction because the unfamiliar environment is not associated with the original habituated experience.

Finally, through this process of conditioning and habituation, a drug user becomes accustomed to unpleasant effects of drug use such as withdrawal symptoms. Such unpleasant effects and experiences may become habituated—neutralized or less severe in their impact—so that the user continues taking drugs without feeling or experiencing the negative effects of the drug.

Social Psychological Learning Theories

Other extensions of reinforcement or learning theory focus on how positive social influences by drug-using peers reinforce the attraction to drugs. Social interaction, peer camaraderie, social approval, and drug use work together as positive reinforcers sustaining drug use (Akers 1992). Thus, if the effects of drug use become personally rewarding, "or become reinforcing through conditioning, the chances of continuing to use are greater than for stopping" (Akers 1992, 86). It is through learned expectations, or association with others who reinforce drug use, that individuals *learn* the pleasures of drug taking (Becker 1963, 1967). Similarly, if the experiences are interpreted as *dis*favorable, as with a frightening LSD trip, then the experience will be negatively perceived and the distinctive appeal of the drug will diminish rapidly.

An example demonstrates how a negative experience can affect favorable drug use attitudes:

> I was tripping for the first time with some friends in my fraternity. I also drank a lot that night and decided to try and sleep for a few hours while drunk and tripping. I had just laid down in bed when I heard a bunch of sounds. After a few minutes, I opened my bedroom door and I saw firemen with axes and hoses and quite a lot of confusion, panic, and noise in the hall. I ran out of the room, down the corridor and kept running and running outside, mostly around the frat house, scared to death that I was going to get caught with the acid in my body and arrested. Since that frightening experience, I have

never wanted to see LSD again. I just am completely afraid of that drug.

From Venturelli's research files, Canadian male senior in college, age 22, residing in a Midwestern town, August 22, 1996

Note that positive reinforcers, such as peers, other friends and acquaintances, family members, and drug advertisements, do not act alone in inciting and sustaining drug use. Learning theory as defined here also relies on some variable amounts of imitation and trial-and-error learning methods.

Finally, **differential reinforcement**—defined as the ratio between reinforcers favorable and disfavorable for sustaining drug use behavior—must be considered. The use and eventual abuse of drugs can vary with certain favorable or unfavorable reinforcing experiences. The primary determining conditions are (1) the amount of exposure to drug-using peers versus non–drug-using peers, (2) the general preference for drug use in a particular neighborhood or community, (3) the age of initial use (younger adolescents are more greatly affected than older adolescents), and (4) the frequency of drug use among peer members.

> **differential reinforcement**
>
> the ratio between reinforcers, both favorable and disfavorable, for sustaining drug use behavior

◢ Sociological Explanations

Sociological explanations for drug use share important commonalities with psychological explanations under social learning theories. The main distinguishing features determining psychological and sociological explanations are that psychological explanations focus more on how the *internal states* of the drug user are affected by social relationships within families, peers, and other more distant relationships. Sociological explanations, in contrast, focus on how factors external to the individual affect drug users. Such outside forces include the types of families, lifestyles of peer groups, or types of neighborhoods and communities in which avid drug users reside. The sociological perspective views the motivation for drug use as largely determined by the types and quality of bonds that the drug user or potential drug user has with significant others or with physical surroundings. The degree of influence and involvement with external factors affecting the individual compared with the influence exerted by internal states distinguishes sociological from psychological analyses.

As previously stated, no one biological and psychological theory can adequately explain why most people use drugs. People differ from one another in terms of such traits as introversion or extraversion and in the outlooks and problems they face, and, as a result, they take drugs for very different reasons. Different theories may emerge partly because of these variations, and partly because the explanations are derived from different perspectives of biology, psychology, and sociology. Explanations may also differ because they simultaneously try to account for individual personality characteristics, unique social influences and situations, and specific circumstances regarding why drugs are used.

Microscopic and macroscopic sociological explanations for drug use are characterized as **social influence theories** and **structural influence theories,** respectively. This section first examines social influence theories and concludes with structural influence theories. The former set of theories is directed toward the roles played by significant others and the impact they have on the individual. In contrast, structural influence theories are based on the assumption that the organizational structure of society has a major impact on the extent of drug use and abuse.

> **social influence theories**
>
> theories that view a persons day-to-day social environment as responsible for drug use
>
> **structural influence theories**
>
> theories that view the organization of a society, group, or subculture as responsible for drug use by its members

Social Influence Theories

The theories presented in this section are known as (1) social learning, (2) the role of significant others in socialization, (3) labeling, and (4) subculture theories. The bases of these theories are that an individual's motivation to seek drugs is caused by social influence or social coercion.

Social Learning Theory

Social learning theory explains drug use as a form of learned behavior. Conventional learning occurs through imitation, trial and error, improvisation, rewarding appropriate behavior, and cognitive mental processes. Social learning theory focuses directly on how drug use and abuse are acquired through interaction with others who use and abuse drugs.

> **social learning theory**
> a theory that asserts that the use of drugs results from early socialization experiences

The theory emphasizes the pervasive influence of *primary groups,* or groups that share a high amount of intimacy and spontaneity and whose members are bonded emotionally. Families and residents of tightly knit urban neighborhoods are examples of primary groups. In contrast, *secondary groups* are groups that share segmented relationships where interaction is based on prescribed role patterns. An example of a secondary group would be the relationship between you and a sales clerk in a grocery store or among a group of employees scattered throughout a corporation.

Social learning theory addresses a type of interaction that is highly specific. This type of interaction involves learning specific motives, techniques, and appropriate meanings that are commonly attached to a particular type of drug.

As the sociologist Howard Becker points out in his well-known article "Becoming a Marijuana User," the novice who is perceived as a first-time user must learn the technique. An example is given from one of the coauthor's of this text:

> The first time I tried smoking weed, nothing much happened. I always thought it was like smoking a cigarette. When the joint came around the first time, I refused it. The next time

it came around, I noticed everyone was looking at me. So, I took the joint and started to inhale, then exhale.

> My friend sitting next to me said something to the effect, "Dude, hold it in; don't waste it. This is good weed and we don't have that much between us." Right after that, we did some "shotguns." This is where someone exhales directly into your mouth—lips to lips. My friend filled my lungs with his exhaled weed breath. After the first comment about holding it in, I started to watch how everyone was inhaling and realized that you really don't smoke weed like an ordinary cigarette; you have to hold in the smoke.

> *From Venturelli's research files, male, age 16, second-year high-school student in a small Midwestern town, February 15, 1997*

A second example of learning theory (also from the author's files):

> I first started using drugs, mostly alcohol and pot, because my best friend in high school was using drugs. My best friend Tim (a pseudonym) learned from his older sister [to use drugs]. Before I actually tried pot, Tim kept telling me how great it was to be high on dope; he said it was much better than beer. I was really nervous the first time I tried pot with Tim and another friend even though I heard so much detail about it from Tim before that first time I tried it. The first time I tried it, it was a complete letdown. The second time (the next day, I think it was), I remember I was talking about a teacher we had and in the middle of the conversation, I remember how everything appeared different. I started feeling happy and while listening to Tim as he poked jokes at the teacher, I started to hear the background music more clearly than ever before. By the time the music ended, and a new CD started, I knew I was high.

> *From Venturelli's research files, 22-year-old male student at a private liberal arts college in the Midwest, February 15, 1997*

A third example illustrates learning theory with another type of drug:

> First time I tried acid (LSD) I didn't know what to expect. Schwa (a pseudonym) told me it was a

very different high from grass (marijuana). After munching on one "square" [one dose of LSD]— after about 20 minutes—I looked at Schwa and he started laughing and said, "Feelin' the effects Ki-ki [interviewee's nickname]?" I said, "Is this it?! Is this what it feels like? I feel weird."

With a devious grin . . . , Schwa said, "Yep. We are now on the runway, ready to take off. Just wait a little while longer, it's going to get better and better. Fasten your seat belts!"

From Venturelli's files, male, age 33, May 6, 1996

Learning to perceive the effects of the drug is the second major outcome in the process of becoming a regular user. Here, the ability to feel the authentic effects of the drug is being learned. The more experienced drug users in the group impart their knowledge to naive first-time users. The coaching information they provide describes how to recognize the euphoric effects of the drug, as illustrated in another excerpt:

I just sat there waiting for something to happen, but I really didn't know what to expect. After the fifth "hit" [a hit consists of deeply inhaling a marijuana cigarette as it is being passed around and shared in a group], I was just about ready to give up ever getting "high."

Then suddenly, my best buddy looked deeply into my eyes and said, "Aren't you 'high' yet?" Instead of just answering the question, I immediately repeated the same words the exact way he asked me. In a flash, we both simultaneously burst out laughing. This uncontrollable laughter went on for what appeared to be over five minutes. Then he said, "You silly ass, it's not like an alcohol 'high,' it's a 'high high.' Don't you feel it? It's a totally different kind of 'high.'"

At that very moment, I knew I was definitely 'high' on the stuff. If this friend would not have said this to me, I probably would have continued thinking that getting 'high' on the hash was impossible for me.

From an interview with a 17-year-old male attending a small, private liberal arts college in the Southeast, conducted by Peter Venturelli on May 15, 1984

Once drug use has begun, continuing the behavior involves learning the following sequence: (1) where and from whom the drug can be purchased, (2) how to acquire a steady supply, (3) how to maintain the secrecy of use from authority figures and casual acquaintances, and (4) how to justify continual use.

Role of Significant Others Once a pattern of drug use has been established, the learning process plays a role in sustaining drug-taking behavior. Edwin Sutherland (1947, 5–9), a pioneering criminologist in sociology, believes that the mastery of criminal behavior depends on the frequency, duration, priority, and intensity of contact with others who are involved in similar behavior (see also Heitzeg 1996, 28, 48). This theory can also be applied to drug-taking behavior.

In applying Sutherland's principles of social learning to drug use, which he calls *differential association theory,* the focus is on how other members of social groups reward criminal behavior and under what conditions this deviance is perceived as important and pleasurable.

Becker and Sutherland's theories explain why adolescents may use psychoactive drugs. Essentially, both theories say that the use of drugs is learned during intimate interaction with others who serve as a primary group. See page 41, "Here and Now" for information on how the role of significant others can determine a child's disposition toward or away from illicit drug use.

Learning theory also explains how adults and the elderly are taught the motivation for using a particular type of drug. This learning occurs through such influences as drug advertising, with its emphases on testimonials by avid users, medical advice, or assurances from actors and actresses portraying physicians or nurses. Listeners, viewers, or readers who experience such commercials promoting particular brand-name over-the-counter drugs are bombarded with the necessary motives, techniques, and appropriate attitudes for consuming drugs. When drug advertisements and medical experts recommend a particular drug for specific ailments, they in effect are authoritatively persuading viewers, listeners, or readers that taking a drug will soothe or cure the medical problem presented.

Symptoms of Drug and Alcohol Abuse

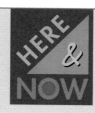

Following are profiles of children who are least likely and more likely, respectively, to use and abuse drugs.

Least Likely

▲ Child comes from a strong family.

▲ Family has a clearly stated policy toward drug use.

▲ Child has strong religious convictions.

▲ Child is an independent thinker, not easily swayed by peer pressure.

▲ Parents know the child's friends and the friends' parents.

▲ Child often invites friends into the house and their behavior is open, not secretive.

▲ Child is busy and productive and pursues many interests.

▲ Child has a good, secure feeling of self.

▲ Parents are comfortable with their own use of alcohol, drugs, and pills, set a good example in using these substances, and are comfortable in discussing their use.

▲ Parents set a good example in handling crisis situations.

▲ Child maintains at least average grades and good working relationships with teachers.

Symptoms Exhibited by the Child Who May Be Using Drugs

EDITOR'S NOTE: A child will usually display more than one of the symptoms below when experimenting with drugs. Please remember that any number of the symptoms could also be the result of a physical impairment or disorder.

▲ Abrupt change in behavior (for example, from very active to passive, loss of interest in previously pursued activities such as sports or hobbies).

▲ Diminished drive and ambition.

▲ Moodiness.

▲ Shortened attention span.

▲ Impaired communication such as slurred speech, jumbled thinking.

▲ Significant change in quality of school work.

▲ Deteriorating judgment and loss of short-term memory.

▲ Distinct lessening of family closeness and warmth.

▲ Suddenly popular with new friends who are older and unknown to family members.

▲ Isolation from family members (hiding in bedroom or locking bedroom door).

▲ Sneaking out of the house.

▲ Sudden carelessness regarding appearance.

▲ Inappropriate overreaction to even mild criticism.

▲ Secretiveness about whereabouts and personal possessions.

▲ Friends who avoid introduction or appearance in the child's home.

▲ Use of words that have odd, underworld connotations.

▲ Secretiveness or desperation for money.

▲ Rapid weight loss or appetite loss.

▲ "Drifting off" beyond normal daydreaming.

▲ Extreme behavioral changes such as hallucination, violence, unconsciousness, and so on that could indicate a dangerous situation close at hand and needing fast medical attention.

▲ Unprescribed or unidentifiable pills.

▲ Strange "contraptions" (e.g. smoking paraphanalia) or hidden articles.

▲ Articles missing from the house. Child could be stealing to receive money to pay for drugs. ■

Sources: L.A.W. Publications, *Let's All Work to Fight Drug Abuse* (Addison, TX: C & L Printing Company, 1985) 38. Used with permission of the publisher. Santa Barbara Alcohol and Drug Program, 1996.

Are Drug Users Socialized Differently? Social scientists—primarily sociologists and social psychologists—believe that many social development patterns are closely linked to drug use. Based on the age when an adolescent starts to consume alcohol, predictions can be made about his or her sexual behavior, academic performance, and other behaviors, such as lying, cheating, fighting, and marijuana use. The same predictions can be made when the adolescent begins using marijuana. Early intense use of alcohol or marijuana represents a move toward less conventional behavior, greater susceptibility to peer influence, increased delinquency, and lower achievement in school. In general, drug abusers have 14 characteristics in common:

1. Their drug use usually follows clear-cut developmental steps and sequences. Use of legal drugs, such as alcohol and cigarettes, almost always precedes use of illegal drugs.

2. Use of certain drugs, particularly habitual use of marijuana, is linked to the **amotivational syndrome,** which causes a general change in personality. This change is characterized by apathy, a lack of interest and/or inability or difficulty in accomplishing goals.* The latest research also clearly shows that marijuana use is often responsible for attention and memory impairment (NIDA 1996).

> **amotivational syndrome**
>
> an intensive state of lethargy coinciding with heavy marijuana use

3. Immaturity, maladjustment, or insecurity usually precede the use of marijuana and other illicit drugs.

4. Those more likely to try illicit drugs, especially before age 12, usually have a history of poor school performance and classroom disobedience.

* Some argue that perhaps a general lack of ambition (also known as *lethargy*) may *precede* rather than *result* from marijuana use, or that aspects of the amotivational syndrome are already present in heavy marijuana users even before the drug is used and that the use of marijuana merely heightens the syndrome. In any case, the steady use of marijuana and the amotivational syndrome often occur together.

5. Delinquent or repetitive deviant activities usually precede involvement with illicit drugs.

6. A set of values and attitudes that facilitates the development of deviant behavior exists before the person tries illicit drugs.

7. A social setting where drug use is common, such as communities and neighborhoods where peers use drugs indiscriminately and where "crack" houses and drug-using gangs dominate, is likely to reinforce and increase the predisposition to drug use.

8. Drug-induced behaviors and drug-related attitudes of peers are usually among the strongest predictors of subsequent drug involvement.

9. Children who feel their parents are distant from their emotional needs are more likely to become drug addicted. (See page 43, "Here and Now" describing how divorce affects adolescent drug use.)

10. The older people are when they start using drugs, the greater the probability of stopping drug use. The period of greatest risk of initiation into illicit drug use is usually over by the early twenties.

11. The family structure has changed, with more than half the women in the United States now working outside the home. How the lack of a stay-at-home parent affects the quality of child care and nurturing is difficult to assess. Also, a higher percentage of children are being raised in single-parent households, due to separation and divorce.

12. Mobility obstructs a sense of permanency, and it contributes to a lack of self-esteem. Often children are moved from one location to another, and their community can easily become nothing more than a group of strangers. There may be little pride in home or community and no commitment to society.

13. Among minority members, a major factor involved in drug dependence is a feeling of powerlessness due to discrimination based on race, gender, social standing, or other attrib-

utes. Groups subject to discrimination have a disproportionately high rate of unemployment and below-average income. The Carnegie Council on Children estimated that 19 million children grow up in poverty every year and feel powerless over their situation. The adults they have as role models are unemployed and powerless. Higher rates of delinquency and drug addiction occur in such settings.

14. Abusers who become highly involved in selling drugs begin by witnessing that drug trafficking is a lucrative business, especially in rundown neighborhoods. In some communities, selling drugs seems to be the only available alternative to real economic success (Blum and Richards 1979; Williams 1989; Wilson 1988; Siegel and Senna 1994, 398–402).

Labeling Theory Although the controversy continues whether labeling is a theory or perspective (Akers 1968, 1992; Plummer 1979; Heitzeg 1996), we take the position that labeling is a theory (Cheron 1992; Hewitt 1994), for it explains something very important with respect to drug use.

Does Divorce Affect Adolescent Drug Use?

As an example of how drug users may be affected by socialization, a study conducted by Dr. Needle (Needle, Su, and Doherty 1990; NIDA 1990; Siegel and Senna 1994) found higher drug use among adolescents whose parents divorce. According to the study, children who are adolescents when their parents divorce are associated with more extensive drug use and experience more drug-related health, legal, and other problems than their peers. This study linked the extent of teens' drug use to their age at the time of their parents' divorce. Teenagers whose parents divorce were found to use more drugs and experience more drug-related problems than two other groups of adolescents: those who were aged 10 or younger when their parents divorced, and those whose parents remained married.

This study has important implications for drug abuse prevention efforts. Basically, it says that not everyone is at the same risk for drug use. People at greater risk can be identified, and programs should be developed to meet their special needs.

In this research project, drug use among all adolescents increased over time. However, drug use was higher among adolescents whose parents had divorced, either when their children were preteens or teenagers. Drug use was highest for those teens whose parents divorced during their children's adolescent years. Such families also reported more physical problems, family disputes, and arrests.

The research results also showed that distinct gender differences existed in the way that divorce affected adolescent drug use, whether the divorce occurred during the offspring's childhood or adolescent years. Males whose parents divorced reported more drug use and drug-related problems than females. Females whose care-taking parents remarried experienced increased drug use after the remarriage. By contrast, males whose care-taking parents remarried reported a decrease in drug-related problems following the remarriage.

The researchers caution that these findings may have limited applicability, as most of the families were white and had middle to high income levels. Dr. Needle also notes that the results should not be interpreted as an argument in favor of the nuclear family. Overall, divorce affects adolescents in complex ways and remarriage can influence drug-using behavior, particularly when disruptions occur during adolescence; such turmoil can "trigger" a desire for extensive recreational licit and illicit drug use, often leading to drug abuse. ■

Labeling theory does not so much explain why initial drug use occurs; it does, however, detail the processes by which many people come to view themselves as socially deviant from others. Note that the terms *deviant* (in cases of individuals) or *deviance* (in cases of behavior), are sociologically defined as involving difference(s) from expected patterns of social behavior. The terms are not used in a judgmental manner, nor are the individuals *judged* to be deviant; instead, the terms refer to norm violators or norm violations. Those who violate expected norms perform deviant behaviors; however, they are not judged as immoral or sick.

Labeling theory says that other people whose opinions we value have a determining influence over our self-image (Best 1994, 237; Goode 1994, 99). (For an example of how labeling theory applies

labeling theory
a theory stressing that other people's impressions have a direct influence over one's self-image

to real-life situations, see page 45, "Case in Point".) Implied in this theory is that we exert only a small amount of control over the image we portray. In contrast, members of society, especially those we consider to be significant others, have much greater power in defining or redefining our image. The image we have of ourselves is vested in the people we admire and look to for guidance and advice. If these people come to define our actions as deviant, then their definition becomes the "fact" of our reality.

We can summarize labeling theory by saying that the labels we use to describe people have a profound influence on their self-perceptions. For example, imagine a fictitious individual known as Billy. Initially, Billy does not see himself (identify) as a compulsive drug user but as an occasional recreational drug user. Billy is very humorous, boisterous, and very outspoken about his drug use and likes to exaggerate the amount of marijuana he smokes on a daily basis. Slowly Billy's friends begin to perceive him as a "real stoner." According to labeling theory, what happens to Billy? As a result of being noticed when "high" and the comments his friends make, he may begin to feel uneasy whenever he is in the company of peers. These uneasy feelings will interfere with Billy's

ability to convey an image of occasional marijuana use. At first Billy may outwardly deny the charge of excessive drug use. Then he may poke fun at others' opinions. Eventually, however, labeling theory predicts that Billy's perception of himself will begin to mirror the consistent perception expressed by his accusers. This final self-perception occurs gradually. If he is unsuccessful in eradicating the addict image or, in this example, the "stoner" image, Billy will reluctantly concur with the label that has been thrust on him. Or, to strive for a self-image as an occasional marijuana user, Billy may abandon his peers so that he can become acceptable once more in the eyes of other people.

An important originator of labeling theory is Edwin Lemert (Lemert 1951, 133–141; Hewitt 1994, 255) who distinguishes between two types of deviance: primary and secondary deviance. **Primary deviance** is inconsequential deviance, which occurs without having a lasting impression on the perpetrator. Generally, most first-time violations of law, for example, are primary deviations. Whether the suspected or accused individual has committed the

primary deviance
inconsequential deviant behavior in which the perpetrator does not identify with the deviance

deviant act does not matter. What matters is whether the individual *identifies* with the deviant behavior.

Secondary deviance develops when the individual begins to identify and perceive himself or herself as deviant. The moment this transition occurs, deviance shifts from being primary to secondary. Many adolescents casually experiment with drugs. If, however, they begin to perceive themselves as drug users, then this behavior is virtually impossible to

secondary deviance
an advanced type of deviant behavior that develops when the perpetrator identifies with the deviant behavior

eradicate. The same holds true with OTC drug abuse. The moment an individual believes that he or she feels better after using a particular drug, the greater the likelihood that he or she will use the drug consistently.

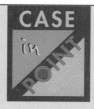

This excerpt, from the author's files, illustrates labeling theory.

After my mom found out, she never brought it up again. I thought the incident was over—dead, gone, and buried. Well, . . . it wasn't over at all. My mom and dad must have agreed that I couldn't be trusted anymore. I'm sure she was regularly going through my stuff in my room to see if I was still smoking dope. Even my grandparents acted strangely whenever the news on television would report about the latest drug bust in Chicago. Several times that I can't ever forget was when we were together and I could hear the news broadcast on TV from my room about some drug bust. There they all were whispering about me. My grandma asking if I "quitta the dope." One night, I overheard my mother reassure my dad and grandmother that I no longer was using dope. You can't believe how embarrassed I was that my own family was still thinking that I was

a dope fiend. They thought I was addicted to pot like a junkie is addicted to heroin! I can tell you that I would never lay such a guilt trip on my kids if I ever have kids. I remember that for two years after the time I was honest enough to tell my mom that I had tried pot, they would always whisper about me, give me the third degree whenever I returned late from a date, and go through my room looking for dope. They acted as if I was hooked on drugs. I remember that for a while back then I would always think that if they think of me as a drug addict, I might as well get high whenever my friends "toke up." They should have taken me at my word instead of sneaking around my personal belongings. I should have left syringes laying around my room!

Source: Interview with a 20-year-old male college student at a private university in the Midwest, conducted by Peter Venturelli on November 19, 1993.

Howard Becker (1963) believes that certain negative status positions (such as alcoholic, mental patient, criminal, drug addict, and so on) are so powerful that they dominate others (see also Pontell 1996). For example, if people who are important to Billy call him a "druggie," this name becomes a powerful label that will take precedence over any other status positions Billy may occupy. This label becomes Billy's **master status**—that of an addicted drug users. Even if Billy is also an above-average biology major, an excellent drummer, and a very likeable individual, those factors become secondary. Furthermore, once a powerful label is attached, it becomes much easier for the individual to uphold the image dictated by members of society. Master status labels distort an individual's public image in that other people expect consistency in role performance.

Once a negative master status has been attached to an individual's public image, labeling theorist Edwin Schur asserts that retrospective interpretation occurs. **Retrospective interpretation** is a form of "reconstitution of individual character or identity" (1971, 52). It largely involves redefining a person's image within a particular social group.

Finally, William I. Thomas's (1923, 203–22) contribution to labeling theory can be summarized in the theorem that "If men define situations as real, they are real in their consequences." Thus, according to this dictum, when someone is perceived as a drug user, the perception functions as a label of that person's character and shapes his or her self-perception (see also Cheron 1992, 31).

master status

the overriding status position in the eyes of others that clearly identifies an individual; e.g. doctor, lawyer, alcoholic

retrospective interpretation

the social psychological process of redefining a person's reputation as a member of a particular group

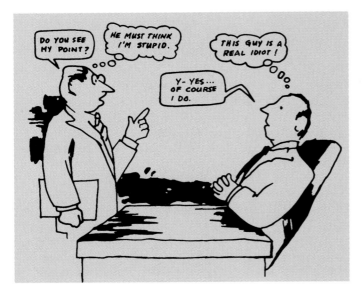

This cartoon illustrates the reflective process in retrospective interpretation that often occurs in daily conversations when we think that our unspoken thoughts are undetectable and hidden. In reality, however, these innermost thoughts are clearly conveyed through body language and nonverbal gestures.

Source: Reproduced with permission of Alex Silvestri.

Subculture Theory

The **subculture theory** speaks to the role of peer pressure and behavior that results from peer group influence(s). In all groups, there are certain members who are very charismatic and, as a result, exert more social influence than other peer members. Often such appealing members are group leaders, task leaders, or emotional leaders, who maintain a strong ability to influence others. Drug use that results from peer pressure demonstrates the extent to which these more popular, charismatic leaders can influence and pressure others to initially use or abuse drugs. These two excerpts from interviews illustrate subculture theory:

> I first started messing around with alcohol in high school. In order to be part of the crowd, we would sneak out during lunchtime at school and get "high." About six months after we started drinking, we moved on to other drugs. . . . Everyone in high school belongs to a clique, and my clique was heavy into drugs. We had a lot of fun being "high" throughout the day. We would party constantly. Basically, in college, it's the same thing.

subculture theory
an explanation that drug use is caused by peer pressure

> *From Venturelli's research files, 19-year-old male student at a small, religiously affiliated private liberal arts college in the Southeast, February 9, 1985*

The second interview illustrates how friendship, coupled with subtle and not-so-subtle peer pressure, influences the novice drug enthusiast:

> There I was on the couch with three of my friends, and as the joint was being passed around everyone was staring at me. I felt they were saying, "Are you going to smoke with us or will you be a holdout again?"

> *From Venturelli's research files, 20-year-old male university student, April 10, 1996*

In sociology, charismatic leaders are viewed as possessing status and prestige, defined as distinction in the eyes of others. In reality, as explained by the eminent sociologist Max Weber, such leaders have power over inexperienced drug users. Members of peer groups are often persuaded to experiment with drug use if leaders say, "Come on, try some, it's great" or "Trust me, you'll love it once you try it." In groups where drugs are consumed, the extent of peer influence with regard to drug use is affected by the more charismatic leaders. Such leaders find that the art of persuasion and camaraderie that drug use entails are very gratifying.

A further extension of subculture theory is the social and cultural support perspective. This perspective explains drug use and abuse in peer groups as resulting from an attempt by peers to solve problems collectively. In the neoclassic book, *Delinquent Boys: The Culture of the Gang* (1955), Cohen pioneered a study that showed for the first time that delinquent behavior is a collective attempt to gain social status and prestige within the peer group (see also Siegel and Senna 1994, 161). Members of certain peer groups are unable to achieve respect within the larger society. Such status-conscious youths find that being able to commit delinquent acts without apprehension by the law is admirable in the eyes of their peers. In effect, Cohen believes, delinquent behavior is a subcultural solution for overcoming status frustration and feelings of low self-esteem largely determined by lower-class frustrations.

Although Cohen's emphasis is on explaining juvenile delinquency, his notion that delinquent behavior is a subcultural solution can easily be applied to drug use and abuse in primarily members of lower-class peer groups. Underlying drug use and abuse in delinquent gangs, for example, results from sharing common feelings of alienation and escape from a society that appears noncaring, distant, and hostile.

Consider the current upsurge in violent gang memberships (see also Chapter 16, "Drug Use Within Subcultures," for more detail on adolescents and gangs). In such groups, not only is drug dealing a profitable venture, but also drug use serves as a collective response to alienation and estrangement from conventional middle-class society. In cases of minority violent gang members, the alienation results from racism, increasing poverty, the effects of migration and acculturation, and the result of minority status in a white-male–dominated society such as the United States (Glick and Moore 1990; Moore 1978; Sanders 1994).

Structural Influence Theories

The focus of these theories is on how the organization of a society, group, or subculture is largely responsible for drug abuse by its members. The belief is that it is not the society, group, or subculture that is causing the behavior—in this case, drug use—but that the organization itself or the lack of an organization determines the resulting behavior.

Social disorganization and social strain theories identify the different kinds of social change that are disruptive and how, in a *general* sense, people are affected by such change. Social disorganization theory asks, what in the social order (the larger social structure) causes people to deviate? Social strain theory asks, as a result of how, for example, family, peer, and employee social structures are organized, what would cause someone to deviate? This theory believes that frustration results from being unable to achieve desired goals. This perceived shortcoming compels an individual to deviate to achieve desired needs.

Overall, social disorganization theory describes a situation where, because of rapid social change, previously affiliated individuals no longer find themselves integrated into a community's social, commercial, religious, and economic institutions. When this isolation occurs, community members that were once affiliated become disaffiliated and lack effective attachment to the social order. As a result, these disaffiliated people begin to gravitate toward deviant behavior.

To develop trusting relationships, stability and continuity are essential for proper socialization. As will be discussed later in this chapter, if identity transformation occurs during the teen years, when drugs are first introduced, a stable environment is very important. Yet in a technological society, destabilizing and disorienting forces often result because technology causes rapid social change.

Although most people have little or no difficulty in adapting when confronted with rapid social change, others perceive this change as beyond their control. For example, consider an immigrant who experienced a nervous breakdown because he was unable to cope with the new society. The following two interviews show how such confusion and lack of control lead to drug use, which is viewed as an attractive alternative to coping with confusion and stress:

Interviewee: The world is all messed up.

Interviewer: Why? In what way?

Interviewee: Nobody gives a damn anymore about anyone else.

Interviewer: Why do you think this is so?

Interviewee: It seems like life just seems to go on and on ... I know that when I am under the influence, life is more mellow. I feel great! When I am "high," I feel relaxed and can take things in better. Before I came to Chalmers College [a pseudonym], I felt home life was one great big mess; now that I am here, this college is also a big pile of crap. I guess this is why I like smoking dope. When I am "high," I can forget my problems. My surroundings are friendlier; I am even more pleasant! Do you know what I mean?

> *Interview with a 19-year-old male marijuana user attending a small, private, liberal arts college in the Southeast, conducted by Peter Venturelli on February 12, 1984*

Similarly, an interview illustrates how a work environment can affect drug use:

> I had one summer job once where it was so busy and crazy that a group of us workers would go out on breaks just to get high. We worked the night shift and our "high breaks" were between 2:00 and 5:00 in the mornings.
>
> *From Venturelli's research files, first-year female college student, age 20, July 28, 1996*

Current Social Change in Most Societies Does social change per se cause people to use and abuse drugs? In response to this question, *social change*—defined as "any measurable change caused by technological advancement that disrupts cultural values and attitudes"—does not by itself cause widespread drug use. In most cases, social change materialistically advances a culture by profoundly affecting how things are accomplished. At the same time, however, rapid social change disrupts day-to-day behavior preserved by tradition, which has a tendency

conventional behavior

behavior largely dictated by custom and tradition and that is often jeopardized by rapid social change

to fragment such conventional social groups as families, communities, and neighborhoods. By **conventional behavior,** we mean behavior that is largely dictated by custom and tradition and thus evaporates or goes into a state of flux under rapid social change.

Examples include the number of youth subcultures that proliferated during the 1960s (Yinger 1982) and other more recent lifestyles and subcultures such as rappers, right to life, prochoice, Mothers Against Drunk Driving (MADD), gay liberation, punk rockers, and the new wave and recent rave subcultures. Furthermore, two other subcultures, teenagers and the elderly, both of whom have become increasingly independent and, in some subgroups, alienated from other age groups in society. These last subgroups are additional examples of groups that have become more distinct subcultures from the past. (See Figure 2.1.)

Simply stated, today's social institutions no longer influence people as much as they did in the past. As a consequence, people are free to explore different means of expression and types of recreation. For most, this occasion is a liberating experience leading to new and exciting outcomes; for others, the freedom to explore involves drug use and abuse.

The following two excerpts, gathered from various interviews, illustrate social disorganization and strain theory:

> These days, everything is rush, rush, rush. There are just not enough hours in the day. I set aside weekends in order to relax. Alcohol and marijuana allow me to relax from the rest of the week.
>
> *Interview with a 22-year-old, female, part-time college student at a public liberal arts college in the Southeast, conducted by Peter Venturelli, April 10, 1986*

I am into my own life because everyone is doing this. I see nearly everyone doing well around here. It's only those who are too stupid to succeed who are poor. I have had a rough time making it lately. Cocaine and speed help, but I know it's not the answer to all my problems. For

Figure 2.1

Levels of technological development and corresponding subcultures

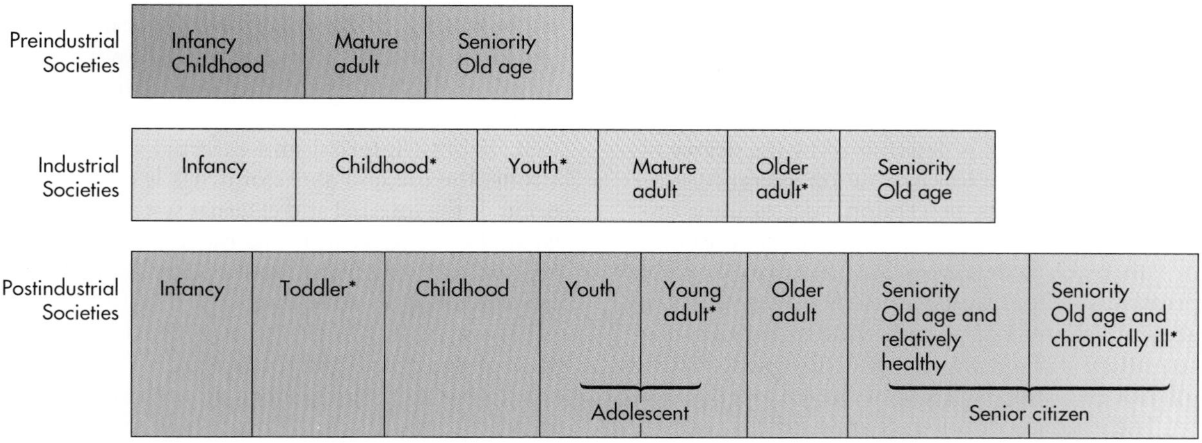

Preindustrial Societies	Infancy Childhood		Mature adult	Seniority Old age			

Industrial Societies	Infancy	Childhood*	Youth*	Mature adult	Older adult*	Seniority Old age	

Postindustrial Societies	Infancy	Toddler*	Childhood	Youth	Young adult*	Older adult	Seniority Old age and relatively healthy	Seniority Old age and chronically ill*

Adolescent   Senior citizen

*Represents a newly developed and separate stage of identification and expression from the prior era.

now, drugs help me to put up with all the shit going on in my life.

> *Interview with a 25-year-old male residing in the Southeast and receiving various forms of welfare, conducted by Peter Venturelli, March 10, 1985*

There is no direct link between social change and drug use. However, plenty of proof exists that certain dramatic changes occur in the organization of society, and many eventually lead certain groups to use and abuse drugs. Figure 2.1 illustrates how the number of life-cycle stages increases, depending on a society's level of technological development. Overall, it implies that, as societies advance from preindustrial to industrial to postindustrial, new subcultures become more likely to develop (see Fischer 1976, for similar thinking). In contrast to industrial and postindustrial societies, preindustrial societies do not have as many separate and distinct periods and cycles of social development. What is implied here is that the greater the number of distinct life cycles, the greater the fragmentation between the members of different stages of development.

"Generation gaps" occur across age groups that are increasingly unable to share differing values and attitudes.

Control Theory This last structural influence theory we are reviewing places most of its primary emphasis on influences outside the self as the primary cause for deviating to drug use and/or abuse. **Control theory** places importance on positive socialization. **Socialization** is defined as "the process by which individuals learn to internalize the attitudes, values, and behaviors needed to become participating members of conventional society." Generally, control theorists believe that human beings can easily become deviant if left without social controls. Thus, theorists who specialize in control theory emphasize the necessity

control theory

a belief that, if left to their own nature, individuals have a tendency to deviate from expected cultural values, norms, and attitudes

socialization

the learning process responsible for becoming human

of maintaining bonds to family, school, peers, and other social, political, and religious organizations.

In the 1950s and 1960s, criminologist Walter C. Reckless (1961; see also Siegel and Senna 1994, 188–190) developed containment theory. According to this theory, the socialization process results in the creation of strong or weak internal and external control systems.

Internal control is determined by the degree of self-control, high or low frustration tolerance, positive or negative self-perception, successful or unsuccessful goal achievement, and either resistance or adherence to deviant behavior. Environmental pressures, such as social conditions, may limit the accomplishment of goal-striving behavior; such conditions include poverty, minority group status, inferior education, and lack of employment.

The external, or outer, control system consists of effective or ineffective supervision and discipline, consistent or inconsistent moral training, positive or negative acceptance, identity, and self-worth. Examples are latchkey children who become delinquent and alcoholic parents who are inconsistent with discipline. They provide another illustration of breakdown in social control.

In applying this theory to the use or abuse of drugs, we could say that, if an individual has a weak external control system, the internal control system must take over to handle external pressure. Similarly, if an individual's external control system is strong from positive socialization based on discipline, moral training, and development of positive feelings of self-worth, then his or her internal control system will not be seriously challenged. If, however, either the internal or external control system is mismatched—one is weak and the other strong—the possibility of drug abuse increases.

If an individual's external and internal controls are both weak, he or she is most likely to use and abuse drugs. Table 2.1 shows the likelihood of drug use resulting from either strong or weak internal and external control systems. It indicates that, if both internal and external controls are strong, the use and abuse of drugs is not likely to occur. If the internal and external systems are both weak, however, drug use is most likely to occur (providing, of course, that drugs are available and presented by trusted friends).

Travis Hirschi (1971, 85, 159), a much respected sociologist and social control theorist, believes that delinquent behavior tends to occur whenever people lack (1) attachment to others, (2) commitment to goals, (3) involvement in conventional activity, and (4) belief in the common value system. If a child or adolescent is unable to become circumscribed within the family setting, school, and the nondelinquent peers, then the drift to delinquent behavior is inevitable.

We can apply Hirschi's theories to drug use as follows:

1. Drug users are less likely than nonusers to be closely tied to their parents.

2. Good students are less likely to use drugs.

3. Drug users are less likely to participate in social clubs and organizations and engage in team sport activities.

Table 2.1 **Likelihood of Drug Use**

Individual Internal Control	External Social Control	
	Strong	**Weak or Nonexistent**
Strong	Least likely (almost never)	Less likely (probably never)
Weak	More likely (probably will)	Most likely (almost certain)

4. Drug users are very likely to have friends whose activities are congruent with their own attitudes.

The following excerpt illustrates how control theory works:

> I was 15 when my mother confronted me with drug use. I nearly died. We have always been very close and she really cried when she found my "dug out"* in her car. My fear was that she would inquire about my drug use with our next-door neighbors, whose children were my best friends. One neighbor residing on the left of our house was one of my high-school teachers who knew me from the day I was born. The neighbor on the right side of our house was our church pastor. For a while after she confronted me, I just sneaked around more whenever I wanted to get high. After a few months, I become so paranoid of how my mother kept looking at me when I would come in at night that I eventually stopped smoking weed. Our family is very close and the town I live in (at that time the population was 400) was filled with gossip. I could not handle the pressure, so I quit.
>
> *From Venturelli's research files, female postal worker, age 22, residing in a smaller Midwestern town, February 9, 1997*

In conclusion, control theory depicts how conformity to conventional groups prevents deviance by demonstrating the relationship between the extent of group conformity and deviant drug use. It suggests that control is either internally or externally enforced by family, school, and peer group expectations. In addition, individuals who are either (1) not equipped with an internal system of self-control reflecting the values and beliefs of conventional society or (2) personally alienated from major social institutions such as family, school, and church may deviate without feeling guilty for their actions, often because of peer pressure resulting in a suspension or modification of internal beliefs.

---

*A "dug out" is a pocket-size wooden box used to store marijuana with a "one hitter." A "one hitter" is also drug paraphernalia designed to load a small amount of marijuana into a metal (usually aluminum) stem that looks like a cigarette. The front portion of the stem has an opening to pack a small amount of this drug at the tip.

◢ Danger Signals of Drug Abuse

How does one know when the use of drugs moves beyond normal use? Many people are prescribed drugs that affect their moods. Using these drugs wisely can be important for both physical and emotional health. Sometimes, however, it may be difficult to decide when use of drugs to handle stress becomes inappropriate.

It is important that your use of drugs does not result in addiction. The following are some danger signals that can help you evaluate your drug use behavior:

1. Do people who are close to you often ask about your drug use? Have they noticed any changes in your moods or behavior?

2. Do you become defensive when a friend or relative mentions your drug or alcohol use?

3. Are you sometimes embarrassed or frightened by your behavior under the influence of drugs or alcohol?

4. Have you ever switched to a new doctor because your regular physician would not prescribe the drug you wanted?

5. When you are under pressure or feel anxious, do you automatically take a sedative, a drink, or both?

6. Do you take drugs more often or for purposes other than those recommended by your doctor?

7. Do you mix drugs and alcohol?

8. Do you drink or take drugs regularly to help you sleep or even to relax?

9. Do you take a drug to get going in the morning?

10. Have you ever seriously thought that you may have a drug addiction problem?

If you answer "yes" to several of these questions, you may be abusing drugs or alcohol. Many places offer help at the local level, such as drug abuse programs in your community listed in the Yellow Pages under "Drug Abuse." Other resources include community crisis centers, telephone hotlines, and the Mental Health Association.

Making Low-Risk Choices

As will become more readily apparent throughout this text, some very real risks are associated with recreational drug use. The term **low-risk choices** refers to both abstinence and consumption of other quantities and frequencies of drug use not associated with increased use. "Low-risk" and "high-risk" are appropriate descriptors because these two concepts allow us to focus on the health and safety issues involved in drug use and acknowledge differences in values, levels of biological risk, and expectations for people at different points in life. Further, the term "low-risk drug use" reduces mixed messages about drug use. The issue is no longer whether to use drugs or to abstain from them, but how to define responsible drug use. The lowest risk is abstinence, of course; research shows that abstainers live longer than people who often use drugs for nonmedical purposes.

> **low-risk choices**
>
> abstinence and consumption of other quantities and frequencies of drug use not associated with increased use

A Five-Step Risk-Reduction Process

This five-step risk-reduction process can be used to help minimize alcohol and drug-related problems:

Step 1: Estimate your level of biological risk for alcoholism or other drug-related problems. This process includes answering such questions as: Do I have a family history of drug addiction? Do I have a parent or grandparent with an addiction problem? By "family," we are referring to blood relatives, not in-laws or step-parents. A strong family history is associated with drug addiction in blood relatives. Thus, the closer the drug-addicted relative is to you, the stronger the family history of addiction.

Another question is: Do I have an unusual early response to the drug I took? Research shows that people who initially exhibit a high tolerance (who are not easily affected by alcohol, for example) have increased risk for developing alcoholism (O'Bryan and Daugherty 1995). Why? In the case of alcohol, it will take more alcohol to create the effect; thus the drinker consumes more alcohol than someone with low tolerance levels. At lower risk for addiction are people who experience a mild flushing (mildly elevated pulse or skin temperature, nausea, and mild discomfort) after drinking one glass of an alcoholic beverage; they are sensitive to alcohol and are known to exhibit low tolerance to the drug in question.

Have I developed significantly increased tolerance? This question looks at current response to alcohol. The rate at which an individual develops higher tolerance is partly determined by genetic factors and partly by the quantity and frequency of alcohol use. People who can drink seven, eight, or even ten drinks before becoming impaired show significantly increased tolerance.

Step 2: Select the correct low-risk guideline. Have you answered "yes" to any of the questions posed in step 1? People who answered "no" to all of these questions do not have any significant biological risk in drug use.

Step 3: Adjust for individual differences to reduce the risk of impairment. The factors that create individual differences are as follows:

▲ Body size—a small person typically becomes more impaired by drug use than a larger person.

▲ Gender—women typically become more impaired than men of the same size, especially with regard to alcohol use.

▲ Age—young children and the elderly become more impaired than adults on the same amount of alcohol.

▲ Other drugs—taking a combination of drugs generally increases the risk of impairment and, in some combinations, accidental death.

▲ Fatigue or illness—fatigue increases impairment from alcohol and increases the risk for impairment.

▲ Empty stomach—an empty stomach increases impairment from most drugs.

Step 4: When consuming drugs, it is important to be aware of laws, fraternity alcohol policies, school policies, job policies, and so on. For example, do I want to risk my security or safety by using a particular drug?

Step 5: Follow through on the drug choice you have made. Follow-through is important on everything for success. Once aware of steps 1 through 4, step 5 completes the behavior.

EXERCISES FOR THE WEB

Exercise 1: SAMHSA

SAMHSA's mission within the nation's health system is to improve the quality and availability of prevention, treatment, and rehabilitation services. SAMHSA focuses on reducing illness, death, disability, and cost to society which result from substance abuse and mental illnesses. The Substance Abuse and Mental Health Services Administration is comprised of three centers [LIST THEM] that carry out the agency's mission of providing substance abuse and mental health services.

Exercise 2: Employee Assistance Programs

The Center for Substance Abuse and Prevention, one of three centers under SAMHSA, was established to lead the federal effort in prevention and intervention of alcohol, tobacco, and other drug abuse (ATOD). CSAP promotes the development of comprehensive prevention systems suited to community, state, national, and international needs. Its programs are designed to connect people and resources with innovative ideas, strategies, and means that encourage efforts to reduce and eliminate substance abuse problems in the United States. CSAP also has information on employee assistance programs. EAPs are designed to help employers maintain the health and wellbeing of their employees. One of the strongest components of an EAP is its strategy for dealing with drug-related problems.

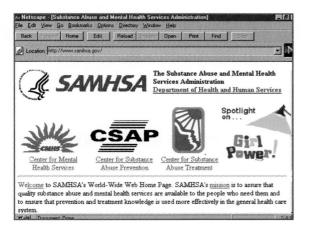

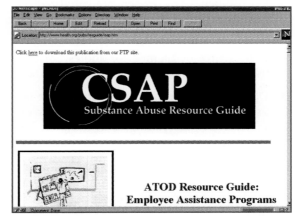

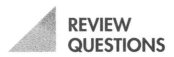 **REVIEW QUESTIONS**

1. In addition to better cultivation techniques, cite several other possible reasons why the potency (THC content) of the average marijuana joint has increased since 1960.

2. Given that over 88% of the U.S. population members are daily drug users of some form, do you think we need to reexamine our strict drug laws, which may be punishing a sizable number of drug users in our society who simply want to use illicit drugs?

3. Is there any way to combine biological and sociological explanations for why people use drugs so that the two perspectives do not conflict? (Sketch out a synthesis between these two sets of theoretical explanations.)

4. What is the relationship between mental illness and drug abuse? Why is this relationship important?

5. Do you accept the "rats in a maze" conception that psychology offers for explaining why people come to abuse drugs? (This view primarily states that humans are like automatons and that reinforcement explains why certain people become addicted to drugs.) Explain your answer.

6. In reviewing the psychological and sociological drug use theories, which theories best explain drug use? Defend your answer.

7. Does differential association theory take into account non–drug-using individuals whose socialization environment was drug-infested?

8. Do you believe drug users are socialized differently and that these alleged differences account for drug use? Defend your answer.

9. Can divorce be blamed for adolescent drug use? Why or why not, and if so, to what extent?

10. Do the current and alarming drug abuse statistics reflect the failure of social change in our society? Why do you agree or disagree with this statement?

11. Why is making low-risk choices regarding drug use a more realistic approach for drug moderation than advocating "just say no" to drug use?

KEY TERMS

sinsemilla
northern lights
Geneva sativa
genetic and biophysiological theories
central nervous system (CNS)

psychoactive effects
neurotransmitters
dopamine
habituation
"addiction to pleasure" theory
differential reinforcement
social influence theories
structural influence theories
social learning theory
amotivational syndrome
labeling theory
primary deviance
secondary deviance
master status
retrospective interpretation
subculture theory
conventional behavior
control theory
socialization
low-risk choices

SUMMARY

1 Drug use is more serious today than in the past because (a) drug use and abuse have increased dramatically since 1960; (b) today, illicit drugs are more potent than in the past; (c) the media presents drug use as rewarding; (d) drug use physically harms members of society; and (e) drug use and dealing by violent gangs are increasing at an alarming rate.

2 Genetic theory suggests that the predisposition to drug use can be found in an individual's gene structure. "Addiction to pleasure" theories indicate that it is biologically normal to continue a pleasure stimulation when drugs give a pleasurable experience.

3 The American Psychiatric Association classifies severe drug dependence as a form of psychiatric disorder. Drug abuse can cause mental conditions that mimic major psychiatric illnesses such as schizophrenia, severe anxiety disorders, and suicidal depression.

4 Introversion and extraversion patterns have been associated with levels of neural arousal in brain stem circuits. These forms of arousal are

closely associated with effects caused by drug stimulants or depressants.

5 Reinforcement or learning theory says that the motivation to use or abuse drugs stems from how the "high" from alcohol and other drugs reduce anxiety, tension, and stress. Positive social influences by drug-using peers also promote drug use.

6 Social influence theories include social learning, the role of significant others, and labeling and subculture theories. Social learning theory explains drug use as a form of learned behavior. Significant others play a role in the learning process involved in drug use and/or abuse. Labeling theory says that other people we consider important can influence whether drug use becomes an option for us. If key people we admire or fear come to define our actions as deviant, then the definition becomes the "facts" of our reality. Subculture theories trace original drug experimentation, use, and/or abuse to peer pressure.

7 There are a number of consistencies in socialization patterns found among drug abusers ranging from: immaturity, maladjustment, and/or insecurity to exposure and belief that selling drugs is a very lucrative business venture.

8 Sociologist Howard Becker believes that first-time drug users become attached to drugs because of three factors: they learn the techniques of drug use; they learn to perceive the pleasurable effects of drugs; and they learn to enjoy the drug experience.

9 *Primary deviance* is deviant behavior that the perpetrator does not identify with; hence, it is inconsequential deviant behavior. *Secondary deviance* is deviance that one readily identifies with.

10 Both internal and external social control should prevail concerning drug use. Internal control deals with internal psychic and internalized social attitudes; external control is exemplified by living in a neighborhood and community where drug use and abuse are severely criticized or not tolerated as a means to seek pleasure or avoid stress and anxiety.

11 Low-risk drug use refers to both abstinence and consumption of other quantities and frequencies of drug use not associated with increased drug use.

REFERENCES

Akers, R. L. "Problems in the Sociology of Deviance: Social Definition and Behavior." *Social Forces* 6 (June 1968): 455–65.

Akers, R. L. *Drugs, Alcohol, and Society: Social Structure, Process, and Policy.* Belmont, CA: Wadsworth, 1992.

American Psychiatric Association. "Substance-Related Disorders." *Diagnostic and Statistical Manual of Mental Disorders,* 4th ed. Allen Frances, Chairperson. Washington, DC: American Psychiatric Association, 1994: 175–272.

Apostolides, M. "Special Report: The Addiction Revolution: Old Habits Get New Choices." *Psychology Today* 29 (September/October 1996): 33–43, 75–6.

Bartels, S., G. Teague, R. Drake, R. Clark, P. Bush, and D. Noordsy. "Substance Abuse in Schizophrenia: Service Utilization and Costs." *Journal of Nervous and Mental Disease* 181 (1993): 227–32.

Becker, H. S. *Outsiders: Studies in the Sociology of Deviance.* New York: Free Press, 1963.

Becker, H. S. "History, Culture, and Subjective Experience: An Exploration of the Social Basis of Drug-Induced Experiences." *Journal of Health and Social Behavior* 8 (1967): 163–76.

Bejerot, N. "Current Problems of Drug Addicted." *Lakartidingen* (Sweden) 62, 50 (1965): 4231–38.

Bejerot, N. *Addiction: An Artificially Induced Drive.* Springfield, IL: Thomas, 1972.

Bejerot, N. "The Biological and Social Character of Drug Dependence." In *Psychiatrie der Gegenwart, Forschung und Praxis* 2nd ed., edited by K. P. Kisker, J. E. Meyer, C. Muller, and E. Stromogrew, 3: 488–518. Berlin: Springer-Verlag, 1975.

Best, J., and D. F. Luckenbill. *Organizing Deviance.* 2nd ed. Englewood Cliffs, NJ: Prentice-Hall, 1994.

Blum, R. H., and L. Richards. "Youthful Drug Use." In *Handbook on Drug Abuse,* edited by R. L. Dupont, A. Goldstein, and J. O. Darnell, 257–69. Washington, DC: National Institute on Drug Abuse, 1979.

Brady, K., and R. Lydiard. "Bipolar Affective Disorder and Substance Abuse." *Journal of Clinical Psychopharmacology* 12 (1992): 178–228.

Carlson, N. *Psychology: The Science of Behavior,* 3rd ed. Boston: Allyn and Bacon, 1990.

Cershon, E., and R. Rieder, "Major Disorders of Mind and Brain." *Scientific American* 267 (September 1992): 127–33.

Chaiken, B. "Felony Defendants in Large Urban Counties, 1992." Washington, DC: U.S. Department of Justice, NCJ-148826, July 1996.

Cheron, J. M. *Symbolic Interactionism: An Introduction, an Interpretation, an Integration,* 4th ed. Englewood Cliffs, NJ: Prentice-Hall, 1992.

Cohen, A. K. *Delinquent Boys: The Culture of the Gang.* Glencoe, IL: Free Press, 1955.

Conrad, P., and J. W. Schneider. *Deviance and Medicalization.* St. Louis, MO: Mosby, 1980.

Cummings, S. "Anatomy of a Wilding Gang." In *Gangs: The Origins and Impact of Contemporary Youth Gangs in the United States,* edited by S. Cummings and D. J. Monti, 49–73. Albany: State University of New York Press, 1993.

Dowieko, H. E. *Concepts of Chemical Dependency,* 3rd ed. Pacific Grove, CA: Brooks/Cole Publishing Co. 1996: 217–18.

Drug Strategies. "Keeping Score: What We Are Getting for Our Federal Drug Control Dollars 1995." Washington, DC: 1995. Available 080/edres/colleges/boss/depts/cesar/drugs/ks1995.

"Epidemiological and Services Research on Mental Disorders that Co-occur with Drug and/or Alcohol Disorders." *Prevention Pipeline* 7 (January–February 1994): 71.

Eysenck, H. J. and M. W. Eysenck. *Personality and Individual Differences: A Natural Science Approach.* New York: Plenum Press, 1985.

Farrar, H., and G. Kearns. "Cocaine: Clinical Pharmacology and Toxicology." *Journal of Pediatrics* 115 (1989): 665–75.

Fischer, C. S. *The Urban Experience.* New York: Harcourt Brace Jovanovich, 1976.

Francis, C. "The Cannabis Cup: Pieces of 8." *High Times,* May 1996: 44–52, 54–56, 62.

Glick, R., and J. Moore, eds. *Drugs in Hispanic Communities.* New Brunswick: Rutgers University Press, 1990.

Goode, E. *Deviant Behavior.* 4th ed. Englewood Cliffs, NJ: Prentice-Hall, 1994.

Gray, J. A. *The Psychology of Fear and Stress,* 2nd ed. Cambridge, UK: Cambridge University Press, 1987.

Grinspoon, L. "Update on Cocaine." *Harvard Mental Health Letter* 10 (September 1993): 1–4.

Halloway, M. "Rx for Addiction." *Scientific American* (March 1991): 94–103.

Heitzeg, N. A. *Deviance: Rulemakers and Rulebreakers.* Minneapolis: West Publishing, 1996.

Hewitt, J. P. *Self and Society: A Symbolic Interactionist Social Psychology,* 6th ed. Boston: Allyn and Bacon, 1994.

Hirschi, T. *Causes of Delinquency,* 2nd ed. Los Angeles: University of California Press, 1971.

Hutchinson, R., and C. Kyle. "Hispanic Street Gangs in Chicago's Public Schools." In *Gangs: The Origins and Impact of Contemporary Youth Gangs in the United*

States, edited by S. Cummings and D. J. Monti, 113–36. Albany: State University of New York Press, 1993.

Imperato, A., A. Mele, M. Serocco, and S. Puglisi-Allegra. "Chronic Cocaine Alters Limbic Extracellular Dopamine Neurochemical Basis for Addiction." *European Journal of Pharmacology* 212 (1992): 299–300.

Izenwasser, S., and C. Kornetsky. "Brain-Stimulation Reward: A Method for Assessing the Neurochemical Basis of Drug-Induced Euphoria." In *Drugs of Abuse and Neurobiology,* edited by R. Watson. Boca Raton, FL: CRC Press, 1992: 1–21.

Jarvik, M. "The Drug Dilemma: Manipulating the Demand." *Science* 250 (1990): 387–92.

Jellinek, E. M. *The Disease Concept of Alcoholism.* New Haven, CT: Hillhouse Press, 1960.

Koob, G. "Drugs of Abuse: Anatomy, Pharmacology and Function of Reward Pathways." *Trends in Pharmacological Sciences* 13 (May 1992): 177–84.

Kumpfer, K. L., and Charles W. Turner, "The Social Ecology Model of Adolescent Substance Abuse: Implications for Prevention," *International Journal of the Addictions* 25, 4A (1991): 433–63.

Kunen, J. S. "Madness in the Heart of the City." *People* (22 May 1989): 107–11.

Lemert, E. M. *Social Psychology: A Systematic Approach to the Theory of Sociopathic Behavior.* New York: McGraw-Hill, 1951.

Mathias, R. "Novelty Seekers and Drug Abusers Tap Same Brain Reward System, Animal Studies Show." *NIDA Notes* 10, 4 (July/August 1995): 1–5.

Mijuriya, T. H., and M. R. Aldrich. "Cannabis 1988: Old Drug, New Dangers—The Potency Question." *Journal of Psychoactive Drugs* 20 (1988): 47–55.

Moore, J. "Gangs, Drugs, and Violence. In *Gangs: The Origins and Impact of Contemporary Youth Gangs in the United States,* edited by S. Cummings and D. J. Monti, 27–46. Albany: State University of New York Press, 1993.

Moore, J. *Homeboys: Gangs, Drugs and Prison in the Barrios of Los Angeles.* Philadelphia: Temple University Press, 1978.

National Institute on Drug Abuse (NIDA). "Study Finds Higher Use Among Adolescents Whose Parents Divorce." *NIDA Notes* 5 (Summer 1990): 10.

National Institute on Drug Abuse (NIDA). "Double Trouble: Substance Abuse and Psychiatric Disorders." *NIDA Notes* 8 (November/December 1993): 20.

National Institute on Drug Abuse (NIDA). "Attention and Memory Impaired in Heavy Users of Marijuana." Rockville, MD: Office of the National Institute on Drug Abuse, February 20, 1996. Available http://www.health.org/pressrel/heavymar/html.

Needle, R. H., S. S. Su, and W. J. Doherty. "Divorce, Remarriage, and Adolescent Substance Use: A Prospective Longitudinal Study." *Journal of Marriage and the Family* 52 (1990): 157–9.

O'Brien, R., S. Cohen, G. Evans, and J. Fine. *The Encyclopedia of Drug Abuse,* 2nd ed. New York: Facts on File, 1992.

O'Bryan, T., and R. Daugherty. *On Campus . . . Talking about Alcohol and Other Drugs.* Lexington, KY: Prevention Research Institute, 1995.

Office of National Drug Control Policy (ONDCP). "Fact Sheet: Drug-Related Crime." Washington, DC: *Drugs and Crime Clearinghouse,* NCJ-149286, September 1994.

Plummer, K. "Misunderstanding Labelling Perspectives." *Deviant Interpretations,* edited by D. Downes and P. Rock, 85–121. London: Robertson, 1979.

Pontell, H. N. *Social Deviance,* 2nd ed. Upper Saddle River, NJ: Prentice-Hall, 1996.

Reckless, W. C. "A New Theory of Delinquency." *Federal Probation* 25 (1961): 42–46.

Rousar, E., K. Brooner, M. W. Regier, and G. E. Bigelow. "Psychiatric Distress in Antisocial Drug Abusers: Relation to Other Personality Disorders." *Drug and Alcohol Dependence* 34 (1995): 149–54.

Sanders, W. B. *Gangbangs and Drive-bys: Grounded Culture and Juvenile Gang Violence.* New York: 1994, Aldine De Gruyter.

Santa Barbara Alcohol and Drug Program. Santa Barbara, CA: July 16, 1996. Available http://www.silcom.com/ 'sbadp/treatment/adoleschecklist.html

Schur, E. M. *Labeling Deviant Behavior.* New York: Harper & Row, 1971.

Siegel, L. J., and J. J. Senna. *Juvenile Delinquency: Theory, Practice and Law.* St. Paul, MN: West Publishing, 1994.

Stolerman, I. "Drugs of Abuse: Behavioral Principles, Methods and Terms." *Trends in Pharmacological Sciences Reviews* 13 (May 1992): 170–76.

Sutherland, E. *Principles of Criminology,* 4th ed. Philadelphia: Lippincott, 1947.

Thomas, W. I., with D. S. Thomas. *The Child in America.* New York: Knopf, 1923.

Uhl, G., K. Blum, E. Noble, and S. Smith. "Substance Abuse Vulnerability and D-2 Receptor Genes." *Trends in Neurological Sciences* 16 (1993): 83–88.

Uhl, G., A. Persico, and S. Smith. "Current Excitement with D-2 Dopamine Receptor Gene Alleles in Substance Abuse." *Archives of General Psychiatry* 49 (February 1992): 157–60.

U.S. Bureau of the Census, U.S. Department of Commerce. *Statistical Abstract of the United States, 1990, The National Data Book,* 110th ed. Washington, DC: U.S. Bureau of the Census, U.S. Department of Commerce, January 1990: 122.

Will, G. "America's Slide into the Sewers." *Newsweek* (30 July 1990): 64.

Williams, T. *The Cocaine Kids.* New York: Addison-Wesley, 1989.

Wilson, W. J. *The Truly Disadvantaged.* Chicago: University of Chicago Press, 1990.

Wilson, M., and S. Wilson. *Drugs in American Life.* New York: Wilson, 1975.

Yinger, M. J. *Countercultures: The Promise and the Peril of a World Turned Upside Down.* New York: Free Press, 1982.

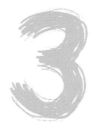

3 Drug Use and the Law

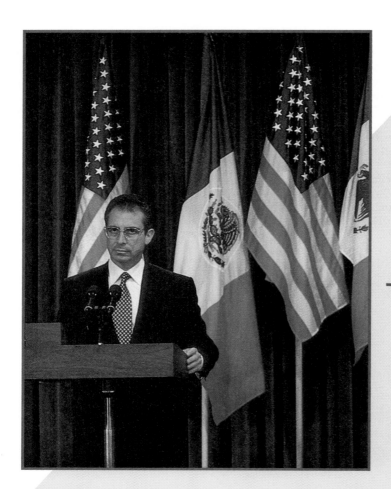

On completing this chapter
you will be able to: ▶

- Before World War II, all drugs, except those classified as narcotics, were available without prescription.
- Enforcement of drug use policies and drug laws differs across different countries.
- Many famous and historical figures in American literature, politics, psychology, and medicine were addicted to both licit and illicit drugs.

- Illicit drug use is much lower in Canada than in the United States, even though U.S. drug laws are more restrictive than Canada's drug laws.
- Despite the publicity and tax dollars spent on fighting the federal government's declared "War on Drugs," teenagers and adults consider drugs and alcohol less harmful and are more tolerant of drug use today than they were three years ago.

- Today it can cost a drug company $500 million and require 10 years of testing before a new drug is approved for marketing.
- The money spent by drug companies to promote their products is more than six times the combined educational budget of all medical schools in the United States.
- Many medical experts consider drug abuse to be a mental disorder.

Learning Objectives

- Identify the two major guidelines for controlling drug development and marketing.
- Identify and explain the Harrison Act of 1914.
- List the principal factors that influence the formation of laws regulating drug abuse.

- Outline the major approaches used to reduce substance abuse.
- Describe the three major strategies for combating drug use and abuse.
- Explain the main arguments for and against legalizing drugs.

- List the most common types of drug testing.
- Describe four major factors required for workable drug policies (pragmatic drug policies).

This chapter examines how and why, acting through democratically elected officials, our society restricts the use of licit drugs and prohibits and legislates against illicit drug use. The primary emphasis is to become familiar with the laws governing the prescription of certain drugs and the prohibition of others and to describe how such laws affect their use.

Society mandates that it maintain control over which drugs are permissible and which drugs are prohibited. Through legislation, enacted by democratically elected members of our society, we decide which drugs are licit and illicit. Thus, drug laws prohibit indiscriminate use of what society defines as a drug. As we saw in chapter 1, licit and illicit drugs produce vastly different effects on both the mental and bodily functions. Chapters 5 and 6 focus on how and why different types of drugs affect our bodies. In this chapter, you will come to better understand how our society attempts to control drug use and abuse.

One respondent gave the following answer to the question, What do you think about the current drug laws in the United States?

Drug use laws? P-l-e-a-s-e don't make me laugh. First of all, a certain percentage of adults, adolescents, and children will keep using drugs [referring here to illicit drugs] no matter what the laws against drug use specify. Second, arresting and putting people through the criminal justice system for a single, solitary possession is asinine! This type of legal social control, which is nothing more than a strong-arm tactical approach, will never stop a rather large percentage of the population from using and selling drugs.

From Venturelli's personal research files, first-year graduate student attending a Midwestern university

While one student may feel that laws that dictate nonuse of drugs are frivolous, others feel they are needed. The difference in perspectives is highlighted by the following comments:

Well, I realize that many people continue to use drugs that are illegal. Can you imagine what our drug use would be like without the laws now in place? At least something is in place [referring to our current drug laws], and if and when some-

one is caught either using or selling drugs, then he or she knows they screwed up and must pay for the consequences. I think stiff penalties for illegal drug use by the dealer are needed.

From Venturelli's personal research files, 31-year-old male juvenile probation officer in a U.S. Midwestern town

These opposing perspectives reflect the diverse opinions about drug use and law enforcement. Obtaining a clear consensus is improbable, if not impossible. Often, drug users or recent users adopt an *insider's* perspective, which views drug use as part of a recent or current lifestyle. Others adopt an *outsider's* perspective, which views drug users and their use of drugs as inappropriate behavior. The topic of drug use rarely evokes mundane or idle talk; opinions are generally emotionally charged in the direction of one perspective or another.

Drug regulation brings to mind numerous questions. For example, why are the laws against drug use so controversial? When were these laws first created? In regulating and prohibiting the free marketing of either licit or illicit drug use, how does U.S. society compare with other societies? Do these other societies have fewer drug users as a result of being more lenient or restrictive toward drug abusers? Do our drug laws coincide with the opinions of most U.S. citizens? Are nonpunitive approaches toward drug use feasible? Do drug laws realistically diminish drug use? What common attitudes prevail regarding the enactment and enforcement of drug laws?

This chapter attempts to respond to many of these questions by delving into the relationship between drug use and law enforcement. We will examine the development of drug regulations in the United States as it applies to both the manufacture of drugs and the control of their use and abuse. Though many of us would think that the regulation of drug manufacturing and drug abuse lie at the opposite ends of the spectrum, regulation of drug manufacturing and drug abuse actually evolved from the same process.

Many assume that laws controlling drug use in the United States and other industrialized nations have developed only recently. By contrasting these approaches with conditions in industrialized and less developed countries, we see that not every society follows U.S. ways of regulating or outlawing drugs. Some seem more repressive, some seem more permissive, and some have raised and imported drugs that other countries have forbidden. As we look at developing societies now in the stage of industrialization that our grandparents experienced in the United States years ago, we can gain insight into how attitudes on drug regulation developed here. We may also appreciate some of the dilemmas that seem so puzzling to us today.

◢ Cultural Attitudes About Drug Use

Currently, the cultural attitudes in the United States regarding the use of mind-altering substances blend beliefs in individuals' rights to live their lives as they desire with society's obligation to protect its members from burdens due to uncontrolled behavior. The history of drug regulation consists of regulatory swings due to attempts by government to balance these two factors while responding to public pressures and perceived public needs. For example, 100 years ago, most people expected the government to protect citizens' rights to produce and market new foods and substances; they did not expect or desire the government to regulate product quality or claims. Instead, the public relied on private morals and common sense to obtain quality and protection in an era of simple technology. Unfortunately, U.S. society had to learn by tragic experience that its trust was not well placed; many unscrupulous entrepreneurs were willing to risk the safety and welfare of the public in order to maximize profits and acquire wealth. In fact, most medicines of these earlier times were not merely ineffective but often dangerous.

Because of the advent of high technology and the rapid advancements society has made, we now rely on highly trained experts and government "watch-dog" agencies for consumer information and protection. Out of this changing environment have evolved two major guidelines for controlling drug development and marketing:

1. *Society has the right to protect itself from the damaging impact of drug use.* This concept is closely aligned with the emotional and highly visible issues of drug abuse, but also includes protection from other drug side effects. Thus, while we expect the government to protect society from drugs that can cause addiction, we also expect it to protect us from drugs that cause cancer, cardiovascular disease, or other threatening medical conditions.

2. *Society has the right to demand that drugs approved for marketing be safe and effective to the general public.* If drug manufacturers promise that their products relieve pain, these drugs should be analgesics; if they promise that their products relieve depression, those drugs should be antidepressants; if they promise that their products relieve stuffy noses, those drugs should be decongestants.

The public, through regulatory agencies and statutory enactments, has attempted to require that drug manufacturers produce *safe* and *effective* pharmaceutical products. Closely linked is the fact that society uses similar strategies to protect itself from the problems associated with the specific drug side effect of dependence or addiction, which is associated with drug abuse.

◢ The Road to Regulation and the FDA

The decline of patent medicines began with the 1906 Pure Food and Drug Act, which required manufacturers to indicate the amounts of alcohol, morphine, opium, cocaine, heroin, and marijuana extract on the label of each container. It became obvious at this time that many medicinal products on the market labeled as "nonaddictive" were, in fact, potent drugs "in sheep's labeling" and could cause severe dependence. However, most government interest at the time centered on regulation of the food industry, not drugs.

Even though federal drug regulation was based on the free-market philosophy that consumers could select for themselves, it was decided that the public should have information on possible dependence-producing drugs to ensure that they understood the risks associated with using these products. The Pure Food and Drug Act made misrepresentation illegal, so that a potentially addicting patent drug could not be advertised as "nonhabit forming." This step marked the beginning of new involvement by governmental agencies in drug manufacturing.

The Pure Food and Drug Act was modified, although not in a consumer-protective manner, by the Sherley Amendment in 1912. The distributor of a cancer "remedy" was indicted for falsely claiming on the label that the contents were effective. The case was decided in the U.S. Supreme Court in 1911. Justice Holmes, writing for the majority opinion, said that, based on the 1906 act, the company had not violated any law because legally all it was required to do was accurately state the contents and their strength and quality. The accuracy of the therapeutic claims made by drug manufacturers was not controlled. Congress took the hint and passed the Sherley Amendment to add to the existing law the requirement that labels should not contain "any statement . . . regarding the curative or therapeutic effect . . . which is false and fraudulent." However, the government had to prove fraud, which turned out to be difficult (and in fact is still problematic). This amendment did not improve drug products, but merely encouraged pharmaceutical companies to be more vague in their advertisements (Temin 1980).

Prescription Versus OTC Drugs

The distinction between prescription and over-the-counter (OTC) drugs is relatively new to the pharmaceutical industry. All nonnarcotic drugs were available OTC prior to World War II. It was not until a drug company unwittingly produced a toxic product that killed over 100 people that the Food and Drug Administration (FDA) was given control over drug safety in the 1938 Federal Food, Drug, and Cosmetic Act (Hunter 1993). The bill had been debated for several years in Congress and showed no promise of passage. Then a pharmaceutical company decided to sell a liquid form of a sulfa drug (the first antibiotic) and found that the drug would dissolve well in a chemical solvent, diethylene glycol (presently used in antifreeze products). The company marketed the antibiotic as Elixir Sulfanilamide without testing the solvent for toxicity. Under the 1906 Pure Food and Drug Act, the company could not be prosecuted for the toxi-

city of this form of drug or for not testing the formulation of the drug on animals first. It could only be prosecuted for mislabeling the product on the technicality that *elixir* refers to a solution in alcohol, not a solution in diethylene glycol. Again, it was apparent that the laws in place provided woefully inadequate protection for the public.

The 1938 act differed from the 1906 law in several ways. It defined drugs to include products that affected bodily structure or function even in the absence of disease. Companies had to file applications with the government for all new drugs showing that they were *safe* (not effective, just safe!) for use as described. And the drug label had to list all ingredients and include the quantity of each, as well as provide instructions regarding correct use of the drug and warnings about its dangers.

Prior to passage of the 1938 act, you could go to a doctor and obtain a prescription for any nonnarcotic drug or go to the pharmacy directly if you had already decided what was needed. The labeling requirement in the 1938 act allowed drug companies to create a class of drugs that could not be sold legally without a prescription. It has been suggested that the actions by the FDA were motivated by the frequent public misuse of two classes of drugs developed prior to passage of the 1938 law: sulfa antibiotics and barbiturates. People often took too little of the antibiotics to cure an infection and too much of the barbiturates and became addicted.

The 1938 Food, Drug, and Cosmetic Act allowed the manufacturer to determine whether a drug was to be labeled prescription or nonprescription. The same product could be sold as prescription by one company and as OTC by another! After the Durham-Humphrey Amendment was passed in 1951, almost all new drugs were placed in the prescription-only class. The drugs that were patented and marketed after World War II included potent new antibiotics and phenothiazine tranquilizers such as Thorazine. Both the FDA and the drug firms thought these products were potentially too dangerous to sell OTC. The Durham-Humphrey Amendment established the criteria, which are still used today, for determining whether a drug should be classified as prescription or nonprescription. Basically, if a drug does not fall into one of the following three categories, it is considered nonprescription:

1. The drug is habit-forming.
2. The drug is not safe for self-medication because of its toxicity.
3. The drug is a new compound that has not been shown to be completely safe.

Senator Kefauver's hearings, which began in 1959, initially were concerned with the enormous profit margins earned by drug companies because of the lack of competition in the market for new, patented drugs. Testimony by physicians revealed that an average doctor in clinical practice often was not able to evaluate accurately the efficacy of the drugs he or she prescribed. The 1938 law did not give the FDA authority to supervise clinical testing of drugs; consequently, the effectiveness of drugs being sold to the public was not being determined. Both the Kefauver and Harris Amendments in the House were intended to deal with this problem but showed no likely signs of becoming law until the **thalidomide** tragedy occurred.

> **thalidomide**
>
> a sedative drug that, when used during pregnancy, can cause severe developmental damage to a fetus

Thalidomide was used in Europe and distributed on a small scale in the United States as a sedative for pregnant women. There are two approximately 24-hour intervals early in pregnancy when thalidomide can alter the development of the arms and legs of an embryo. If a woman takes thalidomide on one or both of these days, the infant could be born with abnormally developed arms and/or legs (called **phocomelia,** from the Greek words for *flippers,* or "seal-shaped limbs").

> **phocomelia**
>
> a birth defect; impaired development of the arms, legs, or both

Although standard testing probably would not have detected this congenital effect of thalidomide and the tragedy would likely have occurred anyway, these debilitated infants stimulated passage of the 1962 Kefauver and Harris Amendments. They strengthened the government's regulation of both the introduction of new drugs and the production and sale of existing drugs. The amendments required, for the first time, that drug manufacturers demonstrate the efficacy as well as the safety of their drug products. The FDA was empowered to withdraw approval of a drug that was already being marketed. In addition, the agency was permitted to regulate and evaluate drug testing by pharmaceutical companies and mandate standards of good drug-manufacturing policy.

The Rising Demand for Effectiveness in Medicinal Drugs

To evaluate the effectiveness of the more than 4000 drug products that were introduced between 1938 and 1962, the FDA contracted with the National Research Council to perform the Drug Efficacy Study. This investigation started in 1966 and ran for three years. The council was asked to rate drugs as either effective or ineffective. Although the study was supposed to be based on scientific evidence, this information often was not available,

Characteristic limb deformities caused by thalidomide

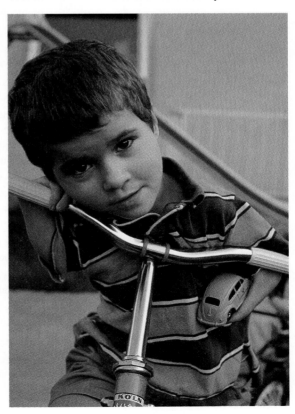

and so conclusions were sometimes founded on the clinical experience of the physicians on each panel; this judgment was not always based on reliable information.

A legal challenge resulted when the FDA took an "ineffective" drug off the market and the manufacturer sued. This action finally forced the FDA to define what constituted an adequate and well-controlled investigation. Adequate, documented clinical experience was no longer satisfactory proof that a drug was safe and effective. Each new drug application now had to include information about the drug's performance in patients compared with the experiences of a carefully defined control group. The drug could be compared with (1) a placebo, (2) another drug known to be active based on previous studies, (3) the established results of no treatment, or (4) historical data on the course of the illness without the use of the drug in question. In addition, a drug marketed before 1962 could no longer be "grandfathered in." If the company could not prove the drug had the qualifications to pass the post-1962 tests for a new drug, it was considered a new, unapproved drug and could not legally be sold. (For more on specific regulatory steps for new drugs, see Appendix 3-2.)

Table 3.1	Federal Laws for the Control of Narcotic and Other Abused Drugs	
Date	Name of Legislation	Summary of Coverage and Intent of Legislation
1914	Harrison Act	First federal legislation to regulate and control the production, importation, sale, purchase, and free distribution of opium or drugs derived from opium
1922	Narcotic Drug Import and Export Act	Intends to eliminate the use of narcotics except for medical and other legitimate purposes
1924	Heroin Act	Makes it illegal to manufacture heroin
1937	Marijuana Tax Act	Provides controls over marijuana similar to those that the Harrison Act provides over narcotics
1942	Opium Poppy Control Act	Prohibits growing opium poppies in the United States except under license
1951	Boggs Amendment to the Harrison Narcotics Act	Establishes severe mandatory penalties for conviction on narcotics charges
1956	Narcotics Control Act	Intends to impose very severe penalties for those convicted of narcotics or marijuana charges
1965	Drug Abuse Control Amendments (DACA)	Adopts strict controls over amphetamines, barbiturates, LSD, and similar substances, with provisions to add new substances as the need arises
1966	Narcotic Addict Rehabilitation Act (NARA)	Allows treatment as an alternative to jail
1968	DACA Amendments	Provides that a drug offender's sentence may be suspended and record be erased if not convicted for another violation for one year
1970	Comprehensive Drug Abuse Prevention and Control Act	Replaces or updates all other laws concerning narcotics and dangerous drugs
1972	Drug Abuse Office and Treatment Act	Provides $1.1 billion over three years to combat drug abuse and start treatment programs
1973	Methadone Control Act	Places controls on methadone licensing
1973	Heroin Trafficking Act	Increases penalties for traffickers and makes bail procedures more stringent

◢ Drug Abuse and the Law

The laws that govern the development, distribution, and use of drugs in general and drugs of abuse in particular are interrelated. There are, however, some unique features concerning the manner in which federal agencies deal with the drugs of abuse that warrant special consideration. A summary of drug abuse laws in the United States is shown in Table 3.1.

Coffee, tea, tobacco, alcohol, marijuana, hallucinogens, depressants (such as barbiturates), and narcotics have been subject to a wide range of controls, varying from none to rigid restrictions. Islamic countries have instituted severe penalties, such as strangulation for smoking tobacco or opium, and strict bans on alcohol. In other countries, these substances have been deemed either legal or prohibited, depending on the political situation and the desires of the population. Historically, laws have been changed when so many people demanded access to a specific drug of abuse that it would have been impossible to enforce a ban (as in the revocation of Prohibition) or because the government needed tax revenues that could be raised by selling the drug (one argument for legalizing drugs of abuse today). A current example is the controversy over decriminalization or legalizing marijuana (see Chapter 14).

Date	Name of Legislation	Summary of Coverage and Intent of Legislation
1973	Alcohol, Drug Abuse, and Mental Health Administration (ADAMHA)	Consolidates NIMH, NIAAA, and NIDA under ADAMHA*
1973	Drug Enforcement Administration (DEA)	Bureau of Narcotics and Dangerous Drugs is remodeled to become the DEA
1974 1978	Drug Abuse Prevention, Control, and Treatment Amendments	Extends the 1972 law
1978	Alcohol and Drug Abuse Education Amendments	Sets up the Office of Alcohol and Drug Abuse Education in the Department of Education; more emphasis on drug abuse in rural areas and on coordination at the federal–state level
1980	Drug Abuse Prevention, Treatment, and Rehabilitation Amendments	Extends prevention education and rehabilitation programs
1984	Drug Offenders Act	Sets up special program for offenders and organizes treatment
1986	Analogue (Designer Drug) Act	Makes illegal the use of substances similar in effects and structure to substances already scheduled
1988	Anti-Drug Abuse Act	Establishes the Office of the National Drug Control Policy to oversee all federal policies regarding research about and control of drugs of abuse.
1990	Crime Control Act of 1990	Doubles the appropriations authorized for drug law enforcement grants to states and localities; expands drug control and education programs aimed at the nation's schools, specific drug enforcement assistance to rural states, and regulation of precursor chemicals used in manufacturing of illegal drugs; provides additional measures aimed at seizure and forfeiture of drug traffickers' assets; sanctions anabolic steroids under the Controlled Substances Act; includes provisions on international money laundering, rural drug enforcement, drug-free school zones, drug paraphernalia, and drug enforcement grants
1992	ADAMHA Reorganization Act	Transfers the three institutes that constitute ADAMHA (NIDA, NIAAA, and NIMH) to NIH, and incorporates ADAMHA's services program into the new Substance Abuse and Mental Health Services Administration (SAMHSA)

(*) National Institute on Mental Health (NIMH), National Institute on Alcohol Abuse and Alcoholism (NIAAA), National Institute on Drug Abuse (NIDA).

The negative experiences that Americans had at the turn of the century with addicting substances such as opium led to the Harrison Act of 1914. It marked the first legitimate effort by the federal government to regulate and control the production, importation, sales, purchase, and distribution of addicting substances.

> **Harrison Act of 1914**
>
> the first legitimate effort by the government to regulate addicting substances

The Harrison Act served as the foundation and reference for subsequent laws directed at regulating drug abuse issues.

Today, the ways in which law enforcement agencies deal with substance abuse are largely determined by the Comprehensive Drug Abuse Prevention and Control Act of 1970. This act divided substances with abuse potential into categories based on the degree of their abuse potential and their clinical usefulness. The classifications, which are referred to as *schedules,* range from I to V.

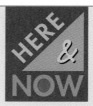

Controlled substances classified as either Schedule I, II, III, IV, or V drugs are described below:

Schedule I

▲ The drug or other substance has a high potential for abuse.

▲ The drug or other substance has no currently accepted medical use in treatment in the United States.

▲ There is a lack of accepted safety for use of the drug or other substance under medical supervision.

Schedule II

▲ The drug or other substance has a high potential for abuse.

▲ The drug or other substance has a currently accepted medical use in treatment in the United States or a currently accepted medical use with severe restrictions.

▲ Abuse of the drug or other substances may lead to severe psychological or physical dependence.

Schedule III

▲ The drug or other substance has less of a potential for abuse than the drugs or other substances in Schedules I and II.

▲ The drug or other substance has a currently accepted medical use in treatment in the United States.

▲ Abuse of the drug or other substance may lead to moderate or low physical dependence or high psychological dependence.

Schedule IV

▲ The drug or other substance has a low potential for abuse relative to the drugs or other substances in Schedule III.

▲ The drug or other substance has a currently accepted medical use in treatment in the United States.

▲ Abuse of the drug or other substance may lead to limited physical dependence or psychological dependence relative to the drugs or other substances in Schedule III.

Schedule V

▲ The drug or other substance has a low potential for abuse relative to the drugs or other substances in Schedule IV.

▲ The drug or other substance has a currently accepted medical use in treatment in the United States.

▲ Abuse of the drug or other substance may lead to limited physical dependence or psychological dependence relative to the drugs or other substances in Schedule IV.   ■

Source: U.S. Code, January 24, 1995.

Schedule I substances have high abuse potential and no currently approved medicinal use; they cannot be prescribed by health professionals. Schedule II drugs also have high abuse potential but are approved for medical purposes and can be prescribed with restrictions. The distinctions between Schedule II through V substances reflect the likelihood of abuse occurring and the degree to which the drugs are controlled by governmental agencies. The least addictive and least regulated of the substances of abuse are classified as Schedule V drugs. (See Table 3.2 and page 66 "Here and Now.")

Drug Laws and Deterrence

As previously discussed, drug laws often do not serve as a satisfactory deterrent against the use of illicit drugs. People have used and abused drugs for thousands of years despite governmental restrictions. (For information on another country's drug control laws, see page 68, "Fighting the Drug War.") It is very likely they will continue to do so (Balabanova et al. 1992) despite stricter laws and greater support for law enforcement.

As the amount of addiction increased during the mid-1960s, many ill-conceived programs and laws were instituted as knee-jerk reactions, with little understanding about the underlying reasons for the rise in drug abuse. Unpopular, restrictive laws rarely work to reduce the use of illicit drugs. Even as laws become more restrictive, they usually have little impact on the level of addiction; in fact, in some cases addiction problems actually have increased. For example, during the restrictive years of the 1960s and 1980s, drugs were sold everywhere to everyone—in high schools, colleges, and probably in every community. In the 1980s especially, increasingly large volumes of drugs were sold throughout the United States. Billions of dollars were paid for those drugs. Although no one knows precisely how much was exchanged, it likely approached $80 to $100 billion per year for all illegal drugs, of which the two biggest categories were an estimated $30 billion for cocaine and $24 billion for marijuana. In fact, it has been claimed that for some states, such as California and Oregon, marijuana is their single largest cash crop.

Because of the large sums of money involved, drugs have brought corruption at all levels. Notorious examples include the loss of millions of dollars of contraband heroin and cocaine held as evidence in police vaults in New York City, as well as other cities and towns throughout the country; the indictment of a number of detectives in the homicide division of the Miami police department for selling

Table 3.2 **Federal Trafficking Penalties**

CSA Schedule	Drugs	Quantity	First Offence	Second Offence
I and **II**	Methamphetamine Heroin LSD	Low quantities	Maximum: 40 years/$2 million	Maximum: life/$4 million
	Cocaine and cocaine base Potent narcotics (Fentanyl)	High quantities	Maximum: life/$4 million	Maximum: life/$8 million
III	All	Any quantity	Maximum: 5 years/$250,000	Maximum: 10 years/$500,000
IV	All	Any quantity	Maximum: 3 years/$250,000	Maximum: 6 years/$500,000
V	All	Any quantity	Maximum: 1 year/$100,000	Maximum: 2 years/$200,000

Source: "Drugs of Abuse," p. 8. Published by the Drug Enforcement Administration, U.S. Department of Justice, Arlington, VA, January 1997; www.usd.gov/dea.

FIGHTING THE DRUG WAR

As in the United States, Canada's federal government has authority over the importing and exporting of alcohol products, alcohol-related excise taxes, and broadcast advertising. In Canada, the control and sale of alcohol is also regulated by legislation in each province. The ten provinces and two territories all have, to varying degrees, monopolies that control the sale of alcohol for off-premises establishments, pricing, minimum drinking age, and transport of alcohol. They also prohibit public consumption, intoxication, and the sale of alcohol to intoxicated persons. In addition, provincial governments exert control over alcohol marketing and advertising. The legal drinking age is 19 in all Canadian provinces and territories, except in Quebec, Manitoba, and Alberta, where the minimum age is 18.

Use of Licit and Illicit Drugs

Regarding alcohol, tobacco, and other drugs, the following are main highlights from a 1993 General Social Survey conducted in Canada:

▲ Some 69.8% of Canadians use aspirin, 8.2% use opiate narcotics, 3.8% use tranquilizers, 4.2% use sleeping pills, and 2.5% use antidepressants.

▲ In 1994, the number of prescriptions written for psychotherapeutic drugs increased by 4% and prescriptions for analgesics increased by 0.7% relative to the number written the previous year.

▲ Between 1989 and 1993, the proportion of Canadians who used cannabis declined from 6.5% to 4.2%; in the United States, 33% of the population were cannabis users. The proportion of Canadians who used cocaine declined from 1.4% to 0.3%; in the United States, approximately 12% of the population were cocaine users.

▲ The proportion of Canadians who used LSD, speed, or heroin was relatively stable (0.4% in 1989 versus 0.3% in 1993).

▲ In 1993, Canadian police forces seized 115,081 kilograms of cannabis, 5285 kilograms of cocaine, and 85 kg of heroin. There were 1321 reported thefts and other losses involving narcotics and controlled drugs; 2170 prescription forgeries were detected.

▲ In 1990–1991, there were 21,746 drug-related cases (78.2 patients per 100,000 population) handled at general and psychiatric hospitals. During the same time period, there were 49,717 defendants convicted in U.S. federal courts of drug-related charges.

▲ In 1991, there were 510 drug-related deaths in Canada. Drug-related mental disorders accounted for 10.8% of these deaths; the remainder involved various types of poisoning.

Other Patterns of Illicit Drug Use in Canada

A substantial proportion of Canadians admit using illicit drugs. As many as one in five adult Canadians, or 4.2 million people, have used an illegal substance at least once in their lifetime.

▲ The most widely used illicit drug is cannabis (marijuana or hashish), used by 20% of adult Canadians compared with 33% of adult Americans.

▲ Three percent have used cocaine or crack; the U.S. percentage is 14%.

▲ Three percent have used LSD; the U.S. percentage is 8%.

▲ Two percent have used amphetamines (speed); the U.S. percentage is 7%.

Finally, young people tend to be the main consumers of illicit drugs in Canada. Illicit drugs are used more often by those between 16 and 17 years old. In the United States, illicit drugs are used more often by those between 18 and 25 years of age. ■

Sources: McKenzie, D., and B. Williams. "Canadian Profile: Alcohol, Tobacco, and Other Drugs." *Canadian Clearinghouse for Substance Abuse,* 1996. Available http://www.ccsa.ca/cpdruge. html. Soloman, R. "The Law Regarding Alcohol, Drugs, and Tobacco in Canada." *Canadian Clearinghouse for Substance Abuse,* 1996. Available http://www.ccsa.ca/cp961aw.html.

drugs and taking large bribes; and the claim that direct links were forged between drug dealers and the governments of Panama, Colombia, and Bolivia. Some law enforcement agencies have said that drugs are the largest export item from these countries. Miami has been known to be the key point of entry into the United States for both cocaine and marijuana, and money is clearly "laundered" in businesses set up as fronts.

Other problems associated with the implementation of drug laws are an insufficient number of law enforcement personnel and inadequate detention facilities; consequently much drug traffic goes unchecked. In addition, the judiciary system gets so backlogged that many cases never reach court. Plea bargaining is almost the rule to clear the court docket. Often dealers and traffickers are back in business the same day that they are arrested. This apparent lack of punishment seriously damages the morale of law enforcers, legislators, and average citizens.

It is estimated that nearly 1 million drug-related arrests occur each year. This problem represents a tremendous cost to society in terms of damaged lives and family relationships; being arrested for drug-related crime seriously jeopardizes the opportunity to pursue a normal life. Drug taking is closely tied to societal problems, and it will remain a problem unless society provides more meaningful experiences to those most susceptible to drug abuse. Improved education and increased support should be given to preteens, because that is the age when deviant behavior starts. In cases where drug education programs have been successful in involving students, the amount of drug taking and illegal activity seems to have decreased (see Chapter 17).

Factors in Controlling Drug Abuse

Three principal issues influence laws on drug abuse:

1. If a person abuses a drug, should he or she be treated as a criminal or as a sick person inflicted with a disease?

2. How is the user (supposedly the victim) distinguished from the pusher (supposedly the criminal) of an illicit drug, and who should be

more harshly punished—the person that creates the demand for the drug or the person who satisfies the demand?

3. Are the laws and associated penalties effective deterrents against drug use or abuse, and how is effectiveness determined?

In regard to the first issue, drug abuse may be considered both an illness and a crime. It is a psychiatric disorder, an abnormal functional state, when a person is compelled (either physically or psychologically—see Chapter 4) to continue using the drug (American Psychiatric Association 1994). It becomes a crime when the law, reflecting social opinion, makes abuse of the drug illegal. Health issues are clearly involved because uncontrolled abuse of almost any drug can lead to physical and psychological damage. Because the public must pay for health care costs or societal damage, laws are created and penalties implemented to prevent or correct drug abuse problems. (See Figure 3.1 on federal trafficking penalties, page 70.)

Concerning the second issue, drug laws have always been more lenient on the *user* than the *seller* of a drug of abuse. Actually, it is often hard to separate user from pusher, as many drug abusers engage in both activities. Because huge profits are often involved, some people may not use the drugs they peddle and are only pushers; the law tries to deter use of drugs by concentrating on these persons but has questionable success. Organized crime is involved in major drug sales, and these "drug rings" have proven hard to destroy.

In regard to the third issue, all available evidence indicates that, in the United States, criminal law has only limited success in deterring drug abuse. Even though there were signs that the use of illicit drugs declined during 1985–1992, since then use of illicit drugs has leveled off. During 1993, approximately 31% of twelfth-graders used an illicit drug; marijuana was used by 26%, LSD by 6.8%, and cocaine by 3.3% (Johnston et al. 1994). The total number of Americans using illegal drugs in 1994 has been estimated by the National Household Survey on Drug Abuse to be 12.5 million (HHS 1995). It is clear that the drug abuse problem is far from being resolved, and many feel that some changes should be made in how we deal with this problem.

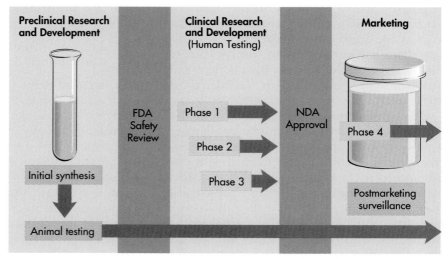

Figure 3.1

Steps Required by the FDA for Reviewing a New Drug

Preclinical Research and Development

Clinical Research and Development (Human Testing)

Marketing

FDA Safety Review

Phase 1

Phase 2

Phase 3

NDA Approval

Phase 4

Initial synthesis

Animal testing

Postmarketing surveillance

Duration: 1–3 years   2–10 years   Variable

◢ Strategies for Preventing Drug Abuse

The U.S. government and the public became concerned about the increasing prevalence of drug use during the 1960s, when demonstrations and nationwide protests against the Vietnam War proliferated as youth (mostly college students) rebelled against what they viewed as an unnecessary and unjust war. During the 1960s and early 1970s, for the first time, large numbers of middle- and upper-middle class youth began using licit and illicit gateway drugs on a massive scale. In response, the government responded with strategies for combating drug use and abuse. The three major strategies it employed were supply reduction, demand reduction, and inoculation strategy (Bennett 1989; HHS Press Office 1996; Heath 1992).

Supply Reduction Strategy

Early attempts at drug abuse prevention included both the Harrison Narcotic Act of 1914 and the Eighteenth (Prohibition) Amendment to the U.S. Constitution (see Table 3.1). Both laws were intended to control the manufacture and distribution of classified drugs, with legislators anticipating that these restrictions would compel people to stop using drugs. The laws enforce **supply reduction,** which involves a lessened, restrictive, or elimination of available drugs.

Supply reduction drug prevention policy attempts to curtail the supply of illegal drugs and exert greater control over other more therapeutic drugs. Part of the supply reduction policy includes **interdiction,** which is defined as decreasing the amount of drugs that are carried across U.S. borders through foreign crop eradication measures and agreements, stiff penalties for trafficking in drugs, and control of alcoholic beverages by licensing.

For example, in 1994 interdiction efforts received more than 60% of all congressional appropriations for drug control. According to the Office

> **supply reduction**
>
> a drug reduction policy aimed at reducing the supply of illegal drugs and controlling other therapeutic drugs

> **interdiction**
>
> the policy of cutting off or destroying supplies of illicit drugs

of National Drug Control Policy (ONDCP), the federal drug control budget increased from $1.5 billion in fiscal 1981 to $13.2 billion in fiscal 1995 (ONDCP 1995). In assessing the effectiveness of supply reduction, the costs of enforcing this form of drug prevention remain problematic. Often, not enough money is appropriated for more effective drug prevention (Woods 1993; ONDCP 1995). Although seizures of large caches of illicit drugs seem to be reported routinely in the national press, there is no indication that the availability of drugs has diminished substantially. One can argue that as long as a strong demand for these psychoactive agents exists demand will be satisfied if the price is right. Even if interdiction is successful in reducing the supply of one drug of abuse, if demand persists, it usually will be replaced by another with similar abuse potential (for example, substitution of amphetamines for cocaine—see Chapter 11).

Demand Reduction Strategy

The **demand reduction** approach attempts to minimize the actual demand for drugs. Through programs and activities often aimed at youth, emphasis is placed on reformulating values, attitudes, skills, and behaviors conducive to resisting drug use. (Chapter 17, Drug Prevention, will provide extensive information on methods and techniques for reducing drug use.) As part of this strategy, support for medical and group drug treatment programs for abusers is encouraged. While this approach does not address the supply of drugs, it does attempt to curb and eventually eliminate the need to purchase drugs by reducing the buyer's demand for drugs.

> **demand reduction**
>
> attempts to decrease individual's tendency to use drugs, often aimed at youth, emphasis on reformulating values and behaviors

Drug abuse is a complex and very individual problem, with many causes and aggravating factors. Even so, experience has shown that prevention and demand reduction are better strategies and, in the long run, less costly than interdiction or penalties administered via the criminal justice system (Goldstein 1994). The following are some suggestions and strategies as to how demand can be reduced:

1. Reduction of demand by youth must be the top priority of any prevention program if it is to provide a long-term solution. Children must be the primary focus in any substance abuse program. To achieve success requires stabilizing defective family structures, implementing school programs that create an antidrug attitude, establishing a drug-free environment, and promoting resistance training to help youth avoid drug involvement. In addition, children should be encouraged to become involved in alternative activities that can substitute for drug-abusing activity. Potential drug abusers need to be convinced that substance abuse is personally and socially damaging and unacceptable.

2. Education about drug abuse must be carefully designed and customized for the population or group to be targeted. For example, as discussed more extensively in Chapter 17, education based on scare tactics is not likely to dissuade adolescents from experimenting with drugs. Adolescents are at a point in their lives when they feel invincible, and graphically depicting the potential health consequences of drug and alcohol abuse has little impact. A discussion about the nature of addiction and the addiction process is more likely to influence their attitudes. Adolescents need to understand why people use drugs to appreciate the behavior patterns in themselves. Other important topics that should be discussed are how drug abuse works and why it leads to dependence. To complement drug education, adolescents also should be taught coping strategies that include proper decision making and problem solving.

3. Attitudes toward drug abuse and its consequence must be changed. The drug use patterns of many people, both young and old, are strongly influenced by peers. If individuals believe that drug abuse is glamorous and contributes to acceptance by friends and

associates, the incidence of drug abuse will remain high. In contrast, if the prevailing message in society is that drug abuse is unhealthy and not socially acceptable, the incidence will be much lower.

4. To indirectly reduce demand, in 1972 the FDA initiated a program to assure that all OTC drugs were safe and effective. Special panels were selected to evaluate more than 700 OTC drug ingredients. Each of these ingredients was classified as follows: category I, those found to be safe and effective and approved for OTC use; category II, those either ineffective or unsafe and removed from OTC medicinal products; and category III, those for which information was insufficient to make a decision.

5. Replacement therapy has shown to be a useful approach to weaning the individual on drugs of abuse. The most common example of this strategy is the use of the narcotic methadone to treat the heroin addict (see Chapter 10). Use of methadone prevents the cravings and severe withdrawal routinely associated with breaking the heroin habit. Unfortunately, most heroin addicts insist that they be maintained on methadone indefinitely. Even though methadone is easier to control and is less disruptive than heroin, one drug addiction has been substituted for another, which draws criticism.

    Replacement therapy certainly is not the entire answer to all drug abuse problems, but it often can provide a window of opportunity for behavioral modification so that a long-term solution to the abuse problem is possible.

6. The FDA is committed to making more effective drugs available in response to public demand for greater self-treatment opportunities and reduced health care costs. The **switching policy** allows the FDA to review prescription drugs and evaluate their suitability as OTC products. (See Appendix B, page 494.)

> **switching policy**
> an FDA policy allowing the change of suitable prescription drugs to over-the-counter status

7. The Harrison Act of 1914 was a principal piece of legislation in defining drug abuse and preventing its occurrence. Specifically, the Harrison Act attempted to regulate the production, importation, sale, purchase, and distribution of addicting substances, such as opium.

Inoculation Strategy

The **inoculation** method of abuse prevention aims to protect drug users by teaching them responsibility. The emphasis is on being accountable, rational, and responsible about drug use, and informing users about the effects of drugs on both mind and bodily function. Responsible drinking that uses designated drivers when consuming alcohol, and nonalcohol parties are outcomes of applying inoculation strategy.

> **inoculation**
> a method of abuse prevention that protects drug users by teaching them responsibility

◢ Current and Future Drug Use and Abuse Regulation

During the Republican administrations of Ronald Reagan and George Bush (1980–1992), the official policy of the U.S. federal government included a "get tough" attitude about drug abuse. Slogans such as "Just say no" and "War on Drugs" reflected the frustration of a public that had been victimized by escalating crime (many incidents were drug-related); personally touched by drug tragedies in families, at work, or with associates and friends; and economically strained by dealing with the cost of the problem. It is no wonder that, in 1989 and 1990, drug abuse was viewed as the number one problem in this country by the majority of its citizens. Consequently, from 1989 to 1991, the National Institute on Drug Abuse dramatically increased its budget directed at improving education and treatment programs in communities and schools. In addition, new research money was earmarked for identifying the causes of abuse and new therapeutic approaches (Halloway 1991).

FIGHTING THE DRUG WAR

The revolutionary drug policy implemented by the Netherlands, which is often subjected to publicity, is becoming more difficult to keep under control. Under this policy, termed a "harm reduction model," the focus is on eliminating strong punishment measures for cannabis use previously advocated by the punitive model of drug control and minimizing financial costs for other citizens. Harm reduction made life safer for drug users by allowing them the use of certain drugs, mainly cannabis-type (marijuana and hashish), in prescribed locations such as coffee shops and cafés and other injectable drugs (such as heroin) in one open-air park. According to S. Trebach, president of the Drug Policy Foundation in Washington, D.C., "Harm reduction is the middle ground between traditional prohibition and full legalization" (Treaster 1993, E5). Overall, the goal is to reduce personal harm, such as stiff jail sentences for drug use, while simultaneously increasing educational programs and treatment and prevention facilities for chronic drug users.

This leniency, say the Dutch, " . . . has given their country one of Europe's lowest and most stable ratios of heroin addiction and deaths" (Simons, May 9, 1994, A7). Crack, here, is nearly nonexistent. The Dutch have termed their stance towards drugs as "normalization." "Possession of small amounts of hard drugs for personal use is tolerated because addiction is seen as a public health problem that is attended by a large network of treatment programs" (Simons 1994, A7). Drug arrests and convictions are still executed, however.

"Normalization [policy] does not mean everything is legal" (Engelsman 1989, 44). Trafficking in drugs or stealing drugs requires punishment. How much punitive action occurs in the Netherlands? Of the prison population, 30% is incarcerated for drug-related reasons, and in Amsterdam and Rotterdam, the percentage is 50%.

The Dutch drug policy of de facto* decriminalization of cannabis products has not encouraged more drug use. In fact, the prevalence of cannabis use in the Netherlands is low. In the age bracket between 10 and 18 years, 4.2 percent have ever used cannabis in their lifetime. Among this group, less than 2 percent are still using occasionally. The number of daily cannabis users appears to be one in 1,000 . . . (Engelsman 1989, 44).

Recently, the Dutch have been invaded by drug users from nearby countries, who flock to the Netherlands, often only for a day, to take advantage of this liberal policy. Maastricht (population 130,000), a town located in the southern tip of the Netherlands, gets "about 1,000 foreign tourists looking for drugs each day" (Simons 1994, A7). The signing of the Maastricht Treaty, which ratified the European Union, by the Netherlands is one reason this tourism is so rampant. In recent years, customs controls in the European Union have disappeared, and so the treaty, " . . . a symbol of togetherness" (Simons 1994, A7), often makes the realization of dramatic policy differences painfully obvious. Several of the "drug cafés" have been closed down recently due to infractions of police policy, which states: " . . . no hard drugs . . . no sales over 30 grams, no noise, no admission for those under 18, and no alcohol" (Simons 1994, A7). An even larger problem is related to the rising street sales of forbidden hard drugs. The Dutch are under pressure from neighboring countries to stifle their liberal policy, while many Dutch feel that their neighbors should "recognize the realities of drugs and similarly decriminalize them" (Simons 1994, A7). One Dutch police chief has been quoted as saying, in a region without borders, " . . . we'll have to search together to find the balance between prevention and repression" (Simons 1994, A7). As far as soft drugs are concerned, he said, " . . . that's a low priority."

* De facto refers to laws that are enforced by government.

Sources: Engelsman E. "The Dutch Model." *New Perspectives Quarterly* 6, 3 (Summer 1989): 44–5. Simons M. "Dutch Swamped by Flood of Drugs." *New York Times* (May 9, 1994): A7.

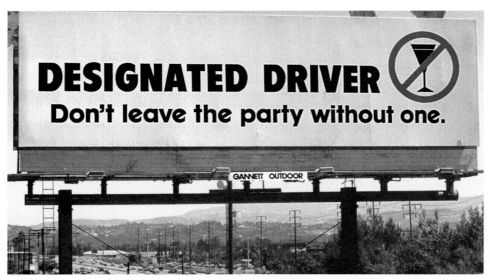

An example of the many public awareness advertisements cautions against drinking and driving.

How successful has the government-declared "War on Drugs" been since its inception during the Reagan years? The Bush administration appropriated more than $32 billion to combat drug abuse and associated problems. During his first year in office, Bush's predecessor Bill Clinton allocated two-thirds of drug funding to enforcement and interdiction. "In the 1995 budget, Clinton proposed substantial increases for prevention and treatment that gives demand reduction 40% of the budget—the largest share since 1980. But congress approved only marginal increases, the Federal drug policy remains primarily focused on supply control efforts" (Drug Strategies 1995, 2). (See "Fighting the Drug War," page 79).

With the "War on Drugs" declared by our government, what has and has not been accomplished?

Has been accomplished:

▲ In 1994, the Violent Crime Control and Law Enforcement Act, known as the Crime Bill, " . . . authorized increased Federal support for drug prevention and treatment programs. . . . The entire appropriations for all crime and drug prevention and treatment programs under the Crime Bill in 1995—its first year of operation—total $92 million, compared with $2.3 billion for police and corrections" (Drug Strategies 1995, 2).

Has not been accomplished:

▲ Since 1981, the federal government has spent more than $60 billion trying to curtail drug supplies; drugs are, however, cheaper and more plentiful today than they were a decade ago. Heroin costs less than half its 1981 street price. Simultaneously, the United States has the highest addiction rate in its history and the highest rate of imprisonment in the world, largely because of drug-related crime (Drug Strategies 1995, 3).

▲ As discussed in Chapter 1, drug use and drug addiction are an equal opportunity affliction, cutting across all social and economic groups. In 1993, the National Household Survey found that 24.4 million Americans—one in eight—used illicit drugs; half this group used drugs at least once per month.

Mixed results:

▲ There are 2.7 million "hard core" drug abusers in the United States, predominantly cocaine addicts—more than triple the number estimated five years ago.

▲ ONDCP estimates that there are 600,000 heroin addicts, a number that has remained constant for a decade.

▲ The federal drug budget allocated $2 billion for prevention, education, and community partnership programs in 1995, up from $1.6 billion in 1994. Nevertheless, teenagers consider drugs and alcohol less harmful today than they did three years ago, and they are more tolerant of drug use. Amazingly, adults maintain similar attitudes, in that a majority see little harm in occasional drug use.

Unfortunately, many more shortcomings in our efforts to win the "War on Drugs" can be listed. The result, however, is that efforts to curb the use of drugs have proved mediocre at best.

The lack of a declared victory in the drug war, inconsistencies in drug laws, and the resulting frustration for both governmental agencies and the general public likely will lead to revised drug policies. In addition, because of enormous governmental budget deficits, diminished money for dealing with drug abuse problems are likely; consequently, creative, less expensive strategies will have to be developed to replace the expensive and often ineffectual approaches. As new approaches for old problems are sought, some issues not yet discussed merit scrutiny.

Drug Legalization Debate

The persistence of the drug abuse problem and the high cost in dollars and frustration of waging the "War on Drugs" helps to energize the ongoing debate of legalizing the use of drugs of abuse. It is argued that legalizing substances of abuse would eliminate law enforcement as a major factor in the control of drug abuse; consequently, if consumption and sale of these substances are decriminalized, individuals would decide for themselves whether to buy and use these addicting drugs, much as they already do for alcohol and tobacco. Proponents of legalization are no longer limited to *libertarians* and so-called *academic intellectuals,* but increasingly include representatives of a dis-

tressed law enforcement system. For example, discontented judges whose courts are swamped with drug cases and police officers who spend much of their on-duty time trying to trap and arrest every drug dealer and user on the street are publicly declaring that the drug laws are wasteful and futile. Even notable public figures such as former secretary of state George Schultz, Nobel Laureate economist Milton Friedman, and the former surgeon general for the Clinton administration, Joycelyn Elders (Buckley 1994) claim that laws against drugs of addiction have been as ineffective as Prohibition against alcohol (Knight-Ridder News Service 1992b; Wilson 1993; Kearns 1993). Although laws against the use and distribution of drugs of addiction have, according to the FBI, resulted in a doubling of drug-related arrests since 1981 (of 1.08 million drug arrests in 1990, 68% were for possession, not selling [Knight-Ridder News Service 1992b]), plenty of people stand ready to replace those dealers imprisoned. Further, 79% of males and females arrested for drug sale/possession in 1993 tested positive for illicit drug use (ONDCP 1994).

Proponents claim that drug legalization would:

1. Allow users to have the right to practice a diversity of consciousness, " . . . the practice of getting high has existed from the dawn of time, and all efforts to eradicate it are based on an incomplete understanding of human nature" (Lenson 1995, 190). Just as diversity of racial, ethnic, sexual orientation, religious, and other varied lifestyles are allowed to be practiced, legalization of drugs permits citizens in our society to alter their consciousness without legal repercussions as long as they do not harm or threaten the safety and security of others.

2. Eliminate dealers' high profit margins by removing the illegality, which drives up the cost of illicit drugs.

3. Reduce drug-related violence by taking drug trade out of the hands of criminals.

4. Decrease law enforcement costs by eliminating the backlog of drug-related court cases and reduce populations in overcrowded prisons (35% of which are for drug-related

crimes [Knight-Ridder News Service 1992b; Nadelman 1993]).

5. Eliminate unfair drug-related laws, which are often accused of being inequitable and biased by racial and socioeconomical factors.

Despite some of the compelling arguments for legalization of drugs of addiction, the majority of law enforcement professionals, politicians, federal agencies, and medical associations oppose legalization of some or all drugs of abuse. In addition, polls indicate that most voters object to legalization or decriminalization of illicit drugs (Knight-Ridder News Service 1992b). A major Gallup survey of public attitudes showed that 54% of respondents opposed drug legalization, and another 31% were moderately opposed to it; only 14% favored it (CNN/USA Today/Gallup Poll 1995).

The opposition to legalization is based on the following concerns (Goldstein 1994; Wilson 1993; Kalant 1992; Goldstein and Kalant 1990):

1. It will increase drug abuse due to greater availability of these substances. Once legitimized, substances such as marijuana, narcotics, and even cocaine may be merchandised and sold like cigarettes and beer.

2. It will increase use due to decreased costs.

3. It will increase use due to perceived social approval that is inherent with legalization. Many "law-abiding" people decide to avoid the use of illicit drugs of abuse because they do not want "trouble with the law."

4. It will increase costs to society due to greater medical and social problems resulting from greater availability and increased use. The two most frequently abused substances, alcohol and tobacco, are both legal and readily available. These two substances cause much greater medical, social, and personal problems than all the illicit drugs of abuse combined. In effect, do we want to legalize additional drugs with abuse potential?

Although arguments for both sides warrant consideration, extreme policies are not likely to be implemented; instead a compromise will most probably be adopted. For example, some areas of compromise include (Kalant 1992) the following:

Selective legalization. Eliminate harsh penalties for those drugs of abuse that are the safest and least likely to cause addiction, such as marijuana.

Control substances of abuse by prescription or through specially approved outlets. Have the availability of the illegal drugs controlled by physicians and trained clinicians, rather than by law enforcement agencies.

Discretionary enforcement of drug laws. Allow greater discretion by judicial systems for prosecution and sentencing of those who violate drug laws. Such decisions would be based on perceived criminal intent.

In conclusion, the drug legalization debate remains a very divisive issue in the United States. Although legalization would lessen the number of drug violators involved in the criminal justice system, the problems associated with legalizing current illicit drugs cause most members in our society to regard this idea with disfavor. As stated in number 4 above, opponents of legalization argue that we already have massive problems with such licit drugs as tobacco and alcohol. According to them, legalizing additional types of drugs would produce substantial increases in the rates of addiction and an increase in the social and psychological problems associated with drug use. Proponents favoring legalization remind us that, despite the current drug laws and severe penalties for drug use, people continue to use illicit drugs.

A compromise between legalization and current criminalization of illicit drug use might include **selective legalization.** Such an approach would probably legalize marijuana, while other drugs such as heroin and cocaine would remain illegal and continue to carry stiff penalties. A second type of compromise would call for controlling drugs by medical practitioners instead of law enforcement agencies. A third compromise might involve discretionary en-

selective legalization

an approach that would legalize marijuana, while other drugs such as heroin and cocaine would remain illegal

forcement of drug laws, which would allow judicial systems to exercise greater discretion in prosecution and sentencing of drug law violators, based largely on perceived criminal intent.

Drug Testing

In response to the demand by society to stop the spread of drug abuse and its adverse consequences, drug testing has been implemented in some situations to detect drug users (Catlin et al. 1992; Jaffe 1995). The most common types of drug testing include breathalyzers and urine, blood, and hair specimens. Urine and blood testing are the preferred samples for testing drug use. Hair specimen testing must overcome a number of technical problems before hair can be used as a definitive proof of drug use, including complications from hair treatment (hair coloring, for example) and environmental absorption (Jaffe 1995).

The drugs of abuse most frequently tested are marijuana, cocaine, amphetamines, narcotics, sedatives, phencyclidine (PCP), and anabolic steroids. Drug testing is mandatory for some professions where public safety is a concern (such as airline pilots, railroad workers, law enforcement employees, medical personnel) or for employees of some organizations and companies as part of general policy (such as the military, many federal agencies, and some private companies). Drug testing is also mandatory for participants in sports at all levels, in high school, college, international, and professional competition (Catlin et al. 1992) in order to prevent unfair advantages that might result from the pharmacological effects of these drugs and to discourage the spread of drug abuse in the athlete population (see Chapter 16). Drug testing is also used routinely by law enforcement agencies to assist in the prosecution of those believed to violate drug abuse laws. Finally, drug testing is used by health professionals to assess the success of drug abuse treatment—that is, to determine if a dependent patient is diminishing his or her drug use or has experienced a relapse in drug abuse habits.

Drug testing to identify drug offenders is usually accomplished by analyzing body fluids, in particular urine, although other approaches (such as analysis of expired air for alcohol) are also used. To understand the accuracy of these tests, several factors should be considered (Catlin et al. 1992; Jaffe 1995).

1. *Testing must be standardized and conducted efficiently.*
   In order to interpret testing results reliably, it is essential that fluid samples be collected, processed, and tested using standard procedures. Guidelines for proper testing procedures have been established by federal regulatory agencies as well as scientific organizations. Deviations from established protocols can result in false positives (a test that indicates a drug is present when none was used), false negatives (a test that is unable to detect a drug that is present), or inaccurate assessments of drug levels.

2. *Sample collection and processing must be done accurately and confidentially.*
   In many cases, drug testing can have punitive consequences (for example, athletes can't compete; employees are fired if results are positive). Consequently, drug users often attempt to outsmart the system. Some individuals have attempted to avoid submitting their own drug-containing urine for testing by filling specimen bottles with "clean" urine from artificial bladders hidden under clothing or in the vagina or by introducing "clean" urine into their own bladders just before the collection (Catlin et al. 1992). To confirm the legitimacy of the specimen, it often is necessary to have the individual strip and the urine collection witnessed directly by a trustworthy observer. To ensure that tampering does not occur with the fluid specimens and confidentiality is maintained, samples should be immediately coded and the movement of each sample from site to site during analysis should be documented and confirmed.

   Just as it is important that testing identify individuals who are using drugs, it is also important that those who have not used drugs not be wrongfully accused. To avoid false positives, all samples that are positive in the screening tests (which are usually fast and inexpensive procedures) should be analyzed again, using more accurate, sensitive, and sophisticated analytical procedures to confirm the results.

3. *Confounding factors can be inadvertently or deliberately present that interfere with the accuracy of the testing.*

   For example, normal dietary consumption of pastries containing poppy seeds is sufficient to cause a positive urine test for the narcotic morphine. The use of bicarbonate alkalinizes the urine and increases the rate of elimination of some drugs, such as methamphetamine, and thereby diminishes the likelihood of a positive test (Catlin et al. 1992). Excessive intake of fluid, or the use of diuretics, increases the volume of urine formed and decreases the concentration of drugs, making them more difficult to detect.

The dramatic increase in drug testing since 1985 has caused experts to question the value of this process in dealing with drug abuse problems. Unfortunately, drug testing often is linked exclusively to punitive consequences, such as disqualification from athletic competition, loss of job, or even fines and imprisonment. Use of drug testing in such negative ways does little to diminish the number of drug abusers or their personal problems. However, drug-testing programs can also have positive consequences by identifying drug users who require professional care. After being referred for drug rehabilitation, the offender can be monitored by drug testing to confirm the desired response to therapy. In addition, tests can identify individuals who put others in jeopardy because of their drug abuse habits as they perform tasks that are dangerously impaired by the effects of these drugs (for example, airline pilots, train engineers, truck drivers, and so forth).

The widespread application of drug testing to control the illicit use of drugs in the general population would be extremely expensive, difficult to enforce, and almost certainly ineffective. In addition, such indiscriminate testing would likely be viewed as an unwarranted infringement on individual privacy and declared unconstitutional. However, the use of drug testing to discourage inappropriate drug use in selected crucial professions, which directly impact public welfare, appears to be publicly tolerated and has been shown to be effective (Bryson 1992). Even so, it is probably worthwhile to periodically revisit the issue of drug testing and analyze its benefits and liabilities relative to "public safety" and "individual privacy" issues.

Pragmatic Drug Policies

Several principles for a **pragmatic drug policy** emerge from a review of past drug policies and an understanding of the drug-related frustrations of today. To create drug policies that work, the following are offered as suggestions:

> **pragmatic drug policy**
> developing drug laws reflecting the desires of the majority of the citizenry; stressing drug education and treatment; developing non-discriminatory policies

1. It is essential that government develops programs that are consistent with the desires of the majority of the population.

2. Given the lack of success and high cost of efforts to prevent illicit drugs from reaching the market, it is logical to deemphasize interdiction and instead stress programs that reduce demand. To reduce demand, drug education and drug treatment must be top priorities.

3. Government and society need to better understand the role played by law in their efforts to reduce drug addiction. Antidrug laws by themselves do not eliminate drug problems; indeed, they may even create significant social difficulties (for example, the Prohibition laws against all alcohol use). Used properly and selectively, however, laws can reinforce and communicate expected social behavior and values (for example, laws against public drunkenness or driving a vehicle under the influence of alcohol).

4. Finally, programs should be implemented that employ "public consensus" more effectively to campaign against drug abuse. For example, antismoking campaigns demonstrate the potential success that could be achieved by programs that alter drug abuse behavior. Similar approaches can be used to change public attitudes about drugs through education without moral judgments and crusading tactics.

The need for more "workable" approaches to control drug use follows from the failure of a "drug war" based primarily on law enforcement to reduce the supply of illegal drugs; this war has not significantly reduced the availability of most drugs. Our society needs to engage in more collaborative programs where drug-using individuals, their families, communities, and helping agencies work together.

FIGHTING THE DRUG WAR

The following is the National Drug Control Strategy as reported by the National Clearinghouse for Drug and Alcohol Information. These five goals and their respective objectives represent a refinement of previous National Drug Control Strategy.

Goal 1: Motivate America's youth to reject illegal drugs and substance abuse.
This strategic goal involves the mobilization of state and local governments, schools, and communities against drug use by American youth. It is to be accomplished through intervention programs involving the family and community and increased public awareness via education.

Goal 2: Increase the safety of America's citizens by substantially reducing drug-related crime and violence.
This strategic goal focuses on the country's law enforcement agents as they attack drug-related crime, especially gang violence, and decrease drug trafficking on both a national and a local level. In addition, rehabilitation and education programs for offenders are involved.

Goal 3: Reduce health, welfare, and crime costs resulting from illegal drug use.
This strategic goal involves the use of treatment, outreach, and education programs to help those addicted to drugs; it also aims to reduce the spread of infectious diseases related to drug use.

Goal 4: Shield America's air, land, and sea frontiers from the drug threat.
This strategic goal focuses on the expansion of law enforcement and intelligence programs designed to decrease the supply of illicit drugs that enters the United States.

Goal 5: Break foreign and domestic drug sources of supply.
The final strategic goal seeks to eliminate drug production at its source through the destruction of major drug trafficking organizations, both foreign and domestic. It includes efforts to strengthen host nation institutions and persuade multilateral organizations to share the international drug control burden. ■

Source: National Clearinghouse for Alcohol and Drug Information. *Strategic Goals and Objectives of the 1996 National Drug Control Strategy.* 1996. Available http://www.health.org/pressrel/goaldrug.html

EXERCISES FOR THE WEB

Exercise 1: Myths

There has been considerable debate on legalizing drugs. More recently, the advocates for legalizing marijuana are being joined by individuals promoting marijuana's medicinal uses. The opponents of legalization claim that permitting drug use will pose serious problems for our society. This page attempts to explain the argument in favor of legalizing drugs and provides rationale for why legalization should not take place.

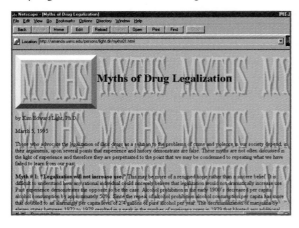

Exercise 3: DEA

The mission of the Drug Enforcement Administration is to demand compliance with the controlled substances laws and regulations of the United States. It brings to the criminal and civil justice system of the United States or any other competent jurisdiction, those organizations, and principal members of organizations, involved in the growth, manufacture, or distribution of controlled substances appearing in or destined for illicit traffic in the United States. Also, the DEA recommends and supports non-enforcement programs aimed at reducing the availability of illicit controlled substances on the domestic and international markets.

Exercise 2: Drug Reform

The Drug Reform Coordination Network (DRCNet) provides information on a variety of issues regarding drugs. Similar to Prohibition in the early 1900s, the "War on Drugs" has created a powerful and pervasive criminal subculture, perpetuated racial injustice, exacerbated the health consequences of drug abuse, corrupted police forces, and undermined respect for law. DRCNet opposes this domestic war that it claims has filled our prisons. This reform network supports intelligent, cost-effective policies that deal with drug abuse as a medical and social issue.

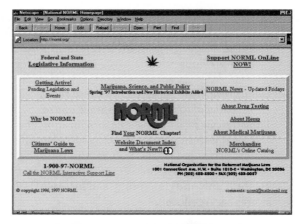

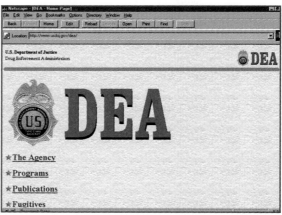

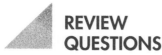

REVIEW QUESTIONS

1. What could account for the vast differences in attitudes and opinions regarding drug use and the law voiced by drug users/abusers and nonusers of drugs?

2. Does society have a right to govern drug use by individuals?

3. What problems arise when a society has unrealistic expectations concerning drug regulation by its government?

4. Would decriminalization of illicit drug use increase or decrease drug-related social problems? Justify your answer.

5. What constitutes the so-called War on Drugs? What changes are needed to win this "war"?

6. How can the supply reduction strategy be used to prevent drug abuse?

7. Why would supply reduction, demand reduction, and inoculation strategies be more effective than interdiction?

8. Do you believe that all potential employees should have a drug test before being hired?

KEY TERMS

thalidomide
phocomelia
Harrison Act of 1914
supply reduction
interdiction
demand reduction
switching policy
inoculation
selective legalization
pragmatic drug policy

SUMMARY

1 Two major guidelines for controlling drug development and marketing are as follows: (a) society has the right to protect itself from the damaging impact of drug use, and (b) society has the right to demand that drugs approved for marketing are safe and effective for the general public.

2 The Harrison Act of 1914 helped to shape public and government awareness of regulation related to all types of drugs, but most particularly those with abuse properties, such as opium and cocaine.

3 Three of the principal factors that influence laws on drug abuse include the following: (a) Should drug abusers be treated as criminals or patients? (b) How can drug users and drug pushers be distinguished from one another? (c) What types of laws and programs are effective deterrents against drug abuse?

4 Controversy exists as to how to best reduce substance abuse. A principal strategy by governmental agencies to achieve this objective is interdiction; the majority of money used to fight drug abuse is spent on trying to stop and confiscate drug supplies. Experience has proved that interdiction is rarely effective. To reduce drug abuse, demand for these substances must be diminished. Youth must be a top priority in any substance abuse program. Treatment that enables drug addicts to stop their habits with minimal discomfort should be provided. Finally, education should be used to change attitudes toward drug abuse and its consequences. Potential drug abusers need to be convinced that substance abuse is personally and socially damaging and is unacceptable.

5 Three major strategies for combating drug use and abuse are as follows: (a) supply reduction, (b) demand reduction, and (c) inoculation strategy. Supply reduction involves using drug laws to control the manufacturing and distribution of classified drugs. Demand reduction strategy aims to reduce the actual demand for drugs by working mainly with youth and teaching them to resist drugs. Inoculation strategy aims to protect drug users by teaching them responsibility and explaining the effects of drugs on bodily and mental functioning.

6 The main arguments for legalizing drugs include the following: (a) people have the right to practice a diversity of consciousness; (b) it will remove the high profits in illicit drug dealing; (c) it will relieve the criminal justice system (federal, state, and local law enforcement, courts, prisons, jails, and correctional institutions) of the burden of lesser violations of drug laws; and (d) it will eliminate drug laws that discriminate on the basis of gender, sexual orientation, and racial or ethnic differences. The main arguments against legalizing drugs are as follows: (a) drugs of abuse will become more available; (b) demand for drugs will rise, at least initially; (c) it will increase use of drugs because of perceived social approval; (d) the fear factor related to drug law violations will dissipate; and (e) increased use of drugs will lead to higher medical costs and more social problems.

7 In response to the demand by society to stop the spread of drug abuse and its adverse consequences, drug testing has been implemented in some situations to detect drug users. Common types of drug testing include breathalyzers and urine, blood, and hair specimens. Urine and blood testing are the preferred samples for testing drug use. Hair specimen testing must overcome a number of technical problems before hair can be used as a definitive proof of drug use. Two major problems related to hair samples arise with hair treatment and environmental absorption.

8 Four major factors must be recognized in order for drug policies to work: (a) government must develop programs that are consistent with the desires of the majority of the population; (b) programs must deemphasize interdiction (seizing of drugs to prevent importation) and stress programs that reduce demand, including drug education and drug treatment; (c) government and society must better understand how laws, used properly and selectively, can reinforce and communicate expected social behavior and values; and (d) programs such as antismoking campaigns should be implemented that employ "public consensus" more effectively.

REFERENCES

Adams, S. H. "The Great American Fraud." *Collier's* 36, 5 (1905): 17–18; 10 (1905): 16–18; 16 (1906): 18–20.

American Psychiatric Association. *Diagnostic and Statistical Manual,* 4th ed. [DSM-IV], A. Frances, chairperson, 175–272. Washington, DC: American Psychiatric Association, 1994.

"A Speedier FDA." *American Druggist* (November 1992): 13.

Associated Press. "Drug Lord Vows to Lead Army Against Bogota." *Salt Lake Tribune* 245 (19 January 1993a): A-2.

Associated Press. "Mexican Cardinal, Six Others Killed in Cross-Fire as Drug Battles Erupt in Guadalajara." *Salt Lake Tribune* 246 (25 May 1993b): A-1.

Austin, G. A. "Perspectives on the History of Psychoactive Substance Use." NIDA Research Issues no. 24. Washington, DC: U.S. Department of Health, Education, and Welfare, 1978.

Balabanova, S., F. Parsche, and W. Pirsig. "First Identification of Drugs in Egyptian Mummies." *Naturwissenschaften* 79 (1992): 358.

Bennett, W. "Introduction." *National Drug Control Strategy.* Washington, DC: U.S. Government Printing Office, (1989): 12–3.

Booth, R., et al. "A Tale of Three Cities: Risk Taking Among Intravenous Drug Users." In *Problems of Drug Dependence.* NIDA Research Monograph Series no 95. Washington, DC: U.S. Department of Health, Education, and Welfare, 1989.

Bryson, R. "Railroads Try to Derail Drug Abuse." *Salt Lake Tribune* 244 (9 June 1992): D-5.

Buckley, B. "Pharmacists Offer Their Views on Reimbursement, Illicit Drugs, Suicide." *Pharmacy Times* (4 April 1994): 43–44.

Catlin, D., D. Cowan, M. Donike, D. Fraisse, H. Oftebro, and S. Rendic. "Testing Urine for Drugs." *Journal of Automated Chemistry* 14 (1992): 85–92.

CNN/USA Today/Gallup Poll. "Drugs and Drug Abuse." *Gallup Poll Survey* G0105147, 9/14-17/95.

Drug Facts and Comparisons. St. Louis: Lippincott, 1991.

Drug Strategies. *Keeping Score: What We Are Getting for Our Federal Drug Control Dollars 1995.* Washington, DC: 1995. Available 080/edres/colleges/boss/depts/cesar/drugs/ks1995

FASEB [Federation of American Societies for Experimental Biology] *Newsletter* 25 (March 1992): 4.

Goldstein, A. "Lessons from the Street." In *Addiction from Biology to Drug Policy.* New York: Freeman, 1994.

Goldstein, A., and H. Kalant. "1990 Drug Policy: Striking the Right Balance." *Science* 249 (1990): 1513–21.

Greenhouse, S. "NIDA Becomes Part of NIH Under Recent ADAMHA Reorganization." *NIDA Notes* (September–October 1992): 1.

Halloway, M. "Rx for Addiction." *Scientific American* (March 1991): 95–103.

Heath, D. B. "U.S. Drug Control Policy: A Cultural Perspective." *Daedalus* (Summer 1992): 269–91.

HHS Press Office. *Substance Abuse—A National Challenge: Prevention, Treatment and Research at HHS.* (May 6, 1996). Available www.os.dhhs.gov/news/press/1996 pres /960506b.html.

Holmstedt, B. "Historical Survey." In *Ethnopharmacological Search for Psychoactive Drugs,* edited by D. H. Efron. Public Health Service Publication no. 1645. Washington, DC: U.S. Government Printing Office, 1967.

Hunter, J. R., D. L. Rosen, and R. DeChristoforo. "How FDA Expedites Evaluation of Drugs." *Welcome Trends in Pharmacy* (January 1993): 2–9.

Hwang, S. "Nicotine Patch Reignites Fight over Drug Ads." *Wall Street Journal* 73 (30 June 1992): B-1.

Jaffe, J. H., ed. *Encyclopedia of Drugs and Alcohol.* New York: Simon and Schuster, MacMillan, 1995.

Johnston, L. *University of Michigan National High School Senior Survey.* Ann Arbor: University of Michigan, 1993.

Kalant, H. "Formulating Policies on the Non-Medical Use of Cocaine." In *Cocaine: Scientific and Social Dimensions,* Ciba Foundation Symposium 166, 261–76. New York: Wiley, 1992.

Kearns, R. "Legalize Drugs? Elders Speaks Firestorm." *Salt Lake Tribune* 247 (9 December 1993): A-18.

Knight-Ridder News Service. "Experts Call War on Drugs a $32 Billion Stalemate." *Salt Lake Tribune* 244 (21 September 1992a): A-3.

Knight-Ridder News Service. "Time to Make Drugs Legal? Many Say Yes." *Salt Lake Tribune* 244 (11 July 1992b): A-1, A-2.

Kokkevi, A., J. Liappas, V. Boukouvala, V. Alevizou, E. Anastassopoulou, and C. Stefanis. "Criminality in a Sample of Drug Abusers in Greece." *Drug and Alcohol Dependence* 31 (1993): 111–21.

Lenson, D. *On Drugs.* Minneapolis, MN: University of Minnesota Press, 1995.

McKenzie, D., and B. Williams. *Canadian Profile: Alcohol, Tobacco and Other Drugs.* Canadian Clearinghouse for Substance Abuse, 1996. Available http://www.ccsa.ca/cpdruge.html.

McShane, L. "Cops Are Crooks in N.Y.'s 30th Precinct." *Salt Lake Tribune* 248 (18 April 1994): A-5.

Millstein, R. "Remarks on the Status of NIDA." Made at the 55th Annual Scientific Meeting of the College on Problems of Drug Dependence, Toronto, Canada, 12 June 1993.

Morgan, H. W. "The Therapeutic Revolution." In *Drugs in America, A Social History, 1800–1980.* Syracuse, NY: Syracuse University Press, 1981.

National Institute on Drug Abuse (NIDA). "Drug Abuse and Aids." *NIDA Capsules.* CAP 04 (July 1990).

National Institute on Drug Abuse (NIDA). "NIDA Plays Key Role in Studying Links Between AIDS and Drug Abuse." *NIDA Notes* 10, 3 (May/June 1995): 1.

Office of National Drug Control Policy (ONDCP). *Fact Sheet: Drug-Related Crime.* Rockville, MD: ONDCP Drugs and Crime Clearinghouse, September 1994.

Office of National Drug Control Policy (ONDCP). *Fact Sheet: Drug Use Trends.* Washington, DC: Drugs and Crime Clearinghouse, NCJ-153518, June 1995.

Office of National Drug Control Policy (ONDCP). *Drugs and Crime Facts,* 1994. Rockville, MD: ONDCP Drugs and Crime Clearinghouse, 1995.

SAMHSA Bulletin. CMHS Office of Public Affairs, Rm 13C-05, 5600 Fishers Lane, Rockville, MD 20857, 1992.

Schuster, C. "Implication for Research of the 1988 Anti-Drug Abuse Act." In *Problems of Drug Dependence.* NIDA Research Monograph Series no. 95. Washington, DC: U.S. Department of Health, Education, and Welfare, 1989.

Siegelman, S. "The Coming Wave of Rx-to-OTC Switches." *American Druggist* (August 1990): 37–42.

Simonsen, L. "Medicines in Development Keep Older Americans Healthy, at Home, Longer." *Pharmacy Times* 59 (1993): 81–85.

Soloman, R. "The Law Regarding Alcohol, Drugs, and Tobacco in Canada." *Canadian Clearinghouse for Substance Abuse (CCSA),* 1996. Available http.//www.ccsa.ca/cp961aw.html.

Temin, P. *Taking Your Medicine: Drug Regulation in the United States.* Cambridge, MA: Harvard University Press, 1980.

U.S. Code. *Title 21—Food and Drugs: Chapter 13—Drug Abuse Prevention and Control. Subchapter 1—Control and Enforcement. Part B—Authority to Control: Standards and Schedules,* January 24, 1995. Available http://www.law.cornell.edu/uscode/21/812.html.

Wallace, I., D. Wallechinsky, and A. Wallace. "Dr. Freud's Magic Nose Powder." *Parade Magazine* (20 September 1981).

Wilson, J. Q., "Against the Legalization of Drugs." In *Taking Sides,* edited by Raymond Goldberg, 15–25. Guilford, CT: Dushkin, 1993.

Wire Services. "Cocaine Kingpin Escapes After Bloody Shootout." *Salt Lake Tribune* 244 (23 July 1992): A-1.

Woods, G. *Drug Abuse in Society: A Reference Handbook.* Santa Barbara, CA: ABC-CLIO Press, 1993.

Woolsey, R. "A Prescription for Better Prescriptions." *Issues in Science and Technology* (Spring 1994): 59–66.

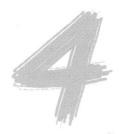

Addictive Behavior and Treating Drug Dependence

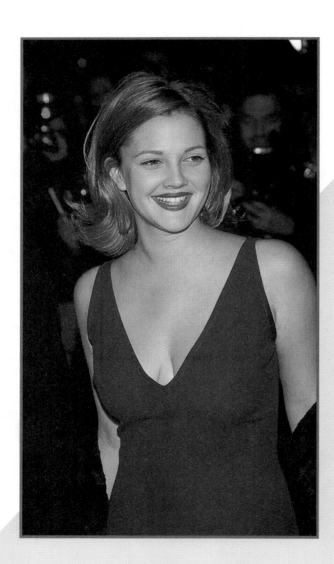

MAMTA

On completing this chapter
you will be able to: ▶

Did You Know?

- Addiction is only one phase of drug use and abuse.
- Prominent drug abuse researchers view some of the major causes of addiction as originating from poverty, affluence, racism, and dysfunctional personalities, families, and communities.
- Drug treatment will not work if the user is unwilling to cease his or her use.
- Rehabilitation cannot succeed if it is not specifically tailored to the individual and the type of drug use.

- Opiate maintenance programs do not eliminate drug addiction; they merely stabilize it.
- Most chemically dependent people deny their dependency.
- The latest criteria suggest that tobacco, which most Americans don't consider a drug, is actually one of the most addictive drugs.
- Alcohol and drug treatment began as self-help movements.
- One of the main reasons that addiction continues and

worsens is that family, friends, and co-workers help the addict avoid facing reality.
- One of the main "treatments" for heroin addiction is methadone, a synthetic drug from the same category.
- Until recently, drug counselors were mostly unlicensed, nonprofessional recovering addicts.
- Month-long, inpatient rehabilitation for alcoholism, an industry standard, is disappearing overnight due to changes in reimbursement.

Learning Objectives

- Provide in your own words a generally accepted definition of addiction.
- Compare and contrast drug abuse and drug dependency.
- Identify and explain two genetic or chemical factors that encourage chemical dependency.

- Identify and explain two social or environmental factors encouraging chemical dependency.
- Identify two models that attempt to explain dependency.
- Describe two vicious cycles in the progression of chemical dependency.
- Identify two models that may be used to treat chemical dependency.

- Describe the important features of Alcoholics Anonymous.
- Describe the important features of therapeutic communities.
- Outline the components of modern chemical dependency treatment.

◢ The Origin and Nature of Addiction

Humans can develop a very intense relationship with chemicals. Most people have chemically altered their mood at some point in their lives, if only by consuming a cup of coffee or a glass of white wine, and a majority do so occasionally. Yet for some individuals, chemicals become the center of their lives, driving their behavior and determining their priorities, even where catastrophic consequences to their health and social well-being ensue. While the word "addiction" is an agreed-upon term referring to such behavior, little agreement exists as to the origin, nature, or boundaries of the concept of addiction. It may be classified as a very bad habit, a failure of will or morality, a symptom of other problems, or a chronic disease in its own right. In addition, while most professional literature limits the definition of addiction to chemical involvements, some seek to include other pathological or compulsive behavior patterns.

Although public perception of drug abuse and addiction as a major social problem has waxed and waned over the past 20 years, the social costs of addiction have not: the total criminal justice, health, insurance, and other costs in the United States are roughly estimated at $80 to $175 billion annually, depending on the source. Despite numerous prevention efforts, the "War on Drugs," and a fall-off in the heavy drug use of the 1960s and 1970s, lessons learned in one decade seem to quickly pass out of awareness. For example, marijuana use among young people, which had declined in every year from 1978 to 1991, has doubled over the past few years, and its use, as well as that of alcohol or cigarettes, is penetrating into younger and younger grades (Drug Strategies 1996, 2–3).

This chapter will introduce facts and ideas to help you better comprehend this persistent social, public health, and safety problem, and critically evaluate claims about old and "newly discovered" addictions.

In asking a student, who represents a segment of the population at large, his view of addiction, he responded:

> Look, everyone is addicted to something. My dad is addicted to TV and snacking. My sister is addicted to the soaps and buying the most expensive makeup, perfumes, and clothes. My brother is addicted to his computer games. I am addicted to drugs. Why is my addiction rated so negative? Because society does not want people who are addicted or constantly walking around high. Why? Because being spaced out on drugs makes you unproductive and there is too much satisfaction with your own happiness. Right now, I know I am addicted to what society says are "no-no's." But really, I don't care what society thinks. Someday I think I will be worried, but I plan to wean myself off these drugs [referring to alcohol, tobacco, marijuana, and occasional use of LSD and psilocybin mushrooms] before I have to check into a drug addiction clinic.
>
> *From Venturelli's research files, 24-year-old male graduate student, July 27, 1996*

To understand addiction, we will explore the nature and characteristics of this phenomenon. As another student reveals:

> Addiction! God, this runs in our family, big time. Especially alcoholism and cigarette smoking. As a family, we are so bad that when we all get together you will find all of us drinking pop. I have so many relatives, uncles, aunts, and cousins that had a whole history of addiction that, when put together, we could have made up a separate chapter of AA [Alcoholics Anonymous]. Most of us are now reformed alcoholics. Addiction is a common affliction in our family. Most of us have gone to hell and back with our addictions.
>
> *From Venturelli's research files, 20-year-old female undergraduate student, July 26, 1996*

These interviews highlight two individuals' strikingly opposing views on their values and attitudes regarding addiction. The first interviewee does not perceive his use of drugs as resulting from addictive behavior. Conversely, the second interviewee is well aware of the relentless grip that addiction has had on her life. The second interviewee's understanding goes beyond her own experience; she sees how other family members have experienced the destructive effects of drug addiction.

In Chapter 1, you became aware of the scope of the substance abuse problem. In Chapter 2, we covered the major theories of why people use or abuse drugs. In Chapter 3, you learned about how drug use and abuse are viewed and regulated by the law.

As the title of this chapter suggests, we will first delve into the nature and outcomes of *addiction* and several views of its meaning and social impact. Following this discussion of addiction, we will explore *addiction treatment* options, such as alternative goals setting and rehabilitation methods.

The American Problem

From the earliest days to the present, different types of drug dependence have plagued American society. At various times, drug dependence has been considered a moral violation, a criminal act, and an illness. Throughout history, the laws that have been passed in the United States have reflected the moral code of the times.

The history of drug addiction shows that, in the early days, alcoholism was rampant, and some pockets of opiate dependence sprung up. The Pilgrims and Puritans, for example, did not forbid drinking, only overindulgence. When the Revolutionary War ended in 1783, people continued to accept heavy drinking as a normal way of life, despite the belief that it was morally wrong to drink to excess. So many Americans were addicted to alcohol that Presidents Washington and Jefferson suggested that people switch from drinking distilled spirits to beer and wine, to reduce the disruptive influence of alcoholism.

Other drug addictions developed as well. From the early 1800s to the early 1900s, opiate and cocaine addiction grew; it was legal to smoke and use these drugs, and they were widely available. Patent medicines, tonics, and elixirs contained liberal amounts of opiates and cocaine as well as alcohol, which compounded the drug dependence. In contrast to later drug abuse patterns, in the late 1800s the typical opiate addict was female, white, rural, and 40 years old.

Barbiturates were also available in the early 1900s. Even though some people became addicted, little attention was given to this problem because supplies were often obtained through medical channels. Amphetamine dependence was also managed medically. Barbiturates and amphetamines were not restricted by federal laws until 1965.

Defining Addiction

Addiction can be characterized as a tremendous attachment, thirst, or desire to *repeatedly* experience the drug of choice. This relentless pursuit to satisfy the need for the drug of choice occurs despite the fact that the drug is usually harmful and injurious to bodily and mental functioning. Oftentimes, the perpetual desire to satisfy an addiction directly interferes with the need to strive for continual self-improvement. As one interviewee revealed:

> It's pleasurable when the drug or drugs are consumed, but it's living hell when trying to quit. An addicted person will lie, cheat, and steal from even family members and friends in order to keep up the "high" from the drug. Never trust an addict about his or her drug use. Addicts are what the word means, addicted! They completely lack self-control. The drug controls them, they don't control the drug.
>
> *From Venturelli's research files, 28-year-old male undergraduate student, August 5, 1996*

In 1964, the World Health Organization (WHO) of the United Nations defined *addiction* as "a state of periodic or chronic intoxication detrimental to the individual and society, which is characterized by an overwhelming desire to continue taking the drug and to obtain it by any means" (World Health Organization 1964, 9–10; see also Eddy et al. 1965, 721–733). Today the WHO prefers the term *drug dependence*, which is indicative of changing views.

In the same definition, specific reference is made to "a particular state of mind that is termed **'psychic dependence'**" (Eddy et al. 1965, 723; Franklin 1995, 39–52). As we proceed in this chapter, you will notice how treatment, education, and prevention programs are geared to either treat, educate against or prevent this psychic dependence. The word *addiction*, derived from the Latin verb *addicere*, refers to the process of binding to things. Today, the word largely refers to a chronic adherence to drugs. In today's definition, we

psychic dependence
the habitual use and need to use a chemical to ameliorate an unwanted emotional state

include physical and psychological dependence. Physical dependence is the body's need to constantly have the drug or drugs, and psychological dependence is the mental inability to stop using the drug or drugs (White 1991). Sociologists Inciardi, Horowitz, and Pottiega state that "addiction entails three characteristics: chronic use, compulsion, plus resulting problems" (1993, 83).

The *Diagnostic and Statistical Manual of Mental Disorders,* published by the American Psychiatric Association, 4th edition (or DSM-IV) (1994), differentiates between intoxication by, abuse of, and addiction to drugs. While "substance abuse" is considered maladaptive, leading to recurrent adverse consequences or impairment (182–183), it is carefully differentiated from true addiction, called "substance dependence" (176–181), the essential feature of which is continued use despite significant substance-related problems known to the user. Many of these features are usually present:

▲ Tolerance: the need for increased amounts, or diminished effect of same amount.

▲ Withdrawal: The characteristic withdrawal syndrome for each substance, which can be avoided by taking closely related substances.

▲ Unsuccessful attempts to cut down.

▲ Increasing time spent in substance-related activities, such as obtaining, using, and recovering from its effects.

Models of Addiction

> No area of medicine is so bedeviled by semantic confusion as is the field of alcoholism. (D. L. Davies 1969)

Various models attempt to describe the essential nature of drug addiction. If we read newspaper accounts of "inebriety" in nineteenth- and early twentieth-century newspapers, we may note an editorializing undertone that looks askance at the poor morals and lifestyle choices followed by the inebriate. This view has been dubbed the **moral model,** and while it may seem outdated from a

moral model

the belief that people abuse alcohol because they choose to do so

modern scientific standpoint, it still characterizes an attitude among many traditionally minded North Americans and members of many other ethnic groups (Andrew Gordon's study of Hispanic subgroup reaction to alcoholism described migrants from Guatemala who categorized drunkenness as "indecente" [Gordon, 1981]).

The prevailing concept or model of addiction in America (and, interestingly, one that is largely limited to English-speaking Americans) is the **disease model.** Furthermore, most proponents of this concept specify addiction to be a chronic and progressive disease, over which the sufferer has no control. This model originated from research performed by one of the founders of addiction studies (Jellinek 1952, 1960) among members of Alcoholics Anonymous; he observed a seemingly inevitable progression in his subjects, which they made many failed attempts to arrest. This philosophy is currently espoused by the recovery fellowships of Alcoholics Anonymous and Narcotics Anonymous, and the treatment field in general. It has even permeated the psychiatric and medical establishments' standard definitions of addiction. There are many variations within the broad rubric of the disease model. This model is still bitterly debated, however, and viewpoints range from fierce adherence to the equally fierce opposition, with intermediate views patronizing the disease concept as a convenient myth (Smith, Milkman, and Sunderwirth 1985).

disease model

the belief that people abuse alcohol because of some biologically caused condition

Those who view addiction as another manifestation of something gone awry with the personality system adhere to the **characterological** or **personality predisposition model.** Every school of psychoanalytic, neophychoanalytic, and psychodynamic psychotherapy has its specific

characterological or personality presidposition model

view of chemical dependency as a symptom of problems in the development or operation of the system of needs, motives, and attitudes within the individual

"take" on the subject of addiction (Frosch 1985). Tangentially, many addicts are also diagnosed with **personality disorders** (formerly known as "character disorders"), such as impulse control disorders and sociopathy. Although few addicts are treated by **psychoanalysis** or psychoanalytic psychotherapy, a characterological type of model was a formative influence on the drug-free, addict-run, "therapeutic community" model, which uses harsh confrontation and time-extended, sleep-depriving group encounters.

> **personality disorder**
>
> a broad category of psychiatric disorders, formerly called "character disorders," that includes the antisocial personality disorder, borderline personality disorder, schizoid personality disorder, and others. These serious, ongoing impairments are difficult to treat.

> **psychoanalysis**
>
> a theory of personality and method of psychotherapy originated by Sigmund Freud, focused on unconscious forces and conflicts and a series of psychosexual stages

Observers concluded that addicts must have withdrawn behind a **"double wall" of encapsulation** in which they failed to grow, making such techniques necessary.

Others view addiction as a "career" —a series of steps or phases with distinguishable characteristics. One career pattern of addiction includes six phases: (1) experimentation or initiation, (2) escalation (increasing use), (3) maintaining or "taking care of business" (optimistic use of drugs coupled with successful job performance), (4) dysfunctional or "going through changes" (problems with constant use and unsuccessful attempts to quit), (5) recovery or "getting out of the life" (arriving at a successful view about quitting and receiving drug treatment), and (6) ex-addict (actually quitting) (Waldorf 1983; also in Clinard and Meier 1992, 206–7).

> **"double wall" of encapsulation**
>
> an adaptation to pain and avoidance of reality, in which the individual withdraws emotionally and further anesthetizes him or herself by chemical means.

Causes of Addiction

In Chapter 2, we reviewed the reasons and motivations for using drugs. We discussed the fact that there are many, perhaps millions, of individuals who use or even occasionally abuse drugs without compromising their basic health, legal, and occupational status and social relationships. Why do a significant minority become caught up in abuse and addictive behavior? To answer this question, we need to cull out some risk factors that have been identified with development of harmful drug use patterns, including addiction. Research on these factors could fill a small library. Table 4.1 represents a compilation of factors identified as complicit in the origin or "etiology" of addiction, taken from the fields of psychology, sociology, and addiction studies. After this review, we will consider vicious cycles that propel at-risk individual abusers further down a path toward chemical dependency, and the stages or phases of this process.

In addition to risk factors for abuse and addiction in our society, an entire subfield of anthropology is devoted to systematically searching for aspects of cultural beliefs and behaviors that result in higher rates of addiction. Some of these factors provide fascinating possibilities. For example, Field (1991) found that degree of drunkenness was statistically related to anxieties about subsistence, or making a living, in tribal-level societies. Might we see a parallel in the United States? Margaret Bacon and her colleagues, researchers in the relationship of culture to personality, found that alcohol abuse was statistically related to developmental conflicts over dependency needs—that is, fostering of dependency needs that are then not indulged or allowed expression (Bacon et al. 1965 a, b; Bacon 1974). The dependent child is, rather suddenly, expected to be self-reliant. One can imagine the deprivation, conflict, and anxiety felt by such inconsistency.

Other "cultural" risk factors for development of abuse include the following:

▲ Drinking at times other than at meals;

▲ Drinking alone;

▲ Same-sex drinking;

Table 4.1	Risk Factors for Addiction

Risk Factor	Leading to this Effect
Biologically Based Factors *(genetic, neurological, biochemical, and so on):*	
▲ A less subjective feeling of intoxication	▲ More use to achieve intoxication (warning signs of abuse absent)
▲ Easier development of tolerance; liver enzymes adapt to increased use	▲ Easier to reach the addictive level
▲ Lack of resilience or fragility of higher (cerebral) brain functions	▲ Easy deterioration of cerebral functioning, impaired judgment, and social deterioration
▲ Difficulty in screening out unwanted or bothersome outside stimuli (low stimulus barrier)	▲ Feeling overwhelmed or stressed
▲ Tendency to amplify outside or internal stimuli (stimulus augmentation)	▲ Feeling attacked or panicked; need to avoid emotion
▲ Attention deficit hyperactivity disorder and other learning disabilities	▲ Failure, low self-esteem, or isolation
▲ Biologically based mood disorders (depression and bipolar disorders)	▲ Need to self-medicate against loss of control or the pain of depression; inability to calm down when manic or to sleep when agitated
Psychosocial/Developmental "Personality" Factors:	
▲ Low self-esteem	▲ Need to blot out pain, gravitate to outsider groups
▲ Depression rooted in learned helplessness and passivity	▲ Need to blot out pain; use of a stimulant as an anti-depressant
▲ Conflicts	▲ Anxiety and guilt
▲ Repressed and unresolved grief and rage	▲ Chronic depression, anxiety, or pain
▲ Post-traumatic stress syndrome (as in veterans and abuse victims)	▲ Nightmares or panic attacks
Social and Cultural Environment	
▲ Availability of drugs	▲ Easy frequent use
▲ Chemical-abusing parental model	▲ Sanction; no conflict over use
▲ Abusive, neglectful parents; other dysfunctional family patterns	▲ Pervasive sense of abandonment, distrust, and pain; difficulty in maintaining attachments
▲ Group norms favoring heavy use and abuse	▲ Reinforced, hidden abusive behavior that can progress without interference
▲ Misperception of peer norms	▲ Belief that most people use or favor use or think it's "cool" to use
▲ Severe or chronic stressors, as from noise, poverty, racism, or occupational stress	▲ Need to alleviate or escape from stress via chemical means
▲ "Alienation" factors: isolation, emptiness	▲ Painful sense of aloneness, normlessness, rootlessness, boredom, monotony, or hopelessness
▲ Difficult migration/acculturation with social disorganization, gender/generation gaps, or loss of role	▲ Stress without buffering support system

▲ Drinking defined as an antistress and antianxiety potion;

▲ Patterns of solitary drinking;

▲ Drinking defined as a rite of passage into an adult role; and

▲ The recent introduction of a chemical into a social group with insufficient time to develop informal social control over its use (Marshall 1979).

It is important to recall that the "mix" of risk factors differs for each person. It varies according to social, cultural, and age groups, and individual and family idiosyncrasies. Most addiction treatment professionals believe that it is difficult, if not impossible, to tease out these factors before treatment, when the user is still "talking to a chemical," or during early treatment, when the brain and body are still recuperating from the effects of long-term abuse. Once a stable sobriety is established, one can begin to address any underlying problems. An exception would be the *mentally ill chemical abuser (MICA),* whose treatment requires special considerations from the outset.

Although we cannot provide an encyclopedic review of risk factors among all groups in society here, we will touch on the life span or developmental dimension, which identifies stressors and conflicts in transitional periods such as adolescence and middle age.

Risk factors that apply especially to adolescents:

▲ Peer norms favoring use

▲ Misperception of peer norms (users set the tone)

▲ Power of age group peer norms versus other social influences

▲ Conflicts, such as dependence versus independence, adult maturational tasks versus fear, new types of roles versus familiar safe roles; conflicts that generate anxiety or guilt

▲ Teenage risk-taking, sense of omnipotence or invulnerability

▲ Cultural definition of use as a rite of passage into adulthood

▲ Cultural definition of use as glamorous, sexy, facilitating intimacy, fun, and so on

Risk factors that apply especially to middle-aged individuals:

▲ Retirement: loss of a meaningful role or occupational identity

▲ Loss, grief, or isolation: loss of parents, divorce, departure of children ("empty nest syndrome")

▲ Loss of positive body image

▲ Disappointment when life expectations do not pan out

Even in each of these age groups, mix of factor is at play. The adolescent abuser might be someone whose risk factors were primary neurological vulnerabilities, such as an adolescent who suffers from undiagnosed attention-deficit hyperactivity disorder; who experiences failure and rejection at school; or who disappoints his parents, and is labeled as odd, lazy, or unintelligent (Kelly and Ramundo 1993).

In response to the information presented in Table 4.1, a student, who was a recovering alcoholic, commented: "You're an alcoholic because you drink!" He had a good point: the mere presence of one, two, or more risk factors by themselves don't create addiction. Drugs must be available, they must be used, and they must become a pattern of adaptation to any of the many painful, threatening, uncomfortable, or unwanted sensations or stimuli that occur in the presence of genetic, psychosocial, or environmental risk factors. Prevention workers often note the presence of multiple messages encouraging use: the medical use of minor tranquilizers to offset any type of psychic discomfort; the marketing of alcohol as sexy, glamorous, adult, and facilitative of social interaction; and so forth. One worker commented:

My dean calls Greeks [fraternities and sororities] "an organized conspiracy dedicated to the consumption of alcohol." Some of these freshmen come from drinking homes, they're scared as hell, and they're pledging in binge-drinking frats. America is an assembly line for alcoholism, and some folks are working very hard on the assembly line. (*Campus Consortium* newsletter 1993)

◢ The Addictive Process

Vicious Cycles

> First the man takes a drink, then the drink takes a drink, then the drink takes the man.
> *(Traditional Chinese proverb)*

Thus far we have identified factors that in combination tend to initiate a pattern of drug abuse, especially when drugs represent a viable pattern of adaptation for that individual. Drug addiction develops as a process, however; it is not a sudden occurrence. In this section we will describe the factors that tend to worsen abuse into true addiction. The body makes simple physiological adaptations to the presence of alcohol and other drugs, as discussed at length in the specific pharmacology chapters of this text:

1. Brain cell tolerance and metabolic efficiency of the liver, develop necessitating consumption of more of the chemical to achieve the desired effect. (Chapters 5 and 6)

2. Physical dependence develops, in which cell adaptations cause withdrawal syndromes to occur in the absence of the chemical. With the development of tolerance, withdrawal syndromes will occur at ever higher levels.

3. Abuse impairs cerebral functioning, including memory, judgment, behavioral organization, ability to plan and solve problems, and motor coordination. Thus, poor decision making, impaired and deviant behavior, and overall dysfunction result in adverse social consequences, such as accidents, loss of earning power and relationships, and impaired health.

4. Adverse social and health consequences cause pain, depression, and lowered self-esteem, which may result in further use as an emotional and physical anesthetic.

5. The addict adapts to the chronically painful situation by erecting a defense system of denial, minimization, and rationalization; this denial of reality may be exacerbated by the chemical blunting of reality. It is unlikely, at this point, that the addict or developing addict will feel compelled to cease or cut back on drug use on his or her own (Tarter et al. 1983).

6. Family, friends, and colleagues unwittingly "enable" the maintenance and progression of addiction by making excuses for addicts, literally and figuratively bailing them out, taking up the slack, denying and minimizing their problems, and otherwise making it possible for addicts to avoid facing the reality and consequences of what they are doing to themselves and others. While they may be motivated by simple naivete, embarrassment, or misguided protectiveness, there are often hidden gains in taking up this role, known popularly as *codependency* (Beattie 1987; Health Communications, 1984). A variety of cultural and organizational factors also operate in the workplace or school so as to deny the existence or severity of abuse or dependency. This triad of personal denial, peer and kin denial and codependency, and institutional denial represents a formidable impediment to successful intervention and recovery (Myers 1990).

Figure 4.1

Processes of Addiction

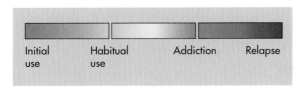

| Initial use | Habitual use | Addiction | Relapse |

Source: Deborah Franklin. "Hooked/Not Hooked. Why Isn't Everyone an Addict?" In *Health* (November–December 1990):41.

Stages of Addiction

Many researchers have attempted to describe identifiable stages or phases in the addictive career. Many of these models show a relentless progression, like an out-of-control baby carriage careening down a staircase. The first was developed by E. M. Jellinek (1952, 1960), an early proponent of the disease concept who suggested that drug addiction develops as a process; it is not a sudden occurrence. Several levels of addiction have been identified (Doweiko 1996, 11–12):

Level 0: Total abstinence. The individual never uses drugs for recreational purposes.

Level 1: Rare social use. The individual rarely uses chemicals during or for recreation.

Level 2: Heavy social use and early problem drug use. The individual is perceived as a frequent user and abuser of drugs. Social, legal, financial, and occupational problems are likely.

Level 3: Heavy problem use-early addiction. The individual is dependent on drugs. Some medical complications will likely occur in the early to middle stages of addiction, followed by more intense medical problems (ulcers, fatty deposits on the liver, hepatitis, pancreatitis, gastritis, and frequent blackouts). The individual at this level may continue to deny dependence.

Level 4: Clear-cut addiction to drugs. The individual is affected by several medical consequences of the dependence and may even be near death. Most friends and family members have experienced a devastating deterioration in their social relations with the addict.

Vernon Johnson, an influential writer on methods of organizing an intervention to get an addict into treatment, has gone into considerable detail on the emotional syndrome involved in the progression of chemical dependency. On a straight line charting the transition from pain to euphoria, future addicts move through a series of 11 stages, which we will condense as follows:

▲ Drug users learn that chemicals can swing them up to euphoria and back with no emotional cost.

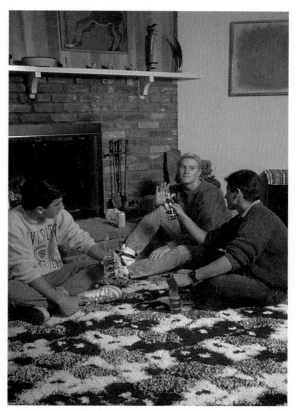

Peer influence. In adolescent groups, the spread of drug abuse usually involves drug/alcohol abuse.

▲ They learn how to control the dose to achieve the desired effect.

▲ They seek the mood swing effect more often.

▲ They start paying an emotional cost by swinging down toward the pain end of the spectrum after usage, which becomes progressively worse.

▲ Addicts begin at a point of chronic depression and pain, and use chemicals to feel somewhat normal. At this point, they are locked in a free-floating mass of anxiety, guilt, shame, and remorse, which they defend with denial and projection (Johnson 1986, 14–36).

Whether chemical use progresses inevitably from abuse to dependency, and onward into worsening dependency, is a matter of controversy.

From the standpoint of observing people who end in treatment or Alcoholics Anonymous, this situation is certainly the case. The addictive "career" also includes individuals who seem to "mature out" of abuse or dependency without addiction-specific help, however, as well as those who bounce around on some level of abuse for their entire life without becoming true addicts.

Both George Valliant's landmark, longitudinal study of alcoholics in Boston (1982) and Marc Shuckit et al.'s more recent research (1993) concluded that there is indeed a tendency toward progression of addiction among many multiple-risk individuals. The studies found, however, that the progression was not inevitable for all, and was anything but an orderly process as Jellinek and others have portrayed it. They characterized the process as being marked by ups and downs in abuse and social functioning.

Thus, a tremendous variety of risk factors exist in the organism, personality, social and cultural context that propel an individual in the direction of chemical abuse. Vicious cycles worsen the syndrome, finally generating a chemical dependency disorder that stands on its own regardless of the original causes. As many prevention workers say, "You started out with three problems; now you have four!"

Examining the Addictive Potential of Drugs

It is important to exercise some independent, critical thinking about drugs. What we believe about the addictive potential of each drug is largely determined by myth or demonization of the substance. In 1938, for example, the film *Reefer Madness* portrayed marijuana as directly causing total insanity, rape, and homicide. Today, student audiences find this film laughable. Crack cocaine, however, has been shown to be highly addictive and is associated with child neglect, and belligerent and paranoid behavior. In other words, this drug acts much like marijuana was portrayed in the 1938 movie. Is crack so different from the cocaine used for decades that is justifies a different legal penalty? According to federal sentencing guidelines, possession of even tiny amounts of crack make the offender liable for huge sentences,

while a person would have to possess 100 times the amount of "regular" cocaine to receive the same sentence. Nevertheless, a recent issue of the *Journal of the American Medical Association* (Hatsukami and Fishman, 1996) reported that crack and regular cocaine are essentially the same pharmacologically. Major differences are that crack is cheaper, more available, sent straight to the brain by smoking, and generally used in communities that are suffering from social disintegration. It is easy to see why the rapid spread of crack—and of related social problems—has been attributed to some addictive property specific to the chemical itself, rather than the context in which it is used.

In contrast to crack, which we endow with mythic properties, nicotine, which is just as addictive as cocaine, is often not considered a drug at all. One prevention worker wrote recently in a campus prevention newsletter that:

> Nicotine is a drug? . . . it's hard to get this idea across. Students say, "*but you don't get high from a cigarette.*" Yes, the mood modification is subtle, not overtly intoxicating, and like booze, it's not deviant behavior to use it. But by the modern criteria of addictiveness—withdrawal, reinforcement, tolerance, dependence, and intoxication—it's very clear: alcohol and heroin are big in terms of intoxication and withdrawal, but nicotine is tops in fostering dependence and tolerance. There are very few "occasional users" of nicotine; they get hooked and stay hooked. (Sorcha Linkard in *Campus Consortium* newsletter 1995) (See Figure 4.2)

Nondrug Addictions?

The addictive disease model and the 12-step recovery model followed by Alcoholics Anonymous and Narcotics Anonymous have seemed so successful to both addictive sufferers and their families and friends that other unwanted syndromes have been added to the list. The degree to which the concept of addiction fits these syndromes varies. Gambling, for example, shows progressive worsening, loss of control, relief of tension from the activity, and continuance despite negative consequences known to the user. Some recovering gamblers even claim to have experienced a form of

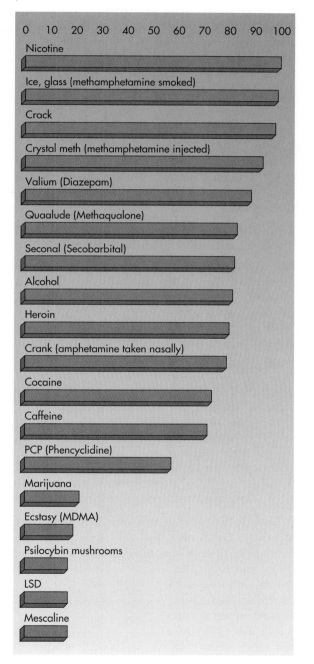

Figure 4.2

Health experts' ratings of how easy it is to become addicted and how difficult it is to stop using the following drugs, with 100 being the highest addiction potential.

withdrawal. Members of Alcoholics Anonymous spun off a separate fellowship, Gamblers Anonymous, which has attracted many non–chemical-abusing members. Clearly, gambling as an activity has much in common with chemical addictions, but it is debatable whether it belongs in the category of addiction (the *DSM-IV* does not include it, for example). Many other groups have followed in Gamblers Anonymous's footsteps, including those related to eating (Overeaters Anonymous) and sexual relationships (The Augustine Fellowship, Sex and Love Addicts Anonymous 1986). In recent years, any excessive or unwanted behaviors, including excess shopping, chocolate consumption, and even Internet use, have been labeled addictions, which has led to satirical coverage in the press. Addictions professionals lament the overdefinition, which they feel trivializes the seriousness and suffering of rigorously defined addictions.

The next section in this chapter will consider individuals for whom engagement in some form of organized recovery work is the route out of addiction.

◢ The Treatment of Addiction

The development of specific techniques, programs, and personnel to treat addiction is a recent enterprise. While psychoanalysis, for example, is a century old, as recently as the 1950s severely intoxicated alcoholics would typically be consigned to a "drunk tank" lockup or mental hospital ward. In the decades that followed, several treatment models evolved, an addiction counseling profession emerged, and governmental and voluntary organizations concerned with addiction proliferated on national, state, and local levels (see Appendix C, page 499).

To best target treatment for an individual, the type and goals of treatment must be determined. Consideration must be given to the fact that both the type and the goals of treatment largely depend on the view one holds on addiction. For example, if the disease model is applied to addiction, total abstinence is required because it views drug abuse as a biological condition that is largely uncontrollable. The user is perceived as "sick" and thus irrational about continued drug use. On the other hand, if responsible drug use is the goal, then occasional and moderate drug use are the intended end-results.

Effective treatment allows addicts to stop abusing drugs, returns former addicts to a drug-free state of existence, and transforms them into employable and productive members of society. Results show that addicts who receive treatment for more than three months remain drug-free a year later; when treatment lasts a year or longer, two-thirds remain drug-free many years later (Drug Strategies 1996). Findings clearly show that treatment is much less expensive than continuing addiction. It costs society $43,200 to let an addict remain untreated, compared with an average of $16,000 for a year of residential care or $1500 in an outpatient program. The Rand Corporation reports that providing treatment for all addicts would save more than $150 billion in social costs over the next 15 years (Drug Strategies 1996).

In the branch of the addictions field that strives for total abstinence from drugs, it is often difficult to separate self-help approaches from professional treatment, as their histories are interwoven. In the next section, we will describe self-help recovery movements, the main treatment modalities that they influenced, and the settings in which drug-free treatment takes place. We will then describe drug maintainance and innovative treatment techniques, and finally conclude with a description of changes in the treatment field.

Alcoholics Anonymous (AA)

Founded in the mid-1930s, AA is now an international organization. The desire to stop drinking is the sole criterion required to join. The original founders of AA were strongly influenced by a religious movement known as the Oxford Group and the psychoanalyst Carl Jung. The "Twelve Steps for Recovery" espoused by AA are cited in the accompanying "Case in Point."

Alcoholics Anonymous calls itself a "fellowship" of recovering alcoholics. It is perhaps the prototype for the self-help group movement, in which nonprofessional, ordinary citizens with problems form a caring community with supportive healing qualities. "Twelve Step" groups offer a simple, concrete program for recovery from addictions. Members always emphasize that they are not "ex-alcoholics," but are merely holding their alcoholic disease in abeyance "a day at a time." Meetings are nonthreatening, nonconfrontational, and noncoercive. AA in particular, and Twelve Step groups in general, have an extremely loose, nonhierarchical organizational structure. Narcotics Anonymous, founded in 1951, is less well known, but has grown tremendously in recent years, particularly in urban communities.

It is difficult to assess AA's success for four reasons:

1. AA insists on anonymity; it does not reveal names of members.

2. Membership is strictly voluntary. Those who want to join become members when they vow to give up drinking. Controlled studies are impossible.

3. Members are a homogeneous group. They tend to be middle class and socially conservative.

4. **Addictionologists** (people who research addiction) are of the opinion that the more severe, "hard-core" alcoholics who refuse to seek help generally do not go to AA, while a smaller percentage of problem drinkers who come to view themselves as addicted to alcohol take this path (see Rudy 1994 for further discussion of this and other related findings). In part, this factor may be responsible for the group's high success rate. Regardless, AA has been, and continues to be, a very important method for treating many recovering alcoholics.

> **addictionologists**
> people who research alcohol and drug addiction

AA has two types of meetings, open and closed meetings. **Open meetings** are open to anyone having an interest in attending and witnessing these meetings, and they last approximately 45 minutes to an hour. **Closed meetings** are for alcoholics having a serious desire to completely stop drinking.

> **open meetings**
> meetings to which anyone having an interest in attending and witnessing is invited

AA's Twelve Steps for Recovery

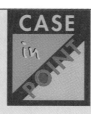

1. We admitted we were powerless over alcohol—that our lives had become unmanageable.

2. Came to believe that a Power greater than ourselves could restore us to sanity.

3. Made a decision to turn our will and our lives over to the care of God *as we understood Him.*

4. Made a searching and fearless moral inventory of ourselves.

5. Admitted to God, to ourselves, and to another human being the exact nature of our wrongs.

6. Were entirely ready to have God remove all these defects of character.

7. Humbly asked Him to remove our shortcomings.

8. Made a list of all persons we had harmed, and became willing to make amends to them all.

9. Made direct amends to such people wherever possible, except when to do so would injure them or others.

10. Continued to take personal inventory and when we were wrong promptly admitted it.

11. Sought through prayer and meditation to improve our conscious contact with God *as we understood Him,* praying only for knowledge of His will for us and the power to carry that out.

12. Having had a spiritual awakening as the result of these steps, we tried to carry this message to alcoholics, and to practice these principles in all our affairs. ■

Source: Alcoholics Anonymous World Services, Inc., *Alcoholics Anonymous: The Story of How Many Thousands of Men and Women Have Recovered from Alcoholism,* 3rd ed. New York: Alcoholics Anonymous (1976): 59–60. Permission to reprint this material does not mean that AA has reviewed or approved the contents of this chapter, nor that AA agrees with the views expressed herein. AA is a program of recovery from alcoholism—use of the Twelve Steps in connection with programs and activities which are patterned after AA, but which address other problems, does not imply otherwise.

---

closed meetings

meetings to which only alcoholics having a serious desire to completely stop drinking are invited

These meetings are not open to viewers or "shoppers." At closed meetings, recovering alcoholics address through testimonials how alcohol has diminished their quality of life.

Some outgrowths of Alcoholics Anonymous include Al-Anon, ACOA (adult children of alcoholics), and Alateen. These are parallel organizations supporting Alcoholics Anonymous. Al-Anon is for spouses and other close relatives of alcoholics, and Alateen is exclusively for teenage children of alcoholic parents. Both relatives and teen members of alcoholic families learn means and methods for coping with destructive behaviors exhibited by alcoholic members.

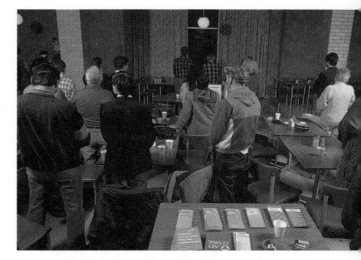

Common alcohol abuse-related problems are shared at AA meetings.

Using Support Groups to Counter Life Stress and Alcohol Abuse

Although Marie was never quite alone with her abuse problem, it took a personal confrontation for her to realize that she needed support. Marie is the adult child of two alcoholics. Her mother died of complications from alcoholism when she was 20, and her father died 15 years later from a similar fate. When she was about 13, Marie began to make the association between the beverages her parents drank and the subsequent moods that followed, and she made a vow that she would never follow that path. As often happens, peer pressure in college changed her position. Weekend keg parties and "booze cruise" road trips seemed to be a part of college life that she could not avoid if she was to be accepted, and more than anything else, deep inside she desired to be accepted.

Growing up as the child of two alcoholic parents, Marie never knew what to expect when she got home from school—in what condition the house would be, or in what state of mind she would find her parents. For this reason, she never invited any friends over for fear that she would be humiliated in front of them because her mother or father was inebriated and abusive. Marie kept to herself, but still longed for the acceptance of friends she felt she could never have while she lived at home. When the time came to go to college, she applied to schools far away. As luck would have it, she was accepted to a school 500 miles away.

Weekend social drinking habits in college became a daily behavior for Marie after graduation. When asked, she would say that she liked the buzz she got from alcohol, but, she said, she was always in control. In her mind, Marie might have been in control, but her body's physiology told a different story. Perhaps her Irish background made her genetically predisposed to alcoholism, perhaps it was a means to be accepted, or perhaps it combined a great many factors. The end-result was that Marie was a full-fledged alcoholic by age 25. Rather than an occasional beer on weekends, she was downing a gallon of vodka every two days, a source of inspiration she kept hidden in her knapsack.

When confronted by her older brother, Marie at first vehemently denied she had a drinking problem. Within hours, however, she admitted she was powerless and needed help—desperately. An alcoholic seizure and subsequent coma the next week made the message abundantly clear. Ironically what attracted her to alcohol, social acceptance, soon became her saving grace—Alcoholics Anonymous. Beginning an alcohol rehabilitation program called Day One, Marie attended her first AA meeting and soon learned that she was not alone with her problem. Although her situation was unique, her predicament was quite common.

Researchers now know that support groups are one of the most effective ways to deal with the stress of life. No matter what the affliction, engaging in the community of friends, colleagues, and even strangers with similar issues, problems, or concerns, diminishes levels of stress. Members of our circle of friends, particularly people who have "been there," tend to help buffer the effects of stress. As Marie will attest, alcoholism is definitely a stressor:

Having something control your life makes you feel powerless, completely helpless. Alcohol offers such an illusion. It makes you think as if you are in complete control, but the truth is, with each sip, you freely give your power away. I was scared shitless with my first AA meeting. It's one thing to admit to yourself that you have a drinking problem. It's quite another when you have to admit to a room full of strangers how weak you are and how much control this substance has over you. But what I learned from AA is that these people don't pass judgment. They accept you as you are. This has made all the difference in my life now. My friends in AA are my new family.

Marie is now happily married with two children. She has been sober for five years. The pieces of her life are firmly back in place after being shattered in her early to late twenties. As she says, "Every day is a struggle, but it's a good struggle. I have been through the dark night of my soul. You only have to do that trip once to realize it's not a place you want to stay very long." As Marie holds her four-year-old daughter on her lap, she beams, "I am very grateful to this family and my family and friends in AA."

One recovering addict explains:

> I'm a community college student. We're not 18-year-olds. In fact, I'm 39 again this year. I have my job, my 12 credits, and, I'm serious, the math professor gets on my last nerve. Well, not my last—that's my daughter, the crazy one. She's out there again [relapsed into addiction], running with her knucklehead [criminally involved] boyfriend, and I had to take the babies. I've been there, done that, got the T-shirt, and I'm too old for another go-round. I'm tired! I'm recovering myself; I have ten years [clean and sober, in Narcotics Anonymous]. I got some help from Al-Anon family groups. They told me, "You didn't cause it, you can't cure it, you can't control it!" They told me to lovingly disengage and get some serenity, not let the addict be the center of my life. Here in Newark we need a *special* support group for burnt-out grandmothers."

> *40-year-old female, African-American Community College student and recovering addict*

Rehabilitation Facilities

The first rehabilitation programs grew out of the work that AA members did with other active alcoholics. Known as Twelfth Stepping, it involves reaching out to others in need and attempting to draw them in. This movement began in the early days of AA, when the organization's founder, Bill W., put up alcoholics trying to dry out at his house in Brooklyn, when "[his] home was stuffed, from cellar to attic, with alcoholics in all stages of recovery" (Al-Anon 1970). It was a natural transition to opening up "drying out" houses in the 1940s and 1950s. Also during the 1950s, **the Minnesota model,** an inpatient rehabilitation model, was developed. It combined the AA philosophy with a multidisciplinary treatment team. A treatment plan was utilized, based

> **Minnesota model**
>
> a major model in the treatment of alcohol and drug abuse, involving a month-long stay in an inpatient rehabilitation facility, a multidisciplinary treatment team, systematic assessment, and a formal treatment plan with long- and short-term goals.

on individual assessment and prioritization of goals. This model, which borrows from social work practice, is still used in treatment programs. Due to the vagaries of insurance reimbursement in Minnesota, the program lasted 28 days; alcoholism programs traditionally were roughly one month long.

The 1970s and 1980s were a golden era for rehabilitation, when many costly, long-term programs flourished. Recently, and in the context of reimbursement concerns, the need for such a length of stay as an inpatient has been questioned in several studies (Holder, Longabaugh, Miller, and Rubonis 1991). Under the pressure of managed care and new insurance guidelines, many inpatient programs have closed or been converted to a new form of treatment.

▲ The *intensive outpatient rehabilitation program* is a partial hospitalization or day program that allows the client to work or attend school, but spend from 15 to 30 hours per week at the treatment center.

▲ *Halfway houses* are residential therapeutic environments in which individuals who have completed a rehabilitation program may live while pursuing employment or while working. They should not be confused with psychiatric halfway houses and board-and-care settings.

▲ *Long-term care* facilities are residential settings for individuals who are socially and psychologically unprepared for self-supporting life in the community. Many are religious in nature, such as the Salvation Army Adult Rehabilitation Programs.

Detoxification Units

Since the 1960s it has been recognized that an alcoholic needs special medical attention and social support to get through the rigors of physical withdrawal. Special facilities known as "detoxes" (detoxification units) evolved to serve this need. Some are hospital-based. Others, called "social detoxes" or "sobering-up stations," are free-standing, nonmedical AA-related units; these units have fallen out of favor in recent years. Finally, such units can be adjuncts to full-fledged rehabilitation programs. Detoxification programs, lasting from three to seven days, are misunderstood as treatment programs or modalities, and are even statistically compared with rehabilitation programs and treatment facilities. Addictionologists and treatment professionals of all persuasions recognize that addiction is a syndrome that often involves relapse, and that an individual may go through treatment more than once. Detoxification is not considered anything more than the first stage of treatment by any chemical dependency professional when attempted and, by itself, will certainly fail (we are not including the heavily involved AA member who undergoes detoxification). Patients typically cycle through the program many times, often at moments of crisis, or, if homeless, during cold weather.

Therapeutic Communities

The other major model of treatment for chemical dependency came from a different branch of the self-help movement. Although the term originated with patient government and other forms of "milieu therapy" in a psychiatric hospital setting, the **therapeutic community** (**TC**) is known today as a residential treatment program for drug dependency that utilizes confrontational methods and groups, hard work, and a status system as rehabilitation aids.

> **therapeutic communities (TCs)**
>
> programs that advocate a complete change in lifestyle, such as complete abstinence from drugs, elimination of deviant behavior, and development of employable skills

The main goal of TCs is a complete change in lifestyle: abstinence from drugs, elimination of criminal behavior, and development of employable skills, self-reliance, personal honesty, and responsibility.

The philosophy behind TCs is that only ex-addicts can truly understand and deal effectively with addicts. Some TCs also employ professionals with training in vocational guidance, education, medicine, and mental health who are paid or who may donate their services. Residents of the traditional TC stay at least 15 months before they return to the community. Several TCs have been experimenting with shorter resident times, ranging from 2 to 9 months, based on individual client needs and progress.

The first therapeutic community for drug addicts was Synanon, which was aimed at psychiatric patients. It was founded in Santa Monica, California, in 1958. Synanon was an AA clubhouse started by Charles E. Dederich, a former alcoholic, that was later expanded to include drug addicts and highly confrontational group sessions. When drug addicts came into the program, the alcoholics left because they felt associating with addicts was degrading.

Many branches of Synanon were founded based on the same philosophy—for example, Daytop Village and Phoenix House. They have been used as models for a number of other programs, with modifications based on the circumstances in each community. TCs have had a major impact on drug abuse treatment.

As of 1994, there were over 400 residential therapeutic communities in the United States serving drug abusers, criminal offenders, and other socially dislocated persons. These programs are quite diverse, ranging in size from 35 to 500 beds, and they serve a variety of clients.

The TC program includes encounter group therapy, educational programs, job assignments within the community, and in the later stages, conventional jobs outside the community. The primary staff are former drug addicts who have been rehabilitated in TC programs. Most TCs use self-government and group pressures, instead of relying on a professional, therapeutic personnel.

More recently, some TCs have been developed to serve criminal justice clients almost exclusively (McNeece and DiNitto 1994, 190). Drug addicts referred to TCs are placed in appropriate settings where delinquent or criminal peers and the adverse effects of crime-ridden neighborhoods, and by extension communities, are physically distant, and where the temptations of peers and environment are excluded.

Outpatient Treatment

The term "outpatient treatment" denotes a nonresidential setting where treatment takes place. It can involve any number of individual, group, or family sessions, in which the client is present one or more times per week, up to about ten hours per week. Treatment may use any of a number of approaches, including Twelve Step-style groups, interactive group therapy, confrontational groups, support and relapse prevention, occupational counseling, and so on. Outpatient treatment in which the client is present 10-30 hours per week is usually called "intensive outpatient treatment," "day treatment," or "partial hospitalization."

If only because it is the least expensive option, most addictions treatment takes place on an outpatient basis. In fact, attendance at an outpatient program can be undertaken for the following purposes:

▲ For initial assessment and referral into inpatient care

▲ As a followup to inpatient or intensive outpatient rehabilitation, called "continuing care"

▲ The entire course of treatment, where addiction is not overly severe

Addiction Treatment versus Psychotherapy

Based on our examination of addiction, some differences between addictions treatment and standard psychotherapy should be clear. The first stage—no easy task—is to get the addict into treatment by hook or by crook; until then, you're "just talking to a chemical." Then, it is necessary to break through the system of denial, rationalization, and minimization. While facilitating a process of recovery, treatment must ensure that the addict does not "fall through the cracks" between detox and rehab, or rehab and halfway house, and develop strategies for the client to avoid relapsing. In accomplishing these tasks, addictions therapy must draw upon skills and interventions from psychotherapy and counseling models, especially in developing communications skills that establish rapport with the client. Treatment that approximates true psychotherapy can only come in a later state of treatment, when stable sobriety is achieved, and painful or threatening issues can be examined without overwhelming the client and triggering a relapse.

Commonalties in Treatment

"Pure" therapeutic communities, Minnesota model rehabs, or other traditional models are becoming a distinct minority. Therapeutic communities, which once focused on graduating "ex-dope fiends," increasingly recognize the need for aftercare, and involve their residents in Narcotics Anonymous. AA-based rehabilitation centers recognize needs of "dual diagnosis" (mentally ill chemical abusing) clients who require medication, previously considered heretical. Federal and state requirements for agency licensure, and certification training of counselors, have also made it possible to describe features that any treatment setting is likely to include.

1. Clients are screened for eligibility and appropriateness for the treatment setting and agency, based on a psychosocial summary, records provided by a referring agency, and standardized tests such as the Michigan Alcoholism Screening Test or the Addiction Severity Index.

2. Clients go through an intake procedure, where they are informed of confidentiality regulations that ensure their privacy. An orientation to the agency and to the treatment process takes place.

A patient receives individual counseling in an alcoholism treatment center.

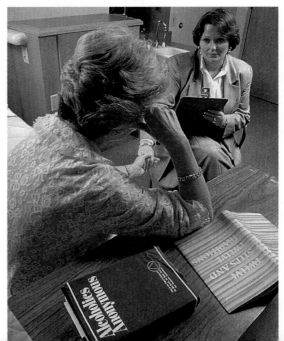

3. Based on an assessment of the client's strengths, weaknesses, and special needs, a treatment plan is drawn up that identifies long- and short-term goals, and prioritizes them in importance. Assessments are continually updated, and adjustments are made to the plan, where necessary.

The following treatment components are usually in place:

4. *Individual counseling* sessions focus on goals and objectives of a treatment plan and strategies for relapse prevention. A generic counseling approach is usually employed (Corey and Corey 1993; Ivey 1994) and elements of eclectic models such as cognitive-behavioral or rational-emotive therapy are frequently borrowed (Ellis et al. 1988) to help clients identify and explore the interaction of their behavior patterns, attitudes and thought processes, and emotions.

5. *Group counseling* sessions facilitate the ability of the client to observe and model the communication of emotions and needs in an open, honest, and direct manner. Groups reduce isolation, provide support, hope, and positive role models, identify with other addicts in the recovery process. Because of their many benefits and cost-effectiveness, most treatment takes place in group settings (Vanicelli 1992).

6. *Family counseling* stops the "enabling" of addiction by kin—the "help" that hurts—and allow the emergence of honest communication patterns within the family system. It also educates the family on the dynamics of addiction (Kaufman 1985).

7. Client education focuses on the nature of addiction, the effects of drugs, and triggers for relapse.

8. Toward the end of the client's stay in this setting, careful planning takes place for the transition to the next stage of treatment, or for the termination of treatment. Vocational and educational goals are stressed for reentry into society. Ongoing participation in recovery support is crucial.

Current Trends in Providing Treatment Services

In the past decade, addictions treatment has moved beyond simplistic implementation of self-help models. It has recognized the unique needs of a variety of populations and subsequently incorporated the concept of "cultural competency." One of the major contributions to cultural competency and ethnic sensitivity has come from the family therapy field (McGoldrick, Pearce, and Giordano 1982). The special needs of addicted women, pregnant women and women with children, and elderly addicts have been addressed with special focus programs.

Certifying Qualified Counselors The separate treatment models that evolved for drug addicts and alcoholics led to separate governmental and certification entities. Over the past decade, most of these bodies have been merged into single chemical dependency or addictions authorities and certification boards, although New York State accomplished this step only in 1995–1996. Most recently, the recognition of the terrible health costs of tobacco consumption has led to the addition of nicotine to the realm of responsibility of addictions authorities and to the knowledge areas required of counselors.

While qualifications for becoming addictions counselors once included merely being a recovering addict and having the enthusiasm, energy, and empathy to work with other addicts, the credentialing requirements became more rigorous in the 1970s. From the mid-1970s on, a credentialing system evolved that demanded increased levels of competency. Today, most states operate certification boards, which are linked in a national consortium, and certification is also provided by the national addiction counselors' association (see Appendix C, page 499).

Certification requirements include educational preparation, passing a written exam, and service experience. The certification consortium requires an oral and written case presentation as well. Although minor variations in the credentialing systems exist, counselors must be able to perform the following tasks:

▲ Screen candidates for eligibility and appropriateness

▲ Follow intake procedures

▲ Handle patient orientation and education

▲ Practice case management

▲ Assess patient strengths and weaknesses

▲ Develop and implement a treatment plan in collaboration with the client

▲ Handle cases involving addiction-specific individual, group, and family counseling

▲ Understand the pharmacology of addictive substances and dynamics of addiction

▲ Maintain ethical practices and patient confidentiality

▲ Understand the role of the addictions counselor and how it differs from that of other professional roles

One of the most important advances in the field has been the development of a subfield for addicts with concurrent psychiatric disabilities (mentally ill chemical abusers, also referred to as MICA) (Kelly and Romando 1993). This field is particularly complex as many symptoms of mental illness share similarities with chemically induced organic brain syndromes (early in the days of crack cocaine, many patients were over-diagnosed with "paranoid schizophrenia" in public hospitals in New York City—especially by newly arrived, out-of-town physicians).

Patient Placement Criteria Today Treatment professionals use **patient placement criteria** to match the severity of the addiction to the level of care needed, ranging from medical inpatient care, nonmedical inpatient care, and intensive outpatient care, to outpatient care (CSAT 1993; 5–8). Unfortunately, the new managed care

> **patient placement criteria**
>
> a system that allows the referring professional to match the assessed level of addictive severity with an appropriate intensity and level of care, ranging from an outpatient clinic to a medical center

guidelines established by many health insurance carriers simply do not allow for treatment beyond outpatient care or brief inpatient detoxification. Moreover, matching the client's profile to a treatment modality is more likely to achieve lasting success. A person with severe attention-deficit hyperactivity disorder, for example, tends to be disorganized and forgetful, and is unsuited for the strict behavioral expectations of therapeutic community. Likewise, an emotionally fragile individual is unsuited to confrontational groups.

Special Focus Programs Programs have been created that are similar to AA and NA, but without the spiritual emphasis, which some potential members find difficult to accept. These programs include *Rational Recovery,* which evolved from Albert Ellis's Rational-Emotive Therapy (Ellis et al. 1988), and similar programs named *Smart Recovery* and *Secular Organizations for Sobriety* (Christopher, 1989). One of the principles behind these programs is early intervention. In contrast to past practices, where the early addict was scooped up off the street (fitting the ideology of the addict "hitting rock bottom"), treatment begins at an earlier phase of addiction.

There has also been a recent shift to mandated or involuntary involvement with treatment. Two components of this practice include the following:

▲ Originally called "industrial alcoholism programs," have existed for some time. Their goal is to identify and refer addicted employees to treatment programs. This model has been adapted for use in school settings (student assistance programs, or SAPs) and in organizational settings such as labor unions or consortia of unions (member assistance programs). Some states now fund SAPs and certify SAP professionals.

▲ The therapeutic community has always counted many court-mandated clients, but the trend accelerated tremendously in the 1990s, with demonstration programs established in Colorado, Texas, and New Mexico for collaborative planning of criminal justice and addictions treatment systems. Many treatment programs have retooled to accommodate convicts paroled or serving out their sentences, and treatment programs have been instituted in prisons (see "Fighting the Drug War" below).

Maintenance Programs Maintenance programs (which offer support to those addicted to morphine, methadone, and heroin) are based on the principle that, if past treatment programs have not been successful, "incurable" addicts should be able to register and receive drugs, such as narcotics, under supervision. Proponents of these programs contend that many addicts are forced into a life of crime to support their habits but would become law-abiding and useful citizens if they received narcotics (usually a less euphoric type, such as methadone) legally. Moreover, it's argued, the illicit narcotics trade would be eliminated due to the loss of these customers. Opponents of maintenance programs say that sufficient treatment programs exist to cure many addicts and that providing addicts with substitute narcotics does not solve the basic problem causing drug dependence.

The concept of maintenance on a **noneuphoric opiate** is now widely accepted in the United States as one way to help treat drug abusers.

Methadone Maintenance. Vincent Dole and Marie Nyswander were the first doctors to use the synthetic narcotic methadone in a rehabilitation program with heroin addicts in the mid-1960s.

Methadone maintenance (MMT) involves replacing street heroin with methadone, a synthetic opiate that allows clients to stabilize themselves physiologically so that they can explore alternative ways of functioning. This type of treatment model is usually provided on an outpatient basis.

> **noneuphoric opiate**
>
> a drug used in maintenance programs that satisfies the craving but does not produce the euphoric effect, such as methadone

There are now 115,000 addicts on methadone maintenance in the United States. Forty thou-

---

FIGHTING THE DRUG WAR

A National Institute on Drug Abuse (NIDA)-funded treatment research program allows offenders imprisoned in the Delaware correctional system to participate in a two-year rehabilitation program. During phase one, the offenders live for 12 months in a therapeutic community in prison, known as KEY, which is separated from the general prison population. During phase two, offenders stay in a therapeutic community for six months, called the CREST outreach center, which is a work-release facility. In the final six-month phase, offenders participate in counseling and group therapy while they are on parole or other supervised release. According to Dr. Peter Delaney of NIDA's Services Research Branch, this program differs from other therapeutic prison treatment in including a work-release component.

The KEY-CREST program has proved effective at reducing both drug use and recidivism in participant offenders. Eighteen months after release from prison, the KEY-CREST participants were 76% drug-free and 71% arrest-free, compared with 19% drug-free and 30% arrest-free for offenders from the general population.

This research demonstrates the importance of a therapeutic prison environment coupled with a community-based work program in preventing additional drug abuse and criminal activity in criminal offenders. ■

Source: Mathias, R. "Correctional Treatment Helps Offenders Stay Drug and Arrest Free." *NIDA Notes* (July/August 1995) http://www.nida.nihgov/NIDA_NOTES

sand of them are in New York state, and about half that many are in California. Methadone is widely employed throughout the world, and is the most effective known treatment for heroin addiction. (Nadelman 1996)

Methadone maintenance is used to reduce illegal heroin use. Although it can be used to detoxify heroin addicts, most such individuals return to heroin. Methadone is most effective when used as an adjunct to reduce or, in a minority of cases, eliminate heroin use by stabilizing addicts as long as it takes to reassemble their lives and avoid returning to previous patterns of drug use. Further, even after 20 to 30 years of methadone use, research shows that " . . . almost no negative health consequences are experienced" (Nadelman 1996).

How successful is methadone treatment? A recent California study found that one dollar spent on treatment saves taxpayers seven dollars. The savings occur as a result of reductions in crime and the need for medical care (Swan 1995). Another study showed that "over a six-month period, the costs to society for an untreated heroin abuser costs $21,500, $20,000 for an imprisoned drug abuser, and $1,750 for someone undergoing methadone maintenance treatment" (Swan 1994).

Once stabilized on methadone, the addict faces a crucial period of adjustment. After being devoted to maintaining a heroin habit 24 hours a day, 365 days a year, the addict must be transformed into a self-supporting, socially acceptable person. Methadone maintenance establishes the potential for such a change, but it is the person's motivation and capabilities that determine the success of the rehabilitation effort. A range of medical, psychiatric, social, and vocational services are usually available during this phase of treatment.

One supervisor of a methadone clinic associated with a Brooklyn, New York, hospital explains the process it employs:

> First of all, we test for alcohol, benzodiazepines [Valium like substances] and other drugs. Clients with positive tox [who text positive for drugs] are administratively discharged. They come in at 6:30 for their dose, and then the vast majority go off to work! Methadone, job counseling, and GED classes allow them to get their lives together. Our goal is to taper them off to zero.

While many criticisms have been levied against the use of methadone, other research findings contradict this skepticism. Recent research findings show that, since the 1980s, 65% to 85% of methadone-treated patients not only remain in treatment for a year or more, but they also dramatically cease or strongly curtail their criminal behavior and have strong records of gainful employment while receiving the drug (Swan 1994). In addition, methadone is reported to reduce the risk of AIDS infection. This benefit alone is believed to lower the costs to society, especially those associated with providing health care to AIDS patients.

The new long-acting methadone analog, levoalpha-acetylmethadol (LAAM), need only be taken three times a week and is being used experimentally in some programs. Initially, addicts participate in intensive daily counseling. Later in the program, they come in for the maintenance drug and follow-up treatment less frequently. Addicts may be treated with daily methadone first to increase the probability that they will at least attend counseling sessions and then be switched to LAAM when they reach an appropriate point in the program. Currently, LAAM is an investigational drug and has not been approved by the U.S. Food and Drug Administration (FDA) for general clinical use.

Opiate Antagonists An **antagonist** is a compound that suppresses the actions of a drug. Narcotic antagonists have properties that make them important tools in the clinical treatment of narcotic drug dependence. For instance, they counteract the central nervous system depressant effects in opioid drug overdoses.

Opiate antagonists are occasionally used as adjuncts to inpatient treatment; they are more typically associated with the emergency treatment of opiate poisoning (overdose), however. Some physicians claim to perform instant detoxification with the use of an opiate antagonist during sedation.

> **antagonist**
> a drug that blocks another drug from producing its effects, often used in detoxification from opiates

Two opiate antagonists, naltrexone and cyclazocine, block heroin from having an effect on the heroin addict. Further, naloxone (Narcan) is often used as an antidote for opioid overdose (commonly known as narcotic poisoning). Narcotic antagonists are generally best suited for opioid-dependent patients who want to leave therapeutic communities and methadone-maintenance treatment programs.

Antagonists were developed as a by-product of research in analgesics. Scientists were interested in dissociating the dependence-producing properties and necessary pain-relieving properties of substances that could replace morphine. This research led to the development of nalorphine, the first specific opiate antagonist. Although its short duration of action and frequent unpleasant side effects limited its clinical usefulness, its properties stimulated further research on this class of drugs (Archer 1981; Palfai and Jankiewicz 1991).

As we will discuss in more detail later, clonidine (Catapres) is useful in treating opiate-dependent people during the difficult withdrawal stages (Ginzburg 1986). Studies thus far show the value of this drug for withdrawal from heroin, morphine, codeine, and methadone. Clonidine is not addictive and does not cause euphoria, but it does block cravings for drugs. It also makes the person feel better compared with the depression experienced by addicts using other methods of withdrawal.

Antabuse, which goes by the trade name Disulfiram, is a drug used for treating alcoholics. This drug is perceived as a deterrent drug—it makes people violently ill if alcohol is used. "Antabuse interferes with the normal metabolism of alcohol, resulting in serious physical reaction if even a small amount of alcohol is ingested" (McNeece and DiNitto 1994, 113). The greatest asset in using this drug is its ability to deter impulsive drinking (McNeece and DiNitto 1994).

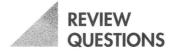

REVIEW QUESTIONS

1. How do modern drug treatment programs differ from those in use 15 years ago?

2. Have people received drug treatment the same way over the past 25 years? How do people actually get into treatment?

3. What treatment options were available to alcoholics in the 1950s?

4. Does drug abuse automatically lead to addiction? Justify your opinion.

5. What are the reasons why chemically dependent parents often have chemically dependent children?

6. Is nicotine really a drug, or is this just a position taken to scare people? Explain your response.

7. Describe the goals of rehabilitation centers for alcohol and drug abuse.

8. Do you agree with the disease model of addiction? Why or why not?

9. Why are adolescents and middle-aged people more at risk for chemical abuse and dependency?

10. Describe the rationale behind a confrontational approach to addiction in the therapeutic community model.

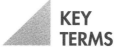

KEY TERMS

psychic dependence
moral model
disease model
characterological or personality predisposition
    model
personality disorders
psychoanalysis
"double wall" of encapsulation
addictionologists
open meetings
closed meetings
Minnesota model
therapeutic community (TC)

EXERCISES FOR THE WEB

Exercise 1: CAAS

Through research, publications, education, and training, the Center's mission is to promote the identification, prevention and effective treatment of alcohol and other drug use problems in our society. The Center, through its affiliation with the Brown Medical School, occupies a unique position within the university. Over sixty faculty and professional staff from eleven university departments and eight affiliated hospitals cooperate as clinicians, scholars, teachers, administrators, and researchers to comprise a single working unit.

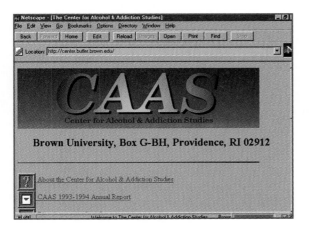

Exercise 2: American Society of Addiction Medicine

The American Society of Addiction Medicine is the nation's medical specialty society dedicated to educating physicians and improving the treatment of individuals suffering from alcoholism or other addictions.

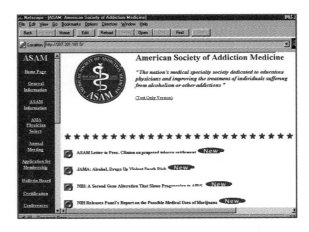

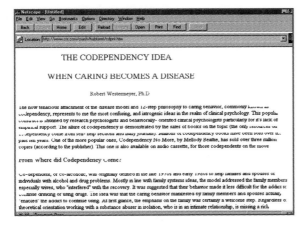

Exercise 3: Co-Dependency

Drug dependency affects more than just the person who is using the drug. Serious effects can be felt by family members, loved ones, or co-workers. A drug dependent can have such an impact on those around him that these "innocent bystanders" often become "victims" in their own right.

patient placement criteria
noneuphoric opiate
antagonist

SUMMARY

1 Chemical dependence has been considered a major social problem throughout U.S. history.

2 People define chemical addiction in many ways. The essential feature is a chronic adherence to drugs despite significant negative consequences.

3 The major models of addiction are the moral model, the disease model, and the characterological or personality predisposition model.

4 Transitional periods, such as adolescence and middle age, are associated with particular sets of risk factors.

5 Addiction is a gradual process in which abusers become caught up in vicious cycles that worsen their situation, cause pain, and increase their drug use. Addiction tends to progress, although this step is not inevitable.

6 Cultural definitions of drugs do not correspond to their chemistry; nicotine, for example, is as addictive as cocaine, but is considered more benign.

7 The earliest real alcoholism recovery effort was Alcoholics Anonymous (AA). Programs modeled on AA, known as Twelve Step fellowships, are a major route to recovery.

8 The most influential model in drug rehabilitation is the therapeutic community, which began in 1958 at Synanon. This addict-run, long-term residential setting features hard work, confrontational groups, and a layered status system.

9 Modern addictions treatment includes screening; intake; assessment; formulation of a treatment plan; individual, group, and family treatment; and vocational reentry.

10 Addiction counseling has now become a true profession, governed by national and state certification.

11 Outside of drug-free treatment such as therapeutic communities, the major approach to heroin and other opiate addiction has involved the provision of methadone, a synthetic opiate.

REFERENCES

Al-Anon *Al-Anon's Favorite Forum Editorials,* New York: An-Anon Family Group Headquarters, 1970

Alcoholics Anonymous World Services. *Alcoholics Anonymous: The Story of How Many Thousands of Men and Women Have Recovered from Alcoholism,* 3rd ed. New York: Alcoholics Anonymous, 1976.

American Psychiatric Association. *Diagnostic and Statistical Manual of Mental Disorders,* 4th ed. Washington, DC: American Psychiatric Association, 1994.

Archer, S. "Historical Perspective on the Chemistry and Development of Naltrexone." In *Narcotic Antagonists: Naltrexone Pharmaco-Chemistry and Sustained-Release Preparations,* edited by R. E. Willette and G. Barnett. NIDA Research Monograph 28. Washington, DC: National Institute on Drug Abuse, 1981.

Augustine Fellowship. *Sex and Love Addicts Anonymous. The Basic Text.* Boston, MA: Fellowship-Wide Services, 1986.

Bacon, M. K. "The Dependency-Conflict Hypothesis and the Frequency of Drunkenness. Further Evidence from a Cross-Cultural Study." *Quarterly Journal of Studies on Alcohol* 35 (1974): 863–76.

Bacon, M. K., H. Barry III, and I. L. Child. "A Cross-Cultural Study of Drinking II: Relations to Other Features of Culture." *Quarterly Journal of Studies on Alcohol,* Supplement 3 (1965a): 29–48.

Beattie, M. *Codependent No More.* San Francisco: Harper, 1987.

Christopher, J. *Unhooked: Staying Sober and Drug-Free.* Buffalo, NY: Prometheus Books, 1988.

Clinard, M. B., and R. F. Meier. *Sociology of Deviant Behavior,* 8th ed. Fort Worth, TX: Harcourt, Brace, Jovanovich, 1992.

Collins, G. B. "Contemporary Issues in the Treatment of Alcohol Dependence." *Psychiatric Clinics of North America* 16 (March 1993).

Corey, M. S., and G. Corey. *Becoming a Helper.* Pacific Grove, CA: Brooks-Cole, 1993.

CSAT *Guidelines for the Treatment of Alcohol and Other Drug-Abusing Adolescents.* Treatment Improvement Protocol (TIP) Series 4, Rockville, MD, U.S. HHS, PHS, SAMHSA, Center for Substance Abuse Treatment.

Davies, D. L. "The Concept of Alcoholism." In *The Medical Annual,* edited by R. Bodley-Scott and Milnes-Walker 29–38. Bristol: Wright, 1969.

Drug Strategies. "Keeping Score: What Are We Getting for Our Federal Drug Control Dollars, 1996," edited by Harvey Milkman and Howard Shaffer, Washington, DC: Drug Strategies, 1996. Available 080/ res/colleges/bsos/depts/cesar/drugs/ks 1996.

Eddy, N. B., H. Halbach, H. Isbell, and M. H. Seevers. "Drug Dependence: Its Significance and Characteristics." *Bulletin of the World Health Organization* 32 (May 1965): 721–33.

Ellis, A., J. F. McInerney, R. DiGiuseppe, and R. J. Yeager. *Rational-Emotive Therapy with Alcoholics and Substance Abusers.* Boston: Allyn and Bacon, 1988.

Evans, K. *Dual Diagnosis—Counseling the Mentally Ill Substance Abuser.* New York: Guilford Press, 1990.

Field, P. B. "A New Cross-Cultural Study of Drunkenness." *Society, Culture, and Drinking Patterns.* New York: John Wiley and Sons, 1962.

Frosch, W. A. "An Analytic Overview of the Addictions." In *The Addictions: Multidisciplinary Perspectives and Treatments,* edited by H. Milkman and H. Shaffer. Lexington, MA: Lexington Books/D. C. Heath, 1985.

Ginzburg, H. M. *Naltrexone: Its Chemical Utility.* Rockville, MD: National Institute on Drug Abuse, 1986.

Gordon, A. J. "The Cultural Context of Drinking and Indigenous Therapy for Alcohol Problems in Three Migrant Hispanic Cultures." *Journal of Studies on Alcohol* Supplement 9 (1981): 217–40.

Health Communications. *Co-dependency, an Emerging Hollywood Issue.* Hollywood, FL: Health Communications, 1984.

Holder, H., R. Longabaugh, W. R. Miller, and A. V. Rubonis. "The Cost Effectiveness of Treatment for Alcoholism: A First Approximation." *Journal of Studies on Alcohol* 52 (1991): 517–40.

Indiardi, J. A., R. Horowitz, and A. E. Pottieger. *Street Kids, Street Drugs, Street Crime.* Wadsworth, 1993.

Ivey, A. E. *Intentional Interviewing and Counseling,* 3rd ed. Pacific Grove, CA: Brooks-Cole, 1994.

Jellinek, E. M. "Phases of Alcohol Addiction." *Quarterly Journal of Studies on Alcohol.* 13 (1952): 673–84.

Jellinek, E. M. *The Disease Concept of Alcoholism.* Highland Park, NJ: Hillhouse Press, 1960.

Johnson, V. *Intervention.* Minneapolis, MN: Johnson Institute, 1984.

Kaufman, E. *Substance Abuse and Family Therapy.* New York: Grune and Stratton, 1985.

Kelly, K., and P. Ramundo. *You Mean I'm Not Lazy, Stupid, or Crazy?!* New York: Scribner, 1993.

Madsen, W. "Alcoholics Anonymous as a Crisis Cult." *Alcohol Health and Research World* (Spring 1974): 32–38.

Marshall, M. "Conclusions." In *Beliefs, Behavior, and Alcoholic Beverages—A Cross-Cultural Survey,* edited by M. Marshall, 451–7. Ann Arbor, MI: University of Michigan Press, 1979.

McGoldrick, M., J. K. Pearce, and J. Giordano. *Ethnicity and Family Therapy.* New York: Guilford Press, 1982.

McNeece, C. A., and D. M. DiNitto. *Chemical Dependency: A Systems Approach.* Englewood Cliffs, NJ: Prentice-Hall, 1994.

Myers, P. L. "Cult and Cult-Like Pathways out of Adolescent Addiction." In *Special Problems in Counseling the Chemically Dependent Adolescent,* edited by E. E. Sweet, 115–35. New York: Haworth Press, 1991.

Myers, P. L. "Sources and Configurations of Institutional Denial." *Employee Assistance Quarterly* 5 (B) (1990): 43–54.

Nadelmann, E. A. *Methadone Maintenance Treatment.* New York: The Lindesmith Center, 1996.

Palfai, T., and H. Jankiewicz. *Drugs and Human Behavior.* Dubuque, IA: Brown, 1991.

Rudy, D. "Perspectives on Alcoholism: Lessons from Alcoholics and Alcohologists." In *Drug Use in America: Social, Cultural, and Political Perspectives,* edited by P. J. Venturelli, 23–29. Boston: Jones and Bartlett, 1994.

Schuckit, M. A., T. L. Smith, R. Anthenelli, and M. Irwin. "Clinical Course of Alcoholism in 636 Male Inpatients." *American Journal of Psychiatry* 150 (1993): 786–92.

Smith, D. E., H. Milkman, and S. Sunderwirth. "Addictive Disease: Concept and Controversy." In *The Addictions: Multidisciplinary Perspectives and Treatments,* edited by H. Milkman and H. J. Shaffer, Lexington, MA: Lexington Books/D. C. Heath, 1985.

Swan, N. "Research Demonstrates Long-Term Benefits of Methadone Treatment." *NIDA Notes* 9 (November/December 1994): http://www.nida.nihgov/NIDA_NOTES.

Swan, N. "California Study Finds $1 Spent on Treatment Saves Taxpayers $7." *NIDA Notes* 10 (March/April 1995): http://www.nida.nihgov/NIDA_NOTES.

Tarter, R. E., A. Alterman, and K. L. Edwards. "Alcoholic Denial: A Biopsychosociological Interpretation." *Journal of Studies on Alcohol* 45 (1983): 214–18.

Valiant, G. *The Natural History of Alcoholism.* Cambridge, MA: Harvard University Press, 1983.

Vannicelli, M. *Removing the Roadblocks—Group Psychotherapy with Substance Abusers and Their Families.* New York: Guilford Press, 1992.

Waldorf, D. "Natural Recovery from Opiate Addiction: Some Social-Psychological Processes of Untreated Recovery." *Journal of Drug Issues* 13 (1983): 237–80.

5 How and Why Drugs Work

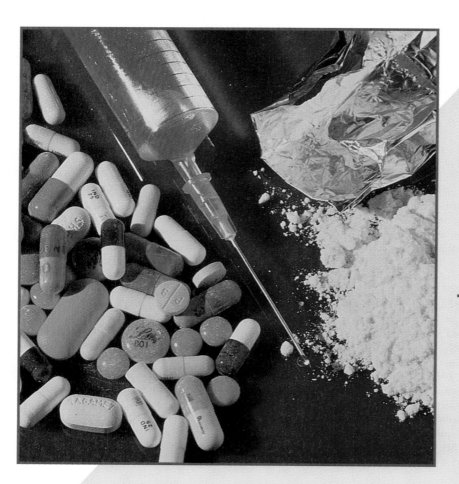

On completing this chapter
you will be able to:

- Twenty percent of the total hospital costs in the United States are due to medical care for health damage caused by substances of abuse.
- Side effects and reactions to prescription drugs send as many as 2 million people to the hospital and kill 140,000 people in the United States each year.
- The same dose of a drug does not have the same effect on everyone.
- In excessive doses, almost any drug or substance can be toxic.
- Sixty-five percent of the strokes among young Americans are related to cigarette, cocaine, or amphetamine use.
- Ninety percent of people who abuse cocaine also abuse alcohol.
- Use of some drugs can dramatically enhance the effects of others.
- Smoking cocaine, methamphetamine, and heroin is as addicting and dangerous as administering these drugs intravenously.
- Many drugs are unable to pass from the blood into the brain.
- Most drugs cross the placental barrier from the mother to the fetus.
- Physical dependence is characterized by withdrawal effects when use of the drug is stopped.
- Tolerance to one drug can often cause tolerance to other similar drugs; this effect is called *cross-tolerance*.
- Placebos can have significant effects in relieving symptoms such as pain.
- The body produces natural narcotic substances called endorphins.
- Hereditary factors may predispose some individuals to becoming psychologically dependent on drugs with abuse potential.

Learning Objectives

- Describe some of the common unintended drug effects.
- Explain why the same dose of a drug may affect individuals differently.
- Explain the difference between potency and toxicity.
- Describe the concept of a drug's margin of safety.
- Identify and give examples of additive, antagonistic, and potentiation (synergistic) drug interactions.
- Identify the pharmacokinetic factors that can influence the effects caused by drugs.
- Cite the physiological and pathological factors that influence drug effects.
- Explain the significance of the blood–brain barrier to psychoactive drugs.
- Define *threshold dose, plateau effect*, and *cumulative effect*.
- Discuss the role of the liver in drug metabolism and the consequences of this process.
- Define *biotransformation*.
- Describe the relationships among tolerance, withdrawal, rebound, physical dependence, and psychological dependence.
- Discuss the significance of placebos in responding to drugs.
- Describe drug craving and how it affects drug abuse.

111

A common belief is that drugs are the solution for life's physical and emotional problems. Although medications are essential to treatment for many diseases, excessive reliance on drugs causes unrealistic expectations that may lead to dangerous, even fatal, consequences. For example, drug addiction and dependence often follow from such unrealistic expectations. Obviously, not every person who uses drugs inappropriately becomes a drug addict, nor are patients who use drugs as prescribed by the doctor immune from being physically and mentally dependent on their medications. In fact, because of individual variability, it is difficult to predict accurately which drug users will or will not have drug problems such as addiction and dependence.

In this chapter we consider the factors that account for the variability of drug responses—that is, what determines how the body responds to drugs and why some drugs work while others do not. First we review the general effects of drugs, both intended and unintended. The correlation between the dose and response of a drug is addressed next, followed by a discussion of how drugs interact with one another. The section on *pharmacokinetic* factors considers how drugs are introduced into, distributed throughout, and eliminated from the body, along with physiological and pathological variables that modify how drugs affect the body. The final sections in the chapter consider concepts important to drug abuse, such as tolerance, physical versus psychological dependence, and addiction.

◢ The Intended and Unintended Effects of Drugs

When physicians prescribe drugs, their objective is usually to cure or relieve symptoms of a disease. Frequently, however, drugs cause unintended effects that neither the physician nor the patient expected.

The intended responses produced by a drug are called **main effects,** whereas those that are unintended

> **main effects**
> intended drug responses

are called **side effects.** The distinction between main and side effects depends on the therapeutic objective. A response that is considered

> **side effects**
> unintended drug responses

unnecessary or undesirable in one situation may, in fact, be the intended effect in another. For example, antihistamines found in many over-the-counter (OTC) drugs have an intended main effect of relieving allergy symptoms, but they often cause annoying drowsiness as a side effect; in fact, their labels include warnings that they should not be used when driving a car. These antihistamines are also included in OTC sleep aids, where their sedating action is the desired main effect because it encourages sleep in people suffering from insomnia.

Side effects can influence many body functions and occur in any organ (see Figure 5.1). Side effects of prescription drugs are estimated to send 2 million people to the hospital and kill 140,000 persons in the United States each year (Combined News Services 1995). The following are basic kinds of side effects that can result from drug use:

Nausea or vomiting. Almost any drug can cause an upset stomach; in fact, this is a common complaint with narcotics.

Changes in mental alertness. Some medications can cause sedation and drowsiness (for example, antihistamines in OTC allergy medications) or nervousness and insomnia (for example, caffeine in OTC stay-awake products).

Dependence. This phenomenon compels people to continue using a drug because they want to achieve a desired effect or they fear unpleasant reaction, called **withdrawal,** that occurs when the drug is discontinued. Dependence has been associated with such apparently benign OTC drugs as nasal decongestant

> **withdrawal**
> unpleasant effects that occur when use of a drug is stopped

sprays and laxatives, as well as more potent drugs such as alcohol (see Chapters 8 and 9), narcotics (see Chapter 10), and stimulants (see Chapter 11).

Figure 5.1

Common side effects with drugs of abuse. Almost every organ or system in the body can be negatively affected by the substances of abuse.

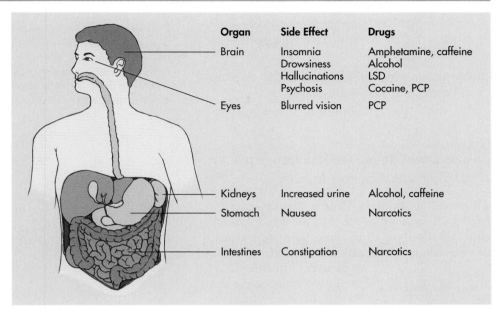

Organ	Side Effect	Drugs
Brain	Insomnia	Amphetamine, caffeine
	Drowsiness	Alcohol
	Hallucinations	LSD
	Psychosis	Cocaine, PCP
Eyes	Blurred vision	PCP
Kidneys	Increased urine	Alcohol, caffeine
Stomach	Nausea	Narcotics
Intestines	Constipation	Narcotics

Allergic reactions (hypersensitive reactions or sensitization). Allergic reactions occur when the body becomes sensitized to a drug and attempts to destroy and dispose of it. During an allergic reaction, the drug can cause tissue reactions such as rashes, hives, and itching or cause very serious conditions such as shock and breathing difficulty.

Changes in cardiovascular activity. Many drugs that are available OTC or by prescription, or are used illicitly, can alter the activity of the heart and change the state of the blood vessels. The results of these side effects include changes in blood pressure, fainting, heart attacks, and strokes.

This partial list of side effects demonstrates the types of risk involved whenever any drug (prescription, nonprescription, or illicit) is used. Consequently, before taking a drug, whether for therapeutic or recreational use, you should understand its potential problems and determine whether the benefits justify the risks. For example, it is important to know that morphine is effective for relieving severe pain, but it also depresses breathing and retards intestinal activity, causing constipation. Likewise, amphetamines can be used to suppress appetite, but they also increase blood pressure and stimulate the heart. Cocaine is a good local anesthetic but can be extremely addicting and can cause tremors or even seizures. The greater the danger associated with using a drug, the less likely the benefits will warrant its use.

Adverse effects of drugs of abuse are particularly troublesome in the United States. Studies have suggested that 20% of the total hospital costs in this country are related to medical care for the health damage caused by alcohol, tobacco, and other drugs of abuse. Other statistics illustrating the major negative health impact of adverse unintended effects caused by drugs of abuse include the following ("Trends, Policy and Research" 1993):

▲ Patients who abuse alcohol, tobacco, and other drugs are hospitalized twice as long as other patients with the same diagnosis.

▲ Seventy-five percent of the chronic pancreatitis (damaged pancreas) cases in the United States are due to alcohol abuse.

▲ Sixty-five percent of the strokes among young Americans are related to cigarette, cocaine, or amphetamine use.

▲ Youth under 15 years of age are hospitalized three to four times longer, regardless of their illness, if they have an alcohol, tobacco, or other drug problem.

▲ More than 50% of the pediatric AIDS cases are the result of injecting drugs of abuse.

◢ The Dose–Response Relationship of Therapeutics and Toxicity

All effects—both desired and unwanted—are related to the amount of drug administered. A small concentration of drug may have one effect, whereas a larger dose may create a greater effect or a different effect entirely. Because some correlation exists between the response to a drug and the quantity of the drug dose, it is possible to calculate **dose–response** curves (see Figure 5.2).

dose–response

the correlation between the amount of a drug given and its effects

Once a dose–response curve for a drug has been determined in an individual, it can be used to predict how that person will respond to different doses of the drug. For example, the dose–response curve for user B in Figure 5.2 shows that 600 mg of aspirin will only relieve 50% of his or her headache. It is important to understand that not everyone responds the same to a given dose of drug. Thus, in Figure 5.2, while 600 mg of aspirin gives 50% relief from a headache for user B, it relieves 100% of the headache for user A and none of the headache for user C. This variability in response makes it difficult to predict the precise drug effect from a given dose.

Many factors can contribute to the variability in drug responses. One of the most important is **tolerance,** or reduced response over time to the same dosage, an effect that is examined carefully in a later section of this chapter. Other factors include the size of the individual, stomach contents if the drug is

tolerance

changes in the body that decrease response to a drug even though the dose remains the same

Figure 5.2

Dose–response curve for relieving a headache with aspirin in three users. User A is the most sensitive and has 100% headache relief at a dose of 600 mg. User B is the next sensitive and gets 50% headache relief with a 600-mg dose. The least sensitive is user C: with a 600-mg dose user, C has no relief from a headache.

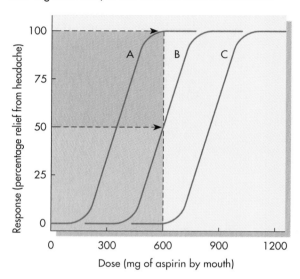

taken by mouth, different levels of enzymatic activity in the liver (which changes the drug via metabolic action), acidity of the urine (which affects rate of drug elimination), the time of day, and the state of a person's health. Such multiple interacting factors make it difficult to calculate accurately the final drug effect for any given individual.

Margin of Safety

An important concept for developing new drugs for therapy, as well as for assessing the probability of serious side effects for drugs of abuse, is called the **margin of safety.** The margin of safety is determined by the difference between the doses necessary to cause the intended (therapeutic or recreational) effects and

margin of safety

the range in dose between the amount of drug necessary to cause a therapeutic effect and that needed to create a toxic effect

toxic unintended effects. The larger the margin of safety, the less likely that serious adverse side effects will occur when using the drug to treat medical problems or even when abusing it. Drugs with relatively narrow margins of safety, such as phencyclidine (PCP) or cocaine, have a very high rate of serious reactions in populations who abuse these substances.

There is no such thing as the perfect drug that goes right to the target, has no toxicity, produces no side effects, and can be removed or neutralized when not needed. Unfortunately, most effective drugs are potentially dangerous if the doses are high enough. Pharmacologists refer to a perfect drug as a "magic bullet"; so far, no "magic bullets" have been developed. Even relatively safe drugs available over the counter can cause problems for some prospective users. Not surprisingly, all drugs of abuse can cause very serious side effects, especially when self-administered by users unfamiliar with the potential toxicities of these substances. The possibility that adverse effects will occur should always be considered before using any drug.

Potency Versus Toxicity

Most of us know that some drugs of abuse are more dangerous than others. For example, it is common knowledge that abuse of the narcotic drug heroin is more likely to be lethal than abuse of another narcotic drug, codeine. One important feature that makes heroin more dangerous than codeine is its high potency. **Potency** is a way of expressing how much of a drug is necessary to cause an effect, whether it be desired or toxic. The smaller the dose required to achieve a drug action, the greater the drug potency.

potency
the amount of drug necessary to cause an effect

The concept of potency can also be used to describe a drug's ability to create a therapeutic effect. More-potent medications require lower doses to be effective. Knowledge of a drug's potency is essential if it is to be used properly and safely.

Toxicity is the capacity of a drug to upset or even destroy normal body functions. Toxic compounds are often called *poisons,* although almost any compound—including sugar, table salt, aspirin, and vitamin A—can be toxic at sufficiently high doses. If a foreign chemical is introduced into the body, it may disrupt the body's normal functions. In many instances, the body can compensate for this disruption, perhaps by metabolizing and rapidly eliminating the chemical, and little effect is noted. Sometimes, however, the delicate balance is altered and the person becomes sick or even dies. If the body's functional balance is already under stress from disease, the introduction of a drug may have a much more serious effect than its use in a healthy person who can adjust to its toxicity.

toxicity
the capacity of a drug to damage or cause adverse effects in the body

A drug with high potency often is toxic even at low doses, so the amount given must be carefully measured and the user closely monitored; if caution is not taken, serious damage to the body or death can occur (see "Here and Now," page 116). Very potent drugs that are abused, such as heroin, are particularly dangerous because they are often consumed by unsuspecting users who are ignorant of the drug's extreme toxicity. Potency depends on many factors, such as absorption of the drug, its distribution in the body, individual metabolism, the form of excretion, the rate of elimination, and its activity at the site of action.

◢ Drug Interaction

A drug's effects can be dramatically altered when other drugs are also present in the body: this effect is known as **drug interaction** (Klaasen 1995). A typical example of multiple drug use occurs when you treat your common cold. Because of your many cold-related symptoms, you may consume an assortment of pain relievers, antihistamines, decongestants, and anticough medications all at the same time.

drug interaction
the presence of a drug alters the action of another drug

Multiple drug use can create a serious medical problem because many drugs

Fatal Consequences of Potent Synthetic Narcotics

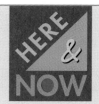

The issues of potency and toxicity are particularly important when dealing with new drugs of abuse that are being created in clandestine laboratories and then sold on the "street." Some of these new pharmacological creations are referred to as *"designer" drugs* and are unexpectedly potent. For example, derivatives of the commonly used narcotic pain reliever fentanyl (see Chapter 11) have been reported to be many times more potent than heroin. One such drug, alpha methylfentanyl, has

been sold on the "street" since 1982 as an illicit synthetic heroin. This drug actually has a potency 3000 to 5000 times greater than that of heroin, and if mistakenly taken as heroin by a narcotic addict, a lethal dose can easily be administered (Henderson 1988). Such mistakes have resulted in scores of fatal narcotic overdoses in the United States.

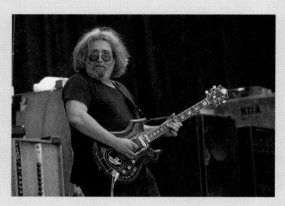

Jerry Garcia, the lead guitarist in the band The Grateful Dead, died in 1995 in a drug treatment center after a long history of abusing potent narcotics. ▶

---

influence the actions of other drugs (Brenner 1994). Even physicians may be baffled by unusual effects when multiple drugs are consumed. Frequently, drug interactions are misdiagnosed as symptoms of a disease. Such errors in diagnosis can lead to inappropriate treatment and serious health consequences. Complications can arise that are dangerous, even fatal. The interacting substance may be another drug, or it may consist of some substance in the diet or in the environment, such as a pesticide. Drug interaction is an area where much more research and public education are greatly needed.

Depending on the effect on the body, drug interaction may be categorized into three types: *additive, antagonistic (inhibitory),* and *potentiative (synergistic).*

Additive Effects

Additive interactions are the combined effects of drugs taken concurrently. An example of an additive interaction results from using aspirin and

additive interactions
effects created when drugs are similar and sum together

acetaminophen (the active ingredient in Tylenol) at the same time. The pain relief provided is equal to the sum of the two analgesics, which could be achieved by a comparable dose of either drug alone. Thus, if a 300-mg tablet of Bayer aspirin were taken with a 300-mg tablet of Tylenol, the relief would be the same as if two tablets of either Bayer or Tylenol were taken instead.

Antagonistic (Inhibitory) Effects

Antagonistic interactions occur when one drug cancels or blocks the effect of another. For example, if you take antihistamines to reduce nasal congestion, you may be able to antagonize some of the drowsi-

antagonistic interactions
effects created when drugs cancel one another

ness often caused by these drugs by using a central nervous system (CNS) stimulant such as caffeine.

It is likely that drug abusers who use two drugs at the same time often are trying to antagonize the unpleasant side effects of the first drug by administering the second. It has been reported that as many as 90% of those currently abusing cocaine also use alcohol (Grant and Harford 1990). The combined use of these two drugs may be a major factor in drug-related problems and death in emergency rooms (Karch 1996). Nevertheless, it appears that some users may coadminister these drugs in order to antagonize the disruptive effects of alcohol with the stimulant action of the cocaine (O'Brien 1995).

Potentiative (Synergistic) Effects

The third type of drug interaction is known as *potentiation,* or **synergism.** Synergism occurs when the effect of a drug is enhanced by the presence of another drug or substance. A common example is the combination of alcohol and Valium (see Table 5.1). It has been estimated that as many as 3000 people die each year from mixing alcohol with CNS depressants such as Valium. Alcohol, like Valium, is a CNS depressant. When depressants are taken together, CNS functions become impaired and the person becomes groggy. A person in this state may forget that he or she has taken the pills and repeat the dose. The combination of these two depressants (or other depressants, such as antihistamines) can depress the CNS to the point where vital functions such as breathing and heartbeat are severely impaired.

Although the mechanisms of interaction among CNS depressants are not entirely clear, these drugs likely enhance one another's direct effects on inhibitory chemical messengers in the brain (see Chapter 6). In addition, interference by alcohol with liver-metabolizing enzymes also contributes to the synergism that arises with the combination of

synergism
the ability of one drug to enhance the effect of another; potentiation

---

Table 5.1 **Common Interactions with Substances of Abuse**

Drug	Combined with	Interaction
Sedatives Valium, Halcion	Alcohol, barbiturates	Increase sedation
Stimulants Amphetamines, cocaine	Insulin Antidepressants	Decrease insulin effect Cause hypertension
Narcotics Heroin, morphine	Barbiturates, Valium Anticoagulant Antidepressants Amphetamines	Increase sedation Increase bleeding Cause sedation Increase euphoria
Tobacco Nicotine	Blood-pressure medication Amphetamines, cocaine	Elevate blood pressure Increase cardiovascular effects
Alcohol	Cocaine	Produces cocaethylene, which enhances euphoria and toxicity

alcohol and some depressants, such as barbiturates (Hobbs, Rall, and Verdoorn 1995).

Dealing with Drug Interactions

Although many drug effects and interactions are not very well understood, it is important to be aware of them. Increasing amounts of evidence indicate that many of the drugs and substance we deliberately consume will interact and produce unexpected and sometimes dangerous effects (see Table 5.1). It is alarming to know that many of the foods we eat and some chemical pollutants also interfere with and modify drug actions. Pesticides, traces of hormones in meat and poultry, traces of metals in fish, nitrites and nitrates from fertilizers, and a wide range of chemicals—some of which are used as food additives—have been shown, under certain conditions, to interact with some drugs.

As the medical community has become aware of the frequent complications arising from multiple drug use, efforts have been made to reduce the incidence as well as the severity of the problem. It is essential that the public be educated about interactions most likely to occur with drugs that are prescribed, self-administered legitimately (for example, OTC drugs), or taken recreationally (for example, drugs of abuse). People need to be aware that OTC drugs are as likely to cause interaction problems as prescription drugs. For example, use of an OTC decongestant (which contains mild CNS stimulants) with potent CNS stimulants, such as cocaine and amphetamines, can cause fatal interactions affecting the heart and brain. If any question arises concerning the possibility of drug interaction, individuals should talk to their physicians, pharmacists, or other health care providers.

Most drug abusers are multiple drug (*polydrug*) users with little concern for the dangerous interactions that could occur. It is common, for example, for drug abusers to combine multiple CNS depressants to enhance their effects or a depressant with a stimulant to titrate a CNS effect (to determine the smallest amount that can be taken to achieve the desired "high") or to experiment with a combination of stimulants, depressants, and hallucinogens just to see what happens.

The effects of such haphazard drug mixing are impossible to predict, difficult to treat in emergency situations, and all too frequently fatal.

Pharmacokinetic Factors That Influence Drug Effects

Although it is difficult to predict precisely how any single individual will be affected by drug use, the following major factors represent different aspects of the body's response that should be considered when attempting to anticipate a drug's effects.

1. How does the drug enter the body? (administration)

2. How does the drug move from the site of administration into the body's system? (absorption)

3. How does the drug move to various areas in the body? (distribution)

4. How and where does the drug produce its effects? (activation)

5. How is the drug inactivated, metabolized, and/or excreted from the body? (biotransformation and elimination)

These issues relate to the **pharmacokinetics** of a drug and are important considerations when predicting the body's response.

> **pharmacokinetics**
> the study of factors that influence the distribution and concentration of drugs in the body

Forms and Methods of Taking Drugs

Drugs come in many forms. Whether a drug is formulated as a solution, powder, capsule, or pill, it may influence the rate of passage into the bloodstream from the site of administration and consequently its efficacy.

The means of introducing the drug into the body will also affect how quickly the drug enters the bloodstream and is distributed to the site of action, as well as how much will ultimately reach its target and exert an effect (Mathias 1994). The principal forms of drug administration include *oral ingestion, inhalation, injection,* and *topical application.*

Oral Ingestion One of the most common and convenient ways of taking a drug is orally. This type of administration usually introduces the drug into the body by way of the stomach or intestines.

Following oral administration, it is difficult to control the amount of drug that reaches the site of action, for three reasons:

1. The drug must enter the bloodstream after passing through the wall of the stomach or intestines without being destroyed or changed to an inactive form. From the blood, the drug must diffuse to the target area and remain there in sufficient concentration to have an effect.

2. Materials in the gut, such as food, may interfere with the passage of some drugs through the gut lining and thus prevent drug action. For example, food in your stomach will diminish the effects of alcohol because it interferes with its absorption.

3. The liver might metabolize orally ingested drugs too rapidly, before they are able to exert an effect. The liver is the major detoxifying organ in the body, which means it removes chemicals and toxins from the blood and usually changes them into an inactive form that is easy for the body to excrete. This function is essential to survival, but it creates a problem for the pharmacologist developing effective drugs. It is especially problematic in the case of oral administration because the substances absorbed from the digestive tract usually go to the liver before being distributed to other parts of the body and their site of action. For this reason, cocaine taken orally is not very effective.

Inhalation Some drugs are administered by inhalation into the lungs through the mouth or nose. The lungs include large beds of capillaries, so chemicals capable of crossing membranes can enter the blood as rapidly as intravenous injection and can be equally as dangerous (Mathias 1994). Ether, chloroform, and nitrous oxide anesthetics are examples of drugs that are therapeutically administered by inhalation. Nicotine from tobacco smoke, cocaine, methamphetamine, and heroin are drugs of abuse that can be inhaled as smoke. One serious problem with inhalation is the potential for irritation to the mucous membrane lining of the lungs; another is that the drug may have to be continually inhaled to maintain the concentration necessary for an effect.

Injection Some drugs are given by injection: **intravenously (IV), intramuscularly (IM),** or **subcutaneously (SC).** A major advantage of administering drugs by IV is the speed of action; the dosage is delivered rapidly and directly, and often less drug is needed because it reaches the site of action quickly. This method can be very dangerous if the dosage is calculated incorrectly. Additionally, impurities in injected materials may irritate the vein; this issue is a particular problem in the drug abusing population, where needle sharing frequently occurs. The injection itself injures the vein by leaving a tiny point of scar tissue where the vein is punctured. If repeated injections are administered into the same area, the elasticity of the vein is gradually reduced, causing the vessel to collapse.

> **intravenous (IV)**
> drug injection into a vein
> **intramuscular (IM)**
> drug injection into a muscle
> **subcutaneous (SC)**
> Drug injection beneath the skin

Intramuscular injection can damage the muscle directly if the drug preparation irritates the tissue or indirectly if the nerve controlling the muscle is damaged. If the nerve is destroyed, the muscle will degenerate (atrophy). A subcutaneous injection may kill the skin at the point of injection if a particularly irritating drug is administered. Another danger of drug injections occurs when contaminated needles are shared by drug users. This danger has become a serious problem in the spread of infectious diseases such as AIDS (acquired immune deficiency syndrome) and hepatitis.

Topical Application Those drugs that readily pass through surface tissue such as the skin, lining of the nose, and mouth can be applied topically, for systemic (whole-body) effects. Although most drugs do not appreciably diffuse across these tissue barriers into the circulation, there are notable exceptions. For example, a product to help quit smoking (Nicoderm) can be placed on the skin; the drug passes through the skin and enters the body to prevent tobacco craving and withdrawal.

Distribution of Drugs in the Body and Time–Response Relationships

Following administration (regardless of the mode), most drugs are distributed throughout the body in the blood. The circulatory system consists of many miles of arteries, veins, and capillaries and includes 5 to 6 liters of blood. Once a drug enters the bloodstream, by passing across thin capillary walls, it is rapidly diluted and carried to organs and other body structures. It requires approximately one minute for the blood, and consequently the drugs it contains, to circulate completely throughout the body.

Factors Affecting Distribution Drugs have different patterns of distribution depending on their chemical properties such as:

▲ Their ability to pass across membranes and through tissues

▲ Their molecular size (large versus small molecules)

▲ Their solubility properties (do they dissolve in water or in fatty—oily—solutions?)

▲ Their tendency to attach to proteins and tissues throughout the body

These distribution-related factors are very important because they determine whether a drug can pass across tissue barriers in the body and reach the site of their action. By preventing the movement of drugs into organs or across tissues, these barriers may interfere with drug activity and limit the therapeutic usefulness of a drug if they do not allow it to reach its site of action. Such barriers may also offer protection by preventing entry of a drug into a body structure where it can cause problems.

Blood is carried to the nerve cells of the brain in a vast network of thin-walled capillaries. Drugs that are soluble in fatty (oily) solutions are most likely to pass across these capillary membranes (known as the **blood–brain barrier**) into the brain tissue. Most psychoactive drugs, such as the drugs of abuse, are able to pass across the blood–brain barrier with little difficulty. However, many water-soluble drugs cannot pass through the fatty capillary wall; such drugs are not likely to cross this biological barrier and affect the brain.

> **blood–brain barrier**
> selective filtering between the cerebral blood vessels and the brain

A second biological barrier, the placenta, prevents the transfer of certain molecules from the mother to the fetus. A principal factor that determines passage of substances across the placental barrier is molecular size. Large molecules do not usually cross the placental barrier, while smaller molecules do. Because most drugs are relatively small molecules, they usually cross from the maternal circulation into the fetal circulation; thus most drugs (including the drugs of abuse) taken by a woman during pregnancy enter the fetus.

Required Doses for Effects Most drugs do not take effect until a certain amount has been administered and a crucial concentration has reached the site of action in the body. The smallest amount of a drug needed to elicit a response is called its **threshold.**

> **threshold**
> the minimum drug dose necessary to cause an effect

The effectiveness of some drugs may be calculated in a *linear* (straight-line) fashion—that is, the more drug that is taken, the more drug distributes throughout the body and the greater the effect. However, many drugs have a maximum possible effect, regardless of dose; it is called the **plateau effect.** OTC medications, in particular, have a limit on their

> **plateau effect**
> the maximum drug effect, regardless of dose

effects. For example, use of the nonprescription analgesic aspirin can effectively relieve your mild to moderate pain, but aspirin will not effectively treat your severe pains, regardless of dose. Other drugs may cause distinct or opposite effects, depending on the dose. For example, low doses of alcohol may act like a stimulant, whereas high doses usually cause sedation.

The Time–Response Factors An important factor that determines responses is the time that has elapsed since a drug was administered and the onset of its effects. The delay in effect after administering a drug often relates to the time required for the drug to disseminate from the site of administration to the site of action. Consequently, the closer a drug is placed to the target area, the faster the onset of action.

The drug response is often classified as immediate, short-term, or **acute,** referring to the response after a single dose. The response can also be **chronic,** or long-term, a characteristic usually associated with repeated doses. The intensity and quality of a drug's acute effect may change considerably within a short period of time. For example, the main intoxicating effects of a large dose of alcohol generally peak in less than one hour and then gradually taper off. In addition, an initial stimulating effect by alcohol may later change to sedation and depression.

The effects of long-term, or chronic, use of some drugs can differ dramatically from their short-term, or acute, use. The administration of small doses may not produce any apparent, immediate, detrimental effect, but chronic use of the same drug (frequent use over a long time) may yield prolonged effects that do not become apparent until years later. Although there is little evidence to show any immediate damage or detrimental response to short-term use of small doses of tobacco, its chronic use has damaging effects on heart and lung functions. Because of these long-term consequences, research on tobacco and

acute

immediate or short-term effects after taking a single drug dose

chronic

long-term effects, usually after taking multiple drug doses

its effects often continues for years, making it difficult to unequivocally prove a correlation between specific diseases or health problems and use of this substance. Thus, the results of tobacco research are often disputed by tobacco manufacturers with vested financial interests in the substance and its public acceptance.

Another important time factor that influences drug responses is the interval between multiple administrations. If sufficient time for drug metabolism and elimination does not separate doses, a drug can accumulate within the body. This buildup of drug due to relatively short dosing intervals is referred to as a **cumulative effect.** Because of the resulting high concentrations of drug in the body, unexpected prolonged drug effects or toxicity can occur when multiple doses are given with short intervals. This situation occurs with cocaine addicts who repeatedly administer the stimulant during "binges," increasing the likelihood of dangerous effects.

cumulative effect

the buildup of a drug in the body after multiple doses taken at short intervals

Inactivation and Elimination of Drugs from the Body

Immediately after drug administration, the body begins to eliminate the substance in various ways. The time required to remove half of the original amount of drug administered is called the **half-life** of the drug. The body will eliminate the drug either directly without altering it chemically or (in most instances) after it has been metabolized (chemically altered) or modified. The process of changing the chemical or pharmacological properties of a drug by metabolism is called **biotransformation. Metabolism** usually (but not always) makes it possible for the body to inactivate,

half-life

the time required for the body to eliminate and/or metabolize half of a drug dose

biotransformation

the process of changing the chemical properties of a drug, usually by metabolism

metabolism

chemical alteration of drugs by body processes

detoxify, and excrete drugs and other chemicals.

The liver is the major organ that metabolizes drugs in the body. It is a complex biochemical laboratory containing hundreds of enzymes that continuously synthesize, modify, and deactivate biochemical substances such as drugs. The healthy liver is also capable of metabolizing many of the chemicals that occur naturally in the body (such as hormones). After the liver enzymes metabolize a drug (the resulting chemicals are called **metabolites**), the products usually pass into the urine or feces for final elimination. Drugs and their metabolites can appear in other places as well, such as sweat, saliva, or expired air.

metabolites

chemical products of metabolism

The kidneys are probably the next most important organ for drug elimination because they remove metabolites and foreign substances from the body. The kidneys constantly eliminate substances from the blood. The rate of excretion of some drugs by the kidneys can be altered by making the urine more acidic or more alkaline. For example, nicotine and amphetamines can be cleared faster from the body by making the urine slightly more acidic, and salicylates and barbiturates can be cleared more rapidly by making it more alkaline. Such techniques are used in emergency rooms and can be useful in the treatment of drug overdosing.

The body may eliminate small portions of drugs through perspiration and exhalation. Approximately 1% of consumed alcohol is excreted in the breath and thus may be measured with a breathalyzer; this technique is used by police officers in evaluating suspected drunk drivers. Most people are aware that consumption of garlic will change body odor because garlic is excreted through perspiration. Some drugs are handled in the same way. The mammary glands are modified sweat glands, so it is not surprising that many drugs are concentrated and excreted in milk during lactation, including antibiotics, nicotine, barbiturates, caffeine, and alcohol. Excretion of drugs in a mother's milk can pose a particular concern during nursing, as the excreted drugs can be consumed by and affect the infant.

Physiological Variables That Modify Drug Effects

As previously mentioned, individuals' responses to drugs can vary greatly, even when the same doses are administered in the same manner. This variability can be especially troublesome when dealing with drugs that have a narrow margin of safety. Many of these variables reflect differences in the pharmacokinetic factors just discussed and are associated with diversity in body size, composition, or functions. They include the following (Nies and Spielberg 1995):

Age Changes in body size and makeup occur throughout the aging process, from infancy to old age. Changes in the rates of drug absorption, biotransformation, and elimination also arise as a consequence of aging. As a general rule, young children and elderly people should be administered lower drug doses (calculated as drug quantity per unit of body weight) due to immature or compromised body processes.

Gender Variations in drug responses due to gender usually relate to differences in body size, composition, or hormones (male versus female types;—for example, androgens versus estrogens). Most clinicians find many more similarities than differences between males and females relative to their responses to drugs.

Pregnancy During the course of pregnancy, unique factors must be considered when administering drugs. For example, the physiology of the mother changes as the fetus develops and puts additional stress on organ systems, such as the heart, liver, and kidneys. This increased demand can make the woman more susceptible to the toxicity of some drugs. In addition, as the fetus develops, it can be very vulnerable to drugs with **teratogenic** (causing abnormal development) properties. Consequently,

teratogenic

something that causes physical defects in the fetus

it is usually advisable to avoid taking any drugs during pregnancy, if possible.

Pathological Variables That Modify Drug Effects

Individuals with diseases or compromised organ systems need to be particularly careful when taking drugs (Nies and Spielberg 1995). Some diseases can damage or impair organs that are vital for appropriate and safe responses to drugs. For example, hepatitis (inflammation and damage to the liver) interferes with the metabolism and disposal of many drugs, resulting in a longer duration of drug action and increased likelihood of side effects. Similar concerns are associated with kidney disease, which causes compromised renal activity and diminished excretion capacity. Because many drugs affect the cardiovascular system (especially drugs of abuse, such as stimulants, tobacco, and alcohol), patients with a history of cardiovascular disease (heart attack, stroke, hypertension, or abnormal heart rhythm) should be particularly cautious when using drugs. They should be aware of those medicines that stimulate the cardiovascular system, especially those that are self-medicated, such as OTC decongestants. These drugs should either be avoided or used only under the supervision of a physician.

◢ Adaptive Processes and Drug Abuse

Your body systems are constantly changing so that they can establish and maintain balance in their physiological and mental functions; such balance is necessary for optimal functioning of all organ systems, including the brain, heart, lungs, gastrointestinal tract, liver, and kidneys. Sometimes drugs interfere with the activity of the body's systems and compromise their normal workings. These drug-induced disruptions can be so severe that they can even cause death. For example, stimulants can dangerously increase the heart rate and blood pressure and cause heart attacks, while CNS depressants can diminish brain activity, resulting in unconsciousness and a loss of breathing reflexes.

To protect against potential harm, the organ systems of the body can adjust to disruption. Of particular relevance to drugs of abuse are adaptive processes known as tolerance and **dependence** (both psychological and physical types) and the related phenomenon of *withdrawal* (see Figure 5.3).

dependence
the physiological and psychological changes or adaptations that occur in response to the frequent administration of a drug

Tolerance and dependence are closely linked, most likely to result from multiple drug exposures, and thought to be caused by similar mechanisms. Tolerance occurs when the response to the same dose of a drug decreases with repeated use (Goldstein 1994). Increasing the dose can sometimes compensate for tolerance to a drug of abuse. For the most part, the adaptations that cause the tolerance phenomenon are also associated with altered physical and psychological states that lead to dependence. These altered states reflect the efforts of the body and brain to reestablish balance in the continual presence of a drug. The user develops dependence in the sense that if the drug is no longer taken, the symptoms of the body become overcompensated and unbalanced, causing withdrawal. In general, withdrawal symptoms are opposite in nature to the direct effects of the drug that caused the dependence (Goldstein 1994).

Although tolerance, dependence, and withdrawal are all consequences of adaptation by the body and its systems, they are not inseparably joined processes. It is possible to become tolerant to a drug without developing dependence and vice versa (see Table 5.2). The following sections provide greater detail about these adaptive drug responses which are very important for many therapeutic drugs and almost all drugs of abuse (O'Brien 1995).

Tolerance to Drugs

The extent of tolerance and the rate at which it is acquired depends on the drug, the person using the drug, and the dosage and frequency of administration. Some drug effects may be reduced more rapidly than others when drugs are used frequently. Tolerance to effects that are rewarding or

Figure 5.3

The relationship and consequences of adaptive processes to drug use. The processes discussed in the text are highlighted in the figure.

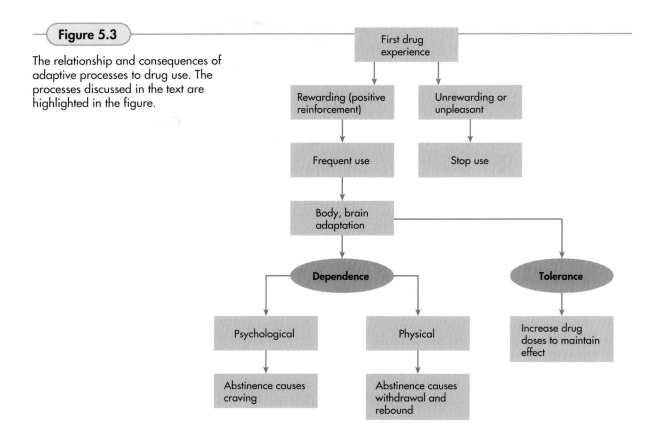

reinforcing often causes users to increase the dosage. Sometimes, abstinence from a drug can reduce tolerance when use of the drug is started again, but with renewed use the tolerance often builds quickly.

The body does not necessarily develop tolerance to all effects of a drug equally. For example, with repeated use, a moderate degree of tolerance develops to most effects of alcohol and barbiturates. A heavy drinker may be able to consume two or three times the alcohol tolerated by an occasional drinker. Little tolerance develops, however, to the lethal toxicity of these drugs. A heavy user of sedatives is just as susceptible to death by overdose as a nontolerant person, even though the heavy user has been forced to increase doses to maintain the relaxing effects of the drug. In contrast, frequent use of opiate narcotics such as morphine can cause profound tolerance, even to the lethal effects of these drugs. Heavy users have been known to use routinely up to 10 times the amount that will kill a nonuser.

The exact mechanisms by which the body becomes tolerant to different drug effects are not completely understood, but as mentioned earlier, may be related to those that cause dependence (Goldstein 1994). Several processes have been suggested. Drugs such as barbiturates stimulate the body's production of metabolic enzymes, primarily in the liver, and cause drugs to be inactivated and eliminated faster. In addition, evidence suggests that a considerable degree of CNS tolerance to some drugs develops independently of changes in the rate of metabolism or excretion. This process reflects the adaptation of drug target sites in nervous tissue, so that the effect of the same concentration of drug decreases. If you were tolerant to alcohol, for example, you would be relatively unaffected by several glasses of wine. This situation may be due to some general molecular adaptation to the

Table 5.2 **Tolerance, Dependence, and Withdrawal Properties of Common Drugs of Abuse**

Drug	Tolerance	Psychological Dependence	Physical Dependence	Withdrawal Symptoms (includes rebound effects)
Barbiturates	■■	■■	■■■	Restlessness, anxiety, vomiting, tremors, seizures
Alcohol	■■	■■	■■■	Cramps, delirium, vomiting, sweating, hallucinations, seizures
Benzodiazepines	■	■■	■■	Insomnia, restlessness, nausea, fatigue, twitching, seizures (rare)
Narcotics (heroin)	■■■	■■	■■■	Vomiting, sweating, cramps, diarrhea, depression, irritability, gooseflesh
Cocaine, amphetamines	■*	■■■	■■	Depression, anxiety, drug craving, need for sleep ("crash"), anhedonia
Nicotine	■	■■	■■	Highly variable; craving, irritability, headache, increased appetite, abnormal sleep
Caffeine	■	■	■	Anxiety, lethargy, headache, fatigue
Marijuana	■	■	■	Irritability, restlessness, decreased appetite, weight loss, abnormal sleep
LSD	■■	■	—	Minimal
PCP	■	■	■	Fear, tremors, some craving, problems with short-term memory

■■■ Intense   ■■ Moderate   ■ Some   — Not significant

* Can sensitize.

drug at the level of the individual nerve cell or it may be caused by a specific brain response that counteracts the sedating effects and maintains normal function (for example, counterbalancing excitatory system is enhanced to compensate for the depression caused by the alcohol).

Another type of drug response that can appear to be tolerance, but is actually a learned adjustment, is called *behavioral compensation*. Drug effects that are troubling may be compensated for or hidden by the drug user. Thus, alcoholics learn to speak and walk slowly to compensate for the slurred speech and stumbling gait they usually experience. To an observer, it might appear as though the pharmacological effects of the drug are diminished, but they are actually unchanged. Consequently, this type of adaptation is not a true form of tolerance.

Other Tolerance-Related Factors The tolerance process can affect drug responses in several ways. We have discussed the effect of tolerance that diminishes the action of drugs and causes the user to compensate by increasing the dose. The following are examples of two other ways that the tolerance process can influence drug responses.

Reverse Tolerance (Sensitization) Under some conditions, a response to a drug is elicited that is the opposite of tolerance. This effect is known as **reverse tolerance,** or sensitization. If you were sensitized, you would have the same response to a lower dose of a drug as you initially did to the

reverse tolerance

an enhanced response to a given drug dose; opposite of tolerance

original, higher dose. This condition seems to occur in users of marijuana, and some hallucinogens, as well as amphetamines and cocaine (O'Brien 1995).

Although the causes of reverse tolerance are still unclear, some researchers believe that its development depends on how often and how much of the drug is consumed. It has been speculated that this heightened response to drugs of abuse may reflect adaptive changes in the nervous tissues (target site of these drugs). The reverse tolerance that occurs with cocaine use may be responsible for the psychotic effects or the seizures caused by chronic use of this drug (O'Brien 1995).

Cross-Tolerance   Development of tolerance to a drug sometimes can produce tolerance to other similar drugs: this phenomenon, known as **cross-tolerance,** may be due to altered metabolism resulting from chronic drug use. For example, a heavy drinker will usually exhibit tolerance to barbiturates, other depressants, and anesthetics because the alcohol has induced (stimulated) his or her liver metabolic enzymes. Cross-tolerance might also occur among drugs that cause similar pharmacological actions. For example, if adaptations have occurred in nervous tissue that cause tolerance to one drug, such changes might also produce tolerance to other similar drugs that exert their effects by interacting with that same nervous tissue site. This type of cross-tolerance has been shown to develop among some of the hallucinogens, such as LSD, mescaline, and psilocybin.

> **cross-tolerance**
> development of tolerance to one drug causes tolerance to related drugs

Drug Dependence

Drug dependence can be associated with either physiological or psychological adaptations. Physical dependence reflects changes in the way organs and systems in the body respond to a drug, while psychological dependence is caused by changes in attitudes and expectations. In both types of dependence, the individual experiences a need (either physical or emotional) for the drug to be present in order for the body or the mind to function normally.

Physical Dependence   In general, the drugs that cause physical dependence also cause a drug withdrawal phenomenon called the **rebound effect.** This condition is sometimes known as the *paradoxical effect* because the symptoms associated with rebound are nearly opposite to the direct effects of the drug. For example, a person taking barbiturates or benzodiazepines will be greatly depressed physically but during withdrawal may become irritable, hyperexcited, nervous, and generally show symptoms of extreme stimulation of the nervous system, even life-threatening seizures. These reactions constitute the rebound effect.

> **rebound effect**
> a form of withdrawal; paradoxical effects that occur when a drug has been eliminated from the body

Physical dependence may develop with high-intensity use of such common drugs as alcohol, barbiturates, narcotics, and other CNS depressants. However, with moderate, intermittent use of these drugs, most people do not become physically dependent. Those who do become physically dependent experience damaged social and personal skills and relationships and impaired brain and motor functions.

Withdrawal symptoms resulting from physical dependency can be prevented by administering a sufficient quantity of the original drug or one with similar pharmacological activity. The latter case, in which different drugs can be used interchangeably to prevent withdrawal symptoms, is called **cross-dependence.** For example, barbiturates and other CNS depressants can be used to treat the abstinence syndrome experienced by the chronic alcoholic. Another example is the use of methadone, a long-acting narcotic, to treat withdrawal from heroin. Such therapeutic strategies allow the substitution of safer and more easily managed drugs for dangerous drugs of abuse and play a major role in treatment of drug dependency.

> **cross-dependence**
> dependence on a drug can be relieved by other similar drugs

Psychological Dependence The World Health Organization (WHO) states that **psychological dependence** instills a feeling of satisfaction and psychic drive that requires periodic or continuous administration of the drug to produce a desired effect or to avoid psychological discomfort. This sense of dependence usually leads to repeated self-administration of the drug in a fashion described as abuse. This type of dependence may be found either independent of or associated with physical dependence.

> **psychological dependence**
>
> dependence that results because a drug produces pleasant mental effects

FINDING a BALANCE

Using Diet and Lifestyle Readjustment to Counter Stress and Caffeine Dependency

When you think about what it takes to get out of bed in the morning, most likely only a few things are strong enough to motivate you to pull back the covers, put your feet on the floor, and stand erect. For most people, it's coffee that does the trick. Wanda is greatly influenced by this motivating force. She lives for coffee, no matter if it's a latte, cappuccino, expresso, or mocha—and we're not just talking about a single cup. Wanda has been known to drink four to eight cups of java before she sits down for a lunch break. Coffee drinking is a passion, a habit, and as Wanda often jokes, an addiction.

Once a habit picked up in college to assist in the effort to pull all-nighters during final exam weeks, Wanda's caffeine addiction now has become a routine part of her every day. An administrative assistant for a busy company, Wanda will admit that she just couldn't function without coffee—let alone get her work done.

"I'll admit at times it appears like a crutch, but I've tried going without it. It just doesn't work." Should she happen to visit a friend's house for a weekend, as she occasionally does, some high octane had better be brewing the next morning or she'll head for the door, get into her car, and drive to the nearest Starbucks.

Recently, Wanda has had to come to terms with what she affectionately refers to as her "affinity for caffeine." Caffeine is a methalated xanthine and activates the neural endings to release epinephrine and norepinephrine, which in essence triggers the stress response. The initial effect is to make one more alert, but the end-result can have some serious consequences on various physiological body functions. For women, drinking high amounts of coffee appears to be strongly correlated with the development of cystic mastitis—cysts in the breast. Wanda was one of these women.

"I went in for a routine exam and lumps were detected in my breasts. I was relieved to find out that it wasn't cancer, but the upshot was that it wasn't healthy either. My doctor asked me if I was a coffee drinker and that's when the connection was made. Immediately, I thought, well great, I'll just switch to decaf. Wrong! I naively thought that decaf was caffeine-free, but this is not the case at all. So now I am faced with a choice."

Making lifestyle readjustments. Wanda's choice is an obvious one, to cut down on her drug of choice. She has switched to decaffeinated coffee (one cup per day) and then drinks caffeine-free tea. "I have to drink something," she explains. Wanda has made another change in her dietary intake by consuming soy products. "As it turns out, I learned that soy products like soy milk and tofu actually help protect against breast cysts. So I have had to make some changes in my diet. But I'll live, and most likely, I'll learn to like it."

Reflecting on her situation, Wanda says, "It's funny. I started drinking coffee to deal with the stress of school, and at the time it helped, but not without its consequences. I may have been drinking caffeine to get revved up, but psychologically speaking, I think I was using coffee as a pacifier for my stress and it backfired. Nutritionally speaking, what we put in our mouths is friend or foe. I have had too many women in my family lose their breasts to cancer. Even though this isn't cancer, it was a wake-up call to me."

Psychological dependence does not produce the physical discomfort, rebound effects, or life-threatening consequences that can be associated with physical dependence. Even so, it does produce intense craving and strong urges that frequently lure former drug abusers back to their habits of drug self-administration. In many instances, psychological aspects may be more significant than physical dependence in maintaining chronic drug use. Thus, the major problem with cocaine or nicotine dependence is not the physical aspects, because withdrawal can be successfully achieved in a few weeks; rather, strong urges often cause a return to chronic use of these substances because of psychological dependence.

How does psychological dependence develop? If the first drug trial is rewarding, a few more rewarding trials will follow until drug use becomes a conditioned pattern of behavior. Continued positive psychological reinforcement with the drug leads, in time, to primary psychological dependence. Primary psychological dependence, in turn, may produce uncontrollable compulsive abuse of any psychoactive drug in certain susceptible people and cause physical dependence. The degree of drug dependence is contingent on the nature of the psychoactive substance, the quantity used, the duration of use, and the characteristics of the person and his or her environment. It is often not possible to draw a sharp line between use and abuse when it comes to developing dependence. Many shades of gray separate the drug user and the drug addict.

Even strong psychological dependence on some psychoactive substances does not necessarily result in injury or social harm. For example, typical dosages of mild stimulants such as coffee usually do not induce serious physical, social, or emotional harm. Even though the effects on the central nervous system are barely detectable by a casual observer, strong psychological dependence on mild stimulants like tobacco and caffeine-containing beverages may develop; however, the fact that their dependence does not typically induce antisocial behavior distinguishes them from most of the forms of dependence-producing drugs.

◢ Psychological Factors

The general effect of most drugs is greatly influenced by a variety of psychological and environmental factors. Unique qualities of an individual's personality, his or her past history of drug and social experience, attitudes toward the drug, expectations of its effects, and motivation for use are extremely influential (see "Case in Point" below). These factors are often referred to collectively as the person's **mental set.** The setting, or total environment, in which a drug is taken may also modify its effect.

mental set

the collection of psychological and environmental factors that influence an individual's response to drugs

---

Researchers Probe Which Comes First, Drug Abuse or Antisocial Behavior?

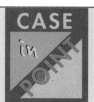

A study conducted by the University of Colorado School of Medicine and directed by Thomas Crowley, a psychiatrist, asked 51 troubled substance-abusing boys, ages 14 to 19, how and when their antisocial behavior began. All the boys were diagnosed with conduct disorders and were enrolled in a Denver residential drug abuse treatment improvement program. Seventy-seven percent of the boys claimed to have engaged in their antisocial behavior (including stealing, truancy, fighting, arson, property destruction, cruelty to people or animals, lying, and running away) 1 to 13 years before regular drug use, suggesting these early problems helped to make these boys more likely to abuse drugs (Swan 1993). ■

The mental set and setting are particularly important in influencing the responses to psychoactive drugs (drugs that alter the functions of the brain). For example, ingestion of LSD, a commonly abused hallucinogen, can cause pleasant, even spiritual-like experiences in comfortable, congenial surroundings. In contrast, when the same amount of LSD is consumed in hostile, threatening surroundings, the effect can be frightening, taking on a nightmarish quality.

The Placebo Effect

The psychological factors that influence responses to drugs, independent of their pharmacological properties, are known as **placebo effects.** The word *placebo* is derived from Latin and means "I shall please." The placebo effect is most likely to occur when an individual's mind-set is susceptible to suggestion. A placebo drug is a pharmacologically inactive compound that the user thinks causes some therapeutic change.

> **placebo effects**
>
> effects caused by suggestion and psychological factors, not the pharmacological activity of a drug

In certain persons or in particular settings, a placebo substance may have surprisingly powerful consequences (Nies and Spielberg 1995). For example, a substantial component of most pain is perception. Consequently, placebos administered as pain relievers and promoted properly can provide dramatic relief. Therefore, in spite of what appears to be a drug effect, the placebo is not considered a pharmacological agent because it does not directly alter any body functions by its chemical nature.

The bulk of medical history may actually be a history of confidence in the cure—a history of placebo medicine—because many effective cures of the past have been shown to be without relevant pharmacological action, suggesting that their effects were psychologically mediated. In fact, even today, some people argue that placebo effects are a significant component of most drug therapy, particularly when using OTC medications. Medical researchers currently are investigating so-called psychological cures, attempting to identify which factors contribute to this interesting phenomenon. It is important when testing new drugs for effectiveness that drug experiments be conducted in a manner that allows a distinction between pharmacological and placebo effects. This study can usually be done by treating with the real drug or a placebo that appears like the drug and then comparing the responses to both treatments.

In some situations, perhaps placebos, or the power of suggestion, activate endogenous systems that help relieve medical problems or associated symptoms (Sherman 1992). This relationship is most likely the explanation for the effectiveness of placebos against pain. A family of *peptides* (called *endorphins*) produced by the body has action similar to that of morphine and other opiate narcotics (Hughes 1975). The endorphins, among other things, are potent endogenous analgesics (substances that block pain) that provide the means for the body to defend itself against the debilitating effects of extreme pain. Research has shown that placebos cause the release of the endorphins to control pain. Other placebo effects may have similar biochemical basis in that they cause the release of endogenous substances that influence the body's functions and alter the course of disease. Just as the placebo effect can alter therapeutic responses, it may also influence responses to drugs of abuse.

◢ Addiction and Abuse: The Significance of Dependence

The term *addiction* has many meanings (see Chapter 2). It is often used interchangeably with *dependence,* either physiological or psychological in nature; other times, it is used synonymously with the term *drug abuse (drug addiction).*

The traditional model of the addiction-producing drug is based on opiate narcotics and requires the individual to develop tolerance and both physical and psychological dependence. This model often is not satisfactory because only a few commonly abused drugs fit its parameters. It is clearly inadequate for many other drugs that can cause serious dependency problems but that produce little tolerance, even with extended use (see Table 5.2).

Because it is difficult to assess the contribution of physical and psychological factors to drug dependency, determining whether all psychoactive drugs truly cause drug addiction poses a challenge. To alleviate confusion, it has been suggested that the term dependence (either physical or psychological) be used instead of addiction. However, because of its acceptance by the public, the term addiction is not likely to disappear from general use.

Some have speculated that the only means by which drug dependence can be eliminated from society is to prevent exposure to those drugs that have potential abuse liability. Because some drugs are such powerful, immediate reinforcers, it is feared that rapid dependence (psychological) will occur when anyone uses them. Although it may be true that most people, under certain conditions, could become dependent on some drug with abuse potential, in reality, most people who have used psychoactive drugs do not develop significant psychological or physical dependence. For example, approximately 87% of those who use alcohol experience minimal personal injury and social consequences. Of those who have used stimulants, depressants, or hallucinogens for illicit recreational purposes, only 10% to 20% become dependent (O'Brien 1995). The following sections discuss some possible reasons for the variability.

Hereditary Factors

The reasons why some people readily develop dependence on psychoactive drugs and others do not are not well understood. One factor may be heredity, which predisposes some people to drug abuse. For example, studies of identical and fraternal twins have revealed that a greater similarity in the rate of alcoholism for identical twins than for fraternal twins occurs if alcohol abuse begins before the age of 20 years (McGue et al. 1992). Because identical twins have 100% of their genes in common while fraternal twins share only 50%, these results suggest that genetic factors can be important in determining the likelihood of alcohol dependence (Uhl et al. 1993). It is possible that similar genetic factors contribute to other types of drug dependence as well.

Drug Craving

Frequently, a person who becomes dependent develops a powerful, uncontrollable desire for drugs during or after withdrawal from heroin, cocaine, alcohol, nicotine, or other addicting substances: this desire for drugs is known as craving. Because researchers do not agree as to the nature of craving, there does not exist a universally recognized scientific definition or an accepted method to measure this psychological phenomenon. Some drug abuse experts claim that craving is the principal cause of drug abuse; others believe that it is not a cause but a side effect of drugs that produce dependence. Craving is often assessed by (1) questioning patients about the intensity of their drug urges; (2) measuring physiological changes such as increases in heart and breathing rates, sweating, and subtle changes in the tension of facial muscles; and (3) determining patients' tendency to relapse into drug-taking behavior (Swan 1993).

Evidence indicates that at least two levels of craving can exist. For example, cocaine users experience an acute craving when using the drug itself, but the ex-cocaine abuser can have chronic cravings that are triggered by familiar environmental cues that elicit positive memories of cocaine's reinforcing effects.

Although it is not likely that craving itself causes drug addiction, it is generally believed that, if pharmacological or psychological therapies could be devised that reduce or eliminate drug craving, treatment of drug dependence would be more successful. Thus, many researchers are attempting to identify drugs or psychological strategies that interfere with the development and expression of the craving phenomenon.

Other Factors

If a drug causes a positive effect in the user's view, it is much more likely to be abused than if it causes an aversive experience (see Figure 5.3). Perhaps genetic factors influence the brain or personality so that some people find taking drugs an enjoyable experience (at least initially), while others find the effects very unpleasant and uncomfortable **(dysphoric).** Other factors that could also contribute significantly to drug use patterns include (1) peer pressure (especially in the initial drug experimentation); (2) home, school, and work environment (Mello and Griffith 1987); and (3) mental state. It is estimated that 20% to 30% of those who abuse drugs, particularly stimulants, are attempting to self-medicate some form of mental disorder; for example, the stimulant cocaine is frequently used to self-treat depression (Weiss et al. 1989; Pagliaro et al. 1992). Consequently, it is not surprising that one treatment for cocaine abuse is the antidepressant desipramine (O'Brien 1995).

It is difficult to identify all specific factors that influence the risk of drug abuse for each individual. (Some of the possible influences are discussed in Chapter 2.) If such factors could be identified, treatment would be improved and those at greatest risk for drug abuse could be determined and informed of their vulnerability.

> **dysphoric**
> characterized by unpleasant mental effects; the opposite of euphoric

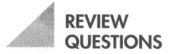

REVIEW QUESTIONS

1. What is the significance of drug "potency" for therapeutic use and abuse of drugs?

2. How can drug interactions be both detrimental and beneficial? Give examples of each.

3. Why would a drug with a relatively narrow "margin of safety" by approved by the FDA for clinical use?

4. What are possible explanations for the fact that you (for example) may require twice as much of a drug to get an effect as does your friend?

5. What significance would the blood–brain barrier have on drugs with abuse potential?

6. Contrary to your advice, a friend is going to spend $20 on a "cocaine buy." What significance will the pharmacokinetic concepts of threshold, half-life, cumulative effect, and biotransformation have on your friend's drug experience?

7. How would the factors of tolerance, physical dependence, rebound, and psychological dependence affect a chronic heroin user?

8. Why would the lack of physical dependence on LSD for some drug abusers make it preferable to cocaine, which does cause physical dependence?

EXERCISES FOR THE WEB

Exercise 1:
Health Source

Health Source is part of the Community Outreach Health Information System (COHIS), a project with two main goals: to promote health and disease prevention using the World Wide Web and to educate and encourage actively the use of this information in under-served communities around Boston. The Boston University School of Medicine COHIS Committee was formed to make these goals attainable.

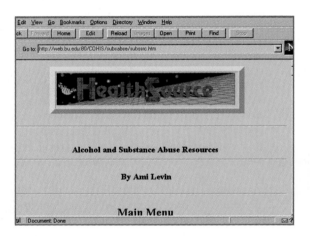

Exercise 2:
NCADI

The National Clearinghouse for Alcohol and Drug Information (NCADI) is the world's largest resource of current information and materials concerning substance abuse prevention. The National Clearinghouse for Alcohol and Drug Information (NCADI) is the information service of the Center for Substance Abuse Prevention, which is part of the U.S. Department of Health & Human Services. Some of NCADI services include: 1) an information services staff equipped to respond to the public's alcohol, tobacco, and illicit drug inquiries (ATID); 2) the distribution of free ATID materials, including fact sheets, brochures, pamphlets, posters, and video tapes from an inventory of over 1,000 items; 3) a repertoire of culturally-diverse prevention materials, tailored for use by parents, teachers, youth, communities, and prevention professionals.

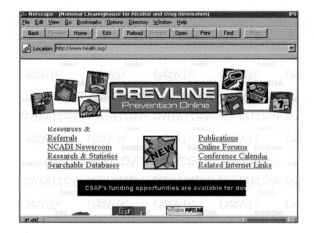

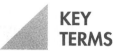

KEY TERMS

main effects
side effects
withdrawal
dose–response
tolerance
margin of safety
potency
toxicity
drug interaction
additive interactions
antagonistic interactions
synergism
pharmacokinetics
intravenous (IV)
intramuscular (IM)
subcutaneous (SC)
blood–brain barrier
threshold
plateau effect
acute
chronic
cumulative effect
half-life
biotransformation
metabolism
metabolites
teratogenic
dependence
reverse tolerance (sensitization)
cross-tolerance
rebound effect
cross-dependence
psychological dependence
mental set
placebo effects
dysphoric

SUMMARY

1 All drugs have intended and unintended effects. The unintended impacts of drugs can include effects such as nausea, altered mental states, dependence, a variety of allergic responses, and changes in the cardiovascular system.

2 Many factors can affect the way an individual responds to a drug: dose, inherent toxicity, potency and pharmacokinetic properties such as the rate of absorption into the body, the way it is distributed throughout the body, and the manner and rate in which it is metabolized and eliminated. The form of the drug as well as the manner in which it is administered can also affect the response to a drug.

3 *Potency* is determined by the amount of a drug necessary to cause a given effect. *Toxicity* is the ability of the drug to affect the body adversely. A drug that is very toxic is very potent in terms of causing a harmful effect.

4 A drug's *margin of safety* relates to the difference in the drug doses that cause a therapeutic or a toxic effect; the bigger the difference, the greater the margin of safety.

5 *Additive* interactions occur when the effects of two drugs are combined; for example, the analgesic effects of aspirin plus acetaminophen are additive. *Antagonistic* effects occur when the effects of two drugs cancel; for example, the stimulant effects of caffeine tend to antagonize the drowsiness caused by antihistamines. *Synergism* (potentiation) occurs when one drug enhances the effect of another; for example, alcohol enhances the CNS depression caused by Valium.

6 Pharmacokinetic factors include absorption, distribution, biotransformation, and elimination of drugs.

7 Many physiological and pathological factors can alter the response to drugs. For example, age, gender, and pregnancy are all factors that should be considered when making drug decisions. In addition, some diseases can alter the way in which the body responds to drugs. Medical conditions associated with the liver, kidneys, and cardiovascular system are of particular concern.

8 In order for psychoactive drugs to influence the brain and its actions, they must pass through the blood–brain barrier. Many of these drugs are fat-soluble and able to pass through capillary walls from the blood into the brain.

9 The *threshold* dose is the minimum amount of a drug necessary to have an effect. The *plateau effect* is the maximum effect a drug can have, regardless of dose. The *cumulative effect* is the buildup of drug concentration in the body due to multiple doses taken within short intervals.

10 The liver is the primary organ for the metabolizing of drugs and many natural occurring substances in the body, such as hormones. By altering the molecular structure of drugs, the metabolism usually inactivates drugs and makes them easier to eliminate through the kidneys.

11 *Biotransformation* is the process that alters the molecular structure of a drug. Metabolism contributes to biotransformation.

12 Drug tolerance causes a decreased response to a given dose of a drug. It can be caused by increasing metabolism and elimination of the drug by the body or by a change in the systems or targets that are affected by the drug.

13 *Physical dependence* is characterized by the adaptive changes that occur in the body due to the continual presence of a drug. These changes are often chemical in nature and reduce the response to the drugs and cause *tolerance.* If drug use is halted after physical dependence has occurred, the body is overcompensated, causing a *rebound* response. Rebound effects are similar to the *withdrawal* that occurs because drug use is stopped for an extended period. *Psychological dependence* occurs because drug use is rewarding, bringing euphoria, increased energy, and relaxation, or because it produces craving.

14 Suggestion can have a profound influence on a person's drug response. Health problems with significant psychological aspects are particularly susceptible to the effects of placebos. For example, because much of pain is related to its perception, a placebo can substantially relieve pain discomfort. This placebo effect may relate to the release of a natural pain-relieving substance, such as endorphins. Other placebo responses may likewise be due to the release of endogenous factors in the body.

15 A powerful, uncontrollable desire (craving) for drugs can occur with chronic use of some drugs of abuse. Although craving by itself may not cause drug addiction, if it can be eliminated, treatment of substance abuse is more likely to be successful.

REFERENCES

Brenner, L. "How Common is Counseling?" *American Druggist* (January 1994): 40.

Combined News Services. "Drug Reactions Can Kill." *Salt Lake Tribune* 249 (Jan. 5, 1995): C–1.

Goldstein, A. *Addiction from Biology to Drug Policy.* New York: Freeman, 1994.

Grant, B., and S. Harford. "Concurrent and Simultaneous Use of Alcohol with Cocaine. Results of National Survey." *Drug and Alcohol Dependence* 25 (1990): 97–104.

Henderson, G. "Designer Drugs: Past History and Future Prospects." *Journal of Forensic Sciences* 33 (1988): 569–75.

Hobbs, W. R., T. Rall, and T. Verdoorn. "Hypnotics and Sedatives: Ethanol." In *The Pharmacological Basis of Therapeutics,* 9th ed., edited by J. Hardman and L. Limbird, 386–96. New York: McGraw-Hill, 1995.

Hughes, J. "Isolation of an Endogenous Compound from the Brain with Pharmacological Properties Similar to Morphine." *Brain Research* 88 (1975): 295–308.

Karch, S. "Cocaine." In *The Pathology of Drug Abuse,* 39–44. New York: CRC Press, 1996.

Klaasen, C. D. "Principles of Toxicology and Treatment of Poisoning." In *The Pharmacological Basis of Therapeutics,* 9th ed., edited by J. Hardman and L. Limbird, 63–75. New York: McGraw-Hill, 1995.

Mathias, R. "Smoking Drugs Creates New Dangers." *NIDA Notes* 9 (February–March 1994): 6.

McGue, M., R. Pickens, and D. Svikis. "Sex and Age Effects on the Inheritance of Alcohol Problems: A Twin Study." *Journal of Abnormal Psychology* 101 (January 1992): 3–17.

Mello, K., and R. Griffith. "Alcoholism and Drug Abuse: An Overview." In *Psychopharmacology: The Third Generation of Progress,* edited by H. Meltzer: 1511–20. New York: Raven Press, 1987.

Nies, A., and S. Spielberg. "Principles of Therapeutics." In *The Pharmacological Basis of Therapeutics,* 9th ed., edited by J. Hardman and L. Limbird, 43–62. New York: McGraw-Hill, 1995.

O'Brien, C. "Drug Addiction and Drug Abuse." In *The Pharmacological Basis of Therapeutics,* 9th ed., edited by J. Hardman and L. Limbird, 557–77. New York: McGraw-Hill, 1995.

Pagliaro, L., L. Jaglalsingh, and A. Pagliaro. "Cocaine Use and Dependence." *Canadian Medical Association Journal* 147 (1992): 1636.

Sherman, M. "The Placebo Effect." *American Druggist* (January 1992): 39–42.

Swan, N. "Despite Advances, Drug Craving Remains an Elusive Research Target." *NIDA Notes* (May–June 1993): 1–4.

"Trends, Policy and Research." *Prevention Pipeline* [Center for Substance Abuse Prevention] (November–December 1993): 27.

Uhl, G., K. Blum, E. Noble, and S. Smith. "Substance Abuse Vulnerability and D-2 Receptor Genes." *Trends in Neurological Sciences* 16 (1993): 83–7.

Weiss, R., M. Griffin, and S. Mirin. "Diagnosing Major Depression in Cocaine Abuser: The Use of Depression Rating Scales." *Psychiatry Research* 28 (1989): 335–43.

Homeostatic Systems and Drugs

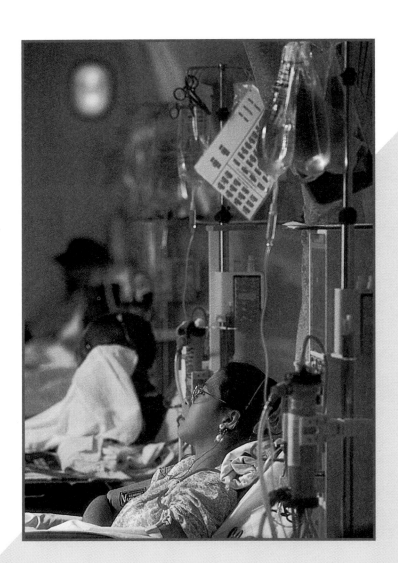

On completing this chapter
you will be able to: ▶

6

6

Homeostatic Systems and Drugs

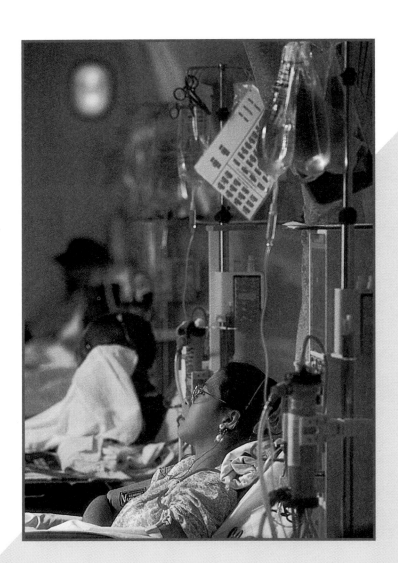

On completing this chapter
you will be able to: ▶

6

Homeostatic Systems and Drugs

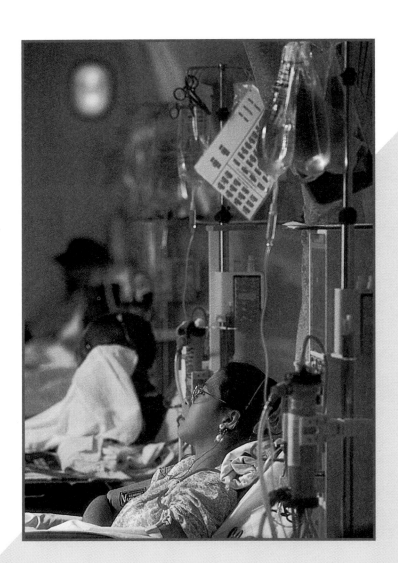

On completing this chapter
you will be able to: ▶

- The brain is composed of over 10 billion neurons that communicate with one another by releasing chemical messengers called *neurotransmitters*.
- Many drugs exert their effects by interacting with specialized protein regions in cell membranes called *receptors*.
- Some natural chemicals produced by the body have the same effect as narcotic drugs; these chemicals are called *endorphins*.
- The body likely produces natural substances that have effects like marijuana and Valium.
- Drugs that affect the neurotransmitter dopamine usually alter both mental state and motor activity.
- The pleasant sensations that encourage continual use of most drugs of abuse are due to stimulation of dopamine activity in the limbic system.
- The hypothalamus is the principal brain region for control of endocrine systems.
- The anabolic steroids often abused by athletes are chemically related to testosterone, the male hormone, and stimulate increased muscle mass.
- Anabolic steroids are considered controlled drugs by the Drug Enforcement Administration (DEA) and have been classified as Schedule III substances.

Learning Objectives

- Explain the similarities and differences between the nervous and endocrine systems.
- Describe how a neuron functions.
- Describe the role of receptors in mediating the effects of hormones, neurotransmitters, and drugs.
- Distinguish between receptor agonists and antagonists.
- Describe the different features of the principal neurotransmitters.
- Outline the principal components of the central nervous system, and explain their general functions.
- Identify which brain areas are most likely to be affected by drugs of abuse.
- Distinguish between the sympathetic and parasympathetic nervous systems.
- Identify the principal components of the endocrine system.
- Explain how and why anabolic steroids are abused and the health impact attributed to abuse.

Why is your body susceptible to the influence of drugs and other substances? Part of the answer is that your body is constantly adjusting and responding to its environment in order to maintain internal stability and balance. This delicate process of dynamic adjustments—**homeostatis**—is necessary to optimize body functions and is essential for survival. These continual compensations help to maintain physiological and psychological balances and are mediated by the release of endogenous regulatory chemicals (such as **neurotransmitters** and hormones). Many drugs exert intended or unintended effects by altering the activity of these regulatory substances, which changes the function of the nervous or endocrine system. For example, all drugs of abuse profoundly influence mental states by altering the chemical messages of the neurotransmitters in the brain, and some alter endocrine function by affecting the release of hormones. By understanding the mechanisms of how drugs alter these body processes, we are able to recognize drug benefits and risks and devise therapeutic strategies to deal with ensuing problems.

This chapter is divided into two sections. The first is a brief overview section to introduce the basic concept of how the body is controlled by nervous systems and explain why drugs influence the elements of these systems. The second section is intended for readers who desire a more in-depth understanding of the anatomical, physiological, and biochemical basis of homeostatic functions. In this section the elements of the nervous system are discussed in greater detail, followed by an examination of its major divisions: the central, peripheral and autonomic nervous systems. The components and operation of the endocrine system are also discussed in specific relation to drugs. The use of anabolic steroids is given as an example.

> **homeostasis**
>
> maintenance of internal stability; often biochemical in nature

> **neurotransmitters**
>
> chemical messengers released by neurons

1: Overview of Homeostasis and Drug Actions

The body continuously adjusts to both internal and external changes in the environment. To cope with these adjustments, the body systems include elaborate self-regulating mechanisms. The name given to this compensatory action is homeostasis, which refers to the maintenance of internal stability or equilibrium. For example, homeostatic mechanisms control the response of the brain to changes in the physical, social, and psychological environments, as well as regulate physiological factors such as body temperature, metabolism, nutrient utilization, and organ functions. The two principal systems that help human beings maintain homeostasis are the nervous system and the endocrine system (described in Section 2, page 140). They greatly influence each other and work together closely.

◢ Introduction to Nervous Systems

All nervous systems consist of specialized nerve cells called **neurons.** The neurons are responsible for conducting the homeostatic functions of the brain and other parts of the nervous system by receiving and sending information. The transfer of messages by neurons includes chemical and electrical processes that consist of the following steps (see Figure 6.1):

> **neurons**
>
> specialized nerve cells that make up the nervous system

▲ The *receiving region* of the neuron (B) is affected by a chemical message (A) that either excites (causes the neuron to send its own message) or inhibits (prevents the neuron from sending a message) it.

▲ If the message is excitatory, an impulse (much like electricity) moves from the receiving region of the neuron,

> **axon**
>
> an extension of the neuronal cell body along which electrochemical signals travel

---

Figure 6.1

The process of sending messages by neurons. The receiving region (B) of the neuron is activated by an incoming message (A) near the neuronal cell body. The neuron sends an electricity-like impulse down the axon to its terminal (C). The impulse causes the release of neurotransmitter from the terminal to transmit the message to the target (D). This is done when the neurotransmitter molecules activate the receptors on the membranes of the target cell (E). The activated receptors then cause a change in intracellular functions to occur (F).

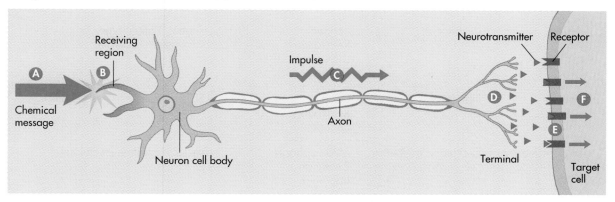

down its wirelike processes (called **axons**) to the *sending region* (called the *terminal*) (C). When the electricity-type impulse reaches the terminal, chemical messengers called neurotransmitters are released (D).

▲ The neurotransmitters travel very short distances and attach to specialized and specific *receiving proteins* called **receptors** on the outer membranes of their target cells (E).

> **receptor**
> a special region in a membrane that is activated by natural substances or drugs to alter cell function

▲ Activation of receptors by their associated neurotransmitters causes a change in the activity of the target cell (F). The target cells can be other neurons or cells that make up organs (such as heart, lungs, kidneys, and so on), muscles, or glands.

Neurons are highly versatile and, depending on their functions, can send discrete excitatory or inhibitory messages to their target cells. Neurons are distinguished by the types of chemical substances they release as neurotransmitters to send

their messages. The neurotransmitters represent a wide variety of molecules that are classified according to their functional association as well as their ability to stimulate or inhibit the activity of target neurons, organs, muscles, and glands. They are discussed in greater detail in Section II.

An example of a common neurotransmitter used by neurons in the brain to send messages is the substance *dopamine.* When released from neurons associated with the *pleasure center* in the brain, dopamine causes substantial euphoria by activating its receptor on target neurons (Goldstein 1994). This effect is relevant to drugs of abuse because most (if not all) of these substances' addictive properties stem from their ability to stimulate dopamine release from these neurons (for example, amphetamine or cocaine) and thus cause pleasant euphoric effects in the user (Uhl et al. 1993).

It is important to understand that many of the effects of **psychoactive** drugs (which alter the mental functions of the brain), such as the drugs of abuse, are due to their abil-

> **psychoactive**
> drugs that affect mood or alter the state of consciousness

> **Table 6.1** **Common Neurotransmitters of the Brain Affected by Drugs of Abuse**

Neurotransmitter	Type of Effect	Major CNS Changes	Drugs of Abuse That Influence the Neurotransmitter (drug action)
Dopamine	Inhibitory–excitatory	Euphoria Agitation Paranoia	Amphetamines, cocaine (activate)
GABA	Inhibitory	Sedation Relaxation Drowsiness Depression	Alcohol, Valium-type, barbiturates (activate)
Serotonin	Inhibitory	Sleep Relaxation Sedation	LSD (activate)
Acetylcholine	Excitatory–inhibitory	Mild euphoria Excitation Insomnia	Tobacco, nicotine (stimulate)
Endorphins	Inhibitory	Mild euphoria Blockage of pain Slow respiration	Narcotics (activate)

ity to alter the neurotransmitters associated with neurons. Some of the most likely transmitter messenger systems to be affected by drugs of abuse are listed in Table 6.1 and are discussed in greater detail in the next section.

2: Comprehensive Explanation of Homeostatic Systems

For those of you who desire a more complete understanding of the consequences of drug effects on the homeostatic systems of the body, this section provides an in-depth discussion of the anatomical and physiological nature and biological arrangements of the nervous and endocrine systems. Because drugs of abuse are most likely to exert their psychoactive effects on neurons and their receptor targets, the nervous system is presented first and in greater depth, followed by a less detailed description of endocrine function.

◢ The Building Blocks of the Nervous System

Your nervous system is composed of your brain, spinal cord, and all the neurons that connect to other organs and tissues of your body (see Figure 6.7). Nervous systems enable you to receive information about your internal and external environment and to make the appropriate responses essential to survival. Considerable money and effort are currently being dedicated to explore the mechanisms whereby the nervous system functions and processes information resulting in frequent new and exciting discoveries.

The Neuron: The Basic Structural Unit of the Nervous System

The building block of the nervous system is the nerve cell, or neuron. Each neuron in the central nervous system (brain and spinal cord) is in close proximity with other neurons, forming a complex network. The human brain contains more than 10 billion neurons, each of which is composed of similar parts but with different shapes and sizes. Neurons do not form a continuous network. They always remain separate, never actually touching, although they are very close. The point of communication between one neuron and another is called a **synapse.** The gap (called the **synaptic cleft**) between neurons at a synapse may be only 0.00002 millimeter, but it is essential for proper functioning of the nervous system (see Figure 6.2).

synapse

site of communication between a message-sending neuron and its message-receiving target cell

synaptic cleft

a minute gap between the neuron and target cell, across which neurotransmitters travel

The neuron has a cell body with a nucleus and receiving regions called **dendrites,** which are short, treelike branches that pick up information from the environment and surrounding neurons.

The axon of a neuron is a threadlike extension that receives information from the dendrites near the cell body, in the form of an electrical impulse; then, like an electrical wire, it transmits the impulse to the cell's terminal. While most axons are less than 1 inch in length, some may be quite long; for example, some axons extend from the spinal cord to the toes.

dendrites

short branches of neurons that receive transmitter signals

Figure 6.2

(A) Each neuron may have many synaptic connections. They are designed to deliver short bursts of a chemical transmitter substance into the synaptic cleft, where it can act on the surface of the receiving nerve cell membrane. Before release, molecules of the chemical neurotransmitter are stored in numerous vesicles, or sacs. (B) A closeup of the synaptic terminals, showing the synaptic vesicles and mitochondria. Mitochondria are specialized structures that help supply the cell with energy. The gap between the synaptic terminal and the target membrane is the synaptic cleft.

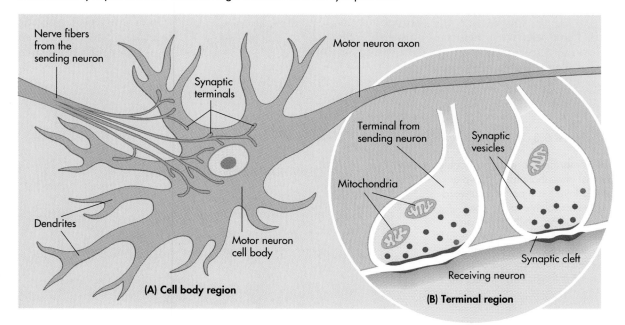

As discussed, at the synapse information is transmitted chemically to the next neuron as shown in Figure 6.1. A similar synaptic arrangement also exists at sites of communication between neurons and target cells in organs, muscles, and glands; that is, neurotransmitters are released from the message-sending neurons and activate receptors located in the membranes of message-receiving target cells.

There are two types of synapses: (1) the excitatory synapse, which initiates an impulse in the receiving neuron when stimulated, thereby causing release of neurotransmitters, or increases activity in the target cell; and (2) the inhibitory synapse, which diminishes the likelihood of an impulse in the receiving neuron or reduces the activity in other target cells. A receiving neuron or target cell may have many synapses connecting it to neurons and their excitatory or inhibitory information (see Figure 6.2, part A). The final cellular activity is a summation of these many excitatory and inhibitory synaptic signals.

The Nature of Drug Receptors

Receptors are special proteins located in the membranes of receiving neurons and other target cells (see Figure 6.3). They help regulate the activity of cells in the nervous system and throughout the body. These selective protein sites on specific cells act as transducers to communicate the messages caused by endogenous messenger substances (chemicals produced and released within the body), such as neurotransmitters and hormones. The receptors process the complex information each cell receives as it attempts to maintain metabolic constancy, or homeostasis, and fulfill its functional role. Many drugs used therapeutically and almost all drugs of abuse exert their effects on the body by directly or indirectly interacting (either to activate or antagonize) with these receptors.

Understanding how receptors interact with specific drugs has led to some interesting results. For example, **opiate receptors** (sites of action by narcotic drugs, such as heroin and morphine) are naturally present in the animal brain (Snyder 1977). Why would human and animal brains have receptors for opiate narcotics, which are plant chemicals? Discovery of the opiate receptors suggested the existence of internal (endogenous) neurotransmitter substances in the body that normally act at these receptor sites and have effects like narcotic drugs, such as codeine and morphine. This finding led to the identification of the body's own opiates, the **endorphins** (Goldstein 1994). Specific receptors have also been found for other drugs such

> **opiate receptors**
> receptors activated by opioid narcotic drugs, such as heroin and morphine

> **endorphins**
> neurotransmitters that have narcotic-like effects

Figure 6.3

Cell membranes consist of a double layer of phospholipids. The water-soluble layers are pointed outward and the fat-soluble layers are pointed toward each other. Large proteins, including receptors, float in the membrane. Some of these receptors are activated by neurotransmitters to alter the activity of the cell.

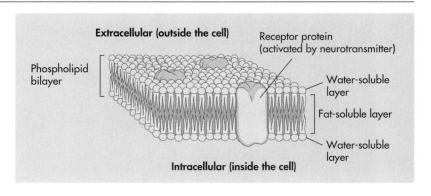

as the central nervous system (CNS) depressant Valium and the active ingredient in marijuana. Because of these discoveries, it is speculated that endogenous substances exist that mimic the effects of Valium and marijuana and help provide natural sedation and relaxation for the body (O'Brien 1995; Hobbs, Rall, and Verdoorn 1995). Presently, several research laboratories are attempting to identify the natural chemical messengers that normally act at the Valium (referred to as the *benzodiazepine receptor*) and marijuana (called the *cannabinoid receptor*) sites of activity.

Much remains unknown about how receptors respond to or interact with drugs. Using molecular biology techniques, many of these receptors have been found to initiate a cascade of linked chemical reactions, which can change intracellular environments to produce either activation or inactivation of cellular functions and metabolism (Linder and Gilman 1992).

Receptors that have been isolated and identified are protein molecules; it is believed that the shape of the protein is essential in regulating a drug's interaction with a cell. If the drug is the proper shape and size and has a compatible electrical charge, it may substitute for the endogenous messenger substance and activate the receptor protein by causing it to change its shape, or conformation. This process is like a "lock-and-key" arrangement, with only certain shapes of chemicals (the keys) being able to interact and activate a receptor (the "lock") (Goldstein 1994).

Agonistic and Antagonistic Effects on Drug Receptors

A drug may have two different effects on a receptor when interaction occurs: **agonistic** or **antagonistic.** As shown in Figure 6.4, an agonistic drug interacts with the receptor and produces some type of cellular response, whereas an antagonistic drug interacts with the receptor but prevents that response. By analogy, using the lock-and-key model, a key can be used to open a lock (agonistic effect), whereas another key that fits in the lock but does not work can jam it (antagonistic effect).

> **agonistic**
> a type of substance that activates a receptor
>
> **antagonistic**
> a type of substance that blocks a receptor

An agonistic drug mimics the effect of a substance (such as a neurotransmitter) that is naturally produced by the body and interacts with the receptor to cause some cellular change. For example, narcotic drugs are agonists that mimic the endorphins and activate opiate receptors. An antagonist has the opposite effect: it inhibits the sequence of metabolic events that a natural substance or an agonist drug can stimulate, without initiating an effect itself. Thus, a drug called *naloxone* is an antagonist at the opiate receptors and blocks the effects of narcotic drugs as well as the effects of the naturally occurring endorphins.

Figure 6.4

Interaction of agonist and antagonist with membrane receptor. When this receptor is occupied and activated by an agonist, it can cause cellular changes.

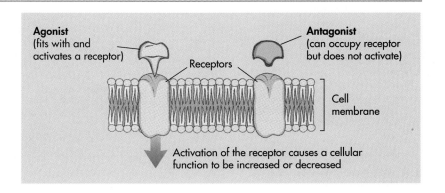

Agonist (fits with and activates a receptor)

Antagonist (can occupy receptor but does not activate)

Receptors

Cell membrane

Activation of the receptor causes a cellular function to be increased or decreased

Neurotransmitters: The Messengers

Many drugs affect the activity of neurotransmitters by altering their synthesis, storage, release, or deactivation. By changing these steps, a drug may modify or block information transmitted by these neurochemical messengers. Thus, by altering the amount of neurotransmitter, such drugs can act indirectly, like agonists and antagonists, even though they do not directly change neurotransmitter receptors.

Experimental evidence shows that many different neurotransmitters exist, although much remains to be learned about their specific functions. These biochemical messengers are released from specific neurons. The transmitters most likely altered by drugs of abuse include acetylcholine, norepinephrine, epinephrine, dopamine, serotonin, gamma-amino-butyric acid (GABA), and the endorphins (peptides). Because of the unique shapes, each neurotransmitter affects only its specific receptors (Bloom 1995). Drugs can also affect these receptors if they are sufficiently similar in shape to the neurotransmitters. Figure 6.5 summarizes some of the important features about the common neurotransmitters.

Acetylcholine   Large quantities of acetylcholine (ACh) are found in the brain. This neurotransmitter is synthesized in the neuron by combining molecules of choline (provided by diet and also manufactured in the body) and acetyl CoA (a product of glucose metabolism). Acetylcholine is

---

Figure 6.5

Features of common neurotransmitters

Acetylcholine
Chemical type: Choline product
Location: CNS—Basal ganglia, cortex, reticular activating system
PNS—Neuromuscular junction, parasympathetic system
Action: Excitatory and inhibitory

Norepinephrine
Chemical type: Catecholamine
Location: CNS—Limbic system, cortex, hypothalamus, reticular activating system, brain stem, spinal cord
PNS—Sympathetic nervous system
Action: Usually inhibitory; some excitation

Epinephrine
Chemical type: Catecholamine
Location: CNS—Minor
PNS—Adrenal glands
Action: Usually excitatory

Dopamine
Chemical type: Catecholamine
Location: CNS—Basal ganglia, limbic system, hypothalamus
Action: Usually inhibitory

Serotonin (S-HT)
Chemical type: Tryptophan-derivative
Location: CNS—Basal ganglia, limbic system, brain stem, spinal cord, cortex
Other—Gut, platelets, cardiovascular
Action: Inhibitory

GABA
Chemical type: Amino acid
Location: CNS—Basal ganglia, limbic system, cortex
Action: Inhibitory

Endorphins
Chemical type: Peptide (small protein)
Location: CNS—Basal ganglia, hypothalamus, brain stem, spinal cord
Other—Gut, cardiovascular system
Action: Inhibitory (narcotic-like effects)

Key: CNS—Central nervous system
PNS—Peripheral nervous system

one of the major neurotransmitters in the autonomic portion of the *peripheral nervous system* (which will be discussed later in the chapter).

Neurons that respond to ACh are distributed throughout the brain. Depending on the region, ACh can have either excitatory or inhibitory effects. The receptors activated by acetylcholine have been divided into two main subtypes based on the response to two drugs derived from plants: muscarine and nicotine. Muscarine (a substance in mushrooms that causes mushroom poisoning) and similarly acting drugs activate **muscarinic** receptors. Nicotine, whether experimentally administered or inhaled by smoking tobacco, stimulates **nicotinic** receptors.

> **muscarinic**
>
> a receptor type activated by ACh; usually inhibitory
>
> **nicotinic**
>
> a receptor type activated by ACh; usually excitatory

Neurotransmitters are inactivated after they have done their job by removal, metabolism (by enzymes), or reabsorption into the neuron. If a deactivating enzyme is blocked by a drug, the effect of the transmitter may be prolonged or intensified. For example, acetylcholine stimulates nicotinic receptors that cause strong contraction of muscles. The acetylcholine is metabolized by the deactivating enzyme, acetylcholinesterase, into the choline and acetate molecules, and the muscles relax. Some nerve gases developed by the military for chemical warfare purposes, for example, block the acetylcholinesterase enzyme. The target receptors in the presence of these drugs continue to be stimulated because the ACh is not inactivated by metabolism. This continual firing of electrical impulses causes muscle paralysis due to the persistent muscle contraction.

Catecholamines **Catecholamines** comprise the neurotransmitter compounds norepinephrine, epinephrine, and dopamine, and have similar chemical structures. Neurons that synthesize catecholamines convert the amino acids phenylalanine or tyrosine to dopamine. In some

> **catecholamines**
>
> a class of biochemical compounds including the transmitters norepinephrine, epinephrine, and dopamine

neurons, dopamine is further converted to norepinephrine, and finally to epinephrine.

Unlike acetylcholine, after acting at their receptors, most of the catecholamines are taken back up into the neurons that released them, to be used over again; this process is called *reuptake*. An enzymatic breakdown system also metabolizes the catecholamines to inactive compounds. The reuptake process and the activity of metabolizing enzymes, especially monoamine oxidase (MAO), can be greatly affected by some of the drugs of abuse. If these deactivating enzymes or reuptake systems are blocked, the concentration of norepinephrine and dopamine may build up in the brain, causing a significantly increased effect. Cocaine, for example, prevents the reuptake of norepinephrine and dopamine in the brain, resulting in continual stimulation of neuron catecholamine receptors.

Norepinephrine and Epinephrine Although norepinephrine and epinephrine are structurally very similar, their receptors are selective and do not respond with the same intensity to either transmitter or to **sympathomimetic** drugs. Just as the receptors to acetylcholine can be separated into muscarinic and nicotinic types, the norepinephrine and epinephrine receptors are classified into the categories of alpha and beta. Receiving cells may have alpha- or beta-type receptors, or both. Norepinephrine acts predominantly on alpha receptors and has little action on beta receptors.

> **sympathomimetic**
>
> agents that mimic the effects of norepinephrine or epinephrine

The antagonistic (blocking) action of many drugs that act on these catecholamine receptors can be selective for alpha, whereas others block only beta receptors. This distinction can be therapeutically useful. For example, beta receptors tend to stimulate the heart, while alpha receptors constrict blood vessels; thus, a drug that selectively affects beta receptors can be used to treat heart ailments without directly altering the state of the blood vessels.

Dopamine As has been mentioned, dopamine is a catecholamine transmitter that is particularly influenced by drugs of abuse (Koob 1992; Uhl et al. 1992; Uhl et al. 1993). Most, if not all, drugs that elevate mood, have abuse potential, or cause psychotic behavior enhance the activity of dopamine in some way, particularly in brain regions associated with limbic structures and mental states. In addition, dopamine is an important transmitter in controlling movement and fine muscle activity, as well as endocrine functions. Thus, because many drugs of abuse affect dopamine neurons, they can also alter all these functions.

Serotonin Serotonin (5-hydroxytryptamine, or 5HT) is synthesized in neurons and elsewhere (for example, in the gastrointestinal tract and platelet-type blood cells) from the dietary source of tryptophan. Tryptophan is an essential amino acid, meaning that humans do not have the ability to synthesize it and must obtain it through diet. Like the catecholamines, serotonin is degraded by the enzyme monoamine oxidase; thus, drugs that alter this enzyme affect levels of not only the catecholamines but also serotonin.

Serotonin is also found in the upper brain stem, which connects the brain and the spinal cord (see Figure 6.6). Axons from serotonergic neurons are distributed throughout the entire central nervous system. Serotonin generally inhibits action on its target neurons. One important role of the

---

Figure 6.6

Functional components of the central nervous system. Limbic structures include the hypothalamus, thalamus, medial forebrain bundle and frontal lobe of the cerebrum and are important for controlling mental states.

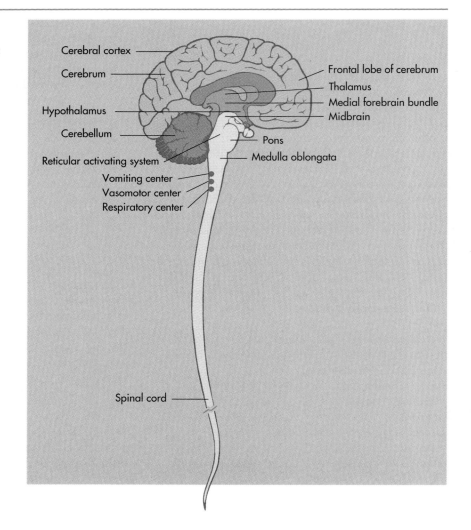

Cerebral cortex
Cerebrum
Hypothalamus
Cerebellum
Reticular activating system
Vomiting center
Vasomotor center
Respiratory center
Frontal lobe of cerebrum
Thalamus
Medial forebrain bundle
Midbrain
Pons
Medulla oblongata
Spinal cord

serotonergic neurons is to prevent overreaction to various stimuli, which can cause aggressiveness, excessive motor activity, exaggerated mood swings, insomnia, and abnormal sexual behavior. Serotonergic neurons also help regulate the release of hormones from the hypothalamus.

Alterations in serotonergic neurons, serotonin synthesis, and degradation have been proposed to be factors in mental illness and to contribute to the side effects of many drugs of abuse. In support of this hypothesis is the fact that drugs such as psilocybin and LSD, which have serotonin-like chemical structures, are frequently abused because of their hallucinogenic properties and can cause psychotic effects (see Chapter 13).

◢ Major Divisions of the Nervous System

The nervous system can be divided into two major components: the central (**CNS**) and peripheral (**PNS**) nervous systems. The CNS consists of the brain and spinal cord (see Figure 6.6), which receive information through the input nerves of the PNS. This sensory information allows the CNS to evaluate the specific status of all organs and the general status of the body. After receiving and processing this information, the CNS reacts by regulating muscle and organ activity through the output nerves of the PNS (Lefkowitz, Hoffman, and Taylor 1995).

CNS
the central nervous system, including the brain and spinal cord

PNS
the peripheral nervous system, including neurons outside the CNS

The PNS comprises neurons whose cell bodies or axons are located outside the brain or spinal cord. It consists of input and output nerves to the CNS. The PNS input to the brain and spinal cord conveys sensory information such as pain, pressure, and temperature, while its output activities are separated into somatic types (control of voluntary muscles) and autonomic types (control of unconscious functions, such as essential organ and gland activity).

The Central Nervous System

The human brain is an integrating (information-processing) and storage device unequaled by the most complex computers. Not only can it handle a great deal of information simultaneously from the senses, but it can evaluate and modify the response to the information rapidly. Although the brain weighs only 3 pounds, its over 10 billion neurons give it the potential to perform a multitude of functions. The following are some important brain regions influenced by drugs of abuse.

The Reticular Activating System The reticular activating system (RAS) is an area of the brain that receives input from all the sensory systems as well as from the cerebral cortex. The RAS is at the junction of the spinal cord and the brain (see Figure 6.6). One of the major functions of the RAS is to control the brain's state of arousal (sleep versus awake).

Because of its complex, diffuse network structure, the RAS is very susceptible to the effects of drugs. The RAS is sensitive to the effects of LSD, potent stimulants such as cocaine and amphetamines, and CNS depressants such as alcohol and barbiturates.

Norepinephrine and acetylcholine are important neurotransmitters in the RAS. High levels of epinephrine, norepinephrine, or stimulant drugs, such as amphetamines, activate the RAS. In contrast, drugs that block the actions of another transmitter, acetylcholine, called **anticholinergic** drugs (for example, antihistamines), suppress RAS activity, causing sleepiness.

anticholinergic
agents that antagonize the effects of acetylcholine

The Basal Ganglia The basal ganglia are the primary centers for involuntary and fine-tuning of motor functions involving, for example, posture and muscle tone. Two important neurotransmitters in the basal ganglia are dopamine and acetylcholine. Damage to neurons in this area may cause Parkinson's disease, the progressive yet selective degeneration of the main dopaminergic neurons in the basal ganglia.

A close association exists between control of motor abilities and control of mental states. Both functions rely heavily on the activity of dopamine-releasing neurons. Consequently, drugs that affect dopamine activity usually alter both systems, resulting in undesired side effects. For example, heavy use of tranquilizers (such as Thorazine, Stelazine, and so on) in the treatment of psychotic patients produces Parkinson-like symptoms. If such drugs are administered daily over several years, problems with motor functioning may become permanent. Drugs of abuse, such as stimulants, increase dopamine activity, causing enhanced motor activity as well as psychotic behavior.

The Limbic System   The limbic system includes an assortment of linked brain regions located near and including the hypothalamus (see Figure 6.6). Besides the hypothalamus, the limbic structures include the thalamus, medial forebrain bundle, and front portion of the cerebral cortex. Functions of the limbic and basal ganglia structures are inseparably linked; drugs that affect one system often affect the other as well.

The primary roles of limbic brain regions include regulating emotional activities (such as fear, rage, and anxiety), memory, modulation of basic hypothalamic functions (such as endocrine activity), and activities such as mating, procreation, and caring for the young. In addition, reward centers are also believed to be associated with limbic structures. It is almost certain that the mood-elevating effects of drugs of abuse are mediated by the limbic systems of the brain.

For example, studies have shown that most stimulant drugs of abuse (such as amphetamines and cocaine) are self-administered by laboratory animals through a cannula surgically placed into limbic structures (such as the medial forebrain bundle and frontal cerebral cortex). This self administration is achieved by linking injection of the drug into the cannula with a lever press by the animal (Koob and Bloom 1988). It is thought that the euphoria or intense "highs" associated with these drugs result from their effects on these brain regions. Some of the limbic system's principal transmitters include dopamine, norepinephrine,

and serotonin; dopamine activation appears to be the primary reinforcement that accounts for the abuse liability of most drugs (Koob and Bloom 1988; Uhl et al. 1993).

The Cerebral Cortex   The unique features of the human cerebral cortex gives humans a special place among animals. The cortex is a layer of gray matter made up of nerves and supporting cells that almost completely surrounds the rest of the brain and lies immediately under the skull (see Figure 6.6). It is responsible for receiving sensory input, interpreting incoming information, and initiating voluntary motor behavior. Many psychoactive drugs, such as psychedelics, dramatically alter the perception of sensory information by the cortex and cause hallucinations that result in strange behavior.

The part of the cortex that has developed most in the evolutionary process is called the *association cortex*. The association areas of the brain do not directly receive input from the environment, nor do they directly initiate output to the muscles or the glands. Instead, these cortical areas may store memories, control complex behaviors, and help to process information. Some psychoactive drugs disrupt the normal functioning of these areas and thereby interfere with an individual's ability to deal with complex issues.

The Hypothalamus   The hypothalamus (see Figures 6.6 and 6.7) is located near the base of the brain. It integrates information from many sources and serves as the CNS control center for the *autonomic nervous system* and many vital support functions. It also serves as the primary point of contact between the nervous and the endocrine systems. Because the hypothalamus controls the autonomic nervous system, it is responsible for maintaining homeostasis in the body; thus, drugs that alter its function can have a major impact on systems that control homeostasis. The catecholamine transmitters are particularly important in regulating the function of the hypothalamus, and most drugs of abuse that alter the activity of norepinephrine and dopamine are likely to alter the activity of this brain structure.

Figure 6.7

Pathways of the parasympathetic and sympathetic nervous systems and the organs affected.

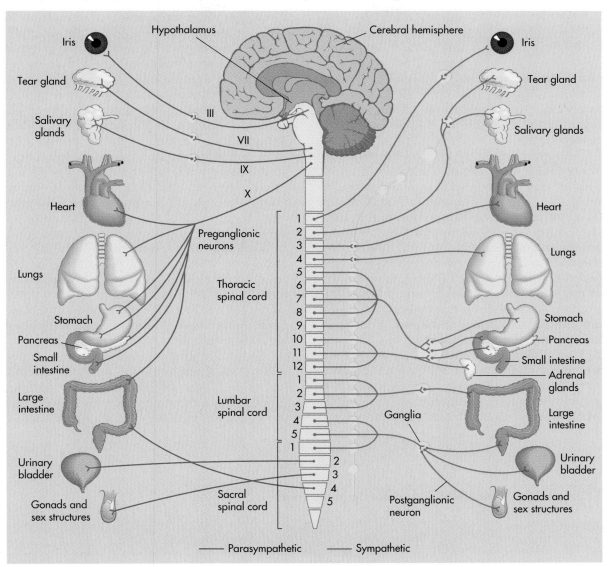

The Autonomic Nervous System

Although the cell bodies of the neurons of the **autonomic nervous system (ANS)** are located within the brain or spinal cord, their axons project outside of the CNS to involuntary muscles, organs, and glands; thus the ANS is considered part of the PNS. The ANS is an integrative, or regulatory, system that does not require conscious control (that is, you do not have to think about it to make it function). It is usually considered primarily a motor or output system. A number of

autonomic nervous system (ANS)

controls the unconscious functions of the body

drugs that cannot enter the CNS because of the blood–brain barrier are able to affect the ANS only. The ANS is divided into two functional components, the sympathetic and the parasympathetic nervous systems (Lefkowitz, Hoffman, and Taylor 1995). Both systems include neurons that project to most visceral organs and to smooth muscles, glands, and blood vessels (see Figure 6.7).

The two components of the ANS generally have opposite effects on an organ or its function. The working of the heart is a good example of sympathetic and parasympathetic control. Stimulation of the parasympathetic nervous system slows the heart rate, whereas stimulation of the sympathetic nerves accelerates it. These actions constitute a constant biological check-and-balance, or regulatory system. Because the two parts of the ANS work in opposite ways much of the time, they are considered physiological antagonists. These two systems control most of the internal organs, the circulatory system, and the secretory (glandular) system. The sympathetic system is normally active at all times; the degree of activity varies from moment to moment and from organ to organ. The parasympathetic nervous system is organized mainly for limited, focused activity and usually conserves and restores energy rather than expends it. For example, it slows the heart rate, lowers blood pressure, aids in absorption of nutrients, and is involved in emptying the urinary bladder. Table 6.2 lists the structures and/or functions of the sympathetic and parasympathetic nervous systems and their effects on one another.

The two branches of the autonomic nervous system use two different neurotransmitters. The parasympathetic branch releases acetylcholine at its synapses, whereas the sympathetic neurons release norepinephrine. An increase in epinephrine in the blood or the administration of drugs that mimic norepinephrine causes the body to respond as if the sympathetic nervous system had been activated. As previously mentioned, such drugs are referred to as *sympathomimetics*. Thus, taking amphetamines (which enhances the sympathetic nervous system by releasing norepinephrine and epinephrine) raises blood pressure, speeds up heart rate, slows down motility of the stomach walls, and may cause the pupils of the eyes to enlarge; other so-called "uppers," like cocaine, have similar effects.

Drugs that affect acetylcholine release, metabolism, or its interaction with its respective receptor are referred to as *cholinergic* drugs. They can either mimic or antagonize the parasympathetic nervous system, according to their pharmacological action.

Table 6.2   **Sympathetic and Parasympathetic Control**

Structure or Function	Sympathetic	Parasympathetic
Heart rate	Speeds up	Slows
Breathing rate	Speeds up	Slows
Stomach wall	Slows motility	Increases
Skin blood vessels (vasomotor function)	Constricts	Dilates
Iris of eye	Constricts (pupil enlarges)	Dilates
Vomiting center	Stimulates	—

◣ The Endocrine System and Drugs

The endocrine system consists of glands, which are ductless (meaning that they secrete directly into the bloodstream) and release chemical substances called **hormones** (see Figure 6.8). These hormones are essential in regulating many vital functions, including metabolism, growth, tissue repair, and sexual behavior, to mention just a few. In contrast to neurotransmitters, hormones tend to have a slower onset and a longer duration of action with a more generalized target. Although a number of tissues are capable of producing and releasing hormones, three of the principal sources of these chemical messengers are the pituitary gland, the adrenal glands, and the sex glands.

hormones

regulatory chemicals released by endocrine systems

Endocrine Glands and Regulation

The pituitary gland is often referred to as the *master gland.* It controls many of the other glands that make up the endocrine system by releasing regulating factors and growth hormone. Besides controlling the brain functions already mentioned, the hypothalamus helps control the activity of the pituitary gland and thereby has a very prominent effect on the endocrine system.

The adrenal glands are located near the kidneys and are divided into two parts: the outer surface, called the *cortex,* and the inner part, called the *medulla.* The adrenal medulla is actually a component of the sympathetic nervous system and releases adrenaline (another name for *epinephrine*) during sympathetic stimulation. Other important hormones released by the adrenal cortex are called *corticosteroids,* or frequently just **steroids.** Steroids help the body to respond appropriately to crises and stress. In addition, small

---

Figure 6.8

Examples of some glands in the endocrine system

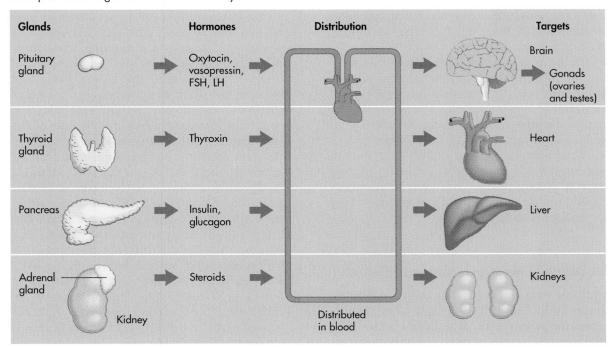

Glands	Hormones	Distribution	Targets
Pituitary gland	Oxytocin, vasopressin, FSH, LH		Brain / Gonads (ovaries and testes)
Thyroid gland	Thyroxin		Heart
Pancreas	Insulin, glucagon		Liver
Adrenal gland / Kidney	Steroids	Distributed in blood	Kidneys

steroids

hormones related to the corticosteroids released from the adrenal cortex

androgens

male sex hormones

amounts of male sex hormones, called **androgens,** are also released by the adrenal cortex. The androgens produce anabolic effects that increase the retention and synthesis of proteins, causing growth in the mass of tissues such as muscles and bones.

Sex glands are responsible for the secretion of male and female sex hormones that help regulate the development and activity of the respective reproductive systems. The organs known as *gonads* include the female ovaries and the male testes. The activity of the gonads is regulated by hormones released from the pituitary gland (see Figure 6.8) and, for the most part, remains suppressed until puberty. After activation, estrogens and progesterones are released from the ovaries and the androgens (principally testosterone) are released from the testes. These hormones are responsible for the development and maintenance of the secondary sex characteristics. They influence not only sex-related body features but also emotional states, suggesting that these sex hormones enter the brain and significantly affect the functioning of the limbic systems.

For the most part, drugs prescribed to treat endocrine problems are intended as replacement therapy. For example, diabetic patients suffer from a shortage of insulin produced by the pancreas, so therapy consists of insulin injections. Patients who suffer from dwarfism receive insufficient growth hormone from the pituitary gland; thus, growth hormone is administered to stimulate normal growth. Because some hormones can affect growth, muscle development, and behavior, they are sometimes abused.

The Abuse of Hormones: Anabolic Steroids

Androgens are the hormones most likely to be abused in the United States (Karch 1996). Testosterone, the primary natural androgen, is produced by the testes. Naturally produced androgens are essential for normal growth and development of male sex organs as well as secondary sex characteristics such as male hair patterns, voice changes, muscular development, and fat distribution. The androgens are also necessary for appropriate growth spurts during adolescence (*Drug Facts and Comparisons* 1996). Accepted therapeutic use of the androgens is usually for replacement in males with abnormally functioning testes. In such cases, the androgens are administered before puberty and for prolonged periods during puberty to stimulate proper male development.

Androgens clearly have an impressive effect on development of tissue (Karch 1996); in particular, they cause pronounced growth of muscle mass and a substantial increase in body weight in young men with deficient testes function. Because of these effects, androgens are classified as **anabolic** (able to stimulate the conversion of nutrients into tissue mass) steroids (they are chemically similar to the steroids).

anabolic steroids

compounds chemically like the steroids that stimulate production of tissue mass

In addition, many athletes and trainers have assumed that, in very high doses, androgens can enhance muscle growth above that achieved by normal testicular function. This conclusion is supported by a recent study that reported that high doses of testosterone for six weeks increased muscle size and strength in both exercising and nonexercising men (Bhasin 1996). Because of this effect, male and female athletes, as well as nonathletes who are into body building, have been attracted to these drugs in hopes of enlarging muscle size and improving their athletic performances and their physiques. Although the androgens might produce some of the desired anabolic effects, they also cause unwanted sex changes. Evidence is mounting that they can create undesirable changes in liver, reproductive system, skin, cardiovascular system, and psychological makeup of the user (*Drug Facts and Comparisons* 1996; Karch 1996). (See "Case in Point," page 153.) The abuse of anabolic steroids by athletes is discussed in greater detail in Chapter 16.

In the 1950s, weight lifters began using androgens to build muscle mass and increase strength as well as improve their physiques. Today, steroid use is widespread throughout all sports, at all levels of competition, and among all ages. Concern about the use of steroids has grown as publicity about the problem has increased.

Neither the short- nor long-term effects of androgen abuse are completely understood (Karch 1996). Nonetheless, many anecdotal stories are told in locker rooms of athletes who experienced dramatic increases in muscle size and strength because of steroid use. Certainly, such testimonials have enhanced the demand for these hormones, whether obtained legally or illegally (Wilson 1990).

The risks caused by androgens are not well understood either (Karch 1996). Most certainly, the higher the doses and the longer the use, the greater the potential damage these drugs can do to the body. However, not everyone involved in sports is convinced that steroid use is dangerous and should be outlawed. Some professional sports trainers even claim that low-dose, intermittent use can enhance athletic performance while causing no health risk (*Morning Edition* 1991).

Several studies have demonstrated that anabolic hormones particularly affect the limbic structures of the brain. Consequently, these drugs can cause excitation and a sense of superior strength and performance in some users. These effects, coupled with increased aggressiveness, could encourage continual use of these drugs. Other CNS effects, however, may be disturbing to the user. Symptoms that may occur with very high doses include uncontrolled rage (referred to as "roid rage"), headaches, anxiety, insomnia, and perhaps paranoia (*Drug Facts and Comparisons* 1996; Karch 1996).

The medical community has become very concerned about the inappropriate use of androgens. Attempts have been made to prevent abuse by implementing education programs, drug screening, and associated penalties when rules are violated. To help prevent abuse, anabolic steroids were classified as controlled drugs by the Drug Enforcement Administration (DEA). The Anabolic Steroids Control Act of 1990 placed these drugs

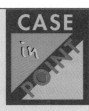

The Risks of Nonmedical Use of Anabolic Steroids

CASE in POINT

A 37-year-old nonsmoking weight lifter was rushed to an emergency room with chest pains, sweating, and shortness of breath, which began midway through his lifting exercises. Although he had a negative medical history, he had used anabolic steroids off and on for seven years. A physical exam revealed normal blood pressure, but his EKG suggested a heart attack accounted for his symptoms (Ferenchick and Adelman 1992). ■

into Schedule III of the Controlled Substances Act, effective February 27, 1991. This act requires anyone who distributes or dispenses anabolic steroids to be registered with the DEA. Persons distributing androgens who are not properly authorized can be imprisoned for not more than five years and be required to pay fines as deemed appropriate. If the offense involves providing drugs to an individual under 18 years of age, the violation is punishable by not more than ten years in prison.

Because of concerns about the effects and detection of anabolic steroids, many athletes are turning to other drugs to enhance their competitive performance by stimulating the endocrine systems. These alternatives include "human growth factor," *erythropoietin,* and *gamma-hydroxybutyrate (GHB);* they are discussed in Chapter 16.

◢ Conclusion

All psychoactive drugs affect brain activity by altering the ability of neurons to send and receive messages. Consequently, drugs of abuse exert their addicting effects by stimulating or blocking the activity of CNS neurotransmitters or their receptors. Thus, to understand why these drugs are abused and the nature of their dependence, you need to study how neurons and their neurotransmitter systems function. In addition, many scientists believe that elucidating how substances of abuse affect nervous systems will lead to new and more effective methods for treating drug addiction.

REVIEW QUESTIONS

1. How are neurotransmitters and hormones alike, and how are they different?

2. Why is it important for the body to have chemical messengers that can be quickly released and rapidly inactivated?

3. Why are "receptors" so important in understanding the effects of drugs of abuse?

4. Why do many drugs of abuse affect motor behavior?

5. What are some mechanisms whereby a drug of abuse can increase the activity of dopamine transmitter systems in the brain?

6. Some drugs of abuse are described as "sympathomimetics" and some as "anticholinergic." What features distinguish these two pharmacological properties?

7. Was classifying anabolic steroids as Schedule III drugs justified? What do you think will be the long-term consequence of this action?

KEY TERMS

homeostasis
neurotransmitters
neurons
receptors
axons
psychoactive
synapse
synaptic cleft
dendrites
opiate receptors
endorphins
agonistic
antagonistic
muscarinic
nicotinic
catecholamines
sympathomimetic
CNS
PNS
anticholinergic
autonomic nervous system (ANS)
hormones
steroids
androgens
anabolic steroids

SUMMARY

1 The nervous and endocrine systems help mediate internal and external responses to the body's surroundings. Both systems release chemical messengers in order to achieve their homeostatic functions. These messenger substances are called *neurotransmitters* and *hormones,* and they exert their functions through receptors. Many drugs exert their effects by influencing these chemical messengers.

2 The neuron is the principal cell type in the nervous system. This specialized cell consists of dendrites, a cell body, and an axon. It communicates with other neurons and organs by releasing neurotransmitters, which can cause either excitation or inhibition at their target sites.

EXERCISES FOR THE WEB

Exercise 1: COHIS

Boston University Medical Center Community Outreach Health Information System has a variety of links associated with maintaining positive health. Pharmacological and/or psychological effects of a particular drug may be ascertained.

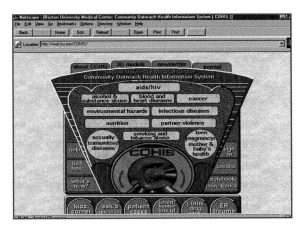

Exercise 2: PharmInfo

PharmInfoNet is a high-volume pharmaceutical information resource on the Internet World Wide Web. This source serves as a recognized entry point to access high-quality, independent assessments of therapeutics and advances in new drug development. Regulatory and clinical users access diverse information through PharmInfoNet, including full text articles from clinical publications, economic data, symposium information from scientific meetings, and can benefit from links to other relevant drug information and pharmaceutical sites. The Pharmaceutical Information Network provides the reader with up-to-date information about medications that they may take.

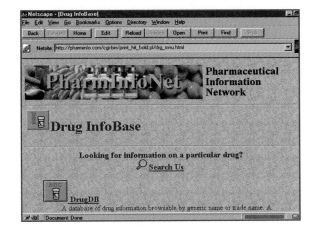

3 The chemical messengers from glands and neurons exert their effects by interacting with special protein regions in membranes called *receptors*. Because of their unique structures, receptors interact only with molecules that have specific configurations. Activation of receptors can initiate a chain of events within cells, resulting in changes in gene expression, enzyme activity, or metabolic function.

4 *Agonists* are substances or drugs that stimulate receptors. *Antagonists* are substances or drugs that attach to receptors and prevent them from being activated.

5 A variety of different substances are used as neurotransmitters by neurons in the body. The classes of transmitters include the catecholamines, serotonin, acetylcholine, GABA, and peptides. These transmitters are excitatory, inhibitory, or sometimes both, depending on which receptor is being activated. Many drugs selectively act to either enhance or antagonize these neurotransmitters and their activities.

6 The central nervous system consists of the brain and spinal cord. Regions within the brain help to regulate specific functions. The hypothalamus controls endocrine and basic body functions. The basal ganglia are primarily responsible for controlling motor activity. The limbic system regulates mood and mental states. The cerebral cortex helps interpret, process, and respond to input information.

7 The limbic system and its associated transmitters, especially dopamine, are a major site of action for the drugs of abuse. Substances that increase the activity of dopamine cause a sense of well-being and euphoria, which encourages psychological dependence.

8 The autonomic nervous system is composed of the sympathetic and parasympathetic systems; neurons associated with these systems release noradrenalin and acetylcholine as their transmitters, respectively. These systems work in an antagonistic fashion to control unconscious, visceral functions such as breathing and cardiovascular activity. The parasympathetic nervous system usually helps conserve and restore energy in the body, while the sympathetic nervous system is continually active.

9 The endocrine system consists of glands that synthesize and release hormones into the blood. Distribution via blood circulation carries these chemical messengers throughout the body, where they act on specific receptors. Some of the principal structures include the pituitary, adrenals, and gonads (testes and ovaries).

10 Anabolic steroids are structurally related to the male hormone testosterone. They are often abused by both male and female athletes trying to build muscle mass and enhance performance. The continual use of high doses of anabolic steroids can cause annoying and dangerous side effects. The long-term effects of low, intermittent doses of these drugs have not been determined. Because of concerns voiced by most medical authorities, anabolic steroids are controlled substances and have been classified as Schedule III substances.

REFERENCES

Bhasin, S., et al. "The Effects of Supraphysiologic Doses of Testosterone on Muscle Size and Strength in Normal Men." *New England Journal of Medicine* 335 (1996): 1–7.

Bloom, F. "Neurotransmission and the Central Nervous System." In *The Pharmacological Basis of Therapeutics,* 9th ed., edited by J. Harman and T. Limbird, 267–93. New York: McGraw-Hill, 1995.

Drug Facts and Comparisons. St. Louis: Lippincott, 1996.

Federal Register 56 (13 February 1991): 3754.

Ferenchick, G., and S. Adelman. "Myocardial Infarction Associated with Anabolic Steroid Use in a Previously Healthy 37-Year-Old Weight Lifter." *American Heart Journal* 124 (August 1992): 507–8.

Goldstein, A. *Addiction from Biology to Drug Policy,* 15–60. New York: Freeman, 1994.

Hobbs, W., T. Rall, and T. Verdoorn. "Hypnotics and Sedatives; Ethanol." In *The Pharmacological Basis of Therapeutics,* 9th ed., edited by J. Hardman and T. Limbird, 361–96. New York: McGraw-Hill, 1995.

Karch, S. "Anabolic Steroids." In *The Pathology of Drug Abuse,* 2nd ed., 409–29. New York: CRC, 1996.

Koob, G. "Drugs of Abuse: Anatomy, Pharmacology and Function of Reward Pathways." *Trends in Pharmacologic Sciences* 13 (1992): 177–84.

Koob, G., and F. Bloom. "Cellular and Molecular Mechanisms of Drug Dependence." *Science* 242 (1988): 715–23.

Lefkowitz, R., B. Hoffman, and P. Taylor. "Neurotransmission, the Autonomic and Somatic Motor Nervous Systems." In *The Pharmacological Basis of Therapeutics,* 9th ed., edited by J. Hardman and T. Limbird, 361–96. New York: McGraw-Hill, 1995.

Linder, M., and A. Gilman. "G Proteins." *Scientific American* (July 1992): 56–65.

Morning Edition. "Sports and Drugs" Series on National Public Radio (14 January 1991, 10 A.M.).

O'Brien, C. "Drug Addiction and Drug Abuse." In *The Pharmacological Basis of Therapeutics,* 9th ed., edited by J. Hardman and T. Limbird, 557–77. New York: McGraw-Hill, 1995.

Pope, H., and D. Katz. "What Are the Psychiatric Risks of Anabolic Steroids?" *Harvard Mental Health Letter* 7 (April 1991): 8.

Snyder, S. H. "Opiate Receptors in the Brain." *New England Journal of Medicine* 296 (1977): 266–71.

Uhl, G., K. Blum, E. Noble, and S. Smith. "Substance Abuse Vulnerability and D-2 Receptor Genes." *Trends in Neurological Sciences* 16 (1993): 83–7.

Uhl, G., A. Persico, and S. Smith. "Current Excitement with D-2 Dopamine Receptor Gene Alleles in Substance Abuse." *Archives of General Psychiatry* 49 (1992): 157–60.

Wilson, J. "Androgens." In *The Pharmacological Basis of Therapeutics,* 8th ed., edited by A. Gilman, T. Rall, A. Nies, and P. Taylor, 1413–30. New York: Plenum, 1990.

CNS Depressants:
Sedative-Hypnotics

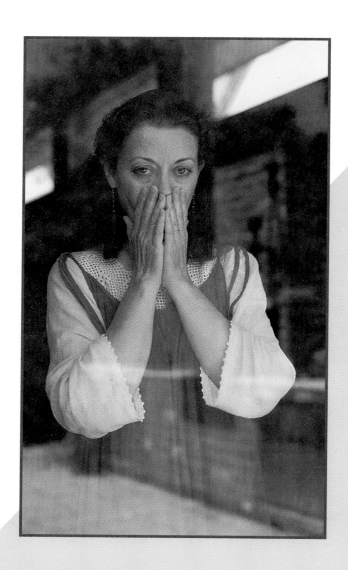

On completing this chapter
you will be able to:

- Alcohol temporarily relieves anxiety and stress because of its CNS depressant effects.
- At low doses a CNS depressant relieves anxiety, and at high doses it becomes a sleep aid.
- The Valium-like benzodiazepines are much safer drugs than the barbiturates.
- Benzodiazepines are by far the most frequently prescribed CNS depressants.

- Most people dependent on benzodiazepines obtain their drugs legally by prescription.
- Long-term users of Valium can experience severe withdrawal symptoms if drug use is stopped abruptly.
- Our bodies probably produce a natural antianxiety substance that is similar to Valium.

- Antihistamines are the principal active ingredients in OTC sleep aids.
- The short-acting CNS depressants are the most likely to be abused.
- GHB (gamma hydroxy butyrate) is a substance naturally present in the body that has been used to treat alcoholism.

Learning Objectives

- Identify the primary drug groups used for CNS depressant effects.
- Explain the principal therapeutic uses of the CNS depressants and how the effects relate to drug dose.
- Explain why CNS depressant drugs are commonly abused.
- Identify the differences and similarities between benzodiazepines and barbiturates.

- Relate how benzodiazepine dependence usually develops.
- Describe the differences in effects between short- and long-acting CNS depressants.
- Describe the CNS depressant properties of antihistamines, and compare their therapeutic usefulness to that of benzodiazepines.

- List the four principal types of people who abuse CNS depressants.
- Identify the basic principles in treating dependence on CNS depressants.
- Explain why GHB is considered to be an alcohol substitute.

Central nervous system (CNS) depressants are some of the most widely used and abused drugs in the United States. Why? With low doses they all produce a qualitatively similar "high" by their disinhibitory effects on the brain. In addition, they relieve stress and anxiety and even induce sleep—effects that appeal to many people, particularly those who are struggling with problems and looking for a break, physically and emotionally. CNS depressants also can cause a host of serious side effects, including problems with tolerance and dependence. Ironically, many individuals who become dependent on depressants obtain them through legitimate means: a prescription given by a physician. In fact, homemakers are often prone to this type of drug abuse. Depressants are also available "on the street," although this illicit source is not the bulk of the problem.

In this chapter, we briefly review the history of CNS depressants, in terms of both development and use, and then discuss the positive and negative effects these drugs can produce. Each of the major types of depressant drugs are then reviewed in detail: *benzodiazepines* (Valium-like drugs), *barbiturates,* and other *minor* categories. We conclude with an examination of abuse patterns of depressant drugs, and discuss how drug dependence and withdrawal are treated.

◢ An Introduction to CNS Depressants

Henry (not his real name) lived with his wife and two children. He claimed to be a nonsmoker and denied any use of illegal drugs; however, he did have a history of daily coffee consumption and admitted to occasionally consuming moderate amounts of alcohol. Despite no history of mental illness, his behavior changed over the course of several months—he experienced insomnia, depression, difficulty concentrating, nightmares, irritability, loss of job, and marital discord. His problems culminated one summer afternoon after drinking beer with a friend, when he got into an argument with the manager of his apartment. Acting in an incoherent manner, Henry picked up

a kitchen knife and small hand ax from his apartment, proceeded to the manager's office, and tried to chop down the door, while yelling at both the manager and witnesses in the hallway. He was apprehended by police and charged with criminal behavior. When questioned, Henry had no recollection of the incident. A medical history revealed that he had been prescribed Rivotril (a Valium-type CNS depressant) for insomnia and stress as well as Anafranil (an antidepressant that can cause CNS depression or excitation). Psychotherapists concluded that his aberrant personal and criminal behavior were directly caused by the effects of the prescribed CNS depressants taken in combination with alcohol. Given the conclusions of the clinicians, the city prosecutor offered Henry a plea bargain to reduce the charge to a misdemeanor and a suspended sentence (Pagliaro and Pagliaro 1992).

This actual case study illustrates several reasons why CNS depressants can be problematic. First, in contrast to most other substances of abuse, CNS depressants are usually not obtained illicitly and self-administered but are prescribed under the direction of a physician. Second, use of CNS depressants can cause very alarming, even dangerous behavior if not monitored closely: most problems associated with these drugs occur due to insufficient professional supervision. Third, several seemingly unrelated drug groups have some ability to cause CNS depression. When these drugs are combined, bizarre and dangerous interactions can result (see Chapter 5 for a discussion on drug interactions). Particularly problematic is the combination of alcohol with other CNS depressants. Finally, CNS depressants can cause disruptive personality changes that are unpredictable and sometimes very threatening.

This chapter will help you to understand the nature of the CNS depressant effects experienced by Henry as well as other important features of these drugs. In addition, the similarities and differences among the commonly prescribed CNS depressant drugs are discussed.

The History of CNS Depressants

Before the era of modern drugs, the most common depressant used to ease tension, cause relaxation, and help people forget their problems was alcohol. These effects undoubtedly accounted for the immense popularity of alcohol and help explain why this traditional depressant is the most commonly abused drug of all time. (Alcohol is discussed in detail in Chapters 8 and 9.)

Attempts to find CNS depressants other than alcohol that could be used to treat nervousness and anxiety began in the 1800s with the introduction of bromides. These drugs were very popular until their toxicities became known. In the early 1900s, bromides were replaced by **barbiturates.**

barbiturates

potent CNS depressants, usually not preferred because of their narrow margin of safety

Like bromides, barbiturates were initially heralded as safe and effective depressants; however, problems with tolerance, dependence, and lethal overdoses became evident. It was learned that the doses of barbiturates required to treat anxiety also could cause CNS depression, affecting respiration and impairing mental functions (Hobbs, Rall, and Verdoorn 1995). The margin of safety for barbiturates was too narrow, so research for a safer CNS depressant began again.

It was not until the 1950s that the first **benzodiazepines** were marketed as substitutes for the dangerous barbiturates. Benzodiazepines were originally viewed as extremely safe and free from the problems of tolerance, dependence, and withdrawal that occurred with the other drugs in this category (Mondanaro 1988). Unfortunately, benzodiazepines also have been found to be less than ideal antianxiety drugs. Although relatively safe when

benzodiazepines

the most popular and safest CNS depressants in use today

used for short periods, long-term use can cause dependence and withdrawal problems much like those associated with their depressant predecessors. These problems have become a major concern of the medical community, as will be discussed in greater detail later in the chapter.

Many of the people who become dependent on CNS depressants such as benzodiazepines began

using the drugs under the supervision of a physician. Some clinicians routinely prescribe CNS depressants for cases of stress, anxiety, or apprehension, without trying nonpharmacological approaches, such as psychotherapy or counseling. This practice sends an undesirable and often detrimental message to patients—that is, CNS depressants are a simple solution to their complex, stressful problems. The following quote illustrates the danger of this practice:

> I am still, unfortunately, lost in "script addiction." . . . I have gone on-line asking for pills. I could really identify with the one posting about doctors who continue to write the 'scripts to increase/continue the patient "flow." This is exactly what is happening with me and my doctor. (From American Online Alcohol and Drug Dependency and Recovery message board)

Consequently, during the 1970s and 1980s, there was an epidemic of prescriptions for CNS depressants. For example, in 1973 100 million prescriptions were written for benzodiazepines alone. Approximately twice as many women as men were taking these drugs at this time; a similar gender pattern continues today. Many homemakers made CNS depressants a part of their household routine, as described in the lyrics of the rock song "Mother's Little Helper" on the Rolling Stones' album *Flowers:*

> Things are different today
> I hear every mother say
> "Mother needs something today to calm her
>   down"
> And though she's not really ill,
> There's a little yellow pill.
> She goes running for the shelter
> Of her "mother's little helper"
> And it helps her on her way,
> Gets her through her busy day.

As the medical community became more aware of the problem, the use of depressants declined ("Top 200 drugs, total Rxs" 1997). Today, efforts are again being made by pharmaceutical companies and scientists to find new classes of CNS depressants that can be used to relieve stress and anxiety without causing serious side effects such as dependence and withdrawal.

The Effects of CNS Depressants: Benefits and Risks

The CNS depressants are a diverse group of drugs that share an ability to reduce CNS activity and diminish the brain's level of awareness. Besides the benzodiazepines, barbiturate-like drugs, and alcohol, depressant drugs also include **antihistamines** and opioid narcotics like heroin (see Chapter 10).

> **antihistamines**
> drugs used to treat allergies that often cause CNS depression

Depressants are usually classified according to the degree of their medical effects on the body. For instance, **sedatives** cause mild depression of the CNS and relaxation. This drug effect is used to treat extreme anxiety and often is referred to as **anxiolytic.**

> **sedatives**
> CNS depressants used to relieve anxiety, fear, and apprehension

CNS depressants can be used as hypnotics to initiate sleep.

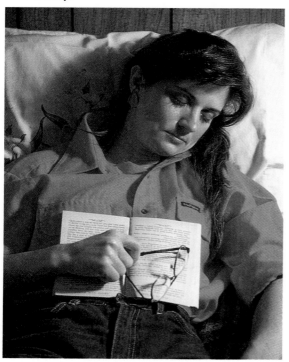

> **anxiolytics**
> drugs that relieve anxiety

Many sedatives also have muscle-relaxing properties that enhance their relaxing effects.

Depressants are also used to promote sleep. **Hypnotics** (from the Greek god of sleep, Hypnos) are CNS depressants that encourage sleep by inducing drowsiness. Often when depressants are used as hypnotics, they produce **amnesiac** effects as well. As already mentioned, the effects produced by depressants can be very enticing and encourage inappropriate use.

> **hypnotics**
> CNS depressants used to induce drowsiness and encourage sleep
>
> **amnesiac**
> causing the loss of memory

The effects of the CNS depressants tend to be dose dependent (see Figure 7.1). Thus, if you were to take a larger dose of a sedative, it might have a hypnotic effect. Often the only difference between a sedative and a hypnotic effect is the dosage; consequently, the same drug may be used for both purposes by varying the dose. By increasing the dose still further, an anesthetic state can be reached. **Anesthesia,** a deep depression of the CNS, is used to achieve a controlled state of unconsciousness so a patient can be treated, usually by surgery, in relative comfort and without memory of an unpleasant experience. With the exception of benzodiazepines, if the dose of most of the depressants is increased much more, coma or death will ensue because the CNS becomes so depressed that vital centers controlling breathing and heart activity cease to function properly (*Medical Letter* 1996).

> **anesthesia**
> a state characterized by loss of sensation or consciousness

As a group, CNS depressant drugs used in a persistent fashion cause tolerance. Because of the diminished effect due to the tolerance, users of these drugs continually escalate their doses. Under such conditions, the depressants alter physical and psychological states, resulting in dependence. The dependence can be so severe that abrupt drug abstinence results in severe withdrawals that include life-threatening seizures (American Psychiatric

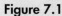

Figure 7.1

Dose-dependent effects of CNS depressants.

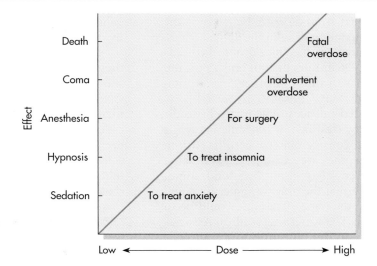

Association 1994). Because of these dangerous pharmacological features, treatment of dependence on CNS depressants must proceed very carefully (Goldstein 1995). This issue is discussed in greater detail at the end of this chapter and in Chapter 5.

Types of CNS Depressants

It is important for you to realize that all CNS depressants are not "created equal." Some have wider margins of safety; others have a greater potential for nonmedicinal abuse. These differences are important when considering the therapeutic advantages of each type of CNS depressant. In addition, unique features of the different types of depressants make them useful for treatment of other medical problems. For example, some barbiturates and benzodiazepines are used to treat forms of epilepsy or acute seizure activity, while opioid narcotics are important in the treatment of many types of pain. Some of these unique features will be dealt with in greater detail when the individual drug groups are discussed. The benzodiazepines, barbiturate-like drugs, antihistamines and the naturally occurring gamma-hydroxybutyrate

(GHB) are discussed in this chapter. Other CNS depressants, such as alcohol and opiates are covered in Chapters 8, 9, and 10.

Benzodiazepines: Valium-Type Drugs

Benzodiazepines are by far the most frequently prescribed CNS depressants for anxiety and sleep. In fact, eight of the top-selling 200 prescription drugs in the United States during 1996 were benzodiazepines; they included Klonopin, Ambien (technically not a benzodiazepine, but related to Xanax), and three generic forms of alprazolam ("Top 200 Drugs" 1997). Because of their wide margin of safety (death from an overdose is rare), benzodiazepines have replaced barbiturate-like drugs for use as sedatives and hypnotics ("Halcion and Other Sleeping Pills" 1992; Goldstein 1995). Benzodiazepines were originally referred to as the *minor tranquilizers,* but this terminology erroneously implied that they had pharmacological properties similar to those of antipsychotic drugs (the *major tranquilizers*), when in fact they are very different. Consequently, the term *minor tranquilizer* is usually avoided by clinicians.

The first true benzodiazepine, Librium, was developed for medical use and marketed about

1960; the very popular drug Valium came on the market about the same time. In fact, Valium was so well received that from 1972 to 1978 it was the top-selling prescription drug in the United States. Its popularity however, has since dropped considerably, and in 1996 its sales did not rank in the top 200 compared with those of other prescription drugs ("Top 200 Drugs" 1997).

Because of dependence problems, the benzodiazepines are now classified as Schedule IV drugs. In recent years, considerable concern has arisen that benzodiazepines are overprescribed because of their perceived safety; it has been said, somewhat facetiously, that the only way a person could die from using the benzodiazpines would be to choke on them. The American Medical Association (AMA) and even consumer organizations ("High Anxiety" 1993) are concerned about this overconfident attitude toward benzodiazepines and have warned patients and doctors against prolonged and unsupervised administration of these drugs.

Medical Uses Benzodiazepines are used for an array of therapeutic objectives, including the relief of anxiety, treatment of neurosis, muscle relaxation, alleviation of lower-back pain, treatment of some convulsive disorders, induction of sleep (hypnotic), relief from withdrawal symptoms associated with narcotic and alcohol dependence, and induction of amnesia usually for preoperative administration (administered just before or during surgery or very uncomfortable medical procedures).

Mechanisms of Action In contrast to barbiturate-type drugs, which cause general depression of most neuronal activity, benzodiazepines selectively affect those neurons that have receptors for the neurotransmitter gamma-aminobutyric acid (GABA) (Hobbs, Rall, and Verdoorn 1995). GABA is a very important inhibitory transmitter in several brain regions: the limbic system, the reticular activating system, and the motor cortex (see Chapter 6). In the presence of benzodiazepines, the inhibitory effects of GABA are increased. Depression of activity in these brain regions likely accounts for the ability of benzodiazepines to alter mood (a limbic function), cause drowsiness (a

reticular activating system function), and relax muscles (a cortical function). The specific GABA-enhancing effect of these drugs explains the selective CNS depression caused by benzodiazepines.

Of considerable interest is the observation that these Valium-like drugs act on specific receptor sites that are linked to the GABA receptors in the CNS. As yet, no endogenous substance has been identified that naturally interacts with this so-called benzodiazepine site. It is very likely, however, that a natural benzodiazepine does exist that activates this same receptor population and serves to reduce stress and anxiety by natural means. Because benzodiazepines have specific target receptors, it has been possible to develop a highly selective antagonist drug, flumazenil (Romazicon). This drug is used to treat benzodiazepine overdoses, but must be used carefully because its administration can precipitate withdrawal in persons taking benzodiazepines (*Medical Letter* 1996).

Types Because benzodiazepines are so popular, and thus profitable, new related drugs are routinely released into the pharmaceutical market. Currently, approximately 14 benzodiazepine compounds are available in the United States.

Benzodiazepines are distinguished primarily by their duration of action (see Table 7.1). As a general rule, the short-acting drugs are used as hypnotics to treat insomnia, thus allowing the user to awake in the morning with few after-effects (such as a hangover). The long-acting benzodiazepines tend to be prescribed as sedatives, giving prolonged relaxation and relief from persistent anxiety. Some of the long-acting drugs can exert a relaxing effect for as long as two to three days. One reason for the long action in some benzodiazepines is that they are converted by the liver into metabolites that are as active as the original drug. For example, Valium (diazepam) has a half-life of 20 to 80 hours and is converted by the liver into several active metabolites, including oxazepam (which itself is marketed as a therapeutic benzodiazepine—see Table 7.1).

Side Effects Reported side effects of benzodiazepines include drowsiness, lightheadedness, lethargy, impairment of mental and physical activ-

Table 7.1	Half-lives of Various Benzodiazepines

Drug	Half-Life (hours)
Alprazolam (Xanax)	12–15
Chlordiazepoxide (Librium)	5–30
Clonazepam (Klonopin)	18–50
Clorazepate (Tranxene)	30–100
Diazepam (Valium)	20–80
Estazolam (Prosom)	10–24
Flurazepam (Dalmane)	2–4
Halazepam (Paxipam)	14
Lorazepam (Ativan)	10–20
Midazolam (Versed)	1–12
Oxazepam (Serax)	5–20
Prazepam (Centrax)	30–100
Quazepam (Doral)	39
Temazepam (Restoril)	10–17
Triazolam (Halcion)	1.5–5.5
Zolpidem (Ambien; not a true benzodiazepine)	2–5

Source: Adapted from W. Hobbs, T. Rall, and T. Verdoorn. "Hypnotics and Sedatives." In *The Pharmacological Basis of Therapeutics,* 9th ed., edited by J. Hardman and L. Limbird, 361–96. New York: McGraw-Hill, 1995.

have less effect on **REM sleep** (rapid eye movement, the restive phase) than do barbiturates. Consequently, sleep under the influence of benzodiazepines is more likely to be restful and satisfying. However, prolonged use of hypnotic doses of benzodiazepines may cause rebound (see Chapter 5) increases in REM sleep and insomnia when the drug is stopped.

> **REM sleep**
> the restive phase of sleep associated with dreaming

On rare occasions, benzodiazepines can have **paradoxical** effects, producing unusual responses such as nightmares, anxiety, irritability, sweating, and restlessness (McEvoy 1994). Bizarre, uninhibited behavior—such as extreme agitation with hostility, paranoia, and rage—may occur as well. One such case was reported in 1988 in Utah. A 63-year-old patient who was taking Halcion (a relatively short-acting benzodiazepine) murdered her 87-year-old mother. The suspect claimed that the murder occurred because of the effects of the drug and that she was innocent of committing a crime. Her defense was successful, and she was acquitted of murder. After her acquittal, the woman initiated a $21 million lawsuit against Upjohn Pharmaceuticals for marketing Halcion, which she claimed is a dangerous drug. The lawsuit was settled out of court for an undisclosed amount. This tragic episode came to a surprising conclusion in 1994 when the daughter committed suicide (Associated Press 1994).

> **paradoxical**
> an unexpected effect

Critics' complaints that Halcion causes unacceptable "amnesia, confusion, paranoia, hostility and seizures" (Associated Press 1994) prompted the FDA to closely evaluate this benzodiazepine. Despite the fact that several other countries have banned Halcion, the FDA concluded that its benefits outweigh the reported risks; however, the FDA also concluded that "In no way should this [the FDA's conclusion] suggest that Halcion is free of side effects. It has long been recognized and emphasized in Halcion's labeling that it is a potent drug that produces the same type of adverse effects as other CNS sedative hypnotic drugs" ("New Halcion Guidelines" 1992; *PDR* 1997). Although the FDA did not require that Halcion be

ities, skin rashes, nausea, diminished libido, irregularities in the menstrual cycle, blood cell abnormalities, and increased sensitivity to alcohol and other CNS depressants (McEvoy 1994). In contrast to barbiturate-type drugs, only very high doses of benzodiazepines have a significant impact on respiration. There are actually few verified instances of death resulting from overdose of benzodiazepines alone (*Medical Letter* 1996).

Almost always, serious suppression of vital functions occurs when these drugs are combined with other depressants, most often alcohol (Hobbs, Rall, and Verdoorn 1995).

There is no clear evidence of permanent, irreversible damage to neurological or other physiological processes, even with long-term benzodiazepine use (Woods et al. 1992). Benzodiazepines

withdrawn, it did negotiate changes in the labeling and package inserts with Halcion's manufacturer, the Upjohn Company. These changes emphasize appropriate Halcion use in treatment of insomnia and additional information about side effects, warnings, and dosage. As a result of these concerns, the sales of Halcion plummeted, causing it to fall from the eighteenth largest-selling prescription drug in 1987 to not even being one of the top 200 most-prescribed drugs in 1995 ("Top 200 Drugs" 1996).

There is no obvious explanation for these strange benzodiazepine-induced behaviors. It is possible that, in some people, the drugs mask inhibitory centers of the brain and allow expression of antisocial behavior that is normally suppressed and controlled.

Related concerns have also been made public about another very popular benzodiazepine, Xanax. In 1990 Xanax became the first drug approved for the treatment of panic disorder (repeated, intense attacks of anxiety that can make life unbearable). Reports that long-term use of Xanax can cause severe withdrawal effects and a stubborn dependency on the drug ("High Anxiety" 1993) have raised public concerns about use of benzodiazepines in general. For example, how many people are severely dependent on these CNS depressants? What is the frequency of side effects such as memory impairment, serious mood swings, and cognitive problems? And how many patients currently using the benzodiazepines would be better served with nondrug psychotherapy? Clearly, use of the benzodiazepines to relieve acute stress or insomnia can be beneficial, but these drugs should be prescribed at the lowest dose possible and for the shortest time possible or withdrawal problems can result, as illustrated in the quote below.

> I was put on alprazolam (Xanax) two and a half years ago by [my] doctor. Now told by another doctor that it is for short-term use only and I am trying to get off slowly, but having difficulty. [I] have never used other drugs and do not have any information on the withdrawal process. (From America Online Alcohol and Drug Dependency and Recovery message board)

Tolerance, Dependence, Withdrawal, and Abuse As with most CNS depressants, frequent, chronic use of benzodiazepines can cause tolerance, dependence (both physical and psychological), and withdrawal (McEvoy 1994). Such side effects are usually not as severe as those of most other depressants, and they occur only after using the drugs for prolonged periods (Hobbs, Rall, and Verdoorn 1995). In addition, for most people the effects of the benzodiazepines are not viewed as reinforcing; thus, compared with other depressants, such as barbiturates, benzodiazepines are not especially addicting (Hobbs, Rall, and Verdoorn 1995; Grinspoon 1996).

Withdrawal can mimic the condition for which the benzodiazepine is given; for example, withdrawal symptoms can include anxiety or insomnia. In such cases, a clinician may be fooled into thinking that the underlying emotional disorder is still present, and may resume drug therapy

---

Table 7.2 Abstinence Symptoms that Occur When Long-term Users of Benzodiazepines Abruptly Stop Taking the Drug

Duration of Abstinence	Symptoms
1–3 days	Often no noticeable symptoms
3–4 days	Restlessness, agitation, headaches, problems in eating, and inability to sleep
4–6 days	The preceding symptoms plus twitching of facial and arm muscles and feeling of intense burning in the skin
6–7 days	The preceding symptoms plus seizures

Source: W. Hobbs, T. Rall, and T. Verdoorn. "Hypnotics and Sedatives." In *The Pharmacological Basis of Therapeutics*, 9th ed., edited by J. Hardman and L. Limbird, 361–96. New York: McGraw-Hill, 1995.

without realizing that the patient has become drug-dependent. In situations where users have consumed high doses of benzodiazepine over the long term, more severe, even life-threatening withdrawal symptoms may occur (Goldstein 1995); depression, panic, paranoia, and convulsions have been reported (see Table 7.2). Severe withdrawal can often be avoided by gradually weaning the patient from the benzodiazepine (Hobbs, Rall, and Verdoorn 1995).

Long-term use of benzodiazepines (periods exceeding three to four months) to treat anxiety or sleep disorders has not been shown to be therapeutically useful for most patients. Even so, this approach is a common indiscriminate practice and has been suggested by some clinicians to be responsible for the largest group of prescription drug-dependent people in the United States. As one user explains:

> I went through a trauma four years ago, and the doctor prescribed a very high dose of Ativan. Well, I soon became addicted, both emotionally and physically . . . How do I get off? . . . This stuff is very addicting and my body can't really function without it. (From America Online Alcohol and Drug Dependency and Recovery message board)

It is very unusual to find nontherapeutic drug-seeking behavior in a patient who has been properly removed from benzodiazepines, unless that individual already has a history of drug abuse. Research has shown that when benzodiazepines are the primary drug of abuse, these CNS depressants are usually self-administered to prevent unpleasant withdrawal symptoms in dependent users. If benzodiazepine-dependent users are properly weaned from the drugs, and withdrawal has dissipated, there is no evidence that craving for the benzodiazepines occurs because people usually do not consider the benzodiazepines particularly pleasant (Woods et al. 1992). An exception to this conclusion appears to be former alcoholics. Many people with a history of alcoholism find the effects of benzodiazepines rewarding; consequently, nearly 21% of prior alcoholics use benzodiazepines chronically (Woods et al. 1992).

Benzodiazepines are commonly used as a secondary drug of abuse and combined with illicit

Temazepam and Drug Addicts

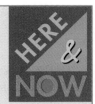

One of the benzodiazepines most frequently used by drug addicts is temazepam, also called *Temazzies* on the street. Stimulant users sometimes turn to Temazzies to get to sleep after a run with their mood enhancer. Hard-core cocaine and crack users turn to Temazzies to soften the crash when the stimulants are gone. Addicts who inject heroin may turn to Temazzies because they cannot afford to *score* (buy heroin) or because their tolerance to narcotics is so high that supplementing their heroin use with temazepam offers a way to regain some of the narcotic effect (McDermott, 1996). ■

drugs (O'Brien 1995) (see "Here and Now" above). For example, narcotic users frequently combine benzodiazepines with weak heroin to enhance the narcotic effect. It is very common to find heroin users who are dependent on depressants as well as narcotics (O'Brien 1995).

Another frequent combination is the use of benzodiazepines with stimulants such as cocaine. Some addicts claim that this combination enhances the pleasant effects of the stimulant and reduces the "crashing" that occurs after using high doses. (More is said about benzodiazepine abuse later in this chapter.)

Barbiturates

Barbiturates are defined as "barbituric acid derivatives used in medicine as sedatives and hypnotics." Barbituric acid was first synthesized by A. Bayer (of aspirin fame) in Germany in 1864. The reason that he chose the name *barbituric acid* is not known. Some have speculated that the compound was named after a girl named Barbara whom

Bayer knew. Others think that Bayer celebrated his discovery on the Day of St. Barbara in a tavern that artillery officers frequented. (St. Barbara is the patron saint of artillery soldiers.)

The first barbiturate, barbital (Veronal), was used medically in 1903. The names of the barbiturates all end in -*al*, indicating a chemical relationship to barbital, the first one synthesized.

Historically, barbiturates have played an important role in therapeutics because of their effectiveness as sedative-hypnotic agents, which allowed them to be routinely used in the treatment of anxiety, agitation, and insomnia. However, because of their narrow margin of safety and their abuse liability, barbiturates have been largely replaced by safer drugs, such as benzodiazepines.

Uncontrolled use of barbiturates can cause a state of acute or chronic intoxication. Initially, there may be some loss of inhibition, euphoria, and behavioral stimulation, a pattern often seen with moderate consumption of alcohol. When taken to relieve extreme pain or mental stress, barbiturates may cause delirium and other side effects that can include nausea, nervousness, rash, and diarrhea. The person intoxicated with barbiturates may have difficulty thinking and making judgments, may be emotionally unstable, may be uncoordinated and unsteady when walking, and may slur speech (not unlike the drunken state caused by alcohol).

When used for their hypnotic properties, barbiturates cause an unnatural sleep. The user awakens feeling tired, edgy, and quite unsatisfied, most likely because barbiturates markedly suppress the REM phase of sleep. (REM sleep is necessary for the refreshing renewal that usually accompanies a good sleep experience.) Because benzodiazepines suppress REM sleep (as do all CNS depressants) less severely than barbiturates, use of these agents as sleep aids is generally better tolerated.

Continued misuse of barbiturate drugs has a cumulative toxic effect on the CNS that is more life-threatening than misuse of opiates. In large doses or in combination with other CNS depressants, barbiturates may cause death from respiratory or cardiovascular depression. Because of this toxicity, barbiturates have been involved in many drug-related deaths, both accidental and suicidal. Repeated misuse induces severe tolerance of and physical dependence on these drugs. Discontinuing use of short-acting barbiturates in people who are using large doses can cause dangerous withdrawal effects such as life-threatening seizures. Table 7.3 summarizes the range of effects of barbiturates and other depressants on the mind and body.

Table 7.3   **Effects of Barbiturates and Other Depressants on the Body and Mind**

	Body	Mind
Low dose	Drowsiness	Decreased anxiety, relaxation
	Trouble with coordination	Decreased ability to reason and solve problems
	Slurred Speech	
	Dizziness	Difficulty in judging distance and time
	Staggering	
	Double vision	Amnesia
	Sleep	
	Depressed breathing	Brain damage
	Coma (unconscious and cannot be awakened)	
	Depressed blood pressure	
High dose	Death	

Concern about the abuse potential of barbiturates caused the federal government to include some of these depressants in the Controlled Substance Act. Consequently, the short-acting barbiturates, such as pentobarbital and secobarbital, are classified as Schedule II drugs, while the long-acting barbiturates, such as phenobarbital, are less rigidly controlled as Schedule IV drugs.

Effects and Medical Uses Barbiturates have many pharmacological actions. They depress the activity of nerves and skeletal, smooth, and cardiac muscles, and impact the CNS in several ways, ranging from mild sedation to coma, depending on the dose. At sedative or hypnotic dosage levels, only the CNS is significantly affected. Higher anesthetic doses cause slight decreases in blood pressure, heart rate, and flow of urine. The metabolizing enzyme systems in the liver are important in inactivating barbiturates; thus, liver damage may result in exaggerated responses to barbiturate use.

Low doses of barbiturates relieve tension and anxiety, effects that give several barbiturates substantial abuse potential. The drawbacks of barbiturates are extensive and severe:

▲ They lack selectivity and safety

▲ They have a substantial tendency for tolerance, dependence, withdrawal, and abuse

▲ They cause problems with drug interaction

As a result, barbiturates have been replaced by benzodiazepines in most treatments; however, they are still included in a number of combination products for the treatment of an array of medical problems, such as gastrointestinal disorders, hypertension, asthma, and pain (Hobbs, Rall, and Verdoorn 1995). Their use in such preparations is very controversial. The long-acting phenobarbital is still frequently used for its CNS depressant activity to alleviate or prevent convulsions in some epileptic patients and seizures caused by strychnine, cocaine, and other stimulant drugs. Thiopental (Pentothal) and other ultrashort- and short-acting barbiturates are used as anesthesia for minor surgery and as preoperative anesthetics in preparation for major surgery.

Mechanism of Action and Elimination The precise mechanism of action for barbiturates is unclear. Like benzodiazepines, they likely interfere with activity in the reticular activating system, the limbic system, and the motor cortex. However, in contrast to benzodiazepines, barbiturates do not seem to act at a specific receptor site; they probably have a general effect that enhances the activity of the inhibitory transmitter GABA. Because benzodiazepines also increase GABA activity (but in a more selective manner), these two types of drugs have overlapping effects. Because the mechanisms whereby they exert their effects are different, it is not surprising that these two types of depressants also have different pharmacological features.

Like the benzodiazepines, barbiturates can be classified in terms of duration of action (see Table 7.4). In general, the more fat-soluble the barbiturate is, the more easily it enters the brain, the faster it will act, and the more potent it will be as a depressant. Barbiturates are eliminated through the kidneys at varying rates. The rate of removal depends primarily on how quickly the barbiturate is metabolized in the liver to a fat-insoluble metabolite. Excretion of barbiturates occurs more rapidly when the urine is alkaline, a characteristic that can be manipulated to treat barbiturate poisoning.

Because barbiturates are not completely removed from the body overnight, even the short-acting ones used for insomnia can cause subtle distortions of mood and impaired judgment and motor skills the following day (Julien 1992). The user may have mild withdrawal symptoms such as hyperexcitability, nausea, and vomiting even after short-term use. The long-acting barbiturates such as phenobarbital are metabolized more slowly and cause an extended drug hangover.

The fat solubility of barbiturates is also an important factor in the duration of their effects. Barbiturates that are the most fat-soluble move in and out of body tissues (such as the brain) rapidly and are likely to be shorter-acting. Fat-soluble barbiturates also are more likely to be stored in fatty tissue; consequently, the fat content of the body can influence the effects on the user. Because women have a higher body–fat ratio than men, their reaction to barbiturates may be slightly different.

Table 7.4   **Details on the Most Frequently Abused Barbiturates**

Drug	Nicknames	Effects
Amobarbital (Amytal)	Blues, blue heavens, blue devils	Moderately rapid action
Pentobarbital (Nembutal)	Nembies, yellow jackets, yellows	Short-acting
Phenobarbital (Luminal)	Purple hearts	A long-acting barbiturate particularly well suited for treatment of epilepsy
Secobarbital (Seconal)	Reds, red devils, red birds, Seccy	Short-acting with a prompt onset of action
Tuinal (50% amobarbital and 50% secobarbital)	Tooeys, double trouble, rainbows	Results in a rapidly effective, moderately long-acting sedative

Continual use of barbiturates results in both tolerance and dependence. Development of physical dependence on barbiturates is a relatively slow process, requiring weeks or months of use before withdrawal symptoms occur during drug abstinence.

Withdrawal from barbiturates after dependence has developed causes hyperexcitability because of the rebound of depressed neural systems. Qualitatively (but not quantitatively), the withdrawal symptoms are similar for all sedative-hypnotics (Goldstein 1995).

Table 7.4 gives details on the barbiturates abused most frequently.

Other CNS Depressants

While benzodiazepines and barbiturates are by far used most frequently to produce CNS depressant effects, many other agents, representing an array of distinct chemical groups, can similarly reduce brain activity. Although the mechanisms of action might be different for some of these drugs, if any CNS depressants (including alcohol) are combined, they will interact synergistically and can suppress respiration in a life-threatening manner. Thus, it is important to avoid such mixtures if possible. Even some over-the-counter (OTC) products such as cold and allergy medications contain drugs with CNS depressant actions.

Nonbarbiturate Drugs with Barbiturate-like Properties   This category of depressants includes agents that are not barbiturates but have barbiturate-like effects. All of these drugs cause substantial tolerance, physical and psychological dependence, and withdrawal symptoms. The therapeutic safety of these CNS depressants more closely resembles that of barbiturates than benzodiazepines; consequently, like barbiturates, these agents have been replaced by the safer and easier-to-manage benzodiazepines.

Because these drugs have significant abuse potential, they are restricted much like other CNS depressants. In this group of depressants, methaqualone is a Schedule II drug; glutethimide and methyprylon are Schedule III drugs; chloral hydrate is a Schedule IV drug. The basis for the classification is the relative potential for physical and psychological dependence. Abuse of Schedule II drugs may lead to severe or moderate physical dependence or high psychological dependence, and abuse of Schedule III drugs may cause moderate physical and psychological dependence. Schedule IV drugs are considered much less likely to cause either type of dependence.

Chloral Hydrate Chloral hydrate (Noctec), or "knock-out drops," has the unsavory reputation of being a drug that is slipped into a person's drink to make him or her unconscious. In the late 1800s, the combination of chloral hydrate and alcohol was given the name "Mickey Finn" on the waterfront of the Barbary Coast of San Francisco when sailors were in short supply. As legend has it, the name of one of the bars dispensing unwanted knockout drops was Mickey Finn's. An unsuspecting man would have a friendly drink and wake up as a crew member on an outbound freighter to China.

Chloral hydrate is a good hypnotic, but it has a narrow margin of safety. This compound is a stomach irritant, especially if given repeatedly and in fairly large doses. Addicts may take enormous doses of the drug; as with most CNS depressants, chronic, long-term use of high doses will cause tolerance and physical dependence (Hobbs, Rall, and Verdoorn 1995).

Glutethimide Glutethimide (Doriden) is another example of a barbiturate-like drug that can be abused and causes severe withdrawal symptoms. It also induces blood abnormalities in sensitive individuals, such as a type of anemia and abnormally low white cell counts. Nausea, fever, increased heart rate, and convulsions occasionally occur in patients who have been taking this sedative regularly in moderate doses. Doriden seems to have a smaller margin of safety than barbiturates. Continual use causes tolerance and physical dependence. Doriden was used more commonly as a "street" drug before it was definitely proved to be addictive and tighter controls were instituted.

Methyprylon Methyprylon (Noludar) is a short-acting nonbarbiturate that is used as a sedative and hypnotic. Its effects are similar to those of Doriden, and it is capable of causing tolerance, physical dependence, and addiction, much like barbiturates.

Methaqualone Few drugs have become so popular so quickly as methaqualone. This barbiturate-like sedative-hypnotic was introduced in India in the 1950s as an antimalarial agent. Its sedative properties, however, were soon discovered. It then became available in the United States as Quaalude, Mequin, and Parest.

After several years of "street" abuse, methaqualone was classified as a Schedule II drug. Since 1985, methaqualone has not been manufactured in the United States because of adverse publicity. It is interesting to note, however, that large amounts of illegal methaqualone are still imported into the United States from Colombia, Mexico, and Canada. It is referred to by "street" names such as *Ludes, Sopors,* or *714s.*

Common side effects of methaqualone include fatigue, dizziness, anorexia, nausea, vomiting, diarrhea, sweating, dryness of the mouth, depersonalization, headache, and paresthesia of the extremities (a pins-and-needles feeling in the fingers and toes). Hangover is frequently reported. High doses of methaqualone can cause psychological and physical dependence and dangerous withdrawal symptoms when drug use is stopped.

Antihistamines Antihistamines are drugs used in both nonprescription and prescription medicinal products. The most common uses for antihistamines are to relieve the symptoms associated with the common cold, allergies, and motion sickness (see Chapter 15). Although frequently overlooked, many antihistamines cause significant CNS depression and are used both as sedatives and hypnotics. For example, the agents hydroxyzine (Visteril) and promethazine (Phenergan) are prescribed for their sedative effects, while diphenhydramine is commonly used as an OTC sleep aid.

The exact mechanism of CNS depression caused by these agents is not totally known but appears to relate to their blockage of acetylcholine receptors in the brain (they antagonize the muscarinic receptor types). This anticholinergic activity (see Chapter 6) helps cause relaxation and sedation and can be viewed as a very annoying side effect when these drugs are being used to treat allergies or other problems.

Therapeutic Usefulness and Side Effects Antihistamines are viewed as relatively safe agents. Compared with other more powerful CNS depressants, antihistamines do not appear to cause significant physical or psychological dependence or addiction problems, although drugs with anticholinergic activity, such as the antihistamines, are sometimes abused, especially by children and teenagers (Carlini 1993). However, tolerance to antihistamine-

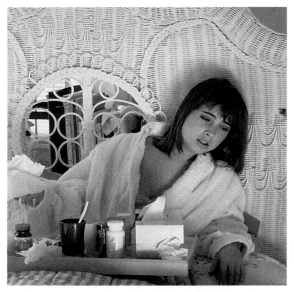

Antihistamines are found in OTC medicines used to relieve cold and allergy symptoms.

induced sedation occurs quite rapidly. Reports of significant cases of withdrawal problems when use of the antihistamines is stopped are rare. This situation may reflect the fact that these agents are used as antianxiety drugs for only minor problems and for short periods of time (often only for a single dose).

One significant problem with antihistamines is the variability of responses they produce. Different antihistamines work differently on different people. Usually therapeutic doses will cause decreased alertness, relaxation, slowed reaction time, and drowsiness. But it is not uncommon for some individuals to be affected in the opposite manner, that is, an antihistamine can cause restlessness, agitation, and insomnia. There are even cases of seizures caused by toxic doses of antihistamine, particularly in children (Serafin and Babe 1995). Side effects of antihistamines related to their anticholinergic effects include dry mouth, constipation, and inability to urinate. These factors probably help to discourage the abuse of these drugs.

Even though antihistamines are relatively safe in therapeutic doses, they can contribute to serious problems if combined with other CNS depressants. Because of this potentially dangerous interaction, patients who have been prescribed other sedative-hypnotics should be aware of consuming drugs that contain antihistamines. For example, many OTC cold, allergy, antimotion, and sleep aid products contain antihistamines and should be avoided by patients using the potent CNS depressants.

GHB (gamma-hydroxybutyrate): The *Natural Depressant* GHB is a natural substance in the body resulting from the metabolism of the inhibitory neurotransmitter, GABA (see Chapter 6). It was first synthesized nearly 30 years ago by a French researcher who intended to study the CNS effects of GABA. Because of its central depressant effects, GHB has been used in Europe as an adjunct for general anesthesia, a treatment for insomnia and narcolepsy (a daytime sleep disorder), and a treatment for alcoholism and alcohol withdrawal (Morgenthaler and Joy 1994). During the 1980s, GHB became available without a prescription in health food stores and was used principally by body builders to stimulate the release of growth hormone with the intent to reduce fat and build muscle (Karch 1996). More recently, this substance has been gaining popularity for recreational use due to what has been described as a pleasant, alcohol-like, hangover-free "high" with aphrodisiac properties (Morgenthaler and Joy 1994).

Because of concerns about apparent GHB abuse, the FDA banned its over-the-counter sale in 1990, although the DEA has yet to classify it as a scheduled substance. Many questions remain regarding the potential risks of GHB (see "Fighting the Drug War," page174). Those who defend its use refer to a "scientific consensus" concerning its benign nature and the fact that no deaths have been reported due to its overdose (Morgenthaler and Joy 1994). In contrast, it has been reported that GHB use can cause significant side effects, such as hormonal problems, sleep abnormalities, drowsiness, nausea, vomiting, and changes in blood pressure (Gallimberti et al. 1989). Both users and clinicians seem to agree that GHB is most dangerous when combined with other drugs, especially other CNS depressants such as alcohol (Gallimberti et al. 1989). Insight into the effects of this unusual substance is expressed by a user who shared her experience over the internet:

I used GHB a number of years back when it had lots of popularity among body builders. I never found it did much for my physique, but it worked great to make me fall asleep. The problem I have with the stuff is that I wake up about two hours after I fall asleep.

> *Source*: Netscape: Newsgroups: alt. psychoactives, alt. psychobiology, sci. med. pharmacy

Because GHB has not been approved for therapeutic purposes by the FDA, it is currently available only through the underground "gray market" as a "bootleg" product manufactured by kitchen chemists, and with suspicious quality and purity (Morgenthaler and Joy 1994). The lack of reliability of these GHB-containing products and the highly variable responses of different people to this substance increase the likelihood of problems when using this depressant. One such incident is recounted by a woman in her late twenties:

I had a brainless acquaintance who thought more must be better and took four scoops of the stuff at once. I ended up over at his house all night when his girlfriend called me because he was behaving like a psychotic. I spent the night there, convincing him that his girlfriend was not his mother and that no one was going to hurt him. This was like witnessing a bad trip. People without good, solid common sense should not play with this stuff.

> *Source*: Netscape: Newsgroups: alt. psychoactives, alt. psychobiology, sci. med. pharmacy

◢ Patterns of Abuse with CNS Depressants

The American Psychiatric Association considers dependence on CNS depressants to be a psychiatric disorder. According to its widely used *Diagnostic and Statistical Manual of Mental Disorders (DSM-IV)*, (American Psychiatric Association 1994), "substance dependence disorder" is present when three of the following criteria are satisfied at any time in a 12-month period:

1. The person needs greatly increased amounts of the substance to achieve the desired effect or experiences a markedly diminished effect with continued use of the substance.

2. Characteristic withdrawal occurs when drug use is stopped, which encourages continued use of the substance to avoid the unpleasant effects.

3. The substance is consumed in larger amounts over a longer period of time than originally intended.

4. The person shows persistent desire or repeated unsuccessful efforts to decrease or control substance use.

5. A great deal of time is spent obtaining and using the substance or recovering from its effects.

6. All daily activities revolve around the substance—important social, occupational, or recreational activities are given up or reduced because of substance use.

7. The person withdraws from family activities and hobbies to use the substance privately or spend more time with substance-using friends.

8. The person continues use of substance despite recognizing that it causes social, occupational, legal or medical problems.

A review of the previous discussion about the properties of CNS depressants reveals that severe dependence on these drugs can satisfy all these *DSM-IV* criteria; thus, according to the American Psychiatric Association, dependence on CNS depressants is classified as a form of mental illness.

The principal types of people who are most inclined to abuse CNS depressants include the following:

1. Those who seek sedative effects to deal with emotional stress, trying to escape from problems they are unable to deal with. Sometimes these individuals are able to persuade clinicians to administer depressants for their problems; at other times, they self-medicate with depressants that are obtained illegally.

2. Those who seek the excitation that occurs, especially after some tolerance has developed; instead of depression, they feel exhilaration and euphoria.

3. Those who try to counteract the unpleasant effect or withdrawal associated with other drugs of abuse, such as some stimulants, LSD, and other hallucinogens.

4. Those who use sedatives in combination with other depressant drugs such as alcohol and heroin. Alcohol plus a sedative gives a faster "high" but can be dangerous because of the

---

FIGHTING THE DRUG WAR

Every era seems to have its "hot" drug—the one that so many people, for one reason or another, just have to have. In the mid-1990s, the drug was Rohypnol (alias flunitrazepam), affectionately known as "Ropies" or the "date-rape drug."

Rohypnol is a depressant (benzodiazepine) that is manufactured legally in Colombia, Mexico, and Switzerland by international pharmaceutical giant Hoffmann-La Roche. It has never been manufactured or marketed legally in the United States, but that detail has not affected its popularity. One of the main attractions for some teenagers and young adults was the substance's purported ability to relax women's resistance to sexual assault—which gave it the "date rape" reputation. Used under the right circumstances, Rohypnol is not always dangerous. When used improperly or in combination with other drugs or alcohol, however, it can be deadly.

Rohypnol tablets, reported to be seven to ten times more potent than Valium, were smuggled into the United States from Mexico and South America. Not surprisingly, traffic in the drug was particularly heavy in Florida, Texas, and California. It was also manufactured illegally in clandestine laboratories in the United States, in locations as disparate as motel rooms and garages, by everyone from high school dropouts to chemists with doctoral degrees.

In 1996, Ropie fervor seemed to be replaced by lust for a newer, liquid substance called gamma-hydroxybutyrate (GHB). That year, more than 100 suspected GHB overdoses were reported in Texas, Florida, and California. Most teenagers appeared to take GHB to get high, likening its effects to an alcohol high without the hangover. But GHB was also known on the street as "Easy Lay," for its reported aphrodisiac effects.

GHB is odorless and nearly tasteless, so it can be slipped into drinks without being detected. It can quickly depress the respiratory system, especially when mixed with alcohol. The major danger is that not enough oxygen gets to the brain, triggering unconsciousness and loss of memory. "A substance that knocks out the victim and leaves her with amnesia makes the perfect agent for date rape," said Michael Ellis, director of the Southeast Texas Poison Center, in *Time* magazine. In 1995, a 17-year-old Texas girl died of a GHB overdose. At the time, police speculated that someone must have slipped the GHB into her soft drink when she was not looking—either as a joke or for more prurient motives.

Like Ropies, GHB is manufactured legally in other countries. It has been used in Europe as an adjunct for general anesthesia, and as a treatment for insomnia, narcolepsy, alcoholism, and alcohol withdrawal. During the 1980s, it was even sold in U.S. health food stores. Concerns about abuse eventually led the FDA to ban OTC sales in 1990 and push for further controls in 1997.

The FDA ban notwithstanding, it hasn't been easy to stop the flow of the drug, which can be brewed at home easily, using instructions found in libraries and over the Internet. Because it is so hard to control the manufacture and distribution of drugs like Rohypnol and GHB, and because the gap between "safe" and lethal doses for both is so narrow, education and prevention should be used as perhaps the most effective weapons in the war against dangerous depressants. ■

Sources: Gorman, C. "A Club Drug Called GHB May Be a Fatal Aphrodisiac." *Time* (September 30, 1996). National Narcotics Intelligence Consumers Committee, Drug Enforcement Administration. "The Supply of Illicit Drugs to the United States." *The NNICC Report 1994* (August 1995).

multiple depressant effects and synergistic interaction. Heroin users often resort to barbiturates if their heroin supply is compromised.

As mentioned earlier, depressants are commonly abused in combination with other drugs (Goldstein 1995). In particular, opioid narcotic users take barbiturates, benzodiazepines, and other depressants to augment the effects of a weak batch of heroin or a rapidly shrinking supply. Chronic narcotic users also claim that depressants help to offset tolerance to opioids, thereby requiring less narcotic to achieve a satisfactory response by the user. It is not uncommon to see joint dependence on both narcotics and depressants.

Another common use of depressants is by alcoholics to soften the withdrawal from ethanol or to help create a state of intoxication without the telltale odor of alcohol. Interestingly, similar strategies are also used therapeutically to help detoxify the alcoholic. For example, long-acting barbiturates or benzodiazepines are often used to wean an alcohol-dependent person away from ethanol. Treatment with these depressants helps to reduce the severity of withdrawal symptoms, making it easier and safer for alcoholics to eliminate their drug dependence.

In general, those who chronically abuse the CNS depressants prefer (1) the short-acting barbiturates, such as pentobarbital and secobarbital, (2) the barbiturate-like depressants, such as glutethimide, methyprylon, and methaqualone; (3) the faster-acting benzodiazepines, such as diazepam (Valium), alprazalam (Xanax), or lorazepam (Ativan). However, most nonabusing people do not find the benzodiazepines particularly reinforcing (Woods et al. 1992).

Dependence on sedative-hypnotic agents can develop insidiously. Often a long-term patient is treated for persistent insomnia or anxiety with daily exposures to a CNS depressant. When an attempt to withdraw the drug is made, the patient becomes agitated, unable to sleep, and severely anxious; a state of panic may be experienced when deprived of the drug. These signs are frequently mistaken for a resurgence of the medical condition being treated and are not recognized as part of a withdrawal syndrome to the CNS depressant. Consequently, the patient is restored to his or her supply of CNS depressant, and the symptoms of

withdrawal subside. Such conditions generally lead to a gradual increase in dosage as tolerance to the sedative-hypnotic develops. The patient becomes severely dependent on the depressant, both physically and psychologically, and the drug habit becomes an essential feature in the user's daily routines. Only after severe dependence has developed does the clinician often realize what has taken place. The next stage is the unpleasant task of trying to wean the patient from the drug (**detoxification**) with as little discomfort as possible.

> **detoxification**
> elimination of a toxic substance, such as a drug, and its effects

Because of the similarities between alcohol and barbiturate-like drugs, it is common to see individuals who abuse both types of depressants. One danger is that these people use both drugs together. Due to the synergism that exists between

Detoxification of patients dependent on CNS depressants can be very unpleasant and even life-threatening.

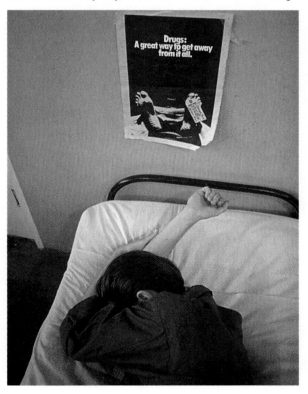

CNS depressants in general, such a mixture can severely suppress respiration and cardiovascular function, often with deadly consequences (Goldstein 1995). Knowledge of this dangerous interaction is quite common among the drug-using population; consequently, many suicide attempts are made by self-administering high doses of barbiturate-like drugs with a chaser of ethanol.

The prevalence of abuse of illicit CNS depressants appeared to peak in the early 1980s for twelfth-graders. Illegal use of these drugs then decreased dramatically until 1992, at which time abuse appears to have rebounded until 1995 (see Table 7.5).

Treatment for Withdrawal

All sedative-hypnotics, including alcohol and benzodiazepines, can produce physical dependence and a barbiturate-like withdrawal syndrome if taken in sufficient dosage over a long period. Withdrawal symptoms include anxiety, tremors, nightmares, insomnia, anorexia, nausea, vomiting, seizures, delirium, and maniacal activity.

The duration and severity of withdrawal depends on the particular drug taken. With short-acting depressants—such as pentobarbital, secobarbital, and methaqualone—withdrawal symptoms tend to be more severe. They begin 12 to 24 hours after the last dose and peak in intensity between 24 and 72 hours later. Withdrawal from longer-acting depressants—such as phenobarbital, diazepam, and chlordiazepoxide—develops more slowly and is less intense; symptoms peak on the fifth to eighth day (Jaffe 1990).

Not surprisingly, the approach to detoxifying a person dependent on a sedative-hypnotic depends on the nature of the drug itself (that is, to which category of depressants it belongs), the severity of the dependence, and the duration of action of the drug. The general objectives of detoxification are to eliminate drug dependence (both physical and psychological) in a safe manner while minimizing discomfort. Having achieved these objectives, it is hoped that the patient will be able to remain free of dependence on all CNS depressants.

Often the basic approach for treating severe dependence on sedative-hypnotics is substitution of either pentobarbital or the longer-acting phenobarbital for the offending, usually shorter-acting CNS depressant. Once substitution has occurred, the long-acting barbiturate dose is gradually reduced. Using a substitute is necessary because abrupt withdrawal for a person who is physically dependent can be dangerous and can cause life-threatening seizures. This substitution treatment uses the same rationale as the treatment of heroin withdrawal by methadone replacement. Detoxification also includes supportive measures such as vitamins, restoration of electrolyte balance, and prevention of dehydration. The patient must be watched closely during this time because he or she will be apprehensive, mentally confused, and unable to make logical decisions (O'Brien 1995).

If the person is addicted to both alcohol and barbiturates, the phenobarbital dosage must be increased to compensate for the double withdrawal. Many barbiturate addicts who enter a hospital for withdrawal are also dependent on heroin. In such

Table 7.5   Lifetime Prevalence of Abuse of CNS Depressants for Twelfth-graders

Year	1980	1985	1990	1992	1995
Any Illicit Drug	65.4%	60.6%	47.9%	40.7%	48.4%
Barbiturates	11.0	9.2	6.8	5.5	7.4
Methaqualone	9.5	6.7	2.3	1.6	1.2
All Depressants (including benzodiazepines)	14.9	11.8	7.5	6.1	7.6

Source: L. Johnston. *Drug Abuse Survey.* Lansing: University of Michigan, 1996.

cases, the barbiturate dependence should be dealt with first because the associated withdrawal can be life-threatening. Detoxification from any sedative-hypnotic should take place under close medical supervision, typically in a hospital (O'Brien 1995).

It is important to remember that elimination of physical dependence does not necessarily result in a cure. The problem of psychological dependence can be much more difficult to handle. If an individual is abusing a CNS depressant because of emotional instability, personal problems, or a very stressful environment, eliminating physical dependence alone will not solve the problem and drug dependence is likely to recur. These types of patients require intense psychological counseling and must be trained to deal with their difficulties in a more constructive and positive fashion. Without such psychological support, benefits from detoxification will only be temporary, and therapy will ultimately fail.

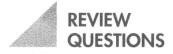

REVIEW QUESTIONS

1. Why have benzodiazepine drugs replaced the barbiturates as the sedative-hypnotic drugs most prescribed by physicians?

2. Which features of CNS depressants give them abuse potential?

3. Why is long-term use of the benzodiazepines more likely to cause dependence than short-term use?

4. Why are some physicians careless when prescribing benzodiazepines for patients suffering from severe anxiety?

5. Currently sleep aid products are available over the counter. Should the FDA also allow sedatives to be sold without a prescription? Support your answer.

6. Are there any real advantages to using barbiturates as sedatives or hypnotics? Should the FDA remove them from the market?

 EXERCISES FOR THE WEB

Exercise 1:
Hypnotics and Sedatives

This "Hypnotics and Sedatives" link gives a pharmacological description of the effects of hypnotics and sedatives. Other topics of interest include addiction and popularity.

Netscape - [COHIS: Hypnotics and Sedatives Abuse]
File Edit View Go Bookmarks Options Directory Window Help
Back Forward Home Edit Reload Images Open Print Find Stop
Location: http://web.bu.edu:80/COHIS/subsabse/hypnotic/hypnotic.htm

HYPNOTICS
and Sedatives

Alcohol and Substance Abuse Menu

Alcohol	Amphetamines	Anabolic Steroids	Caffeine	Cocaine (Crack)	Hallucinogens	HealthSource Substance Abuse
Heroin	Hypnotics/Sedatives	Inhalants	Marijuana (Cannabis)	Morphine	Prescription Drugs	Substance Abuse Menu

7. What types of people are most likely to abuse CNS depressants? Suggest ways to help these people avoid abusing these drugs.

8. What is the appeal for using GHB?

9. What dangers are associated with treating individuals who are severely dependent on CNS depressants?

KEY TERMS

barbiturates
benzodiazepines
antihistamines
sedatives
anxiolytic
hypnotics
amnesiac
anesthesia
REM sleep
paradoxical
detoxification

SUMMARY

1 Several unrelated drug groups cause CNS depression, but only a few are actually used clinically for their depressant properties. The most frequently prescribed CNS depressants are benzodiazepines, which include drugs such as Klonepin, Ambien, and Xanax. Barbiturates once were popular but, because of their severe side effects, they are no longer used by most clinicians. Much like barbiturates, drugs such as chloral hydrate, glutethimide, and methaqualone are little used today. Finally, some antihistamines, such as diphenhydramine, hydroxyzine, and promethazine, are still occasionally used for their CNS depressant effects.

2 The clinical value of CNS depressants is dose-dependent. At low doses, these drugs relieve anxiety and promote relaxation (sedatives). At higher doses, they can cause drowsiness and pro-

mote sleep (hypnotics). At even higher doses, some of the depressants cause anesthesia and are used for patient management during surgery.

3 Because CNS depressants can relieve anxiety and reduce stress, they are viewed as desirable by many people. If used frequently over long periods, however, they can cause tolerance that leads to dependence.

4 The principal reason benzodiazepines have replaced barbiturates in the treatment of stress and insomnia is that benzodiazepines have a greater margin of safety and are less likely to alter sleep patterns. Benzodiazepines enhance the GABA transmitter system in the brain through a specific receptor, while the effects of barbiturates are less selective. Even though benzodiazepines are safer than barbiturates, dependence and significant withdrawal problems can result if the drugs are used indiscriminately.

5 Often benzodiazepine dependence occurs with patients who suffer stress or anxiety disorders and are under a physician's care. If the physician is not careful and the cause of the stress is not resolved, drug treatment can drag on for weeks or months. After prolonged therapy, tolerance develops to the drug, so that when benzodiazepine use is stopped, withdrawal occurs, which itself causes agitation. A rebound response to the drug might resemble the effects of emotional stress, so use of benzodiazepine is continued until the patient becomes severely dependent.

6 The short-acting CNS depressants are preferred for treatment of insomnia. These drugs help the patient get to sleep and then are inactivated by the body; when the user awakes the next day, he or she is less likely to experience residual effects than with long-acting drugs. The short-acting depressants are also more likely to be abused because of their relatively rapid onset and intense effects. In contrast, the long-acting depressants are better suited to treating persistent problems such as anxiety and stress. The long-acting depressants are also used to help wean dependent people from their use of short-acting compounds such as alcohol.

7 Although at one time very popular, methaqualone is no longer legally available in the United States due to abuse problems. Even so, it continues to be found on the "street" because it is

smuggled across the Mexican and Canadian borders into the United States.

8 Many antihistamines cause sedation and drowsiness due to their anticholinergic effects. Several of these agents are useful for short-term relief of anxiety and are available in OTC sleep aids. The effectiveness of these CNS depressants is usually less than that of benzodiazepines. Because of their anticholinergic actions, antihistamines can cause some annoying side effects. These agents are not likely to be used for long periods; thus, dependence or abuse rarely develops.

9 The people most likely to abuse CNS depressants include individuals who (a) use drugs to relieve continual stress; (b) paradoxically feel euphoria and stimulation from depressants; (c) use depressants to counteract the unpleasant effects of other drugs of abuse, such as stimulants; and (d) combine depressants with alcohol and heroin to potentiate the effects.

10 The basic approach for treating dependence on CNS depressants is to detoxify in a safe manner while minimizing discomfort. This state is achieved by substituting a long-acting barbiturate or benzodiazepine, such as phenobarbital or Valium, for the offending CNS depressant. The long-acting drug causes less severe withdrawal symptoms over a longer period of time. The dependent person is gradually weaned from the substitute drug until depressant-free.

REFERENCES

American Medical Association (AMA), Committee on Alcoholism and Addiction, Dependence on Barbiturates, and Other Sedative Drugs. *Journal of the American Medical Association* 193 (1965): 673–77.

American Psychiatric Association. "Substance Related Disorders." In *Diagnostic and Statistical Manual of Mental Disorders,* 4th ed. *[DSM-IV],* Allen Frances, chairperson, 175–272. Washington, DC: American Psychiatric Association, 1994.

Associated Press. "Woman Who Used Halcion Defense Hangs Self." *Salt Lake Tribune* 248 (1994):D3.

Carlini, E. "Preliminary Note: Dangerous Use of Anticholinergic Drugs in Brazil." *Drug and Alcohol Dependence* 32 (1993): 1–7.

Gallimberti, L., N. Gentile, M. Cibin, F. Fadda, G. Canton, M. Ferri, S. Ferrara, and G. Gessa. "Gamma-Hydroxy-butyrate for Treatment of Alcohol Withdrawal Syndrome." *Lancet* 30 (1989): 787–9.

Goldstein, A. "Pharmacological Aspects of Drug Abuse." In *Remington's Pharmaceutical Sciences,* 19th ed., edited by A. R. Gennaro, 780–793. Easton, PA: 1995.

Grinspoon, L. "Benzodiazepine Dependence." *Harvard Medical Letter* 12 (1996): 7.

"High Anxiety." *Consumer Reports* (January 1993): 19–24.

Hobbs, W., T. Rall, and T. Verdoorn. "Hypnotics and Sedatives." In *The Pharmacological Basis of Therapeutics,* 9th ed., edited by J. Hardman and L. Limbird, 361–396. New York: McGraw-Hill, 1995.

Julien, R. "General Nonselective Central Nervous System Depressants." In *A Primer of Drug Action,* 6th ed., 51–70. New York: Freeman, 1992.

Karch, S. "Anabolic Steroids." In *The Pathology of Drug Abuse,* 2nd ed., 409–29. New York: CRC, 1996.

McDermott, P. "McDermott's Guide to the Depressant Drugs." Available http://www.hyperreal.com/drugs/depressants/mcdermotts.guide.1996.

McEvoy, G., ed. *American Hospital Formulary Service Drug Information.* Bethesda, MD: American Society of Hospital Pharmacists, 1994.

Miller, L., and D. Greenblatt. "Neurochemistry of the Benzodiazepines." In *Drugs of Abuse and Neurobiology,* edited by Ronald Watson, 175–83. Ann Arbor, MI: CRC Press, 1992.

Mondanaro, J. *Chemically Dependent Women.* Lexington, MA: Lexington Books/Heath, 1988.

Morgenthaler, J., and D. Joy. *Special Report on GHB.* Petaluma, CA: Smart Publication, 1994.

"New Halcion Guidelines." *American Druggist* (January 1992): 14.

O'Brien, C. "Drug Addiction and Drug Abuse." In *The Pharmacological Basis of Therapeutics,* 9th ed., edited by J. Hardman and L. Limbird, 557–77. New York: McGraw-Hill, 1995.

Pagliaro, L., and A. Pagliaro. "Drug Induced Aggression." *Medical Psychotherapist* (Newsletter of the American Board of Medical Psychotherapists) 8 (Fall 1992): 1.

PDR (Physician's Desk Reference). 50th ed., Montvale, NJ: Medical Economics, 1997.

Serafin, W., and Babe, K. "Histamine, Bradykinin and Their Antagonists." In *The Pharmacological Basis of Therapeutics,* 9th ed., edited by J. Hardman and L. Limbird, 581–600. New York: McGraw-Hill, 1995.

"Top 200 Drugs of 1992." *Pharmacy Times* (April 1993): 30–32.

"Top 200 drugs, total Rxs." Pharmacy Times (April 1997) 30–34.

Woods, J., J. Katz, and G. Winger. "Benzodiazepines: Use, Abuse and Consequences." *Pharmacological Reviews* 44 (1992): 155–323.

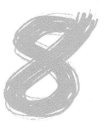

Alcohol (Ethanol):

Pharmacological Effects

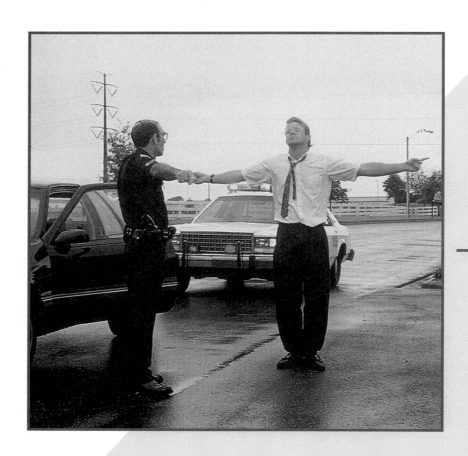

On completing this chapter
you will be able to: ▶

- Ethanol is the only alcohol used for human consumption; the other alcohols are poisonous.
- Some wild animals and insects become drunk after seeking out and consuming alcohol-containing fermented fruit.
- The first recorded beer brewery was in existence in 3700 B.C.

- In some communities, malt liquors are called "liquid crack."
- Women reach a higher blood alcohol level than men when consuming the same amount of alcohol.
- The lethal level of alcohol is between 0.4% and 0.6% by volume in the blood.
- The liver metabolizes alcohol at a constant rate unaffected by the amount ingested.

- Among alcoholics, liver disorders are the most common causes of death.
- Fetal alcohol syndrome (FAS) is characterized by facial deformities, growth deficiencies, and mental retardation.
- The incidence of FAS is one in three infants born to alcoholic mothers.
- Alcoholic beverages are high in calories, but contain no other nutrients.

Learning Objectives

- Explain why common alcohol (ethanol) is a drug.
- Identify three types of poisonous alcohols and name the fourth type, which is used in alcoholic beverages.
- Explain the pharmacokinetic properties of alcohol.
- Describe the factors that affect the concentration of alcohol in the blood.

- Name the short-term physical effects of drinking alcohol at low and moderate doses.
- Name the possible physical effects of prolonged heavy ethanol consumption.
- Describe fetal alcohol syndrome and its effects.
- Explain how prolonged consumption of alcohol affects the brain and

nervous system, liver, digestive system, blood, cardiovascular system, sexual organs, endocrine systems, and kidneys, and how it leads to mental disorders and damage to the brain as well as to fetuses.
- Explain why malnutrition is so common in alcoholics.

In this chapter and the next, we will examine several aspects of alcohol use. This chapter focuses on how alcohol affects the body from a pharmacological perspective. Chapter 9 studies the social effects of this drug—mainly, the effects and consequences of alcohol on an individual's social life.

As a licit drug, alcohol is not only extensively promoted socially through advertising, but more important, drinking is perceived as acceptable. The popularity of this drug was recently shown by the 1996 *National Survey Results on Drug Use:* In 1994, 88% of U.S. college students had used alcohol sometime during their life; 83% used it during the preceding year; 68% used it during the preceding month; 4% used it daily; and 40% consumed at least five drinks in a row sometime during the preceding two weeks (Johnston et al. 1996).

Most adolescents use alcohol because they want to experience new sensations, relieve peer pressure, or enhance a social setting with chemistry.

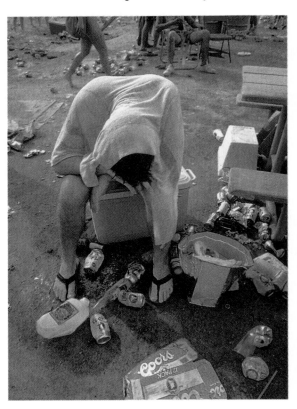

This chapter focuses on the many adverse effects of alcohol on the human body. Overall, it will provide you with a foundation to understand the pharmacological nature of alcohol. We hope that such an understanding of how this drug affects the various organ systems of the body will lead to more responsible use and less abuse of alcohol.

The Nature and History of Alcohol

Alcohol has been part of human culture since the beginning of recorded history. The technology for alcohol production is ancient. Several basic ingredients and conditions are needed: sugar, water, yeast, and warm temperatures.

The process of making alcohol, called **fermentation,** is a natural one. It occurs in ripe fruit and berries and even in honey that wild bees leave in trees. These substances contain sugar and water and are found in warm climates, where yeast spores are transported through the air. Animals such as elephants, baboons, birds, wild pigs, and bees will seek and eat fermented fruit. Elephants under the influence of alcohol have been observed bumping into one another and stumbling around. Intoxicated bees fly an unsteady beeline toward their hives. Birds eating fermented fruit become so uncoordinated that they cannot fly, or if they do, they crash into windows or branches. In fact, fermented honey, called **mead,** may have been the first alcoholic beverage.

fermentation

the biochemical process in which yeast converts sugar to alcohol

mead

fermented honey often made into an alcoholic beverage

The Egyptians had breweries 6000 years ago; they credited the god Osiris with introducing wine to humans. The ancient Greeks used large quantities of wine and credited a god, Bacchus (or Dionysus), with introducing the drink. Today, we use the words *bacchanalia* and *dionysian* to refer to revelry and drunken events. The Hebrews were also heavy users of wine. The Bible mentions that Noah, just nine generations removed from Adam, made wine and became drunk.

Alcohol is produced by a single-celled microscopic organism, one of the yeasts, which breaks down sugar by a metabolic form of combustion, thereby releasing carbon dioxide and forming water and ethyl alcohol as a waste product. Carbon dioxide creates the foam on a glass of beer and the fizz in champagne. Fermentation continues until the sugar supply is exhausted or the concentration of alcohol reaches the point at which it kills the yeast (12% to 14%). Thus, 12% to 14% is the natural limit of alcohol found in fermented wines or beers.

The **distillation** device, or *still,* was developed by the Arabs around A.D. 800 and was introduced into medieval Europe around A.D. 1250. By boiling the fermented drink and gathering the condensed vapor in a pipe, a still increases the concentration of alcohol, potentially to 50% or higher. Because distillation made it easier for people to get drunk, it greatly intensified the problem of alcohol abuse. However, even before the arrival of the still, alcoholic beverages had been known to cause problems in heavy users that resulted in severe physical and psychological dependence.

> **distillation**
>
> heating fermented mixtures of cereal grains or fruits in a still to evaporate and be trapped as purified alcohol

◢ Alcohol as a Drug

Alcohol (more precisely designated as **ethanol**), as a natural product of fermentation, is an extremely popular social beverage and the second most widely used and abused of all the psychoactive drugs (next to caffeine). This psychoactive substance depresses the central nervous system while influencing almost all major organ systems of the body. Alcohol is also an addictive drug in that it may produce a physical and behavioral dependence. ("Centerpiece" 1993). Although tradition and

> **ethanol**
>
> the consumable type of alcohol that is the psychoactive ingredient in alcoholic beverages; often called *grain alcohol*

attitude are important factors in determining the use patterns of this substance, the typical consumer rarely appreciates the diversity of pharmacological effects caused by alcohol, the drug. The pharmacological action of alcohol accounts for both its pleasurable and CNS effects as well as its hazards to health and public safety.

Alcohol as a Social Drug

Why is alcohol often perceived as an acceptable adjunct to such celebrations as parties, birthdays, weddings, and anniversaries, and as a way of relieving stress and anxiety? Social psychologists refer to the perception of alcohol as a **social lubricant.** This term implies that drinking is misconceived as a safe drug activity promoting conviviality and social interaction, and as an activity that bolsters confidence by repressing inhibitions and strengthening extraversion. Why do many people have to be reminded that alcohol is a drug like marijuana or cocaine? Four reasons explain this misconception: (1) the use of alcohol is legal; (2) through widespread advertising, the media promote the notion that alcohol consumption is as normal and safe as drinking fruit juices and soft drinks; (3) the distribution or the sale of alcoholic beverages is widely practiced; and (4) alcohol use has a long tradition of use, dating back to 30,000 B.C. (Royce 1989, 28).

> **social lubricant**
>
> the belief that drinking (misconceived as safe) that represses inhibitions and strengthens extraversion leads to increased sociability

Impact of Alcohol

Although many consider the effects of alcohol enjoyable and reassuring, the adverse pharmacological impact of this drug is extensive and its effects are associated with more than 100,000 deaths each year in the United States. It is estimated that at some time during their lives, almost 50% of all Americans will be involved in an alcohol-related traffic accident ("Centerpiece" 1993). The pharmacological effects of alcohol abuse cause severe dependence, which is classified as a psychiatric disorder according to *DSM IV* criteria (Hoffman and Tabakoff 1996); disrupt personal, family, social, and professional functioning; and frequently result in multiple illnesses and accidents, violence, and crime (Eronen et al. 1996). Alcohol consumed during pregnancy can lead to devastating damage to offspring and is the principal cause of mental retardation in newborns. Next to tobacco, alcohol is the leading cause of premature death in America. Experts have estimated that in the United States approximately $140 billion is spent annually dealing with social and health problems resulting from the pharmacological effects of alcohol (Samson and Harris 1992). However, such estimates fall short of assessing the emotional upheaval and human suffering caused by this drug ("Centerpiece" 1993).

Despite all of the problems that alcohol causes, our free society has demanded that access to this drug be preserved. However, it is unthinkable to ignore the tremendous negative social impact of this drug. There are no simple answers to this dilemma, yet clearly governmental and educational institutions could do more to protect members of society against the dangers of alcohol. The best weapons we have against the problems of alcohol are education, prevention, and treatment (see Chapter 17).

◢ The Properties of Alcohol

Technically alcohol is a chemical structure that has a hydroxyl group (OH, for one oxygen and one hydrogen atom) attached to a carbon atom. Of the many types of alcohol, several are important in this context. The first is **methyl alcohol** (methanol, or wood alcohol), so called because it is made from wood products. Its metabolites are poisonous. Small amounts (4 ml) cause blindness, affecting the retina, and larger amounts (80 ml to 150 ml) are usually fatal (Klaasen 1995). Methyl alcohol is added to ethyl alcohol (ethanol or grain alcohol, the drinking type) intended for industrial use so that people will not drink it. A similar

> **methyl alcohol**
> wood alcohol or methanol

mixture is also sometimes added to illegally manufactured ("bootleg") liquor.

Another type of poisonous alcohol, **ethylene glycol,** is used in antifreeze, and a third type, **isopropyl alcohol,** is commonly used as rubbing alcohol and as an antiseptic (a solution for preventing the growth of microorganisms). They are also poisonous if consumed. Pure ethyl alcohol (ethanol) is recognized as an official drug in the U.S. Pharmacopoeia, although the various alcoholic beverages are not listed for medical use.

> **ethylene glycol**
> alcohol used as antifreeze
> **isopropyl alcohol**
> rubbing alcohol, sometimes used as an antiseptic

Alcohol can be used as a solvent for other drugs or as a preservative. It is used to cleanse, disinfect, and harden the skin and to reduce sweating. A 70% alcohol solution is an effective bactericide. However, it should not be used on open wounds because it will dehydrate the injured tissue and worsen the damage. Alcohol may be deliberately injected in or near nerves to treat severe pain; it causes local anesthesia and deterioration of the nerve. For the elderly or convalescent who enjoys it, a drink of ethanol before meals may improve appetite and digestion (Ritchie 1980). In small amounts, ethanol alcohol is recommended by some physicians as a CNS depressant or sedative for convalescent and geriatric patients.

In all alcoholic beverages—beer, wine, liqueurs or cordials, and distilled spirits—the psychoactive agent is the same, but the amount of ethanol varies (see Table 8.1). The amount of alcohol is expressed either as a percentage by volume or, in the older proof system, as a measurement based on the military assay method. To make certain that they were getting a high alcohol content in the liquor, the British military would place a sample on gunpowder and touch a spark to it. If the alcohol content exceeded 50%, it would burn and ignite the gunpowder. This test was "proof" that the sample was at least 50% alcohol. If the distilled spirits were "under proof," the water content would prevent the gunpowder from igniting. The percentage of alcohol volume is one-half the proof number. For example, 100-proof whiskey has a 50% alcohol content.

Table 8.1	The Concentration of Ethanol in Common Alcoholic Beverages

Type of Beverage	Concentration of Ethanol
U.S. beers	4–6%
Wine coolers	10–12%
Cocktail and dessert wines	17–20%
Liqueurs	22–50%
Distilled spirits	40–50%

◢ The Physical Effects of Alcohol

How does alcohol affect the body? Figure 8.1 graphically illustrates how alcohol is absorbed into the body. After a drink, alcohol has direct contact with the mouth, esophagus, stomach, and intestine, acting as an irritant and an **anesthetic** (blocking sensitivity to pain). In addition, alcohol influences almost every organ system in the body after entering the bloodstream. Alcohol diffuses into the blood rapidly after consumption by passing (absorption process) through gastric and intestinal walls. Once the alcohol is in the small intestine, its absorption is largely independent of the presence of food, unlike in the stomach, where food retards absorption.

anesthetic
a drug that blocks sensitivity to pain

The effects of alcohol on the human body depend on the amount of alcohol in the blood, known as the BAC (blood alcohol concentration). This concentration largely determines behavioral and physical responses to alcoholic beverages. Relative to behavior, circumstances in which the drinking occurs, the drinker's mood, and his or her attitude and previous experience with alcohol all contribute to the reaction to drinking. People demonstrate individual patterns of psychological functioning that may affect their reactions to alcohol, as well. For instance, the time it takes to empty the stomach may be either reduced or accelerated as a result of anger, fear, stress, nausea, and the condition of the stomach tissues.

The blood alcohol level produced depends on the presence of food in the stomach, the rate of alcohol consumption, the concentration of the alcohol, and the drinker's body composition. Fatty foods, meat, and milk slow the absorption of alcohol, allowing more time for its metabolism and reducing the peak concentration in the blood. When alcoholic beverages are taken with a substantial meal, peak BACs may be as much as 50% lower than they would have been had the alcohol been consumed by itself. When large amounts of alcohol are consumed in a short period, the brain and other organs are exposed to higher peak concentrations. Generally, the more alcohol in the stomach, the greater the absorption rate. There is, however, a modifying effect of very strong drinks on the absorption rate. The absorption of drinks stronger than 100 proof is inhibited. This effect may be due to blocked passage into the small intestine or irritation of the lining of the stomach, causing mucus secretion, or both.

Diluting an alcoholic beverage with water helps to slow down absorption, but mixing with carbonated beverages increases the absorption rate. The carbonation causes the stomach to empty its contents into the small intestine more rapidly, causing a more rapid "high." The carbonation in champagne has the same effect.

Once in the blood, distribution occurs as the alcohol uniformly diffuses throughout all tissues and fluids, including fetal circulation in pregnant women. Because the brain has a large blood supply, its activity is quickly affected by a high alcohol concentration in the blood. Body composition—the amount of water available for the alcohol to be dissolved in—is a key factor in blood alcohol concentration and distribution. The greater the muscle mass, the lower the blood alcohol concentration that will result from a given amount of alcohol. This relationship arises because muscle has more fluid volume than does fat. For example, the blood alcohol level produced in a 180-pound man drinking 4 ounces of whiskey will be substantially lower than that in an equally muscular 130-pound man drinking the same amount over the same period. The heavier man will show fewer effects. A woman of a weight

Figure 8.1

How alcohol is absorbed in the body

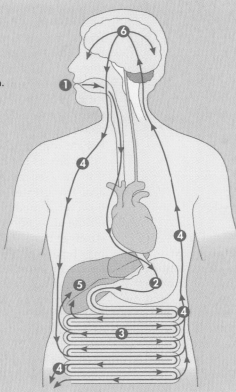

1. **Mouth**—Alcohol is drunk.

2. **Stomach**—Alcohol goes right into the stomach. A little of the alcohol passes through the wall of the stomach and into the bloodstream. Most of the alcohol continues down into the small intestine.

3. **Small intestine**—Alcohol goes from the stomach into the small intestine. Most of the alcohol is absorbed through the walls of the intestine and into the bloodstream.

4. **Bloodstream**—The bloodstream then carries the alcohol to all parts of the body, such as the brain, heart, and liver.

5. **Liver**—As the bloodstream carries the alcohol around the body, it passes through the liver. The liver changes the alcohol to water, carbon dioxide, and energy. The process is called *oxidation*. The liver can oxidize (change into water, carbon dioxide, and energy) only about one-half ounce of alcohol an hour. Thus, until the liver has time to oxidize all of the alcohol, the alcohol continues passing through all parts of the body, including the brain.

6. **Brain**—Alcohol goes to the brain almost as soon as it is consumed. Alcohol continues passing through the brain until the liver oxidizes all the alcohol into carbon dioxide, water, and energy.

Source: National Institute on Alcohol Abuse and Alcoholism. *Alcohol Health and Research World.* Washington, DC: U.S. Department of Health and Human Services, 1988.

equivalent to a given man will have a higher blood alcohol level because women generally have a higher percentage of fat. Thus, they will be affected more by identical drinks.

Alcoholic beverages contain almost no vitamins, minerals, protein, or fat—just large amounts of carbohydrates. Alcohol cannot be used by most cells; it must be metabolized by an enzyme, **alcohol dehydrogenase,** that is found almost exclusively in the liver. Alcohol provides more calories per gram than carbohydrate or protein and only slightly less

alcohol dehydrogenase
the principal enzyme that metabolizes ethanol

than pure fat. Because it can provide many calories, the drinker's appetite may be satisfied, and he or she may not eat properly, causing malnutrition (Achord 1995). The tolerance that develops to alcohol is comparable to that of barbiturates (see Chapter 7). Some people have a higher tolerance for alcohol and can more easily disguise intoxication.

Alcohol and Tolerance

Repeated use of alcohol results in tolerance and in a reduction in many of alcohol's pharmacological effects. As with other psychoactive drugs, tolerance to alcohol encourages increased consumption to regain its effects and can lead to severe physical and psychological dependence (O'Brien 1995). Tolerance to alcohol is similar to that seen with CNS depressants, such as the barbiturates and benzodiazepines. It consists of both an increase in the rate of alcohol metabolism (due to stimulation of metabolizing enzymes—see Chapter 5) and a reduced response by neurons and transmitter systems (particularly by increasing the activity of the inhibitory neurotransmitter, GABA) to this drug. Development of tolerance to alcohol is extremely variable, allowing some users to consume large quantities of this drug with minor pharmacological effects. The tolerance-inducing changes caused by alcohol can also alter the body's response to other drugs (referred to as *cross-tolerance;* see Chapter 5) and can specifically reduce the effects of some other CNS depressants (O'Brien 1995).

Many chronic alcohol users learn to compensate for the motor impairments of this drug by modifying their patterns of behavior. These adjustments are referred to as **behavioral tolerance.** An example of this adjustment would be when individuals alter and slow their speech, walk more deliberately, or move more cautiously to hide the fact that they have consumed debilitating quantities of alcohol.

> **behavioral tolerance**
>
> compensation for motor impairments by chronic alcohol users through behavioral pattern modification

Alcohol Metabolism

Almost 95% of the consumed alcohol is inactivated by liver metabolism. The liver metabolizes alcohol at a slow and constant rate and is unaffected by the amount ingested. Thus, if one can of beer is consumed each hour, the **blood alcohol level (BAL)** will remain constant without resulting in intoxication. If, however, more alcohol is

> **blood alcohol level (BAL)**
>
> the concentration of alcohol found in the blood, often expressed as a percentage

consumed per hour, the BAC will rise proportionately because large amounts of alcohol that cannot be metabolized spill over into the bloodstream.

Polydrug Use

It is a common practice to take alcohol with other drugs; this mode of consumption is known as **polydrug use.** Mixing alcohol with other types of drugs can intensify intoxication. For example, alcohol combined with other depressant drugs, such as barbiturates and benzodiazepines, have produced lethal results.

> **polydrug use**
>
> using multiple drugs concurrently

A common practice is to use alcohol with substances of abuse. Some surveys show that as many as 50% to 60% of the young adults who use marijuana also consume alcohol (Golub and Johnson 1994), while 30% to 60% of cocaine-dependent persons have a concurrent alcohol use disorder (Brady et al. 1995). In a recent report from the Drug Enforcement Administration, almost one-third of the emergency cases due to an overdose of methamphetamine also had consumed large quantities of alcohol (DEA 1996).

The reasons why individuals combine alcohol with other drugs of abuse are not always apparent. The following explanations have been proposed: (1) alcohol enhances the reinforcing properties of other CNS depressants; (2) it decreases the amount of an expensive and difficult-to-get drug required to achieve the desired effect; or (3) it helps to diminish unpleasant side effects of other drugs of abuse, such as the withdrawal caused by CNS stimulants (NIAAA 1993). Clearly, coadministration of alcohol with other substances of abuse is a common practice that can be very problematic and result in dangerous interactions.

Short-Term Effects

The impact of alcohol on the CNS is most similar to that of sedative-hypnotic agents such as barbiturates. Alcohol depresses CNS activity at all doses, producing definable results.

At low to moderate doses, **disinhibition** occurs; this loss of conditioned reflexes reflects a depression of inhibitory centers of the brain. The effects on behavior are variable and somewhat unpredictable. To a large extent, the social setting and mental state determine the individual's response to such alcohol consumption. For example, alcohol can cause one person to become euphoric, friendly, and talkative but can prompt another to become aggressive and hostile. Low to moderate doses also interfere with motor activity, reflexes, and coordination. Often this impairment is not apparent to the affected person.

> **disinhibition**
>
> the loss of conditioned reflexes due to depression of inhibitory centers of the brain

In moderate quantities, alcohol slightly increases the heart rate; slightly dilates blood vessels in the arms, legs, and skin; and moderately lowers blood pressure. It stimulates appetite, increases production of gastric secretions, and markedly stimulates urine output.

At higher doses, the social setting has little influence on the expression of depressive actions of the alcohol. The CNS depression incapacitates the individual, causing difficulty in walking, talking, and thinking. These doses tend to induce drowsiness and cause sleep. If large amounts of alcohol are consumed rapidly, severe depression of the brain system and motor control area of the brain occurs, producing uncoordination, confusion, disorientation, stupor, anesthesia, coma, and even death.

The lethal level of alcohol is between 0.4% and 0.6% by volume in the blood. Death is caused by severe depression of the respiration center in the brain stem, although the person usually passes out before drinking an amount capable of producing this effect. Though an alcoholic person may metabolize the drug more rapidly, the alcoholic toxicity level of alcohol stays about the same. In other words, it takes approximately the same amount of alcohol to kill a nondrinker as to kill someone who drinks on a regular basis. The amount of alcohol required for anesthesia is very close to the toxic level, which is why it would not be a useful anesthetic. See Table 8.2 for a summary of the psycho-logical and physical effects of various blood alcohol concentration levels.

As a rule, it takes as many hours as the number of drinks consumed to sober up completely. Despite widely held beliefs, drinking black coffee, taking a cold shower, breathing pure oxygen, and so forth will not hasten the process. Stimulants such as coffee may help keep the drunk person awake but will not improve judgment or motor reflexes to any significant extent.

The Hangover A familiar aftereffect of over-indulgence is fatigue combined with nausea, upset stomach, headache, sensitivity to sounds, and ill temper—the hangover ("Centerpiece" 1993). These symptoms are usually most severe many hours after drinking, when little or no alcohol remains in the body. No simple explanation exists for what causes the hangover. Theories include accumulation of acetaldehyde (a metabolite of ethanol), dehydration of the tissues, poisoning due to tissue deterioration, depletion of important enzyme systems needed to maintain routine functioning, an acute withdrawal (or rebound) response, and metabolism of the impurities in alcoholic beverages.

The body loses fluid in two ways through alcohol's **diuretic** action, which sometimes results in dehydration: (1) the water content, such as in beer, will increase the volume of urine, and (2) the alcohol depresses the center in the hypothalamus of the brain that controls release of a water conservation hormone (antidiuretic hormone). With less of this hormone, urine volume is further increased. Thus, after drinking heavily, especially the highly concentrated forms of alcohol, the person is thirsty. However, this effect by itself does not explain the symptoms of hangover.

> **diuretic**
>
> a drug or substance that increases the production of urine

The type of alcoholic beverage you drink may influence the hangover that results. Some people are more sensitive to particular alcohol impurities than others. For example, some drinkers have no problem with white wine but an equal amount of some red wine will give them a hangover.

Table 8.2   **Psychological and Physical Effects of Various Blood Alcohol Concentration Levels**

Number of Drinks*	Blood Alcohol Concentration	Psychological and Physical Effects
1	0.02–0.03%	No overt effects, slight mood elevation
2	0.05–0.06%	Feeling of relaxation, warmth; slight decrease in reaction time and in fine muscle coordination
3	0.08–0.09%	Balance, speech, vision, hearing slightly impaired; feelings of euphoria, increased confidence; loss of motor coordination
	0.10%	Legal intoxication in most states; driving is illegal with this level
4	0.11–0.12%	Coordination and balance becoming difficult; distinct impairment of mental faculties, judgment
5	0.14–0.15%	Major impairment of mental and physical control; slurred speech, blurred vision, lack of motor skills
7	0.20%	Loss of motor control—must have assistance in moving about; mental confusion
10	0.30%	Severe intoxication; minimum conscious control of mind and body
14	0.40%	Unconsciousness, threshold of coma
17	0.50%	Deep coma
20	0.60%	Death from respiratory failure

Note: For each hour elapsed since the last drink, subtract 0.015% blood alcohol concentration, or approximately one drink.
(*) One drink = one beer (4% alcohol, 12 oz) or one highball (1 oz whiskey).
Source: Modified from data given in Ohio State Police Driver Information Seminars and the National Clearinghouse for Alcohol and Alcoholism Information, 5600 Fishers Lane, Rockville, MD 85206.

Whiskeys, scotch, and rum may cause worse hangovers than vodka or gin, given equal amounts of alcohol, because vodka and gin have fewer impurities. There is little evidence that mixing different types of drinks per se produces a more severe hangover. It is more likely that more than the usual amount of alcohol is consumed when various drinks are sampled.

A common treatment for a hangover is to take a drink of the same alcoholic beverage that caused the hangover. This practice is called "taking the hair of the dog that bit you" (from the old notion that the burnt hair of a dog is an antidote to its bite). This treatment might help the person who is physically dependent, in the same way that giving heroin to a heroin addict will ease the withdrawal symptoms. The "hair of the dog" method may work by depressing the centers of the brain that interpret pain or by relieving a withdrawal response. In addition, it may impact the psychological factors involved in having a hangover; distraction or focusing attention on something else may ease the effects.

Another remedy is to take an analgesic compound like an aspirin-caffeine combination before drinking. This treatment is based on the belief that aspirin will help control headache; the caffeine may help counteract the depressant effect of the alcohol. In reality, however, these ingredients have no effect on the actual sobering-up process. In fact, products such as aspirin, caffeine, and Alka-Seltzer can irritate the stomach lining to the point where the person feels worse.

Dependence

Because of the disinhibition, relaxation, and sense of well-being mediated by alcohol, some degree of psychological dependence often develops, and the use of alcoholic beverages at social gatherings may become routine. Unfortunately, many people become so dependent on the psychological influences of alcohol that they become compulsive, continually consuming it. These individuals can be severely handicapped because of their alcohol dependence and often become unable to function normally in society. People who have become addicted to this drug are called *alcoholics.*

Because of the physiological effects, physical dependence also results from the regular consumption of large quantities of alcohol. This consequence becomes apparent when ethanol use is abruptly interrupted and withdrawal symptoms result. For example, during abstinence alcohol-dependent individuals can experience periods of rebound hyperexcitability marked by anxiety, agitation, confusion, insomnia, and delirium. The excitation might progress to convulsions and death (O'Brien 1995). Short-term, intermittent episodes of mild to moderate alcohol consumption appear to exert only reversible and transient effects on the CNS. However, the extended use of large quantities of alcohol has been associated with permanent

brain damage and dementia (destruction of thinking capabilities).

Effects of Alcohol on Organ Systems and Bodily Functions

As mentioned earlier, blood alcohol concentration depends on the size of the person, presence of food in the stomach, rate of drinking, amount of carbonation, and the ratio of muscle mass to body fat. Furthermore, we mentioned that alcohol has pervasive effects on the major organs and fluids of the body (Hobbs, Rall, and Verdoorn 1995). The pervasive effects of alcohol on bodily organs are discussed in greater detail in the next section.

Brain and Nervous System

Every part of the brain and nervous system is affected and can be damaged by alcohol (Figure 8.2). "Initially, alcohol depresses subcortical inhibitions of the control centers of the cerebral

---

Figure 8.2

The principal control centers of the brain affected by alcohol consumption. Note also that all areas of the brain are interconnected.

● Brain regions influenced by moderate doses of alcohol

▲ Brain region suppressed by moderately high doses of alcohol

■ Brain regions suppressed by very high doses of alcohol

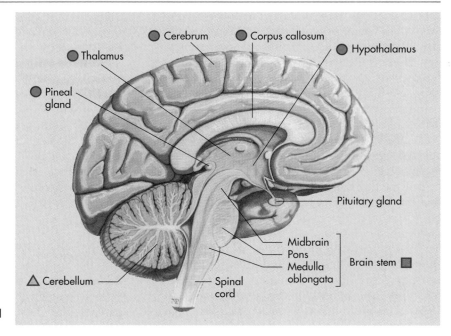

cortex, resulting in disinhibition. In higher doses, alcohol depresses the cerebellum, resulting in slurred speech and staggering gait. In very high doses, alcohol can depress the respiratory centers of the medulla, resulting in death" (Levin 1990, 23). Furthermore, alcohol impairs the production and functioning of transmitters such as dopamine, serotonin, GABA, and brain endorphins (Grinspoon 1995). These neurochemical effects contribute to the fact that alcohol consumption can aggravate underlying psychiatric disorders such as depression and schizophrenia ("Centerpiece" 1993).

Heavy drinking over many years may result in serious mental disorders and permanent, irreversible damage to the brain and peripheral nervous system, leading to compromised mental function and memory.

Liver

Among alcoholics, liver disorders are the most common causes of death (Hall 1985; Hobbs, Rall, and Verdoorn 1995). There are three stages of alcohol-induced liver disease. The first stage is known as *alcoholic fatty liver*, where liver cells increase the production of fat, resulting in an enlarged liver (Achord 1995). This direct toxic effect on liver tissue is known as the **hepatotoxic effect.** This effect is reversible and can disappear if alcohol use is stopped. Several days of drinking five or six drinks of alcoholic beverages produce fatty liver in males. For females, as little as two drinks of hard liquor per day several days in a row can produce the same condition (Achord 1995). After several days of abstaining from alcohol, the liver will return to normal.

The second stage develops as the fat cells continue to multiply. Generally, irritation and swelling that result from

> **hepatotoxic effect**
>
> when liver cells increase the production of fat, resulting in an enlarged liver

> **alcoholic hepatitis**
>
> the second stage of alcohol-induced liver disease in which chronic inflammation occurs; reversible if alcoholic consumption ceases

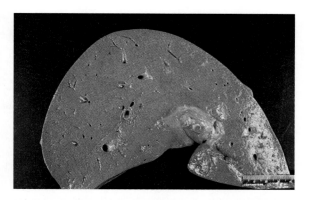

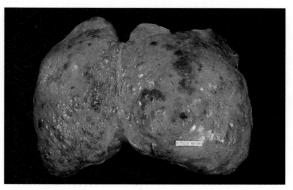

A normal liver *(top)* as it would be found in a healthy human body. An abnormal liver *(bottom)* that exhibits the effects of moderate to heavy alcohol consumption.

continued alcohol intake causes **alcoholic hepatitis.** At this stage, chronic inflammation sets in and can be fatal. This second stage is also reversible if the intake of alcohol ceases.

Unlike stage 1 and 2, stage 3 is not reversible. Scars begin to form on the liver tissue during this stage. These scars are fibrous, and they cause hardening of the liver as functional tissue shrinks and deteriorates. This condition of the liver is known as **cirrhosis.** Cirrhosis is a leading cause of death among alcoholics and the third leading cause of death in males aged 25-65 (Royce 1989, 63); it affects approximately 15% of the alcoholic population (see "Case in Point," page 192).

> **cirrhosis**
>
> scarring of the liver and formation of fibrous tissues; results from alcohol abuse; is irreversible

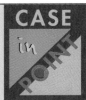

Mickey Mantle Dies from Complications of Alcoholism

Mickey Mantle, the legendary centerfielder for the New York Yankees, died August 14, 1995, at the age of 63, from complications of alcoholism. During his heyday as a baseball star, his heavy drinking was discreetly hidden from adoring fans. It wasn't until well after his retirement from baseball that Mantle checked himself into a treatment clinic and admitted publicly that he had been severely dependent on alcohol for most of his life. He sought professional treatment only after doctors warned Mantle that his drinking habits had almost destroyed his liver. Despite heroic attempts to save Mantle's life with a liver transplant in June of the same year, a cancer from the diseased liver spread rapidly, resulting in death only two months later. ▪

Source: Knight-Ridder/Tribune News Service, Aug. 14, 1995, p. 814K6829.

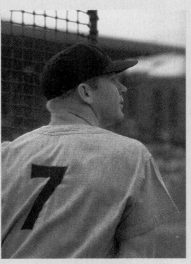

Mickey Mantle

Digestive System

The digestive system consists of gastrointestinal structures involved in processing and digesting food and liquids; it includes the mouth, pharynx, esophagus, stomach, and small and large intestines. As alcohol travels through the digestive system, it irritates tissue and can even damage the tissue lining as it causes acid imbalances, inflammation, and acute gastric distress. Often the result is gastritis (an inflamed stomach) and heartburn. The more frequently consumption takes place, the greater the irritation; one out of three heavy drinkers suffers from chronic gastritis. Furthermore, the heavy drinker has double the probability of developing cancer of the mouth and esophagus as alcohol passes these two organs on the way to the stomach.

Prolonged heavy use of alcohol may cause ulcers, hiatal hernia, and cancers throughout the digestive tract. The likelihood of cancers in the mouth, throat, and stomach dramatically increases (15 times) if the person is also a heavy smoker ("Centerpiece" 1993). The pancreas is an-other organ associated with the digestive system that can be damaged by heavy alcohol consumption. Alcohol can cause pancreatitis, pancreatic cirrhosis, and alcoholic diabetes ("Centerpiece" 1993).

Blood

High concentrations of alcohol diminish the effective functioning of the hematopoietic (blood-building) system. They decrease production of red blood cells, white cells, and platelets. Problems with clotting and immunity to infection are not uncommon among alcohol abusers. Often the result is lowered resistance to disease. Heavy drinking appears to affect the bone marrow, where various blood cells are formed. The suppression of the bone marrow can contribute to anemia, in which red blood cell production cannot keep pace with the need for those cells. Heavy drinkers are also likely to develop alcoholic bleeding disorders because they have too few platelets to form clots (Hobbs, Rall, and Verdoorn 1995).

Cardiovascular System

The effects of ethanol on the cardiovascular system have been extensively studied, but much remains unknown. Ethanol causes dilation of blood vessels, especially in the skin. This effect accounts for the flushing and sensation of warmth associated with alcohol consumption.

The long-term effects of alcohol on the cardiovascular system are dose-dependent. Recent studies have demonstrated that regular light to moderate drinking (two drinks or less of wine a day) actually reduces the incidence of heart diseases such as heart attacks, strokes, and high blood pressure. The type of alcoholic beverage consumed does not appear to be important as long as the quantity of alcohol consumed is moderate (1 to 2.5 ounces per day) (Klatsky 1995). Although the precise explanation for this coronary benefit is not known, it appears to be related to the effects of moderate alcohol doses in relieving stress and increasing the blood concentration of high-density lipoproteins (HDL). HDL is a molecular complex used to transport fat through the bloodstream, and its levels are negatively correlated with cardiovascular disease. In contrast, heavy drinking has been shown to *cause* heart disease.

Chronic intense use of alcohol changes the composition of heart muscle by replacing it with fat and fiber, resulting in a heart muscle that becomes enlarged and flabby. Congestive heart failure from **alcoholic cardiomyopathy** often occurs when heart muscle is replaced by fat and fiber. Other results of alcohol abuse that affect the heart are irregular heartbeat or arrhythmia, high blood pressure, and strokes. A common example of damage is "holiday heart," so called because people drinking heavily over a weekend turn up in the emergency room with a dangerously irregular heartbeat. Chronic excessive use by people with arrhythmia causes congestive heart failure. Malnutrition and vitamin deficiencies associated with prolonged heavy drinking also contribute to cardiac abnormalities (Klatsky 1995).

alcoholic cardiomyopathy

congestive heart failure due to the replacement of heart muscle with fat and fiber

Sexual Organs

Although alcohol lowers social inhibition, its use interferes with sexual functioning. As Shakespeare said in *Macbeth,* alcohol "provokes desire, but it takes away the performance." Continued alcohol use causes prostatitis, which is an inflammation of the prostate gland. This condition directly interferes with the male's ability to maintain an adequate erection during sexual stimulation. Another frequent symptom of alcohol abuse is atrophy of the testicles, which results in lowered sperm count and diminished hormones in the blood.

Endocrine System

As mentioned in Chapter 6, endocrine glands release hormones into the bloodstream. The hormones function as messengers that directly affect cell and tissue function throughout the body. Alcohol abuse alters endocrine functions by influencing the production and release of hormones, and affects endocrine regulating systems in the hypothalamus, pituitary, and gonads. Because of alcohol abuse, levels of testosterone (the male sex hormone) may decline, resulting in sexual impotence, breast enlargement, and loss of body hair in males. Females experience menstrual delays, ovarian abnormalities, and infertility.

Kidneys

Frequent abuse of alcohol can also severely damage the kidneys. The resulting decrease in kidney function diminishes this organ's ability to screen blood and properly form urine and can result in serious metabolic problems. Another consequence of impaired kidney function in alcoholics is that they tend to experience more urinary tract infections than do nondrinkers or moderate drinkers.

Mental Disorder and Damage to the Brain

Long-term heavy drinking can severely affect memory, judgment, and learning ability.

Wernicke-Korsakoff's syndrome

psychotic condition associated with heavy alcohol use and associated vitamin deficiencies

Wernicke-Korsakoff's syndrome is a characteristic psychotic condition caused by alcohol use and the associated nutritional and vitamin deficiencies. Patients who are brain-damaged (Hobbs, Rall, and Verdoorn 1995) cannot remember recent events and compensate for their memory loss with confabulation (making up fictitious events that even the patient accepts as fact).

The Fetus

In pregnant women, alcohol easily crosses the placenta and often damages the fetus in cases of moderate to excessive drinking. It can also cause

Fetal alcohol syndrome (FAS) is characterized by facial deformities, as well as growth deficiency and mental retardation.

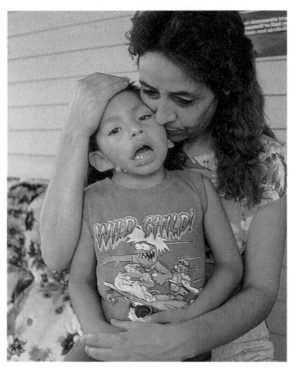

spontaneous abortions due to its toxic actions. Another tragic consequence of high alcohol consumption during pregnancy is **fetal alcohol syndrome (FAS),** which is characterized by facial deformities, growth deficiency, mental retardation, and joint and limb abnormalities (Hobbs, Rall, and Verdoorn 1995). The growth deficiency occurs in embryonic development, and the child usually does not "catch up" after birth. The mild to moderate mental retardation does not appear to im-

fetal alcohol syndrome (FAS)

a condition affecting children born to alcohol-consuming mothers that is characterized by facial deformities, growth deficiency, and mental retardation

prove with time, apparently because the growth impairment affects the functional development of the brain as well.

The severity of FAS appears to be dose-related: the more the mother drinks, the more severe the fetal damage. A safe lower level of alcohol consumption has not been established for pregnant women ("Centerpiece" 1993). Birthweight decrements have been found at levels corresponding to about two drinks per day, on average. Clinical studies have established that alcohol itself clearly causes the syndrome; it is not related to the effects of smoking, maternal age, parity (number of children a woman has borne), social class, or poor nutrition. The incidence of FAS is one in three infants born to alcoholic mothers actively consuming during pregnancy (Hobbs, Rall, and Verdoorn 1995).

Malnutrition

As previously mentioned, malnutrition is a frequent and extremely serious consequence of severe alcoholism that tends to occur most often in less-affluent alcoholics. It has been suggested that malnutrition exaggerates the damage that alcohol causes to the body's organs, especially the liver (Achord 1995). Malnutrition apparently arises so frequently in this population because many alcoholics find it difficult to eat a balanced diet with adequate calorie intake. Many alcoholics consume between 300 and 1000 kilocalories per day (approximately 2000 kilocalories per day is considered normal for an average adult male). In addition, most of the calories consumed by alcoholics come from alcohol, which contains 7 kilocalories/gram (compared with fat, which contains 9 kilocalories/gram). The malnutrition problem is aggravated because alcohol's calories are *empty*—that is, alcohol does not contain other nutrients such as vitamins, minerals, proteins, or fat (Achord 1995). Because alcoholics may be deriving 50% or more of their usual calorie intake from alcoholic beverages, profound deficiencies in important nutrients result, leading to serious degeneration of health.

 EXERCISES FOR THE WEB

Exercise 1:
NIAAA

This link discusses some of the government's efforts to help prevent alcoholism and alcohol abuse. The National Institute of Alcohol Abuse and Alcoholism provides information on its role in combating alcohol abuse and alcoholism in this country.

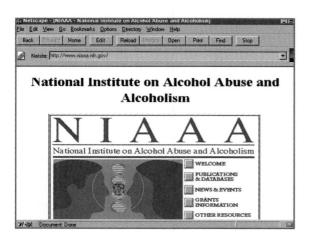

Exercise 2:
Fetal Alcohol Syndrome

Over the past 20 years medical research has identified that any alcohol consumed while pregnant could lead to serious complications on a developing fetus. This movie on fetal alcohol syndrome can be found on the web. It is an informative movie, highlighting the risks of alcohol consumption during pregnancy.

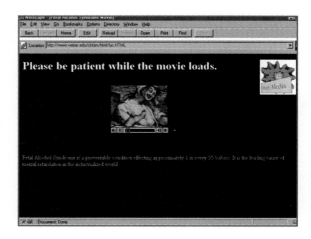

REVIEW QUESTIONS

1. What evidence indicates that alcohol is a drug like marijuana, cocaine, or heroin?

2. Explain how alcohol is manufactured.

3. In the Western world, alcohol use has a long history. List and discuss some of these historical events.

4. Explain how alcohol affects the mouth, stomach, small intestine, brain, liver, and bloodstream.

5. List at least five factors that affect the absorption rate of alcohol in the bloodstream.

6. List three short-term effects of alcohol abuse.

7. Describe the symptoms and causes of a hangover.

8. What characterizes fetal alcohol syndrome?

9. Why is malnutrition a common occurrence in alcoholics, and what are its consequences?

KEY TERMS

fermentation
mead
distillation
ethanol
social lubricant
methyl alcohol
ethylene glycol
isopropyl alcohol
anesthetic
alcohol dehydrogenase
behavioral tolerance
blood alcohol level (BAL)
polydrug use
disinhibition
diuretic
hepatotoxic effect

alcoholic hepatitis
cirrhosis
alcoholic cardiomyopathy
Wernicke-Korsakoff's syndrome
fetal alcohol syndrome (FAS)

SUMMARY

1. Alcohol is a drug because it is a central nervous system (CNS) depressant, and it affects both mental and physiological functioning.

2. Three types of poisonous alcohols are methyl alcohol, made from wood products; ethylene glycol, used as antifreeze; and isopropyl alcohol, used as an antiseptic. A fourth type, ethanol, is the alcohol used for drinking purposes.

3. The blood alcohol level (BAL) produced depends on the presence of food in the stomach, the rate of alcohol consumption, the concentration of alcohol, and the drinker's body composition.

4. Alcohol depresses CNS activity at all doses. Low to moderate doses of alcohol interfere with motor activities, reflexes, and coordination. In moderate quantities, alcohol slightly increases heart rate; slightly dilates blood vessels in the arms, legs, and skin; and moderately lowers blood pressure. It stimulates appetite, increases production of gastric secretions, and at higher doses markedly stimulates urine output. The CNS depression incapacitates the individual, causing difficulty in walking, talking, and thinking.

5. Long-term heavy alcohol use directly causes serious damage to nearly every organ and function of the body.

6. Prolonged heavy drinking causes various types of muscle disease and tremors. Heavy alcohol consumption causes irregular heartbeat. Heavy drinking over many years results in serious mental disorders and permanent, irreversible damage to the brain and peripheral nervous system. Memory, judgment, and learning ability can deteriorate severely.

7. Women who are alcoholics or who drink heavily during pregnancy have a higher rate of spontaneous abortions. Infants born to drinking

mothers have a high probability of being afflicted with fetal alcohol syndrome. These children have characteristic patterns of facial deformities, growth deficiency, joint and limb irregularities, and mental retardation.

8 Alcohol has pervasive effects on the major organs and fluids of the body. Every part of the brain and nervous system is affected and can be damaged by alcohol. Among alcoholics, liver disorders include alcoholic fatty liver, alcoholic hepatitis, and cirrhosis. Alcohol also irritates tissue and damages the digestive system. Heavy use of alcohol seriously affects the blood, heart, sexual organs, the endocrines, and kidneys.

9 Malnutrition is a common occurrence in severe alcoholism. It is the result of decreased calorie intake by alcoholics and the diminished consumption of essential nutrients due to the nutritional deficiency of alcoholic beverages.

REFERENCES

Achord, J. L. "Alcohol and the Liver." *Scientific American and Medicine* 2 (1995): 16–25.

Brady, K., S. Sonne, C. Randall, B. Adinoff, and R. Malcolm. "Features of Cocaine Dependence with Concurrent Alcohol Abuse." *Drug and Alcohol Dependence* 39 (1995): 69–71.

"Centerpiece: Alcohol in Perspective." *Wellness Letter* 9 (February 1993): 4–6.

Doweiko, H. *Concepts of Chemical Dependency.* Pacific Grove, CA: Brooks/Cole, 1990.

Drug Enforcement Administration (DEA). Internet address: http//www.usdoj.gov/dea/deahome.htm (1996).

Eronen, M. J., J. Tiihonen, and P. Hakola. "Schizophrenia and Homocidal Behavior." *Schizophrenia Bulletin* 22 (1996): 83–89.

Golub, A., and B. Johnson. "The Shifting Importance of Alcohol and Marijuana as Gateway Substances Among Serious Drug Users." *Journal of Study of Alcohol* 55 (1994): 607–14.

Grinspoon, L. "What Are the Uses of Naltrexone in the Treatment of Alcoholism." *Harvard Mental Health Letter* 12 (1995): 8.

Hall, P., ed. *Alcoholic Liver Disease: Pathology, Epidemiology, and Clinical Aspects.* New York: Wiley, 1985.

Hobbs, W. T., Rall, and T. Verdoorn. "Hypnotics and Sedatives; Ethanol." In *The Pharmacological Basis of Therapeutics,* 9th ed. edited by J. Hardman and L. Limbird, 361-96. New York: McGraw-Hill, 1995.

Hoffman, P. L., and B. Tabakoff. "Alcohol Dependence: A Commentary on Mechanisms." *Alcohol and Alcoholism* 31 (1996): 333–40.

Johnston, L. D., P. O'Malley, and J. Bachman. *National Survey Results on Drug Use from the Monitoring the Future Study, 1975–1994.* National Institute on Drug Abuse, NIH Publication #96-4027, Bethesda, MD. 1996.

Klaasen, C. "Nonmetallic Environmental Toxins." In *The Pharmacological Basis of Therapeutics,* 9th ed., edited by J. Hardman and L. Limbird, 1673-96. New York: McGraw-Hill, 1995.

Levin, J. D. *Alcoholism: A Bi-Psycho-Social Approach.* New York: Hemisphere, 1990.

Margen, S. "Ask the Expert." *Wellness Letter* 9 (1993): 8.

National Institute on Drug Abuse (NIDA). *NIDA Capsules.* Capsule 18. U.S. Department of Health and Human Services. Rockville, MD: NIDA, April 1988.

NIAAA. (National Institute on Alcohol Abuse and Alcoholism) *8th Special Report to Congress on Alcohol and Health.* (Sept. 1993): 121.

O'Brien, C. "Drug Addiction and Drug Abuse." In *The Pharmacological Basis of Therapeutics,* 9th ed. edited by J. Hardman and L. Limbird, 557–77. New York: McGraw-Hill, 1995.

Ritchie, J. M. "The Aliphatic Alcohols." In *The Pharmacological Basis of Therapeutics,* 6th ed., edited by G. Gilman, L. S. Goodman, and A. Gilman. New York: Macmillan, 1980.

Royce, J. E. *Alcohol Problems and Alcoholism: A Comprehensive Survey.* New York: Free Press, 1989.

Samson, H., and R. Harris. "Neurobiology of Alcohol Abuse." *Trends in Pharmacological Sciences* 13 (1992): 206–11.

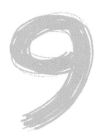

9 Alcohol: A Behavioral Perspective

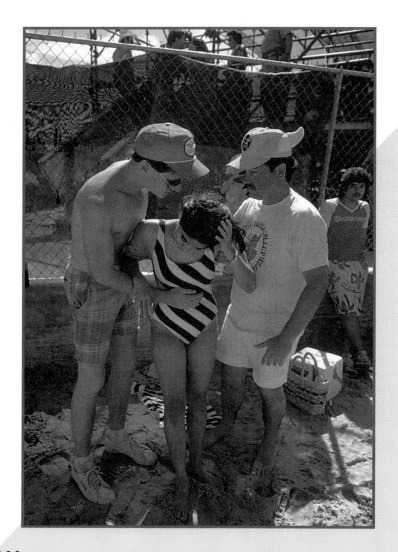

- Alcohol kills over 100,000 people annually.
- Approximately 100 million Americans drink alcohol, and between 10 and 15 million are alcoholics.
- Problem drinking and alcoholism cost the United States well over $70 billion yearly.
- In 85% of homicides, either the attacker, the victim, or both had been drinking.
- In 50% of motor vehicle crashes, alcohol was involved.
- In the United States, consumption of hard liquor has dropped sharply since 1981.
- Women are less likely to drink than men.

- In a recent National Institute on Drug Abuse (NIDA) study, 54% of eighth-graders, 72% of tenth-graders, and 77% of twelfth-graders reported drinking in the past year.
- African Americans have high rates of abstinence from alcohol.
- Of all U.S. minority groups, Asian Americans have the highest rates of abstinence, the lowest rates of heavy drinking, and the lowest levels of drinking-related problems.
- Most people who consume alcohol do not develop into problem drinkers.

- Children of alcoholics are two to four times more likely to develop alcoholism.
- Anthropologists have observed "pseudointoxication" (people acting drunk when they barely drank at all) in many societies.
- Americans consumed twice as much alcohol in 1830 than they do now.
- Spouses of alcoholics can play 10 types of roles.
- People have complained about fraternity drinking since 1840.
- Two-thirds of Americans drink.
- Poorer people drink less than more affluent individuals.

Learning Objectives

- Discuss the ways in which ethanol use is costly for our society.
- Discuss how beer, wines, rum, and whiskey relate to American history.
- Discuss the main events of the temperance movement and the Prohibition era.
- Name four different positions that cultures may take regarding alcohol consumption. Give examples of cultures that exemplify each attitude toward drinking.
- List the major findings regarding alcohol consumption in America by social class and by religious, regional, gender, age, and youth groups.
- Define *alcoholism,* and cite the general characteristics of a typical alcoholic.
- Define and explain *codependency* and *enabling.*
- Describe children of alcoholics, and explain why these children are important to study.
- Understand the relationship of alcohol to sexuality.
- Critically discuss the concept of "binge drinking" and its relationship to social problems, in a cross-cultural context and on U.S. college campuses.

I know one customer who comes in here every morning and like clockwork buys two half-pint bottles of vodka before going to work every day. She tells me that she drinks one bottle on her way to work in the car and drinks the other bottle during her lunch break. Plus, she tells me that three or four nights a week she goes to bars until early morning hours. No one could ever tell she drinks so much by just looking at her. She looks like a regular person about 30 years old. I am just amazed that she can hold her liquor so well.

From Venturelli's research files, interview with a 51-year-old liquor store clerk in a small Midwestern town, September 1, 1996

The Alcoholic Society

Alcohol has always been part of American society. The quote above illustrates how an individual can consume medically dangerous amounts of a psychoactive, addicting substance, without necessarily coming to the attention of anyone except a lone liquor-store employee. In addition, this same depressant chemical is barely considered a drug by many Americans: It is considered more a *social substance.*

According to a Gallup poll (McAneny 1994), 70% of men and 60% of women identify themselves as drinkers, or roughly two-thirds of the population. This figure includes many extremely light drinkers. Among the 65% of the population that does drink, according to the latest statistics from the National Clearinghouse for Alcohol and Drug Information's Website, approximately 111 million persons aged 12 or older drank in the last month, or 52% of all Americans aged 12 or older.

teetotaler

Individual who drinks no alcoholic beverages whatsoever; a term in common usage in decades past

The pyramid shown in Figure 9.1 has a base of 35% who are **teetotalers,** then a layer of about 13% who occasionally drink, and a top half (actually 52%) who drink fairly regularly. Some 11 million Americans, or 5.5%

of Americans aged 12 or older, had five or more drinks on the same occasion at least five different days in the past month, which is one possible definition of heavy drinking. If we define "heavy drinking" differently—for example, as more than two drinks per day—we come up with a much larger slice of the pyramid—three times as large! See Figure 9.1.

A pyramid can be constructed based on the amount of alcohol consumed, the pattern of drinking (Figure 9.1 combines these two approaches), or along a "problem" or "illness" dimension—that is, by attempting to calculate what proportion of Americans are "abusers" or "dependent" (the criteria for each were discussed in Chapter 4). The gray areas immediately expand. The young woman who was the subject of the interview at the beginning of the chapter is a prime example: She probably imbibes about one quart per day, which by some definitions is a clear diagnostic criterion for a diagnosis of alcoholism. Yet she is apparently fully functional, or at least manages to create such an appearance. Later in this chapter, we will discuss rowdy, heavy drinking collegians who crash cars, fight, and kick in dorm-room walls.

Drinking is scarcely confined to adults: 10 million individuals under age 21 drank in the last month. Of those individuals, 4.4 million had five or more drinks at one sitting and 1.7 million had five or more drinks on at least five different days. These 1.7 million heavy drinkers aren't even legally allowed to drink! In the 1994 National Institute of Drug Abuse (NIDA) study, 13% of eighth-graders reported having consumed five or more drinks in a row in the two weeks prior to the survey. Alcohol abuse and alcoholism can and do occur at all ages. However, the prevalence of alcohol abuse is most typical among young adults, as shown in Figure 9.2.

In 1995, Caucasians had the highest rate of alcohol use (56%), while 45% of Hispanics and 41% of African Americans consumed this drug.

In contrast to common assumptions, the higher the level of educational attainment, the more likely is the current use of alcohol. In 1995, 68% of adults with college degrees were current drinkers, compared with only 42% of Americans having less than a high school diploma.

Drinking is also commonly assumed to be associated with poverty, yet according to a Gallup poll (Gallup 1995), there are proportionally more drinkers in households with relatively high incomes.

The costs to society from alcohol abuse are tremendous: According to the National Council on Alcoholism and Drug Dependency (information flyer "The Hidden Costs of Alcoholism" 1996), alcohol-related costs to society were at least $100 billion when we consider health, insurance, criminal justice, and treatment costs, as well as lost productivity. Alcohol is officially linked to at least half of all highway fatalities, and that figure includes only legal intoxication. In most states, that level is 0.1% of blood alcohol level. Single-vehicle fatal crashes where the driver was legally intoxicated on weekend nights approach 70% (Wagenaar 1994). Interestingly, this single issue has been the only alcohol problem striking a spark for change: MADD (Mothers Against Drunk Driving) and SADD (Students Against Drunk Driving) are the largest prevention organizations in the nation.

Figure 9.1

Broad distribution of drinking behaviors.

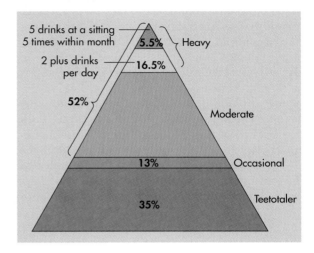

Figure 9.2

Alcoholics and alcohol abusers, United States: resident, noninstitutionalized population, 1985–1995

Source: G. D. Williams et al., "Demographic Trends, Alcohol Abuse and Alcoholism, 1985–1995," *Alcohol Health and Research World* 11, no. 3 (1987): 80–83.

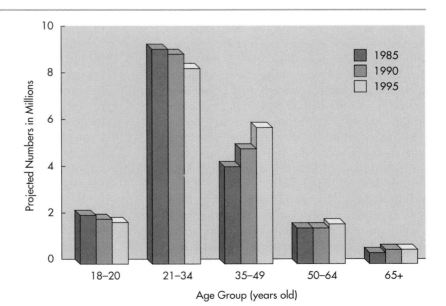

◢ Alcohol in America

From a peak in 1830, when the amount of alcohol ingested in all alcoholic beverages by the average drinking-age American was 7.1 gallons, use declined continuously until 1871–1880, when the average was 1.72 gallons, then rose to a high in 1906–1910 of 2.6 gallons, and fell to a low again, of 1.96 gallons just *before* Prohibition, 1916–1919. Under Prohibition, less than a gallon of absolute alcohol per person was consumed on average. In the last half of the twentieth century, alcohol consumption has stayed fairly constant, within the 2–3 gallon range. Wine and beer have gained as factors in producing this absolute alcohol rate, while "spirits" (hard liquor) have declined in popularity (Lender 1985, 205–6).

Historical Considerations

Alcoholic beverages have played an important role in the history of the United States.

Rum, the alcoholic essence of fermented molasses, was probably invented by the first European settlers in the West Indies. The manufacturing of rum became New England's largest and most profitable industry in the so-called triangle trade. Yankee traders would sail with a cargo of rum to the west coast of Africa, where they bargained the "demon" for slaves. From there, they sailed to the West Indies, where they bartered the slaves for molasses. They took the molasses back to New England, where it was made into rum, thus completing the triangle. For many years, New England distilleries flourished and the slave trade proved highly lucrative. This process continued until 1807, when an act of Congress prohibited the importation of slaves.

The period of heaviest drinking in America began during Jefferson's term of office (1800–1808). The nation was going through uneasy times, trying to stay out of the war between Napoleon and the British allies. The transient population increased, especially in the seaport cities, and the migration westward had begun. Heavy drinking had become a major form of recreation and a "social lubricant" at elections and public gatherings. Thus, the temperance move-

ment began with the goal of *temperance* in the literal sense: "moderation." In the 1830s, at the peak of this early campaign, temperance leaders (many of whom drank beer and wine) recommended abstinence only from distilled spirits.

African Americans were preeminent promoters of temperance. The temperance movement was closely tied into the abolitionist movement as well as the African-American church. Frederick Douglass stated that "it was as well to be a slave to master, as to whisky and rum. When a slave was drunk, the slaveholder had no fear that he would plan an insurrection; no fear that he would escape to the north. It was the sober, thinking slave who was dangerous, and needed the vigilance of his master to keep him a slave" (Douglass 1867).

Over the next decades, partly in connection with religious revivals, the meaning of *temperance* was gradually altered from "moderation" to "total abstinence." All alcoholic beverages were attacked as being unnecessary, harmful to health, and inherently poisonous. Over the course of the nineteenth century, the demand gradually arose for total prohibition (Austin 1978).

Almost every civilized country has passed prohibition laws, but few have worked for long. Attempts to control, restrict, or abolish alcohol have been made in the United States, but they have all met with abysmal failure. From 1907 to 1919, 34 states passed prohibition laws. Finally, in 1919, the Eighteenth Amendment to the Constitution was ratified in an attempt to stop the rapid spread of alcoholic addiction. As soon as such a widely used substance became illegal, criminal activity to satisfy the huge demand for alcohol flourished. Illegal routes were developed for purchasing liquor. Numerous not-so-secret "speakeasies" developed as illegal places where people could buy alcoholic beverages, and "bootlegging" was a widely accepted activity. In effect, then, such developments filled the vacuum for many drinkers during Prohibition.

Both Prohibitionists and critics of the law were shocked by the violent gang wars that broke out between rivals seeking to control the lucrative "black market" in liquor. More important, a general disregard for the law developed. Corruption among law enforcement agents was widespread. Organized crime was born and grew to be an enormous "business." In reaction to these developments, political support rallied against Prohibition, resulting in its repeal in 1933 by the Twenty-First Amendment. Early in the twentieth century, women suffragettes had been prominent temperance organizers; paradoxically, women of the "flapper" era organized against Prohibition and were the vital factor in gathering the signatures for repeal.

Defining Alcoholics

As we discussed in Chapter 4 and at the beginning of this chapter, creating absolute definitions or categories of behavioral syndromes is virtually impossible, because all behaviors fall on a continuum, and because we can never agree on precisely what the criteria should be. An alcoholic, in the minds of many Americans, is a derelict who frequents skid rows and bus terminals; yet that stereotypical alcoholic represents only a few percent of the millions of Americans who qualify as "alcoholic" by any of the accepted medical definitions. The more typical alcoholic, in fact, is the young woman mentioned at the beginning of this chapter.

> Even definitions of "problem drinker" differ from one culture to the next. In Poland, loss of productivity tend to demonstrate a "problem," while Californians emphasize drunk driving as a key indicator. Some methods of assessing problem drinking look to behavior that leads to a brush with the law. However, drunkenness may or may not lead to disruptive behavior, as we will discuss later in the chapter . . . In the Netherlands, alcoholic beverage consumption is similar to that in Finland and Poland, but there is much less disruptive or public drinking. In these nations, arrest figures do not mirror the actual amount consumed, nor the consequence to physical health. Secondly, the social response to drunkenness may not be arrest and conviction. Ireland, for example, has traditionally used psychiatric institutions to control drunkenness. (Osterberg 1986)

Estimates vary, but it is believed that approximately three-fourths of problem drinkers are men and one-fourth are women. The proportion of women has risen in recent years, partly because they are increasingly willing to acknowledge the problem and seek treatment. Female problem drinkers may therefore now be more visible as well as more numerous.

For defining alcoholism, we turn to models that speak to the state of addiction. *Alcoholism* is a state of physical and psychological addiction to a psychoactive substance, ethanol. It was once viewed as a vice and dismissed as "sinful," but over the years, there has been a shift from this perspective to one that views alcoholism as a disease. The "sinfulness" perspective failed to focus on the fact that alcoholism is an addiction—an illness—and not the result of a lack of personal discipline and morality.

Attempts to expand the basic definition of alcoholism to include symptoms of the condition and psychological and sociological factors have been difficult; no one definition satisfies everyone. The World Health Organization defines the *alcohol dependence syndrome* as a state, psychic and usually also physical, resulting from taking alcohol and characterized by behavioral and other responses that include a compulsion to take alcohol on a continuous or periodic basis to experience its psychic effects and sometimes to avoid the discomfort of its absence; tolerance may or may not be present (NIAAA 1980).

The following are two other widely accepted definitions of alcoholism:

> Alcoholism is a chronic behavioral disorder manifested by repeated drinking of alcoholic beverages in excess of the dietary and social uses of the community, and to an extent that interferes with the drinker's health or his social or economic functioning. (Keller 1958)
>
> Alcoholism is a chronic, primary, hereditary disease that progresses from an early, physiological susceptibility into an addiction characterized by tolerance changes, physiological dependence, and loss of control over drinking. Psychological symptoms are secondary to the physiological disease and not relevant to its onset. (Gold 1991, 99)

For many years, people with drinking problems were lumped together under the label *alcoholic,* and all were assumed to be suffering from the same illness.

Types of Alcoholics

A personality type theory or system demarking the types of alcoholics is described by Jellinek (1960). The categories are as follows:

Alpha alcoholism. Mostly a psychological dependence on alcohol to bolster an inability to cope with life. The alpha type constantly needs alcohol and becomes irritable and anxious when it is not available.

Beta alcoholism. Mostly a social dependence on alcohol. Often this type is a heavy beer drinker who continues to meet social and economic obligations. Some nutritional deficiencies can occur, including organic damage such as gastritis and cirrhosis.

Gamma alcoholism. The most severe form of alcoholism. This type of alcoholic suffers from emotional and psychological impairment, Jellinek believed that this type of alcoholic suffered from a true disease and progressed from a psychological dependence to physical dependence. Loss of control over when alcohol is consumed, and how much is taken, characterizes this latter phase of this type of alcoholism.

Delta alcoholics. Called the *maintenance* drinker (Royce 1989). The person loses control over drinking and cannnot abstain for even a day or two. Many wine-drinking countries such as France and Italy contain delta-type alcoholics who sip wine throughout most of their waking hours. Being "tipsy" but never completely inebriated is typical of the delta alcoholic.

Epsilon alcoholic. This type of alcoholic is characterized as a binge drinker. The epsilon-type drinker drinks excessively for a certain period, then abstains completely from alcohol until the next binge period. The dependence on alcohol is both physical and psychological. Loss of control over the amount consumed is another characteristic of this type of alcoholic.

Zeta alcoholic. This type was added to Jellinek's types to typify the moderate drinker who becomes abusive and violent. Although this type is also referred to as a pathological drinker or "mad drunk," zeta types may not be drinkers addicted to alcohol.

Other classifications differentiate alcoholics by their reaction to the drug as quiet, sullen, friendly, or angry types. Finally, another method is to classify alcoholics according to drinking patterns: people with occupational, social, escape, and emotional disorders.

◢ Culture and Alcohol

In this section, we will consider the pervasive role of culture in thought, attitudes, values, beliefs, and behavior regarding alcohol.

Maps and Definitions of Chemicals

Q: Do you consider yourself a heavy drinker?

A: No, I only drink beer.

Counselor: You were drunk when you came in here last week.

A: No, we only had a few beers.

These interviews illustrate a mental map shared by many Americans, which places beer almost outside of the domain of alcoholic beverages, as merely a step above soda. A prevention message aimed at modification of that mental map is "when you drink a lot of beer, you drink a lot!" (That is, a beer has the same amount of alcohol as a shot of bourbon).

"I would never use drugs. I only drink." That kind of statement could be made by a large proportion of Americans, probably a majority, who place alcohol in a different category from drugs. The abbreviation AODA (alcohol and other drug abuse) tries to establish a different map.

Evaluation of Alcohol

In the 1930s, American college students acquired a "reverence for strong drink" (Room 1984). Although college students "majored in drinking" for decades, during the 1930s they grew to consider heavy use as romantic and adult, resonating with the "romantic," heavy-drinking expatriate community of writers in Paris, such as Ernest Hemingway. American culture in general evaluates ethanol-containing beverages as sexy, mature, sophisticated, facilitating socializing, and enhancing status.

Culture and Disinhibited Behavior

It is necessary to stand outside of our culture, and see how people behave when intoxicated in a variety of cultures, to understand the real relationship of alcohol to human beings. A major contribution to our knowledge of intoxicated behavior comes from the field of cultural anthropology, with the concept of "drunken comportment," first formulated by McAndrew and Edgerton (1969). Alcohol *is* a **disinhibitor,** a chemical that depresses cerebral cortex functions that would impose rational or thoughtful constraints on impulsive behavior. But when consumed, it is also a signal for a "time out" in which, as in Christmas parties, one can engage in noncustomary behaviors. A review of various ethnographic studies (Marshall 1983, 190–1) reveals "pseudointoxicated" behavior among Tahitians, Rarotongans, Chippewa, Dakota, Pine Ridge and Teton Sioux, Aleuts, Baffin Island Inuits, and Potawatomi—that is, people acting drunk before, or seconds after the bottle is opened, or as the drink goes down. The frequency of use, or the amount consumed, have less effect on how drinkers comport themselves, but rather the cultural values, beliefs, mental maps, and norms cause a particular behavioral outcome. Using the terminology of psychology, we would say that it is not the biochemical effects on the brain alone that account for disinhibitory behavior, but the *belief* that one has been drinking a substance that has a disinhibitory effect; that is, the cognitive appraisal of the physiological state as disinhibition allows disinhibited behavior. Using the terminology of sociology, rewriting the sociological axiom that "what we believe to be true (or

> **disinhibitor**
>
> a psychoactive chemical, which, by depressing thought and judgment functions in the cerebral cortex, has the effect of allowing relatively unrestrained behavior, alcohol being a major example

define as true) is true in social consequences" to say "if we believe we are drunk, we act in ways that we believe drunk people act."

Cultural Rules State How Much One Can Drink, and Where

For example, many cultures, such as traditional Italian and Jewish cultures, permit moderate drinking within the family, especially at meals, but disapprove of "drunken" behaviors (although many differences separate these groups; for example, Italians use wine as if a food, whereas it has only ritual value among Orthodox Jews). In one study of Scandinavian nations, by contrast, drinking was considered absolutely separated from work. Where such behavior was permitted, however, it was allowed to go on to the point of intoxication (Makela 1986). Finnish, Polish, and Russian cultures are associated with binge drinking, while French culture is linked with sipping. In the United States, we encounter a vast variety of subgroups: some heavy drinkers may live in a community where it is not considered excessive to drink with their friends out of paper bags, on the street in the morning. Some people may belong to a "workplace culture of drinking" at a post office, construction site, or law firm where "three martini lunches" are not unheard of. Perhaps this type of drinking is not much different from the habits of peers; thus, to be "treated" for this behavior might seem as strange as going into rehab for eating birthday cake!

Cultures Provide Ceremonial Meaning to Alcohol Use

The first notable work on ceremonial use and ethnicity of alcohol use was undertaken by Robert Bales (1946), who attempted to explain the different rates of drinking among Jews (low) and Irish (high) in terms of symbolic and ceremonial meanings. For Jews, drinking had familial and sacramental significance, whereas for the Irish it represented male convivial bonding.

A high rate of heavy drinking was observed among Irish in the 1800s. It was said that these individuals drank because they were Irish. Today, some Irish-descent persons continue to live up to the stereotype; for them, it represents Irishness—they are Irish because they drink. A button on sale on St. Patrick's Day proclaimed, "Today I'm Irish, Tomorrow I'm hung over," and a *New York Post* supplement declared this event to be "Three Days of Drinking and Revelry." Jews, on the other hand, think that Jews cannot be "alcoholic." That is, they believe that if a person is Jewish, even though he or she drinks a lot, true alcoholism is impossible. If the individual gives up denial, however, and admits alcoholism, then he or she can't be Jewish (Blume, Dropkin, and Sokolow 1980)!

Culture Provides a Model of Alcoholism

In Chapter 4, we discussed models of addiction, such as the disease model. U.S. citizens define alcoholism as a disease far more often than French Canadians or French (Babor et al. 1986). Some South Bronx Hispanics have ascribed alcoholism to "spells," spirits (Garrison 1981), the evil eye (mal ojo), or witchcraft (brujeria). The entire addiction may also be ignored or bypassed; ulcers, divorce, or car accidents that an alcohol counselor may recognize as alcoholism-based may instead be traced directly to supernatural influence. One way or another, if it is attributed to a supernatural cause, a supernatural solution may be called upon to cure this problem. Thus, many seek the help of a folk curer (espiritista, santero, and so on). Some African Americans interpret their problems as a punishment from God, and may also often subscribe to a moral model that conflicts with a disease or other psychiatric or addictive model.

Culture Shapes the Alcoholic Patient Career

African Americans may progress into extremely heavy "gamma" alcoholism at an earlier age. As psychiatrists think it unlikely that a 35-year-old can incur alcohol organic brain syndrome, "schizophrenic" misdiagnoses of African-American alcoholics occur frequently (Bell et al. 1985).

Statements That Describe the Behavior of a Cultural Group as a Whole May Be Misleading

"Black" drinking patterns run the gamut from middle-class cocktail lounges (as seen in liquor ads in *Ebony*), to (Irish-like) "blue collar" wakes and birthday parties, to the "bottle-gang" of homeless poor. By class, African-American female middle-class drinkers are not dramatically different from white middle-class female drinkers, who are typically "moderate" drinkers, with few nondrinkers and heavy drinkers. Poorer African-American female groups have a larger proportion of nondrinkers; among those who do drink, more are heavy drinkers. Breaking it down further, being married, older, and church-affiliated has also been associated with nonacceptance of heavy drinking (Gary and Gary 1985).

Andrew Gordon, who studied a Connecticut city in 1981, examined three Hispanic groups, all new to the United States and all "blue-collar." In this group, Dominicans drank less after migration. They emphasized "suave" or sophisticated drinking, and saw drunkenness as "indecente" (without respect). Alcoholics were seen as "sick," perhaps from some tragic experience. Guatemalans drank substantially more after migration: one-third of males were often drunk and binged most weekends. Being drunk was considered glamorous and sentimentalized—like Humphrey Bogart under the hanging lightbulb, alone in a hotel room. These individuals boasted of hangovers, even when they did not have one. The Guatemalan AA group was alien to Puerto Ricans. Puerto Ricans broke down into middle-class American-style moderate drinkers, depressed and wife-abusing alcoholic welfare recipients, and various sorts of polydrug abusers, including those who entered into the mainland "druggie" youth culture (Gordon 1981).

Howard Blane (1977) surveyed Italian-American drinking patterns, comparing recent arrivals, born abroad but living in the United States for more than 10 years, children of immigrants, and grandchildren of immigrants. Among males, the percentage of daily drinkers declined from 92% to 15% as one moved through the generations, as did wine and cordial consumption. Any heavy use (five drinks at one sitting) rose from one-fifth to three-fifths, and once-a-week heavy use went from one-eighth to one-third. With women, daily drinking declined from 73% to 9%, wine and cordial use was more than halved (although still significantly "Italian"), occasional heavy use rose from 6% to 32%, and weekly heavy use increased from 3% to 10% (Blane 1977, 1339).

As information on cultural differences in alcohol use and abuse has become known throughout the alcohol abuse field, administrative agencies have attempted to incorporate these insights into professional standards of practice, under the rubric of "cultural competence." Prevention and treatment programs are to be evaluated from the standpoint of their competence in providing services to the cultural populations they serve. To avoid stereotyping, these considerations include understanding of such variables as ethnic acculturation and skills at eliciting information on the cultural background of clients (OSAP 1992). Prevention issues such as consumption of "gateway drugs" and media advocacy have been refined to target ethnic at-risk populations. For example, urban African-American youths are bombarded with aggressive marketing of 40-ounce malt liquors, known as "40's." Consumption of "40's" is celebrated in rap lyrics such as "Tap the Bottle." The alcohol content of malt liquors ranges from 5.6% to 8%, compared with 3.5% for regular beers. This large, cheap bottle of potent brew offers a cheap, trendy high, often leading to alcohol abuse. Moreover, in the mid-1990s, "40's" drinking increasingly became associated with marijuana smoking, going together "like cookies and milk," used before school or in "hooky parties" (*New York Times*, 1993).

Attitudes Regarding Drinking in the United States

Although cultures often maintain generalized (normative) attitudes regarding alcohol use and abuse, significant attitude differences also exist *within* cultures (Arkin and Funkhouser 1992; Inciardi 1992; Siegel 1989). As mentioned previously, the United States is characterized as culturally ambivalent regarding alcohol use. This fragmentation occurs because of dichotomies in the culture such as urban versus rural communities, and religious and ethnic differences. Other factors that contribute to diversity in attitudes include social upbringing, peer group dynamics, social class, income, education, and occupational differences.

What specific impact do such attitudes have on drinking? Attitudes are responsible for making alcohol consumption acceptable or unacceptable—or even relished as a form of behavior! For example, in one segment of impoverished African-American groups, alcohol use and abuse is so common that it has become accepted behavior (Primm 1987). The following excerpt describes an accepted use of alcohol consumption:

> A party without liquor or a street rap without a bottle is often perceived as unimaginable. These attitudes about drinking are shaped as youth grow up seeing liquor stores in their communities next to schools, churches, and homes. Liquor stores and bootleg dealers frequently permeate the black residential community, where in traditionally white communities they are generally restricted to commercial or business zones. With liquor stores throughout the fabric of black residential life, black youth grow up seeing men drinking in the streets and relatives drinking at home. (Harper 1986)

Contrast this attitude with orthodox religious and fundamentalist lifestyle communities where the use of alcohol and other drugs is strictly prohibited:

> I was raised in a very religious, Seventh-Day Adventist family. My father was a pretty strong figure in our little church of 18 members. My mother stayed home most of the time, living in a way like an Old Testament kind of biblical life, so to speak. We were strict vegetarians, and all of us in the family had to be very involved with church life. The first time I ever saw alcohol outside of always hearing how corrupting it was to the mind and the body, was when I was 7. One day the father of a friend of mine—the only non-Adventist family friend I was allowed to play with—was drinking a beer in the kitchen when we walked in. I asked, "What's that?" The father's reply was "This is beer, dear John." I looked strangely at him and pretended to be amused at the father's answer. Actually, inside I remember being very surprised and scared at the same time for I was always told that people who drink alcohol were not doing what God wanted them to do in life. (Interview with an eighteen-year-old undergraduate second-year male university student, conducted by Peter Venturelli, on May 21, 1993.)

From these contrasting examples, we can see that the values expressed through group and family attitudes regarding drug use are very significant for determining the extent of alcohol consumption.

Alcohol Abuse Among College and University Students

Alcohol has distinguished itself among college students in that usage patterns have remained steady over the years, even as marijuana use, for example, has dramatically risen, fallen, and then risen again. The CORE survey is a validated survey instrument that has been administered to more than 1 million students—by far, the largest sample of college students surveyed. The latest available figures from the CORE Institute survey (Presley, Meilman, and Lyerla 1995) indicate that college students across the nation consume an average of 4.3 drinks per week, with males averaging 6.7 drinks and females consuming 3.7 drinks weekly.

For college men, alcohol consumption was inversely related to the size of the institution, almost in a direct, algebraic relationship. That is, male students at smaller institutions consumed far more than those at larger institutions.

FIGHTING THE DRUG WAR

According to a number of studies conducted in the early to mid-1990s, binge drinking is widespread among U.S. college students—particularly in the Northeast, at Midwestern schools with big athletic programs, and at schools where fraternities and sororities account for much of the social life. As national awareness of the dangers of alcohol consumption has increased, and tolerance for drinking and driving has decreased, many college campuses are acting to try to reduce the number and extent of alcohol-related problems. So far, however, these efforts have not produced significant results.

For the purpose of the studies, binge drinking was defined as taking five or more drinks at one sitting. In 1994, 40% of college students reported such consumption at least once within two weeks of being surveyed. The age range of undergraduates, from 18 to 21, represents the period of heaviest alcohol consumption for most drinkers in the United States. According to psychology professor John Schulenberg, of the University of Michigan, "On the path to adulthood, most people pause to get drunk. It's kind of like one of the fruits of adulthood." Within this age group, surveys showed binge drinking to be more prevalent among college students than nonstudents.

The implications of this problem are enormous. Beyond the danger to drinkers' health, excessive alcohol consumption on campuses has widespread secondary consequences. For example:

▲ Students who binge-drink are more likely to damage property, have trouble with authorities, miss classes, have hangovers, and experience injuries than students who do not engage in this behavior.

▲ Binge drinkers appear to engage in more unplanned sexual activity and to abandon safe sex techniques more often than those who do not drink excessively.

▲ Students who live on campuses with higher proportions of binge drinkers experience more incidents of assault and unwanted sexual advances as a result of their peers' drinking than students who live on campuses with lower proportions of binge drinkers. They also report having their studies disturbed by drinkers or having to take care of drunken students.

Alcohol abuse prevention and treatment programs exist on many college campuses, but not many have proved effective. Some schools sponsor alcohol awareness events and classroom lectures,

"Binge Drinking" Binge drinking, defined as consumption of five or more drinks in one sitting, is a major concern at colleges and universities (see page 208, "Fighting the Drug War"). The widely reported study by Henry Wechsler and colleagues (1994) brought this issue to the public's attention. This report, which surveyed 17,592 students at 140 campuses, revealed that 44% engaged in binge drinking, which impacted on many areas of students' lives—both their own and those of others whose lives were disrupted by this behavior (giving rise to the term **"second-hand drinking"**). This issue had been worrisome to college student affairs and health professionals for decades, however. The CORE survey had collected information on collegiate binge drinking for several years before the Wechsler report and, in fact, was the source of the five-drink binge drinking definition.

binge drinking
consumption of five or more drinks in one sitting

second-hand drinking
effects of drunken behavior on associates and peers, analogizing from the term "second-hand smoking"

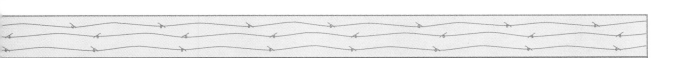

and distribute information about alcohol use. While most of these programs succeed in raising students' awareness of issues surrounding alcohol use, many do not appear to have a significant effect on drinking or the rates of alcohol-related problems. Programs that offer behavioral intervention have been more effective than education programs. The Alcohol Skills Training Program, for example, gives students the cognitive behavioral skills they need to monitor and moderate their own drinking.

In 1996, the American Medical Association (AMA) and the Robert Wood Johnson Foundation decided to fund innovative projects aimed at curbing binge drinking. The University of Wisconsin–Madison and the University of Iowa were among ten schools that launched new programs to address a "bad attitude" problem toward binge drinking. In awarding the grants, AMA Board Chair Nancy W. Dickey said, "Binge drinking is a high-risk behavior that disrupts institutions of higher education, endangers the drinkers, and victimizes their fellow students . . . You cannot drink and think. The AMA is extremely pleased to be working with universities and national leaders in the fight to reduce underage drinking."

Aspects of the Wisconsin and Iowa programs involve more enforcement of laws prohibiting sales to minors in bars, implementation of formal and informal campus policies affecting drinking, and greater availability of recreational alternatives to drinking. To address both attitudes and behavior, the programs mobilize business leaders and government officials to develop policies focused on high-risk drinking issues, using mass media to educate the community about the potentially devastating effects of alcohol abuse in a learning community. Whether the new college programs can make a dent on attitudes on the same scale as MADD efforts in high schools remains to be seen.

Sources:
American Medical Association (AMA). *AMA Forms Partnerships with Six Universities,* October 8, 1996.
Drosner, C. "UW students having a 'smashing' time." *Cardinal* (U. Wisconsin) (January 15, 1995).
Gordis, E. "College Students and Drinking—A Commentary." *Alcohol Alert* (National Institute on Alcohol Abuse and Alcoholism and National Institute on Drug Abuse) No 29 PH 357 (July 1995).
Harvard School of Public Health. "College Alcohol Study." 1993. Quoted in *Join Together* (alcohol hotline Web site service), December 6, 1994. Available at: http://www.niaaa.nih.gov.
Robinson, A. "Binge Drinking in Youth May Not Lead to Later Habits." *Michigan Daily Online News* (April 9, 1996).
Wiese, H. "Binge Drinking Survey Claims That Midwest Schools Are Among the Worst." *Iowa State Daily* (December 1, 1995).

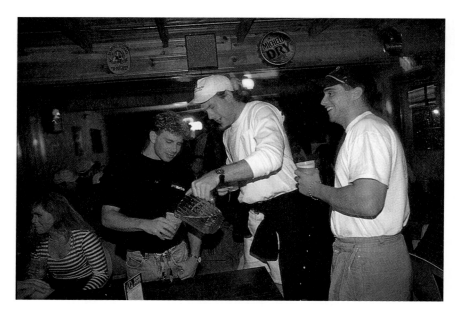

Alcohol consumption is routine at many social activities for college students.

One may question whether all five-drink episodes qualify as binge drinking, a term that calls to mind a weekend of drinking, or Jellinek's "epsilon" alcoholism. However, 11.1% of males and 7.4% of females reported three or more episodes of memory loss during the past year due to drug or alcohol use, of which the overwhelming majority were alcohol-related, both because alcohol is the major drug consumed by students, and because it produces amnesiac episodes. Amnesiac episodes are accepted as symptoms of problem drinking behavior.

Almost 15% of students (22.6% of males and 9.5% of females) reported so-called binge drinking on at least three occasions during the previous two weeks (Presley, Meilman, and Lyerla 1995). Community college students were less likely to engage in binge drinking: 29.9% had binged in the past two weeks compared with 40.4% of their peers at four-year schools. Approximately one-fourth of all males enrolled at four-year colleges reported three or more binge episodes during the past two weeks.

"On-campus" students were more likely to binge overall, and also more frequently, than off-campus students: older, working, off-campus students are less likely to engage in such behavior, lowering their scores in this regard, relative to the standard college student. Some 12.1% of on-campus students suffered three or more memory losses, compared with 7.3% of off-campus students (this last figure is not broken down by gender). These data are corroborated by the observation that 30.3% of students under age 21 had memory losses during the year, as opposed to 20.1% of those over age 21.

Native-American students had the highest frequency of drinking episodes, binge drinking, and memory loss, followed by Caucasian, Hispanic, African-American, and finally Asian students.

Gender and Collegiate Alcohol Use The findings from the CORE survey consistently indicated greater frequency of male drinking, male binge drinking, and consequences of drinking. In a review of the literature concerning gender and student drinking patterns, Berkowitz and Perkins (1987) found a historic pattern of male-dominated college drinking patterns. The transition into college is associated with a doubling of the percentages of those who drink for both genders. Both men and women drink to enhance sociability or social interaction, to escape negative emotions or release otherwise unacceptable ones, and to simply get drunk. "Drinking to get drunk" was considered more of a male pursuit. Indeed, males are more frequently associated with binge drinking and negative public consequences.

Severe drunkenness and a customary "rowdiness," or "drunken comportment", is normative for male drinkers who binge, including fighting, property damage, and troubles with authorities. The latter were twice as likely to be male problems.

Drinking is, unsurprisingly, inversely related to grades. With heavier drinkers, grades suffered, both for male and female students (see Table 9.1).

According to the studies cited by Berkowitz and Perkins (1987) for binge drinkers, the impact on impaired academic performance is just as great for women drinkers. More recent information (De Jong 1995) corroborates this finding, and also shows similar consequences among male and female binge drinkers in terms of health problems, personal injury, and unplanned sexual activity. Over the past few decades, however, some convergence between men and women has occurred in drinking patterns of all sorts.

Women Drinkers in the General Population

As a group, alcohol-abusing women tend to drink alone or at home. High incidence of alcohol abuse is found in women who are unemployed and looking for work, while less alcohol abuse is likely to occur with women employed part-time outside the home. Divorced or separated women, women who never marry, and those who are unmarried and living with a partner are more likely to use and abuse alcohol. Other high-risk groups are women in their twenties and early thirties and women with heavy-drinking husbands or partners. Wilsnack and others (1986) found that women who experience depression or reproductive problems also demonstrate heavier drinking behavior.

Looking at specific age groups, the following conclusions were drawn by the National Institute on Alcohol Abuse and Alcoholism (1990):

1. Women in the 21- to 34-year-old age group were least likely to report alcohol-related problems if they had stable marriages and were working full-time. Thus, young mothers with full-time occupations reported less reliance on alcohol in comparison to childless women without full-time work.

| Table 9.1 | Grade Averages of Heavy-Drinking Collegians |

Grade Average	Male	Female	All Heavy Drinkers
A	4.9	2.1	3.1
B	6.7	2.8	4.4
C	8.0	3.3	5.6
D or F	11.6	5.2	9.5

Source: C. Presley, P. Meilman, and R. Lyerla. *Alcohol and Drugs on American College Campuses*, Vol. II, 1990–1992. Carbondale, IL: CORE Institute, Student Health Programs, Southern Illinois University at Carbondale, 1995.

2. In the 35- to 49-year-old age group, the heaviest drinkers were divorced or separated women without children in the home.

3. In the 50- to 64-year-old age group, the heaviest drinkers were women whose husbands or partners drank heavily.

4. Women 65 years and older comprised less than 10% of drinkers with drinking problems.

More alcohol consumption is also found in women who closely perform so-called masculine gender roles, such as female executives and women in traditional blue-collar occupations.

In April 1995, former First Lady Betty Ford made the following statement: "Today we know that when a woman abuses alcohol or other drugs, the risk to her health is much greater than it is for a man. Yet there is not enough prevention, intervention, and treatment targeting women. It is still much harder for women to get help. That needs to change." In fact, women risk serious health consequences when they choose to use alcohol and other drugs. Alcohol, in particular, can often be devastating to women's health.

The Substance Abuse and Mental Health Services Administration of the Public Health Service, U.S. Department of Health and Human Services (SAMHSA) stated, in 1995, that "women become more intoxicated than men when drinking identical amounts of alcohol." As you learned in Chapter 8, women have lower water and higher fat content in their bodies; therefore, alcohol is less diluted and has a greater impact on women than men. Also, SAMHSA explains that enzymes that help metabolize alcohol in the body are less efficient in women than in men" (SAMHSA 1995). Consequently, not only does alcohol have a greater immediate effect on women, but its long-term risks are more dangerous as well. For example, cirrhosis of the liver (one result of chronic alcohol consumption) develops in women drinkers much faster than in men with similar drinking habits.

Some surveys now show that more alcohol consumption occurs among females 12–17 years old than among males at the same age. This factor places young women at a risk in delaying the onset of puberty, a condition that can wreak havoc in terms of adolescent maturation. Finally, women are more likely to combine alcohol with prescription drugs than men. When the use of other drugs enters into the equation, these adverse effects are more likely to occur. Ovulation may become inhibited and fertility adversely affected. Women also risk early menopause when they consume alcohol.

The Role of Alcohol in Domestic Violence

Much attention has been focused on domestic violence issues through high-profile criminal cases like those involving the Menendez brothers and O. J. Simpson. The increased emphasis on fighting this problem has inspired much research into the causes and effects of domestic violence, as well as into common traits of abusers. Recent studies have found a significant relationship between the incidence of battering and the abuse of alcohol; furthermore, the abuse of alcohol " . . . consistently emerges as a significant predictor of marital violence" (Kantor 1993; CSAP 1995). A study of 2000 American couples conducted in 1993 discovered that rates of domestic violence were as much as 15 times higher in households where the husband was described as "often" being drunk, as opposed to "never" drunk (Collins and Messerschmidt 1993). The same study found that alcohol was present in more than half of all reported incidences of domestic abuse.

Domestic violence also creates significant problems for its victims later in life. A study of 472

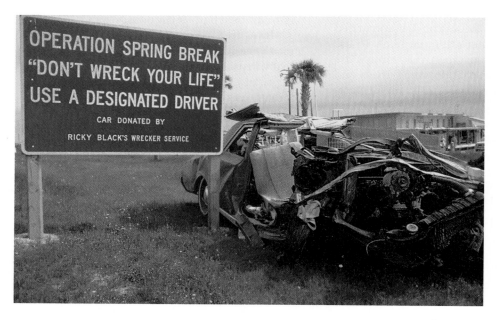

Alcohol-related traffic fatalities have fallen under 50% due to major educational and enforcement efforts over the past decade.

women by the Research Institute on Addictions found that 87% of female alcoholics had been physically or sexually abused as children (Miller and Downs 1993). The insidiousness of domestic violence may lie in the consistent abuse of alcohol that is associated with both abusers and victims. Given these disturbing statistics, the need for more research and counseling programs focused on the prevention of alcoholism and subsequent domestic violence becomes apparent. As one reformed alcoholic explains:

> . . . I had gone too far. I had abused my family, I had beaten my wife. I had driven them off, all for a drink . . .
>
> *From P. Venturelli files, 50-year-old male, 1995*

Alcohol and Sexuality

Alcohol use is linked to an overwhelming proportion of unwanted sexual behaviors, including acquaintance and date rape, unplanned pregnancies, and sexually transmitted disease, including AIDS (Abbey 1990). Factors that come immediately to mind include disinhibition concerning restraints on sexuality, poor judgment, and unconsciousness or helplessness on the part of victims. The links between unwanted sex and substance abuse are more subtle than many imagine, however. Although disinhibition, impulsivity, and helplessness are certainly major considerations, other considerations come into play:

▲ The "drunken comportment" thesis was introduced in the section on alcohol and culture. Some non-religious ceremonial drinking settings incorporate expectations of disinhibited behaviors, such as at office parties at holiday times. Drinking is a signal or cue that it is acceptable to be amorous, even sexually aggressive, and that the intoxicated object of one's affections will not object and is disinhibited.

▲ Intoxicated people are not as capable of attending to multiple cues. When cues are ambiguous, drunken men are be more likely to miss the ambiguity and to interpret cues as meaning that sex will occur and should be initiated (men are generally more likely to interpret friendly cues as sexual signals, but intoxication makes this misun-

derstanding more likely). In addition, possible dangers implicit in a private setting, on a date, with a drunken male will not be picked up as often by the intoxicated and potentially victimized female (Abbey 1990).

Alcohol and the Family: Destructive Support and Organizations for Victims of Alcoholics

Co-dependency and Enabling Co-dependency and enabling generally occur together. Co-dependency (which some call *coalcoholism*) refers to a relationship pattern, and enabling refers to a set of specific behaviors (Doweiko 1990). **Co-dependency** is defined as the behavior displayed by the non-addicted family members (codependents) who identify with the alcohol addict and cover up the excessive drinking behavior.

> **co-dependency**
> a relationship with an addict that is unhealthy for both individuals, helping the addiction to continue and letting it affect the "co-dependent's" life.

Enablers are those close to the alcohol addict who deny or make excuses for enabling the excessive drinking. Often both co-dependency and enabling are done by the same person. An example is the husband who calmly conspires and phones his wife's place of employment and reports that his wife has a stomach flu when the addicted spouse is too drunk or hungover to even realize it's Monday morning.

Such a husband is both co-dependent and an enabler. He lies to cover up his wife's addiction and enables her not to face the irresponsible drinking behavior. In this example, the husband is responsible for perpetuating the spouse's addiction. Even quiet toleration of the alcoholic's addiction enables the drinker to continue.

Children of Alcoholics (COAs) and Adult Children of Alcoholics (ACOAs) It is estimated that there are 28.6 million COAs in the United States, and 6.6 million are under the age of 18 (NCADI 1992). The children of alcoholics are at a high risk

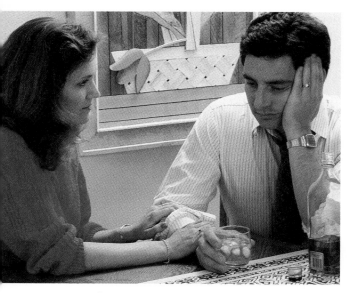

Even after the alcoholic is ready for rehabilitation, the other family members will also need treatment and support.

5. Small children of alcoholics exhibit an excessive amount of crying, bed wetting, and sleep problems, such as nightmares.

6. Teenagers display excessive perfectionism, hoarding, staying by themselves (loners), and excessive self-consciousness.

7. Phobias develop, and difficulty with school performance is not uncommon.

◀ Treatment of Alcoholism

Chapter 4 provided an overview of treatment and rehabilitation of addicts. While treatment of alcoholism and other addictions have somewhat separate historical roots and consequently gave rise to separate treatment systems, governmental authorities, and counselor certifications, they have now merged in most states in the United States. In addition to recognizing that alcohol is a drug addiction, it is also true that, epidemiologically, few "pure" alcoholics and drug addicts exist any more. Most addicts drink in addition to their other addictions, many alcoholics abuse other drugs, and some move through stages of heroin, methadone, and alcohol use, in that order. Alcoholism and its treatment have a few special features:

1. While all addicts may remain in denial, the socially acceptable nature of drinking, or even of heavy drinking, makes it easier to maintain denial as a psychological defense. It is harder to stay in denial of crack addiction, for example.

2. While all addictions are **relapsing syndromes,** and any addict may relapse, the social environment that permits or even encourages drinking and the ready availability of alcohol make it easy to relapse without a radical shift in lifestyle. Again, the alcoholic is "buffered" within a sociocultural cloud of use. Alcoholics Anonymous remains particularly vigilant for signs of relapse, advising the alcoholic to "keep the memory

> **relapsing syndrome**
> a condition from which an individual goes into remission, but which may later return

of developing the same attachment to alcohol. Alcoholics are more likely than nonalcoholics to have an alcoholic father, mother, sibling, or other relative.

Within the last decade, both COAs and ACOAs have been studied extensively. Here are some findings concerning these two groups:

1. Children of alcoholics are two to four times more likely to develop alcoholism. In addition, both COAs and ACOAs are more likely to marry into families where alcoholism is prevalent.

2. Research studies show that approximately one-third of alcoholics come from families where one parent was or is an alcoholic (NCADI 1992).

3. Both physiological and environmental factors appear to place COAs and ACOAs at a greater risk of becoming alcoholics.

4. COAs and ACOAs exhibit more symptoms of depression and anxiety than do children of nonalcoholics.

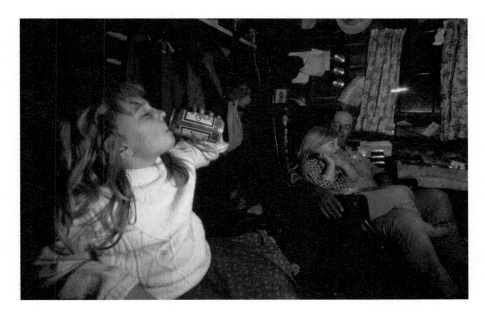

Family adjustment to addiction may encourage its persistence.

green," HALT (don't get too hungry, angry, lonely, or thirsty/tired, as these are possible relapse triggers), and not to become "isolated" from others, but to stay in the support system, making phone calls and attending "90 meetings in 90 days."

3. Alcohol rehabilitation differs from other addiction treatments mainly in its medical ramifications. Alcoholism is devastating to the liver, muscles, nutritional system, gastrointestinal system, and brain. Alcoholics that have become "dry" only recently may still suffer from pancreatitis, weakness, impaired cognitive capacities, and so forth. The fact that treatment is so structured, simplified, and sloganized ("Don't drink and go to meetings," "Keep coming: it works") reflects the bleary and confused mental status of the recently dried-out alcoholic (an AA term for this condition is "mokus"). While the cognitive impairment tends to clear up somewhat over a period of six months (unless clear cortical wasting has occurred, a condition known as "wet brain"), the alcoholic is often physically ravaged to an extent that requires years to mend the damage, if ever.

4. The alcoholic is typically more emotionally fragile than other addicts in treatment, a fact that may reflect "street" identities of many narcotics or stimulant addicts, rather than any inherent feature of alcohol addiction.

5. The other major medical ramification is withdrawal. Withdrawal from alcohol and withdrawal from barbiturate addiction are the two most severe withdrawal syndromes. Prior to modern medical management techniques, many individuals succumbed to **acute alcohol withdrawal syndrome.**

> **acute alcohol withdrawal syndrome**
> symptoms that occur when an individual who is addicted to alcohol does not maintain his/her usual blood alcohol level

Getting Through Withdrawal An alcoholic who is well nourished and in good physical condition can go through withdrawal with reasonable safety as an outpatient. However, an acutely ill alcoholic needs medically supervised care. A general hospital ward is best for preliminary treatment.

The alcohol withdrawal syndrome is quite similar to that described in Chapter 7 for barbiturates and other sedative hypnotics. Symptoms typically appear within 12 to 72 hours after total cessation of drinking but can appear whenever the blood alcohol level drops below a certain point. The alcoholic experiences severe muscle tremors, nausea, and anxiety. In extremely acute alcohol syndromes, a condition known as **delirium tremens** occurs, where the individual hallucinates, is delirious, and suffers from a high fever and rapid heartbeat. Delirium tremens, commonly called DTs, is a fairly uncommon, but life-threatening condition.

The syndrome reaches peak intensity within 24 to 48 hours. About 5% of the alcoholics in hospitals and perhaps 20% to 25% who suffer the DTs without treatment die as a result. Phenobarbital, chlordiazepoxide (Librium), and diazepam

delirium tremens (DTs)

the most severe, and even life-threatening form of alcohol withdrawal, involving hallucinations, delirium, and fever

---

Information Seeking as a Way to Counter Life Stress and Alcohol Dependency

Skip's first exposure to alcohol came when he was about 10 years old; a buddy and he discovered the liquor cabinet in his mother's house and, like two crazy chemists in a laboratory, they concocted drinks that no bartender has ever heard of—and then proceeded to swallow them. In Skip's words, "The end-result was not a pretty sight. Oh boy, was I sick." His next drinking venture occurred in the Boy Scouts, roughly a year later. "It was a rite of passage you might say," Skip remembers. "No one really said anything, even the leaders. I guess it was kind of expected." By the age of 15, Skip had tried pot; by 16, he had done his first (and last) can of Freon gas. "It was the stupidest thing I have ever done," he admitted one day. "The end-result was not a happy place to be. It took 30 days to clear my head." Curiosity led him on to try shrooms (psychedelic mushrooms), cocaine, speed, and Ecstasy, yet these drugs never had quite the same lure as alcohol.

Skip admits that alcohol is, by far, the drug that has caused the most problems in his life. "I don't drink often. I am more of a binge drinker, you might say. As a result I am a bad drunk. I don't drink to escape from my problems, I enjoy alcohol as a means to celebrate getting though exams, papers, and assignments." At the age of 21, Skip's encounters with alcohol hit an all-time low. After several shots of liquor, Skip became rowdy—a behavior that then turned into a civil disturbance. "I guess I was mouthing off and walked into an area I shouldn't have. It's all so blurry, because I don't really remember much, which is what typically happens. So I got arrested for trespassing and thrown in jail."

Seeking another way. Information seeking is a very common stress-management technique. In this method, the individual seeks out information about a situation or circumstance to get a better handle on it, such as asking a professor what the next exam is going to be like or asking an accountant how to prepare for a tax audit. In Skip's case, he didn't actually seek out information about the consequences of drinking; it sought him out—with a vengeance. He was given a choice: go to jail or attend an alcohol awareness class. The choice became a turning point for him. In essence, the month-long series of informative alcohol classes brought some sense back to Skip. "I knew I didn't have a drinking problem, not like the other people in that class. But I took a look around at these guys and it was a complete wasteland. I mean, these people had real life problems; I was just a college student. I knew I had more potential than any one of them; I have so much more going for me. So now I'm aware of my behaviors. I enjoy a buzz every now and then, but that's where it stops."

"My binge drinking was really stupid," Skip admits. "When you get to a point where you don't remember anything, you become very vulnerable and there is no way to protect yourself. You become a laughing stock. I cannot do that anymore!" ∎

(Valium) are commonly prescribed to prevent withdrawal symptoms. Simultaneously, the alcoholic may need treatment for malnutrition and vitamin deficiencies (especially the B vitamins). Pneumonia is also a frequent complication (Jaffe 1980).

Once the alcoholic patient is over the acute stages of intoxication and withdrawal, administration of CNS depressants may be continued for a few weeks, with care taken not to transfer dependence on alcohol to dependence on the depressants. Long-term treatment with sedatives (such as Librium or Valium) does not prevent a relapse of drinking or assist with behavioral adaptation. A prescription of disulfiram (Antabuse) may be offered to encourage patients to abstain from alcohol; it blocks metabolism of acetaldehyde, and drinking any alcohol will result in a pounding headache, flushing, nausea, and other unpleasant symptoms. The patient must decide about two days in advance to stop taking Antabuse before he or she can drink. Antabuse is an aid to other supportive treatments, not the sole method of therapy.

◢ Helping the Alcoholic Family Recover

Alcoholism is a pervasive family disease. The family is a system, not of planets or subatomic particles, but of people who affect one another, and who play certain roles, all maintaining a balance in the system. We are all familiar with the sterotype of families in which an oldest child is the "hero," the middle child is "forgotten," and the youngest is the "baby." Whatever the roles of the individuals, when the family includes an alcoholic, it means that a member of the system is ill. The system adapts to dysfunction by rearranging itself around the problem. The family is like a mobile, a sculpture with interdependent parts that revolve around one another. We are not talking about adjusting to a person with a broken leg or diabetes, but someone who is in denial—manipulative, lying, and blaming other family members. By adjusting around the addiction, they enable the addict to progress further along the disease path. Roles become exaggerated and distorted. Persons

may be blamed, scapegoated, or lost and forgotten. One major adaptation is related to the person who "takes up the slack" by assuming extra responsibilities and taking on the role of a parent or even spouse.

Early family therapy systems research described how the family often acts as a unit. It focused on the disturbed communication patterns within families, and the process by which the family throws up a scapegoat, often in the form of a child who is presented as the "identified patient" (Kolevson and Green 1985; Satir 1964;) The concept of the "super-responsible one" was first described by Virginia Satir (1964). In modern, popular writing on addiction in the family and codependent roles of children that are carried into adulthood, all of these roles are depicted as especially characteristic of *addicted* families (Wegscheider 1981). Because such roles are so common, many individuals may identify with them and ascribe a variety of ills to their being addict offspring. Many individuals do suffer tremendously from the legacy of family addiction, and some have indeed been cast in one of these roles as a by-product of addiction in the family. Acting as if only one kind of family, or one kind of addicted family, existed that transcended cultural backgrounds is not much better than saying that all languages or religions are the same. For example, "executive authority" over younger children can be the normal role of an eldest female child in African-American families as part of a broader pattern of role flexibility (Brisbane 1985a; Brisbane and Womble 1985). When an older child plays a "parental" part in the family, it may represent culturally routine behavior or it may be indicative of a response to addiction in the family.

There is some gain or perceived benefit to the person playing a role, and to the system as a whole in the individual's actions, although this gain may seem very indirect and, in fact, injurious in the long run. While the person may be overburdened and resentful, he or she also feels important, heroic, and capable. Over a period of time this role solidifies. Perhaps the "hero" becomes unable to remember or imagine it any other way. If the alcoholic enters or promises to enter into recovery, it may threaten the benefits to the family member. One of many examples is a wife in a traditionally

"The Top Tens" of Helping Alcoholics and Their Families

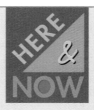

10 "Don'ts"

Don't "persecute" the addict. Confront lovingly.

Don't have the goal of "saving the family."

Don't start sentences with "you never," or "you always."

Don't live in the past or in the future.

Don't make excuses for the alcoholic.

Don't let the alcoholic be the center of your life.

Don't clean up after the alcoholic (literally or figuratively).

Don't protect the alcoholic from the consequences of his or her behavior.

Don't blame, excuse, justify, or rationalize.

Don't join in drinking.

10 "Do's"

Set limits, using "I" words (I need to stop).

Set limits empathetically (I know, you want me to _____, but I can't).

Detach, lovingly, from the addict's problems.

Teach parenting skills.

Concentrate on the here and now.

Talk about violence and abuse.

Remember that you didn't cause it, you can't cure it, and you can't control it!

Take life a day at a time.

Give "self" assignments, taking care of yourself.

Accept the right to have your feelings, and for others to have their feelings.

Source: Inservice Training Program, Essex County, New Jersey, Professional Advisory Committee on Alcohol and Drug Abuse. November 1993. Prepared by Peter L. Myers, Ph.D.

10 Alcoholic Family Self-Statements

In an actively alcoholic family:
"Don't talk" (about how you feel, about what's going on).
"Don't trust."
"Don't feel."
"Alcoholism isn't the cause of our problems."
"Keep the status quo at all costs."

Where the family is having a hard time getting used to sobriety:
"We liked you better drunk."
"You're always away at AA meetings."
"Who are these people you're always having coffee with?"
"I felt important feeding my brothers and sisters, Mom."
"I felt important going to the school on Open School Night, Dad."

10 Roles for Spouses of Alcoholics
Rescuer
Long-suffering martyr
Blamer, conscience
Fellow drinker
Placater
Overextended, superresponsible one
Composed computer
Sick hypochondriac
Scapegoat ("it's all your fault")
Avoider

10 Roles for Children of Alcoholics
Family hero*
Scapegoat*
Lost child*
Mascot*
Placater
Sick role
Parental child or pseudoparent to younger children
Pseudoparent to alcoholic parent
Pseudospouse to sober parent
Place of refuge (for younger children)

*Wegscheider 1991.

subservient role who relishes at some level the power, control, and authority she has had with an alcoholic husband, or the recognition she received in martyrdom—perhaps her only recognition in life. Another example is the child who is given executive authority, prematurely, in the family. Without knowing it, the family members may resist change, not only for what they may have to give up, but also because change is always feared and the "devil" is a known quantity. Thus they may undermine recovery.

Role systems found in alcoholic families can be "enmeshed," so that everyone is hyperresponsive to and dependent on one another, "disorganized," chaotic, or exploded into nothingness. The old-fashioned middle-class alcoholic family is more commonly enmeshed. If religion represents a barrier to divorce, and hence removal of the alcoholic, this situation is even more likely to arise.

A family counselor can help the family members understand the roles they are playing, and start a process of change. This recognition allows family members to develop their own identities separate from the roles they have been playing. Two of the techniques used in understanding roles and relationships are **psychodrama** (or **role playing**) and the **genogram,** a kind of family tree in which behavioral relationships as well as biological relationships are explored.

> **psychodrama**
>
> a family therapy system developed by Jacques Moreno, in which significant interpersonal and intrapersonal issues are enacted in a focused setting using dramatic techniques
>
> **role playing**
>
> a therapeutic technique in which group members play assigned parts to elicit emotional reactions

The family counselor can help the family figure out their patterns of thinking, which involves certain modes of information processing. In the alcoholic family, these patterns typically involve denial, minimization, rationalization, shame, blame, and projection. They also rely on certain "self-statements" (see "Here and Now," page 218).

> **genogram**
>
> a family therapy technique that records information about behavior and relationships on a type of family tree to elicit persistent patterns of dysfunctional behavior

In addition, the family counselor can help the family understand their patterns of communication. Alcoholic family communication will almost certainly be a type of abnormal communication, characterized by either simple absence of communication (chaotic, destructive, manipulative, blaming) or a combination of communication methods. What the family does in the public view, visible to the outside world (front stage), differs from what goes on "back stage." Some individuals may be "cut off" from communication or embroiled in endless argument and acrimony. Teaching people how to communicate their feelings and opinions in a direct, honest, and nonhurtful way will begin the healing process.

The alcoholic family is injured, traumatized, often in debt, and collectively suffering from **post-traumatic stress disorder.** Impacted grief, loss, pain, and rage are present. Healing will not take place overnight, and will not occur just because the alcoholic stops drinking. The child, in particular, may have been wounded by violence, neglect, and inconsistent parenting, and may have been witness to sex, violence, or depression.

> **post-traumatic stress disorder**
>
> a psychiatric syndrome in which an individual who has been exposed to a traumatic event or situation, experiences persistent psychological stress that may manifest itself in a wide range of symptoms, including reexperiencing the trauma, numbing of general responsiveness, and hyperarousal

EXERCISES FOR THE WEB

Exercise 1: AA

There are many ways to help an individual deal with his or her alcoholism. Self-help groups are one of the most popular approaches. The Alcoholics Anonymous Home Page is the location of one of the world's oldest and most effective self-help groups.

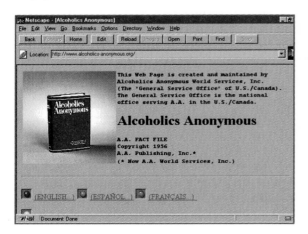

Exercise 2: Alcohol Self-Check

Visit the Self-Check web site. There is a self-scoring alcohol check. Go through the assessment and complete the questions. Have the results analyzed to determine your level of dependency on alcohol. Discuss whether or not you think this assessment is accurate.

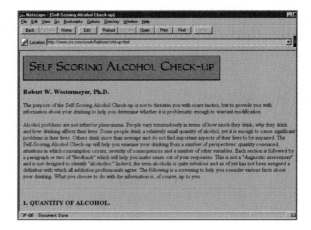

 REVIEW QUESTIONS

1. Why do you think alcohol remains a legal drug despite the tremendous costs to our society?

2. Would a temperance movement and/or prohibition on alcohol be successful today? Why or why not? Give at least three reasons in support of your position.

3. Do you personally believe that the setting can have a stronger effect on the alcohol user than the ethanol itself? In other words, do you think that nonalcoholic beer, for example, could possibly cause people to actually believe and act as if they were inebriated?

4. Review the reasons cited regarding the decrease of alcohol consumption since 1981.

Which single reason do you believe is the most important for the decrease? Why?

5. Review the major findings regarding alcohol consumption among social class, religious, regional, gender, age, and youth groups. Describe two groups where the findings contradicted your commonsense expectations.

6. What theory discussed in Chapter 2 do you think best explains the reasons why racial and ethnic minorities, gays, and the homeless are prone to abuse so much alcohol?

7. From the views and theoretical explanations given for alcoholism in this chapter, which view or theoretical explanation best explains the causes of alcoholism? Why does the view or theory you selected provide more explanatory power than the others?

8. What specific factors do you think make the children of alcoholics and adult children of alcoholics more likely to develop drinking problems?

KEY TERMS

teetotaler
disinhibitor
binge drinking
second-hand drinking
co-dependency
relapsing syndrome
acute alcohol withdrawal syndrome
delirium tremens (DTs)
psychodrama
role playing
genogram
post-traumatic stress disorder

SUMMARY

1 Ethanol is the psychoactive ingredient found in alcoholic beverages. The ill effects of its misuse exceed those of any other legal or illicit drugs.

2 In response to the heaviest drinking period in America during Jefferson's turn in office (1800–1808), the *temperance movement* occurred. The original goal of this movement was to promote moderate use of alcohol. Largely because it was unsuccessful, the temperance movement began advocating "total abstinence." Over the course of the nineteenth century, total prohibition was enacted into law. Shortly after Prohibition laws were created making alcohol use illegal, organized crime involved itself in producing and selling alcohol as an illicit drug.

3 Cultures vary in the use of alcohol. Abstinent cultures strictly prohibit alcohol use. Ambivalent cultures have contradictory views on alcohol consumption. Permissive cultures promote alcohol consumption, and over-permissive cultures encourage alcohol use.

4 Groups in our society vary in their consumption of alcohol. The higher the household income, the greater is the percentage who drink.

Women are less likely to drink than men, although the percentage of women drinking has been increasing in recent years. People over age 50 drink the least, while those under 30 through 49 drink the most. Although in the last few years the percentage of youth drinking alcohol has begun to decline, a disturbing percentage—well over 60% of all youth—continue to drink alcohol.

5 There are several accepted definitions of alcoholism. Alcohol addiction involves both physical and psychological dependence on ethanol. Most definitions include chronic behavioral disorders, repeated drinking to the point of loss of control, health disorders, and difficulty functioning socially and economically.

6 Children of alcoholics (COAs) and adult children of alcoholics (ACOAs) are of particular interest in the study of alcoholism because research shows that these children and adults are two to four times more likely to develop alcoholism.

7 Prevention differs from treatment in that it involves delaying or preventing alcohol consumption. Treatment involves stopping the ongoing consumption of alcohol. Primary prevention techniques are aimed at nonusers and early experimenters. Secondary prevention techniques address experimenters or early users of alcohol.

8 The system of roles in families of alcoholics often includes scapegoats, overresponsible ones, "lost children," placaters, and other types.

9 College student binge drinking has deleterious effects in many areas.

10 Culture provides definitions of alcohol abuse and alcoholism, its causes, problems associated with it, and appropriate behavior while intoxicated (drunken comportment).

11 Alcoholism treatment must take into consideration physical withdrawal and denial.

REFERENCES

Abbey, A. "Sex and Substance Abuse: What Are the Links." *Eta Sigma Gamman*, 22 (Fall 1990): 16–18.

Akers, R. L. *Deviant Behavior: A Social Learning Approach*, 3d ed. Belmont: CA: Wadsworth, 1985.

Akers, R. L. *Drugs, Alcohol, and Society: Social Structure, Process, and Policy.* Belmont, CA: Wadsworth, 1992.

"Alcoholism," *Academic American Encyclopedia* (Electronic database on CARL system at the University of Colorado, Boulder). Grolier Electronic Publishing, no date.

Arkin, E. B., and J. E. Funkhouser, eds. *Communicating About Alcohol and Other Drugs: Strategies for Reaching Populations at Risk,* OSAP Prevention Monograph 5. Rockville, MD: Office of Substance Abuse Prevention, U.S. Department of Health and Human Services, 1992.

Aronow, L. *Alcoholism, Alcohol Abuse, and Related Problems: Opportunities for Research.*Washington, DC: National Academy Press, 1980.

Austin, G. A. *Perspectives on the History of Psychoactive Substance Use.* National Institute on Drug Abuse Research Issues 23. Washington, DC: U.S. Department of Health, Education, and Welfare, 1978.

Barbor, T. F. "Alcohol, Economics and Ecological Fallacy: Toward an Integration of Experimental and Quasi-Experimental Research." In *Public Drinking and Public Policy,* edited by E. Single and T. Storm, 161–89. Proceedings of a Symposium on Observation Studies held at Banff, Alberta, 26–28 April 1984. Toronto: Addiction Research Foundation, 1985.

Babor, T. F., M. Hesselbrock, S. Radouce-Thomas, L. Feguer, J.-P. Ferrant, and K. Choquette "Concepts of Alcoholism Among American, French-Canadian, and French Alcoholics." In *Alcohol and Culture: Comparative Perspectives from Europe and America.* NY, New York Academy of Sciences. Edited by T. F. Babor (1986): 98–109.

Baker, S. P., B. O'Neil, and R. Karpf. *Injury Fact Book.* Lexington, MA: D. C. Heath, 1984.

Bales R. F. "Cultural Differences in Rates of Alcoholism." *Quarterly Journal of Studies on Alcohol* 6 (1946): 489–99.

Becker, H. S. *Outsiders: Studies in the Sociology of Deviance.* New York: Free Press, 1966.

Bell, C. C., J. P. Thompson, D. Lewis, J. Redd, M. Shears, and B. Thompson. "Misdiagnosis of Alcohol-Related Organic Brain Syndromes: Implications for Treatment. *Alcoholism Treatment Quarterly* 2 (1985): 45–65.

Berg, G., and A. Skutle. "Early Intervention with Problem Drinkers." In *Treating Addictive Behaviors Processes of Change,* edited by W. R. Miller and N. Heather, 205–20. New York: Plenum, 1986.

Berkowitz, A. D., and H. W. Perkins. "Recent Research on Gender Differences in Collegiate Alcohol Use." *Journal of American College Health* 36 (September 1987): 12–15.

Blane, H. "Acculturation and Drinking in an Italian American Community." *Journal of Studies on Alcohol* 38 (1977): 1324–44.

Blume, S., D. Dropkin, and L. Sokolow. "The Jewish Alcoholic: A Descriptive Study." *Alcohol, Health, and Research World* 4 (1980): 21–6.

Bower, B. "Gene in the Bottle" A controversial Alcoholism Gene Gets a New Twist." *Science News* 140 (21 September 1991): 392–93.

Brisbane, F. L. "Understanding the Female Child Role of Family Hero in Black Alcoholic Families." *Bulletin of the NY State Chapter of the National Black Alcoholism Council.* 4 April 1985a.

Brisbane, F. L. "A Self-Help Model for Working with Black Women of Alcoholic Parents." *Alcoholism Treatment Quarterly* 2 (Fall 1985b/Winter 1986): 47–53.

Brisbane, F. L., and M. Womble. "Afterthought and Recommendations." *Alcoholism Treatment Quarterly* 2 (Fall 1985/Winter1986): 54–58.

Catanzaro, R. J. "Psychiatric Aspects of Alcoholism." In *Alcoholism,* edited by D. J. Pittman. New York: Harper & Row, 1967.

Center for Substance Abuse Prevention (CSAP). *Making the Link: Impaired Driving, Injury, and Trauma and Alcohol and Other Drugs.* Substance Abuse and Mental Health Services Administration, Rockville, MD. ML004, spring 1995.

Chan, A. W. K. "Racial Differences in Alcohol Sensitivity." *Alcohol and Alcoholism* 21 (1986): 93–104.

Chi, I., H. H. L. Kitano, and J. E. Lubben. "Male Chinese Drinking Behavior in Los Angeles." *Journal of Studies on Alcohol* 49 (1988): 21–5.

Colasanto, D., and J. Zeglarski. "Alcoholic Beverages: Alcohol Consumption at Lowest Level in 30 Years." *Gallup Report* 288 (September 1989).

Collins, J. J., and M. A. Messerschmidt. "Epidemiology of Alcohol-Related Violence." U.S. Department of Health and Human Services, National Institute on Alcohol Abuse and Alcoholism. *Alcohol, Health, and Research World* 17 (1993): 93–100.

De Jong. "Scope of the Problem: Gender and drinking." *Catayst* (Higher Education Center for Alcohol and Other Drug Prevention) 1 (spring 1995): 1.

Desmond, E. W. "Out in the Open: Changing Attitudes and New Research Give Fresh Hope to Alcoholics." *Time* (30 November 1987): 42–50.

Douglass, Frederick. *Life and Times of Frederick Douglass.* New York. Collier Books. (1967 edition) 1892: 147–8.

Dowdall, G. W., and H. Wechsler. "Binge Drinking on Campus: The Harvard School of Public Health College Alcohol Study." Conference paper prepared for presentation to the Society for the Study of Social Problems, New York, 1996.

Doweiko, H. E. *Concepts of Chemical Dependency.* Monterey, CA: Brooks/Cole, 1990.

Frankana, M., M. Cohen, T. Danill, L. Ehrlich, N. Greenspun, and D. Kelman. "Alcohol Advertising, Consumption and Abuse." In *Recommendations of the Staff of the Federal Trade Commission: Omnibus Petition for Regulation of Unfair and Deceptive Alcoholic Beverage Marketing Practices,* edited by staff. Docket no. 290–346. Washington, DC: Federal Trade Commission, 1985.

Freud, Sigmund. "Dostoyevsky and Parricide." *The Standard Edition of the Complete Works of Sigmund Freud,* edited by J. Strachey, 340–86. London: Hogarth Press and Institute of Psychoanalysis, 1961.

Gallup, G., Jr. *The Gallup Poll: Public Opinion 1994.* Wilmington, DE: Scholarly Resources, Inc., 1995.

Gallup, G., Jr. *The Gallup Poll: Public Opinion 1994.* Wilmington, DE: Scholarly Resources, 1994.

Gallup, G., Jr., and F. Newport. "Americans Now Drinking Less Alcohol." *Gallup Poll Monthly* (December 1990).

Gallup Report. No. 276 (September 1988).

Garrison, V., and J. Podell. "Community Support Systems Assessment for Use in Clinical Interviews." *Schizophrenia Bulletin* 7 (1981): 1.

Gary, L. E., and R. B. Gary. "Treatment Needs of Black Alcoholic Women." *Alcoholism Treatment Quarterly* 2 (1985): 97–113.

Gfroerer, J. "Preliminary Estimates from the 1994 National Household Survey on Drug Abuse." Advance Report Number 10. Rockville, MD: U.S. Department of Health and Human Services, Substance Abuse and Mental Health Services Administration (SAMHSA), September 1995.

Gold, M. S. *The Good News About Drugs and Alcohol.* New York: Villard Books, 1991.

Gomberg, E., and S. Lisansky. "Historical and Political Perspective: Women and Drug Use." In *Drug Use and Misuse: A Reader,* edited by T. Heller, M. Gott, and C. Jeffery. New York: Wiley, 1989.

Gordon, A. J. "The Cultural Context of Drinking and Indigenous Therapy for Alcohol Problems in Three Migrant Hispanic Cultures." *Journal of Studies on Alcohol* supplement 9 (1981): 217–40.

Greeley, Andrew M., W. C. McCreedy, and G. Theison. *Ethnic Drinking Subcultures.* New York: Praeger, 1980.

Harper, F. "Research and Treatment with Black Alcoholics." *Alcohol, Health, and Research World* 4 (summer 1980): 10–6.

Harper, F. D. *The Black Family and Substance Abuse.* Detroit: Detroit Urban League, 1986.

Horton, D. "The Functions of Alcohol in Primitive Societies: A Cross-Cultural Study." *Quarterly Journal of Studies on Alcohol* 4 (1943): 199–320.

Inciardi, J. A. *The War on Drugs II.* Mountain View, CA: Mayfield, 1992.

"In These Times." Chicago, IL: 18–24 October 1989.

Jaffe, J. H. "Drug Addiction and Drug Abuse." In *The Pharmacological Basis of Therapeutics,* 6th ed., edited by A. G. Gilman, L. S. Goodman, and A. Gilman, 494–534. New York: Macmillan, 1980.

Jellinek, E. M. *The Disease Concept of Alcoholism.* New Haven, CT: College and University Press, 1960.

Jennison, K. M. "The Impact of Stressful Life Events and Social Support on Drinking Among Older Adults: A General Population Survey." *International Journal of Aging and Human Development* (1992): 991–1023.

Jensen, M. A., T. L. Peterson, R. J. Murphy, and D. A. Emmerling. "Relationship of Health Behaviors to Alcohol and Cigarette Use by College Students." *Journal of College Students Development* 33 (1992): 170.

Johnston, L. D., P. O'Malley, and J. G. Bachman. "Smoking, Drinking, and Illicit Drug Use Among American Secondary School Students, College Students, and Young Adults, 1975–1991." In *Drugs, Society and Behavior 93/94,* edited by E. Goode. Sluice Dock, Guilford, CT: Dushkin, pp. 87–91 Publishing Group, Inc. 1993.

Johnston L. D., P. M. O'Malley, and J. G. Bachman. "Monitoring the Future Study," *Vol. 1, Secondary School Students.* Rockville, MD: National Institute on Drug Abuse, 1994.

Kantor, G. K. "Refining the Brushstrokes in Portraits of Alcohol and Wife Assaults." *Alcohol and Interpersonal Violence. Fostering Multidisciplinary Perspectives.* Research monograph 24. Rockville, MD: National Institute on Alcohol Abuse and Alcoholism, 1993.

Keller, M. "Alcoholism: Nature and Extent of the Problem." *Understanding Alcoholism, Annals American Academy Political and Social Science* 315 (1958): 1–11.

Kilbourne, J., ed. "Advertising Addiction: The Alcohol Industry's Hard Sell." *Multinational Monitor* (Washington, DC) 10 (June 1989): 13–6.

Kolevzon, M. S., and R. G. Green. *Family Therapy Models.* New York: Springer, 1985. "Spirituality: A Tool in the Assessment and Treatment of Black Alcoholics and Their Families" *Alcoholism Treatment Quarterly* 2: 3/4 pp. 31–44 F 1985/W 1986.

Lee, H. *How Dry We Were: Prohibition Revisited.* Englewood Cliffs, NJ: Prentice-Hall, 1963.

Leerhsen, C., with T. Namuth. "Alcohol and the Family." *Newsweek* (18 January 1988): pp. 62–68

Lender, M. E. *Drinking in America.* New York: Free Press, 1985.

Levin, J. D. *Alcoholism: A Bio-psychosocial Approach.* New York: Hemisphere, 1990.

Lewis, G. R., and S. M. Jordan. "Treatment of the Gay or Lesbian Alcoholic." In *Alcoholism and Substance Abuse in Special Populations,* edited by G. W. Lawson and A. W. Lawson, 165–203. Gaithersburg, MD: Aspen, 1989.

Liska, K. *Drugs and the Human Body,* 3rd ed. New York: Macmillan, 1990.

Little, C. B. *Deviance and Control: Theory, Research, and Social Policy.* Itasca, IL: Peacock, 1989.

Lumeng, L., and Li, T.-K. "The Development of Metabolic Tolerance in the Alcohol-Preferring P Rats: Comparison on Forced and Free-Choice Drinking of Ethanol." *Pharmacological Biochemical Behavior* 25 (1986): 1013–20.

MacAndrew, C., and R. B. Edgerton. *Drunken Comportment: A Social Explanation.* Chicago: Aldine, 1969.

Makela, K. "Attitudes Towards Drinking and Drunkenness in Four Scandinavian Countries." *Alcohol and Culture:*

Comparative Perspectives from Europe and America, (1986). *Annals of the New York Academy of Sciences,* NY, New York Academy of Sciences. vol. 472, edited by T. F. Babor.

Marriott, M. "For Minority Youths, 40 Ounces of Trouble," *New York Times,* April 16, 1993, 1.

Marshall, M. "Four Hundred Rabbits": An Anthropological View of Ethanol as a Disinhibitor." In *Alcohol and Disinhibition: Nature and Meaning of the Link.* Washington, DC: U.S. HHS, PHS, ADAMHA, National Institute on Alcohol Abuse and Alcoholism Research Monograph 12, 1983.

McAneny, Leslie, "Alcoholism in America: Number of Drinkers Holding Steady but Drinking Less." *Gallup Poll News Service* 59 (17 June 1994): 1–4.

McKirnan, D. J., and P. L. Peterson. "Psychosocial and Cultural Factors in Alcohol and Drug Abuse: An Analysis of a Homosexual Community." *Addictive Behaviors* 14 (1989): 555–63.

Merrill, D. S. "The Changing Homeless Population." *U.S. News and World Report* (15 January 1990): 27.

Miller, B. A., and W. R. Downs, "The Impact of Family Violence on the Use of Alcohol by Women." *Alcohol, Health, and Research World* 17 (1993): 137–43.

Minuchin, S. *Families and Family Therapy* Cambridge, Harvard University Press, 1974.

Moskowitz, J. M. "The Primary Prevention of Alcohol Problems: A Critical Review of the Research Literature." *Journal of Studies on Alcohol* 50 (1989): 54–88.

Nathan, P. E. "Integration of Biosocial and Psychosocial Research on Alcoholism." *Alcoholism: Clinical and Experimental Research* 14 (1990): 368–74.

Nathan, P. E., and A. H. Skinstad. "Outcomes of Treatment for Alcohol Problems: Current Methods, Problems, and Results." *Journal of Consulting Clinical Psychology* 55 (1987): 332–40.

National Clearinghouse for Alcohol and Drug Information (NCADI). *The Fact Is . . . Alcoholism Tends to Run in Families.* Rockville, MD: NCADI, October 1991.

National Clearinghouse for Alcohol and Drug Information (NCADI). *The Fact Is . . . Alcoholism Tends to Run in Families.* OSAP Prevention Resource Guide. Rockville, MD: NCADI, 1992.

National Highway Traffic Safety Administration (NHTSH), National Center for Statistics and Analysis. *Drunk Driving Facts.* Washington, DC: NHTSA, 1988.

National Institute on Alcohol Abuse and Alcoholism (NIAAA). *Facts About Alcohol and Alcoholism.* Washington, DC: U.S. Government Printing Office, 1980.

National Institute on Alcohol Abuse and Alcoholism (NIAAA). *Apparent Per Capita Alcohol Consumption: National, State and Regional Trends, 1977–1987.* Surveillance report no. 13. Washington, DC: U.S. Government Printing Office, 1989.

National Institute on Alcohol Abuse and Alcoholism (NIAAA). *Seventh Special Report to the U.S. Congress on Alcohol and Health.* 1990.

National Institute on Alcohol Abuse and Alcoholism (NIAAA). *Alcohol Alert: Moderate Drinking.* Rockville, MD: U.S. Department of Health and Human Services, no. 16, PH 315m, April 1992.

National Institute on Alcohol Abuse and Alcoholism (NIAAA). *Alcohol Alert: Estimating the Economic Cost of Alcohol Abuse.* Rockville, MD: U.S. Department of Health and Human Services, Alcohol Abuse and Mental Health Administration, no. 11, PH293, January 1995.

National Institute on Drug Abuse (NIDA). "Presenter's Comments." In *Alcohol and Disinhibition: Nature and Meaning of the Link.* Washington, DC: U.S. HHS, PHS, ADAMHA, National Institute on Alcohol Abuse and Alcoholism Research Monograph 12, 1983.

NIDA Notes. Available at http://www.nida.nigov/ NIDA_NOTES

National Institute on Drug Abuse (NIDA). *National Survey Results on Drugs from the Monitoring the Future Study, 1975–1992. Vol. 1: Secondary School Students,* 137. Rockville, MD: NIDA, 1993.

Novello, A. C. "Alcohol and Kids: It's Time for Candor." *Christian Science Monitor* (26 June 1992): 19.

Nusbaumer, M. R. "Governmental Control of Deviant Drinking: The Manipulation of Morals and Medicine." *Drug Use in America: Social, Cultural and Political Perspectives,* edited by P. J. Venturelli, 13–22. Boston: Jones and Bartlett, 1994.

OSAP. *Cultural Competence for Evaluators.* Washington, DC: Office for Substance Abuse Prevention, U.S. HHS, PHS, ADAMHA, DHHS publication no. (ADM) 92-1884, 1992.

Osterberg, E. "Alcohol-Related Problems in Cross-National Perspective." In *Alcohol and Culture: Comparative Perspectives from Europe and America.* Annals of the New York Academy of Sciences, vol. 472, (1986), 10–21.

Parrish, K., S. Higuchi, F. S. Stinson, et al. "Genetic or Cultural Determinants of Drinking: A Study of Embarrassment at Facial Flushing Among Japanese and Japanese-Americans." *Journal of Substance Abuse* 2 (1990): 439–47.

Peele, S., and A. Brodsky with M. Arnold. *The Truth About Addiction and Recovery.* New York: Simon & Schuster, 1991.

Pernanen, K. "Causal Inferences About the Role of Alcohol in Accidents, Poisonings and Violence." In *Drinking and Casualties: Accidents, Poisonings and Violence in an International Perspective,* edited by N. Giesbrecht, R. Gonzalez, M. Grant, E. Osterberg, R. Room, I. Rootman, and L. Towle. New York: Tavistock/Routledge, 1989.

Pittman, D. J., ed. *Alcoholism.* New York: Harper & Row, 1967.

Presley, C., P. Meilman, and R. Lyerla. *Alcohol and Drugs on American College Campuses,* vol. II, 1990–1992. Carbondale, IL: CORE Institute, Student Health Programs, Southern Illinois University at Carbondale, 1995.

Primm, B. J. "Drug Use: Special Implications for Black Americans." In *The State of Black America, 1987,* edited by J. Dewart, 145–66. New York: National Urban League, 1987.

Riechmann, D. "Drug, Alcohol Use Up Among College Students." *Associated Press International,* (April 21, 1995).

Room, R. "'A Reverence for Strong Drink': The Lost Generation and the Elevation of Alcohol in American Culture." *Journal of Studies on Alcohol* (1984): 540–45.

Ropers, R. H., and R. Bayer. "Homelessness as a Health Risk." *Alcohol, Health, and Research World* 11, (1987): 38–41.

Royce, James E. *Alcohol Problems and Alcoholism,* rev. ed. New York: Free Press, 1989.

Rudy, D. R. *Becoming Alcoholic: Alcoholics Anonymous and the Reality of Alcoholism.* Carbondale: Southern Illinois University Press, 1986.

Satir, V. *Conjoint Family Therapy.* Palo Alto, CA: Science and Behavior Books, 1964.

Schaler, J. A. "Drugs and Free Will." *Society* (September–October 1991): 42–49.

Schuckit, M. A., and V. Rayes. "Ethanol Ingestion: Differences in Blood Acetaldehyde Concentrations in Relatives of Alcoholics and Controls." *Science* 203 (1979): 54–55.

Siegel, R. K. *Intoxication: Life in the Pursuit of Artificial Paradise.* New York: Dutton, 1989.

Substance Abuse and Mental Health Services Administration (SAMHSA). *1994 Household Survey: Good and Bad News.* Rockville, MD: U.S. Department of Health and Human Services, vol. II, no. 3, Summer 1994.

Substance Abuse and Mental Health Services Administration (SAMHSA). *Making the Link: Alcohol, Tobacco, and Other Drugs and Women's Health.* Rockville, MD: U.S. Department of Health and Human Services, ML011, spring 1995.

Sutherland, Edwin H. *Principles of Criminology.* Philadelphia: Lippincott, 1947.

Trice, H. M. "Job-Based Alcohol and Drug Abuse Programs: Recent Program Developments and Research." In *Handbook on Drug Abuse,* edited by R. L. DuPont, A. Goldstein, and J. O. O'Donnell, 181–91. Washington, DC: National Institute on Drug Abuse, 1979.

Ullman, A. D. "Sociocultural Backgrounds of Alcoholism." In *Understanding Alcoholism, Annals American Academy Political and Social Science,* vol. 315, edited by S. D. Bacon, 48–54. 1958.

U.S. Department of Health and Human Services. *Facts About Alcohol and Alcoholism.* Rockville, MD: National Institute on Alcohol Abuse and Alcoholism, 1980.

U.S. Department of Health and Human Services. *Sixth Special Report to the U.S. Congress on Alcohol and Health from the Secretary of Health and Human Services.* Rockville, MD: National Institute on Alcohol Abuse and Alcoholism, 1987.

U.S. Department of Health and Human Services (USDHHS). *Preliminary Estimates on Drug Abuse.* Rockville, MD: Substance Abuse and Mental Health Services Administration, advance report no. 7, July 1994.

Wagenaar, A. C. "Protecting Our Future: Options for Preventing Alcohol-Impaired Driving Among Youth." In *Drug Use in America: Social, Cultural and Political Perspectives,* edited by P. J. Venturelli, 193–202. Boston: Jones and Bartlett, 1994.

Watson, D., and L. A. Clark. "Negative Affectivity: The Disposition to Experience Aversive Emotional States." *Psychological Bulletin* 96 (1984): 465–90.

Watts, D. W., Jr. *The Psychedelic Experience: A Sociological Study.* Beverly Hills, CA: Sage, 1971.

Wechsler, H., A. Davenport, G. Dowdall, B. Moeykens, and S. Castillo. "Health and Behavioral Consequences of Binge Drinking in College: A National Survey of Students at 140 Campuses." *Journal of the American Medical Association* 272 (December 7, 1994).

Wegscheider, S. *Another Chance.* Palo Alto, CA: Science and Behavior Books, 1981.

Whitman, D., with D. Friedman and L. Thomas. "The Return of Skid Row: Why Alcoholics and Addicts Are Filling the Street Again." *U.S. News and World Report* (15 January 1990): 27–9.

Williams, G. D., F. S. Stinson, D. A. Parker, T. C. Harford, and V. Noble. "Demographic Trends, Alcohol Abuse and Alcoholism, 1985–1995." Epidemiologic Bulletin no. 15. *Alcohol, Health, and Research World* 11 (1987): 80–3.

Wilsnack, S. C., R. W. Wilsnack, and A. D. Klassen. "Epidemiological Research on Women's Drinking, 1978–1984." In *Women and Alcohol: Health-Related Issues.* Research Monograph no. 16. DHHS Pub. no. (ADM). Washington, DC: U.S. Government Printing Office, 1986.

Woods, G. *Drug Abuse in Society: A Reference Handbook.* Santa Barbara, CA: ABC-CLIO, 1993.

Wright, J. D., J. W. Knight, E. Weber-Burdin, and J. Lam. "Ailments and Alcohol: Health Status Among the Drinking Homeless." *Alcohol, Health, and Research World* 11 (1987): 22–7.

Zinberg, N. E. *Drug, Set, and Setting: The Basis for Controlled Intoxicant Use.* New Haven, CT: Yale University Press, 1984.

Zinberg, N. E., and J. A. Robertson. *Drugs and the Public.* New York: Simon & Schuster, 1972.

10

Narcotics
(Opioids)

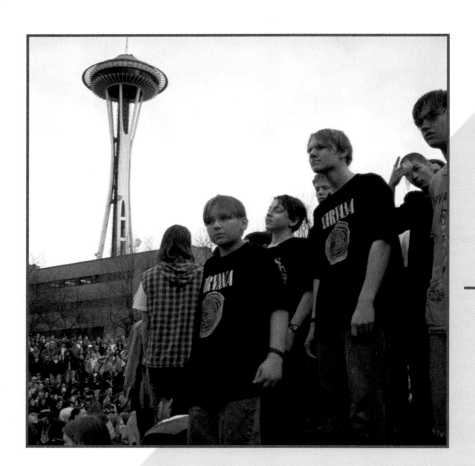

On completing this chapter
you will be able to: ▶

- The release of natural substances called *endorphins* can mimic the effects of narcotics such as heroin.
- By the end of the nineteenth century, almost 1 million Americans were addicted to opiates, primarily due to the use of patent medicines that contained opium products.
- Narcotics are the most potent analgesics available today.
- A narcotic antagonist has been shown to effectively reduce craving for alcohol in some alcoholics.

- Extreme tolerance to the narcotics can develop with continual use, causing as much as a 35-fold increase in dosage to maintain the effects.
- About 75% of the heroin addicts seeking treatment use needles.
- Almost one-half of all heroin addicts have been exposed to the AIDS virus.
- Heroin supplies in the 1990s are more potent and cheaper than those available in the 1980s.

- Many young people believe that heroin is safe as long as it is not injected.
- One designer drug, made from the narcotic fentanyl, is 6000 times more potent than heroin.
- Some heroin addicts have to be treated with the narcotic methadone for the rest of their lives.
- One contaminant of illegal narcotic manufacturing, called MPTP, can cause irreversible, severe Parkinson's disease in a matter of days.

Learning Objectives

- Describe the principal pharmacological effects of narcotics and their main therapeutic uses.
- Identify the major side effects of the narcotics.
- Identify the abuse patterns for heroin.
- Outline the stages of heroin dependence.
- Describe the association of AIDS with heroin abuse.

- List the withdrawal symptoms that result from narcotic dependence, and discuss the significance of tolerance.
- Describe the use of methadone and other long-acting narcotics in treating narcotic addiction.
- Identify the unique features of fentanyl that make it appealing to illicit drug dealers but dangerous to narcotic addicts.

- Describe how "designer" drugs have been associated with the narcotics.
- Distinguish among the narcotic agents fentanyl, morphine, codeine, pentazocine, and propoxyphene.

The term *narcotic* in general means central nervous system (CNS) depressants that produce insensibility or stupor. The term has also come to designate those drugs and substances with pharmacological properties related to opium and its drug derivatives. All opioid narcotics activate opioid receptors and have abuse potential. In addition, the narcotics are effective pain relievers (**analgesics**) and anticough medications, and are effective in the treatment of diarrhea.

analgesics

drugs that relieve pain without affecting consciouness

In this chapter we introduce the opioid narcotics with a brief historical account. The pharmacological and therapeutic uses of these drugs are discussed, followed by a description of their side effects and problems with tolerance, withdrawal, and addiction. Narcotic abuse is presented in detail, with special emphasis on heroin. In addition, treatment approaches for narcotic addiction and dependence are included. This chapter concludes with descriptions of other commonly used opioid narcotics.

The opium poppy

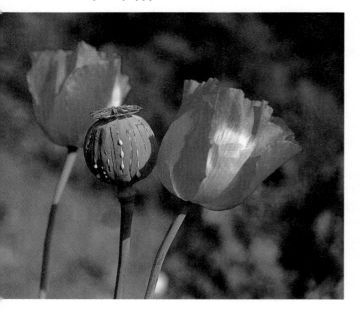

What Are Narcotics?

The word *narcotic* has been used to label many substances, from opium to marijuana to cocaine. The translation of the Greek word *narkoticos* is "benumbing or deadening." The term *narcotic* is sometimes used to refer to a CNS depressant, producing insensibility or stupor, and at other times to refer to an addicting drug. Most people would not consider marijuana among the narcotics today, although for many years it was included in this category. Although pharmacologically cocaine is not a narcotic either, it is still legally so classified. Perhaps part of this confusion is due to the fact that cocaine, as a local anesthetic, can cause a numbing effect.

For purposes of the present discussion, the term *narcotic* will be used to refer to those naturally occurring substances derived from the opium poppy and their synthetic substitutes. These drugs are referred to as the **opioid** (or opiate) narcotics because of their association with opium. They have similar pharmacological features, including abuse potential, pain-relieving

opioid

relating to the drugs that are derived from opium

effects (referred to as analgesics), cough suppression, and reduction of intestinal movement often causing constipation. Some of the most commonly used opioid narcotics are listed in Table 10.1

The History of Narcotics

The opium poppy, *Papaver somniferum,* from which opium and its naturally occurring narcotic derivatives are obtained, has been cultivated for millenia. A 6000-year-old Sumerian tablet has an ideograph for the poppy shown as "joy" plus "plant," suggesting that the addicting properties of this substance have been appreciated for many centuries. The Egyptians listed opium along with approximately 700 other medicinal compounds in the famous Ebers Papyrus (about 1500 B.C.).

The Greek god of sleep, Hypnos, and the Roman god of sleep, Somnus, were portrayed as

Table 10.1   Commonly Used Opioid Narcotic Drugs and Products

Narcotic Drugs	Common Product Name(s)	Most Common Use(s)
Heroin	Horse, smack, junk (street names)	Abuse
Morphine	(Several)	Analgesia
Methadone	Dolophine	Treat narcotic dependence
Meperidine	Demerol	Analgesia
Oxycodone	Percodan	Analgesia
Propoxyphene	Darvon	Analgesia
Codeine	(Several)	Analgesia, antitussive
Loperamide	Imodium A-D	Antidiarrheal
Diphenoxylate	Lomotil	Antidiarrheal
Opium tincture	Paregoric	Antidiarrheal

carrying containers of opium pods, and the Minoan goddess of sleep wore a crown of opium pods.

During the so-called Dark Ages that followed the collapse of the Roman Empire, Arab traders actively engaged in traveling the overland caravan routes to China and to India, where they introduced opium. Eventually, both China and India grew their own poppies.

Opium in China

The opium poppy had a dramatic impact in China, causing widespread addiction (Karch 1996b). Initially, the seeds were used medically, as was opium later. However, by the late 1690s, opium was being smoked and used for diversion. The Chinese government, fearful of the weakening of national vitality by the potent opiate narcotic, outlawed the sale of opium in 1729. The penalty for disobedience was death by strangulation or decapitation.

Despite these laws and threats, the habit of opium smoking became so widespread that the Chinese government went a step further and forbade its importation from India, where most of the opium poppy was grown. In contrast, the British East India Company (and later the British government in India) encouraged cultivation of

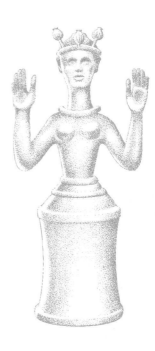

Minoan goddess of sleep, wearing a headband of opium poppies

opium. British companies were the principal shippers to the Chinese port of Canton, which was the only port open to Western merchants. During the next 120 years, a complex network of opium smuggling developed in China with the help of local merchants, who received substantial profits, and local officials, who pocketed bribes to ignore the smugglers.

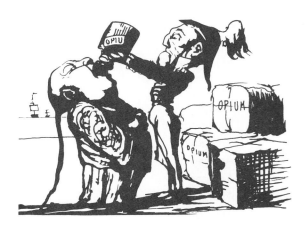

Famous cartoon, showing a British sailor shoving opium down the throat of a Chinese man, which dates back to the Opium War of 1839–1842.

Everyone involved in the opium trade, particularly the British, continued to profit until the Chinese government ordered the strict enforcement of the edict against importation. Such actions by the Chinese caused conflict with the British government and helped trigger the Opium War of 1839 to 1842. Great Britain sent in an army, and by 1842, 10,000 British soldiers had won a victory over 350 million Chinese. Because of the war, the island of Hong Kong was ceded to the British, and an indemnity of $6 million was imposed on China to cover the value of the destroyed opium and the cost of the war. In 1856, a second Opium War broke out. Peking was occupied by British and French troops, and China was compelled to make further concessions to Britain. The importation of opium continued to increase until 1908, when Britain and China made an agreement to limit the importation of opium from India (Austin 1978).

American Opium Use

Meanwhile, in 1803, a young German named Frederick Serturner extracted and partially purified the active ingredients in opium. It was ten times more potent than opium itself and was named *morphine* after Morpheus, the Greek god of dreams. This discovery increased worldwide interest in opium, and by 1832, a number of different active substances had been isolated from the raw material. In 1832, the second compound was purified and named *codeine,* after the Greek word for "poppy capsule" (Maurer and Vogel 1967).

The opium problem was aggravated further in 1853, when Alexander Wood perfected the hypodermic syringe and introduced it in first Europe and then America. Christopher Wren and others had worked with the idea of injecting drugs directly into the body by means of hollow quills and straws, but the approach was never successful or well received. Wood perfected the syringe technique with the intent of preventing an addiction to morphine by injecting the drug directly into the veins rather than by oral administration (Golding 1993). Unfortunately, just the opposite happened: Injection of morphine increased the potency and the chance of dependence (Maurer and Vogel 1967).

The hypodermic syringe was used extensively during the Civil War to administer morphine for treating pain, dysentery, and fatigue. A large percentage of the men who returned from the war were addicted to morphine. Opiate addiction became known as the "soldier's disease" or "army disease."

By 1900, an estimated 1 million Americans were dependent on the opiates (Abel 1980). This drug problem was made worse because of (1) Chinese laborers, who brought with them to the United States opium to smoke (it was legal to smoke opium in the United States at that time); (2) the availability of purified morphine and the hypodermic syringe; and (3) the lack of controls on the large number of patent medicines that contained opium derivatives (Karch 1996b).

Until 1914, when the Harrison Narcotic Act was passed (regulating opium, coca leaves, and their products), the average opiate addict was a middle-aged, Southern, white woman who functioned well and was adjusted to her role as a wife and mother. She bought opium or morphine legally by mail order from Sears, Roebuck or at the local store, used it orally, and caused very few problems. A number of physicians were addicted as well. One of the best-known morphine addicts was William Holsted, a founder of Johns Hopkins

Medical School. Holsted was a very productive surgeon and innovator, although secretly an addict for most of his career. He became dependent on morphine as a substitute for his cocaine dependence (Brecher 1972).

Looking for better medicines, chemists found that modification of the morphine molecule resulted in a more potent compound. In 1898, diacetylmorphine was placed on the market as a cough suppressant by Bayer. It was to be a "heroic" drug, without the addictive potential of morphine—it thus received the name *heroin.*

Heroin was first used in the United States as a cough suppressant and to combat addiction to other substances. However, its inherent abuse potential was quickly discovered. When injected, heroin is more addictive than other narcotics because of its ability to enter the brain rapidly and cause a euphoric surge (DiChiara and North 1992). Heroin was banned from U.S. medical practice in 1924, although it is still used legally as an analgesic in other countries (Karch 1996b).

The Vietnam War was an important landmark for heroin use in the United States. It has been estimated that as many as 40% of the U.S. soldiers serving in Southeast Asia at this time used heroin to combat the frustrations and stress associated with this unpopular military action. Although only 7% of the soldiers continued to use heroin after returning home, those who were addicted to this potent narcotic became a major component of the heroin-abusing population in this country (Golding 1993).

◢ Pharmacological Effects

Even though opioid narcotics have a history of being abused, they continue to be important therapeutic agents.

Narcotic Analgesics

The most common clinical use of the opioid narcotics is as analgesics to relieve pain. These drugs are effective against most varieties of pain, including visceral (associated with internal organs of the body) and somatic (associated with skeletal mus-

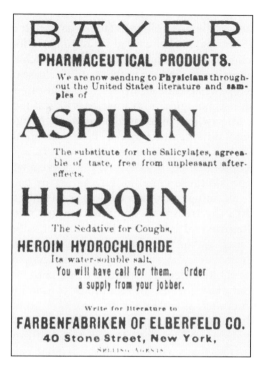

Bayer Pharmaceutical introduced two new products in the late 1800s: aspirin and heroin.

cles, bones, skin, and teeth) types. Used in sufficiently high doses, narcotics can even relieve the intense pain associated with some types of cancer (Nowak 1992; Reisine and Pasternak 1995).

The opioid narcotics relieve pain by activating the same group of receptors that are controlled by the endogenous substances called *endorphins.* As discussed in Chapter 6, the endorphins are peptides (small proteins) that are released in the brain and spinal cord and from the adrenal glands in response to stress and painful experiences. When released, the endorphins serve as transmitters and stimulate receptors designated as an opioid type. Activation of opioid receptors by either the naturally released endorphins or administration of the narcotic analgesic drugs blocks the transmission of pain through the spinal cord or brain stem and alters the perception of pain in the "pain center" of the brain. Because the narcotics work at all three levels of pain transmission, they are potent analgesics against almost all types of pain.

Interestingly, the endorphin system appears to be influenced by psychological factors as well. It is possible that pain relief caused by administration of placebos or nonmedicinal manipulation such as acupuncture is due in part to the natural release of endorphins. This relationship suggests that physiological, psychological, and pharmacological factors are intertwined in pain management through the opioid system, which makes it impossible to deal with one without considering the others.

Although the narcotics are very effective analgesics, they do cause some side effects that are particularly alarming; thus their clinical use usually is limited to the treatment of moderate to severe pain (Reisine and Pasternak 1995). Other, safer drugs, such as the aspirin-type analgesics (see Chapter 15), are preferred for pain management when possible. Often the amount of narcotic required for pain relief can be reduced by combining a narcotic, such as codeine, with aspirin or acetaminophen (the active ingredient in Tylenol): such combinations reduce the chance of significant narcotic side effects while providing adequate pain relief (Reisine and Pasternak 1995).

Morphine is a particularly potent pain reliever and often is used as the analgesic standard by which other narcotics are compared. With continual use, tolerance develops to the analgesic effects of morphine and other narcotics, sometimes requiring a dramatic escalation of doses to maintain adequate pain control (Reisine and Pasternak 1995).

Because pain is expressed in different forms with many different diseases, narcotic treatment can vary considerably. Usually the convenience of oral narcotic therapy is preferred but often is inadequate for severe pain. For short-term relief from intense pain, narcotics are effective when injected subcutaneously or intramuscularly. Narcotics can also be given intravenously for persistent and potent analgesia or administered by transdermal patches for sustained chronic pain (Karch 1996b). Despite the fact that most pains can be relieved if enough narcotic analgesic is properly administered, physicians frequently underprescribe narcotics. Because of fear of causing narcotic addiction or creating legal problems with federal agencies such as the Drug Enforcement Administration (DEA), it is estimated that less than 50% of

the cancer patients in the United States receive enough narcotics for adequate pain relief (Nowak 1992). An important rule of narcotic use is that adequate pain relief should not be denied because of concern about the abuse potential of these drugs (Reisine and Pasternak 1995). In fact, addiction to narcotics is rare in patients receiving these drugs for therapy unless they have a history of drug abuse or have an underlying psychiatric disorder (Pfefferbaum and Hagberg 1993).

Other Therapeutic Uses

Opioid narcotics are also used to treat conditions not related to pain. For example, these drugs suppress the coughing center of the brain, so they are effective **antitussives.** Codeine, a natural opioid narcotic, is commonly included in cough medicine. In addition, opioid narcotics slow the movement of materials through the intestines, a property that can be used to relieve diarrhea or can cause the

antitussive
drugs that block coughing

side effect of constipation. Paregoric contains an opioid narcotic substance and is commonly used to treat severe diarrhea.

When used carefully by the clinician, opioid narcotics are very effective therapeutic tools. Some precautions for avoiding unnecessary problems with these drugs include the following (Way and Way 1992):

1. Before beginning treatment, therapeutic goals should be clearly established.

2. Doses and duration of use should be limited as much as possible while permitting adequate therapeutic care.

3. If other, safer drugs (for example, nonnarcotic analgesics such as ibuprofen or aspirin) adequately treat the medical condition, narcotics should be avoided.

Mechanisms of Action

As mentioned, the opioid receptors are the site of action of the endorphin peptide transmitters and are found throughout the nervous system, intestines, and other internal organs. Because narcotic drugs such as morphine and heroin enhance the endorphin system by stimulating opioid receptors, these drugs have widespread influences throughout the body.

For example, the opioid receptors are present in high concentration within the limbic structures of the brain. Stimulation of these receptors by narcotics causes release of the transmitter, dopamine, in limbic brain regions. This effect contributes to the rewarding actions of these drugs and leads to dependence and abuse (Reisine and Pasternak 1995).

Side Effects

One of the most common side effects of the opioid narcotics is constipation. Other side effects of these drugs include drowsiness, mental clouding, respiratory depression (suppressed breathing is usually the cause of death from overdose), nausea and vomiting, itching, inability to urinate, a drop in blood pressure, and constricted pupils ("Opioids" 1996). This array of seemingly unrelated side effects is due to widespread distribution of the opioid receptors throughout the body and their involvement in many physiological functions (O'Brien 1995). With continual use, tolerance develops to some of these undesirable narcotic responses (Reisine and Pasternak 1995).

Drugs that selectively antagonize the opioid receptors can block the effects of natural opioid systems in the body and reverse the effects of narcotic opiate drugs. When an opioid antagonist such as the drug naloxone is administered alone, it has little noticeable effect. The antiopioid actions of naloxone become more apparent when the antagonist is injected into someone who has taken a narcotic opioid drug. For example, naloxone will cause (1) a recurrence of pain in the patient using a narcotic for pain relief, (2) the restoration of consciousness and normal breathing in the addict who has overdosed on heroin, and (3) severe withdrawal effects in the opioid abuser who has become dependent on the narcotics ("Opioids" 1996).

An interesting recent use of opioid antagonists is in the treatment of alcohol dependence. The FDA has approved the use of naltrexone (a narcotic antagonist) to relieve the craving of alcoholics for excessive alcohol consumption (*Facts and Comparisons* 1995). Early research suggests that this drug may have a dramatic effect on the future therapeutic approach for alcoholism. Only time and experience will reveal whether the benefits are truly as dramatic as originally thought. These findings suggest that the natural opioid (endorphin) system likely contributes to the dependence seen in alcoholics.

◢ Abuse, Tolerance, Dependence, and Withdrawal

All the opioid narcotic agents that activate opioid receptors have abuse potential and are classified as scheduled drugs (see Table 10.2). An estimated 2.5 million people in the United States abuse heroin or other narcotics (DiChiara and North 1992). Their patterns of abuse are determined by the ability of these drugs to cause tolerance, dependence, and withdrawal effects.

Table 10.2   Schedule Classification of Some Common Narcotics

Narcotic	Schedule*
Heroin	I
Morphine	II, III
Methadone	II
Fentanyl	II
Hydromorphone	II
Meperidine	II
Codeine	II, III, V
Pentazocine	IV
Propoxyphene	IV
Narcotics combined with nonsteroidal anti-inflammatory drugs	III

(*) According to Drug Enforcement Administration (DEA) classification, Controlled Substances Act (CSA).

The process of tolerance literally begins with the first dose of a narcotic, but does not become clinically evident until after two to three weeks of frequent use (either therapeutic- or abuse-related). Tolerance occurs most rapidly with high doses given in short intervals. Doses can be increased as much as 35 times so as to regain the narcotic effect. Physical dependence invariably accompanies severe tolerance (Reisine and Pasternak 1995). Psychological dependence can also develop with continual narcotic use because these drugs can cause euphoria and relieve stress. Such psychological dependence leads to compulsive use (Way and Way 1992). Because all narcotics affect the same opioid systems in the body, developing tolerance to one narcotic drug means the person has cross-tolerance to all drugs in this group.

The development of psychological and physical dependence makes breaking the narcotic habit very difficult. Abstinence from narcotic use by a long-term addict can cause severe withdrawal effects such as exaggerated pain responses, agitation, anxiety, stomach cramps and vomiting, joint and muscle aches, runny nose, and an overall flu-like feeling. Although these withdrawal symptoms are not fatal, they are extremely aversive and encourage continuation of the narcotic habit (Reisine and Pasternak 1995; Colapinto 1996). Overall, the narcotics have similar actions; there are differences, however, in their potencies, severity of side effects, likelihood of being abused, and clinical usefulness.

Heroin Abuse

Heroin is currently classified as a Schedule I drug by the DEA. It is not approved for any clinical use in the United States and is the most widely abused illegal drug in the world (Best et al. 1996). Heroin also was illicitly used more than any other drug of abuse in the United States (except for marijuana) until 15 years ago, when it was replaced by cocaine (DiChiara and North 1992), although a recent resurgence in its use has caused great concern with the authorities (Weiss 1995; "Heroin '96" 1996).

From 1970 through 1976, most of the heroin reaching the United States originated from the Golden Triangle region of Southeast Asia, which includes parts of Burma, Thailand, and Laos.

During that period, the United States and other nations purchased much of the legal opium crop from Turkey in order to stop opium from being converted into heroin. From 1975 until 1980, the major heroin supply came from opium poppies grown in Mexico. The U.S. government furnished the Mexican government with helicopters, herbicide sprays, and financial assistance to destroy the poppy crop. Changes in political climates have shifted the source of supply back to the Golden Triangle, and much of these supplies are currently brought into the United States by Chinese criminal societies (Maas 1994) or Mexican drug organizations (Leland 1996) (See page 235, "Fighting the Drug War.")

Heroin Combinations Pure heroin is a white powder. Other colors, such as brown Mexican heroin, result from unsatisfactory processing of morphine or from adulterants. Heroin is usually "cut" (diluted) with lactose (milk sugar) to give it bulk and thus increase profits. When heroin first enters the United States, it may be up to 95% pure, but by the time it is sold to users, its purity may be as low as 3% or (recently) as high as 60%. If addicts are unaware of the variance in purity and do not adjust doses accordingly, the results can be extremely dangerous and occasionally fatal (Leland 1996).

Heroin has a bitter taste, so sometimes it is "cut" with quinine, a bitter substance, to disguise the fact that the heroin content has been reduced. Quinine can be a deadly adulterant. Part of the "flash" from direct injection of heroin may be caused by this contaminant. Quinine is an irritant, and it causes vascular damage, acute and potentially lethal disturbances in heartbeat, depressed respiration, coma, and death from respiratory arrest. Opiate poisoning causes acute pulmonary edema as well as respiratory depression. Heroin plus quinine has an unpredictable additive effect (Bourne 1976). To counteract the constipation caused by heroin, sometimes mannitol is added for its laxative effect.

Another potentially lethal combination is when heroin is laced with the much more potent artificial narcotic fentanyl. This adulterated heroin is known on the streets as *Tango and Cash* or *Goodfellas* and can be extremely dangerous due to its unexpected potency (Treaster and Halloway

FIGHTING THE DRUG WAR

In a remote mountainous area in the Shan hills of northeast Burma, the world's most powerful opium dealer, Khun Sa, has run a clearinghouse for Southeast Asia's heroin trade for nearly 30 years. His operation controls as much as 60% of the heroin that flows from that region to the rest of the world. For years, the governments of Burma, Thailand, and the United States have been trying to stop him, but to no avail.

In a January 1996 *Time* magazine article, it was reported that the powerful drug lord may have struck a deal with the military junta known as the State Law and Order Restoration Council (SLORC), which has ruled the Union of Myanmar (Burma) since 1988. While no details of the agreement were made public, SLORC's pattern of dealing with rebel movements has been to buy military control by offering economic freedom—essentially "turning the other cheek" to even the most blatantly illegal businesses. Assistant Secretary of State Robert Gelbard was quoted in *Time* as saying, "We've been concerned that SLORC is engaged in an effort to reach agreements with these groups and end their insurgency, as opposed to destroying their narcotics-production capabilities." In fact, the Burmese government has already been subjected to maximum international pressures: the United States has restricted trade with SLORC as a "noncooperating" regime for its failure to curb drug traffic, and the United Nations has protested numerous civil rights abuses in the country. Unfortunately, the United States and other Western countries have little leverage that they can exert in Burma.

Similar scenarios are being played out in Southwest Asia, particularly in Afghanistan and Pakistan, where unstable political climates give rise to byzantine intrigue, as well as ethnic and other power struggles in which the lucrative drug trade becomes a valuable pawn. Afghanistan, the world's second-largest producer of heroin, is the primary supplier of heroin to Europe, and a major supplier to the United States—though it has been hard to measure the extent to which Southwest Asian and Middle Eastern drug traffickers supply ethnic Southwest

Asian and Middle Eastern heroin users residing in the United States. Much of the heroin produced in Afghanistan is exported to the West through Russia.

By late 1996, the Taliban, a powerful Islamic militia movement in Afghanistan, had gained military control over the southern half of the country, bidding for legitimacy with a strong program of morality and strict religious observance. From time to time the Taliban forces appeared to be cracking down on participants in the thriving Afghan narcotics trade, but said little about an antinarcotic program. Meanwhile, the rival religious regime in Iran has accused the Taliban of actually *encouraging* the drug trade in western Afghanistan, on the Iranian border. In its rise to power, the Taliban also received help from neighboring Pakistan, which has also served as a major conduit for heroin flowing into the United States. Faced with drug trafficking in such a chaotic mix of competing interests, the United States and other Western powers could do little but wait for a clearer picture to emerge.

Unable to stop heroin production in Southeast and Southwest Asia, Western powers can only boycott, ostracize, and try to contain the traffic. Inside the United States and Europe, most Southwest Asian heroin-trafficking groups are very tight-knit and difficult to penetrate, based as they are on ethnic, familial, religious and tribal relationships. The heroin traffickers and wholesalers rarely do business with outsiders, and tend to be more active in cities with large Near Eastern ethnic populations—such as Chicago, Detroit, and New York in the United States. Trying to stem the flow—by blocking passage for these geographically scattered, yet well-organized traffickers—is a task that, unfortunately, is much easier said than done. ∎

Sources:
NNIC Report (August 1995).
"Deal of the Decade." [On-line]. *Time International* (January 15, 1996).
"Afghan Taliban Seize Heroin from Air Passengers." [On-line]. *Reuters* (November 1, 1996).
Bradlee, B., Jr. "Afghanistan's Fight to the Finish: A Nation Dissolves into Tribal War." [On-line]. *Boston Globe* (November 3, 1996).

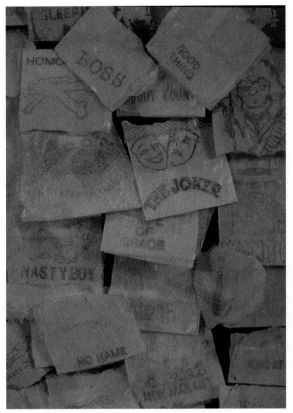

Types of heroin packaging sold in the streets.

smoking a heroin and crack mixture called *moon rock* or *parachute rock* ("Heroin '96" 1996). It also has been reported that street heroin addicts use cocaine to withdraw or detoxify themselves from heroin by gradually decreasing amounts of heroin while increasing amounts of cocaine. This drug combination is called **speedballing,** and addicts claim the cocaine provides relief from the unpleasant withdrawal effects that accompany heroin abstinence in a dependent user. A possible explanation for this effect is that cocaine, like heroin, stimulates the natural endorphin systems of the brain (Kreek 1987).

> **speedballing**
> combining heroin and cocaine

Profile of Heroin Addicts There are an estimated 500,000 to 750,000 heroin addicts in the United States, a figure that has remained relatively stable despite changes in the number of infrequent and moderate users (Leland 1996). Heroin addicts are always searching for a better and purer drug; however, if they do find an unusually potent batch of heroin, there is a good chance they will get more than they bargained for. Addicts are sometimes found dead with the needle still in the vein after injecting heroin (Thompson 1995). In such cases, as described earlier, the unsuspecting addict may have died in reaction to an unusually concentrated dose of this potent narcotic. Approximately 3000–4000 deaths occur annually in the United States from heroin overdoses (Leland 1996). Death associated with heroin injection is usually due to concurrent use of alcohol or barbiturates, and not the heroin alone.

It is typical for hard-core addicts to have a common place where they can stash supplies and equipment for their heroin encounters. These locations, called "shooting galleries," serve as gathering places for addicts. Shooting galleries can be set up in homes, but are usually located in less-established locations such as abandoned cars, cardboard lean-tos, and in weed-infested vacant lots. An entrance charge often is required of the patrons. Conditions in shooting galleries are notoriously filthy, and these places are frequented by IV heroin users with blood-borne infections that can cause AIDS or hepatitis. Because of needle sharing

1994). In February 1991, a batch of heroin cut with fentanyl sold for $10 a bag in a South Bronx neighborhood and killed 22 people, while sending more than 200 other users to area hospitals (Greenhouse 1992).

Frequently, heroin is deliberately combined with other drugs when self-administered by addicts (Darke and Hall 1995). According to the NIDA-sponsored Drug Abuse Warning Network (DAWN) survey of emergency rooms in the United States, 41% of the reported heroin abuse cases included other drugs of abuse in combination with this narcotic. Heroin was most frequently used with alcohol, but also frequently was combined with CNS stimulants, such as cocaine. Some crack cocaine smokers turn to heroin to ease the jitters caused by the CNS stimulant (Leland 1996). Such users often "chase the dragon" by

Heroin paraphernalia is usually simple and crude but effective: a spoon on which to dissolve the narcotic and a makeshift syringe with which to inject it.

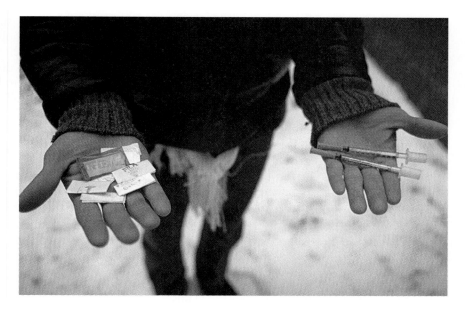

and other unsanitary practices, shooting galleries have become a place where serious communicative diseases are spread to a wide range of people of different ages, races, sexes, and socioeconomic status (Bearak 1992). Some addicts become resigned to their fate, such as one user who, after testing positive for the human immunodeficiency virus (HIV), responded, "I've seen lots of guys die already. They turned into skeletons and their teeth fell out . . . I hope I die before I get that far. Maybe I'll be lucky and just die one night up in the gallery" (Bearak 1992).

The heroin in shooting galleries is typically prepared by adding several drops of water to the white powder in an improvised container (such as a metal bottle cap) and lightly shaken while heating over a small flame to dissolve the powder. The fluid is then drawn through a tiny wad of cotton to filter out the gross contaminants into an all-too-often used syringe ready for injection (Bearak 1992).

Some addicts become fixated on the drug's paraphernalia, especially the needle. They can get a psychological "high" from playing with the needle and syringe. The injection process and syringe plunger action appear to have sexual overtones for them. As one reformed user explained, "I think what I miss more than heroin sometimes is just the ritual of shooting up." A current user con-

curred, explaining, "You get addicted to the needle . . . Just the process of sticking something into your vein, having such a direct involvement with your body . . . ("Mary" 1996).

Heroin and Crime In 1971, the Select Committee on Crime in the United States released a report on methods used to combat the heroin crisis that arose in the 1950s and 1960s. This report was a turning point in setting up treatment programs for narcotic addicts. The report stated that drug arrests for heroin use had increased 700% since 1961, that there were as many as 4000 deaths per year from heroin, and that the cost of heroin-related crimes was estimated to exceed $3 billion per year. Other studies since that time have linked heroin addiction with crime (Hall et al. 1993).

Although many young heroin addicts come from affluent, middle-class families (Weiss 1995), research shows most heavy heroin users are poorly educated with minimal social integration. Because of these disadvantages, heroin addicts often have a low level of employment, exist in unstable living conditions, and socialize with other illicit drug users (Hall et al. 1993). Clearly such undesirable living conditions encourage criminal activity; however, three other factors also likely contribute to the association between heroin use and crime. (1) The use of heroin and its pharmacological effects encourage antisocial behavior that is crime-related. Depressants such as heroin diminish inhibition and cause people to engage in activities they normally would not. The effects of heroin and its withdrawal makes addicts self-centered, demanding, impulsive, and governed by their "need" for the drug. (2) Because heroin addiction is expensive, the user is forced to resort to crime to support the drug habit (Weiss 1995). (3) A similar personality is driven to engage in both criminal behavior and heroin use. Often heroin addicts start heroin use about the same time they begin to become actively involved in criminal activity. In most cases the heroin user has been taking other illicit drugs, especially marijuana, years before trying heroin (Hall et al. 1993). These findings suggest that for many heroin addicts the antisocial behavior causes the criminal behavior rather than resulting from the heroin use. Thus, the more a drug such as heroin is perceived as being illegal, desirable, and addictive, the more likely it will be used by deviant criminal populations. One user explained how he got caught up in criminal activity to support his addiction:

> I lost everything, financially and emotionally . . . I was literally walking up and down Hollywood Boulevard with one pair of tennis shoes, looking to steal a handbag off some old lady to get another fix. [*Newsweek* (August 26, 1996): 54]

Patterns of Heroin Abuse   It has become apparent that problems with narcotics are no longer confined to the inner cities, but have infiltrated suburban areas and small towns and afflict both rich and poor. Although the use of heroin appeared to decline each year from 1989 to 1991 (see Table 10.3), several disturbing trends have since caused authorities to become concerned. These trends include the following:

▲ Heroin use is increasing in almost every part of the United States and among all age groups ("Heroin '96" 1996; see Table 10.3).

▲ Heroin has become purer (60% to 70% purity) and cheaper ($0.37 per milligram) than ever before (Leland 1996).

▲ With greater purity, new users are able to administer heroin in less efficient ways, such as smoking and snorting, and avoid the dangers of IV use (Leland 1996).

▲ Many youth believe that heroin can be used safely if it is not injected ("Heroin '96" 1996).

▲ The volume of heroin imported into the United States has doubled to 10–15 metric tons per year since the mid-1980s (Shoemer 1996).

▲ Because of its association with popular fashions and entertainment (see the Here and Now box), heroin is viewed as glamorous and chic, especially by many young people, despite its highly publicized lethal consequences ("Heroin '96" 1996; Kennedy 1996).

▲ Emergency room visits due to narcotic overdoses increased from approximately 38,000 in

Table 10.3   Prevalence of Heroin and Other Opioid Abuse in High School Seniors

High School Seniors	Annual Use		Lifetime Use	
	Heroin	Other Opiods	Heroin	Other Opiods
1989	0.6%	4.4%	1.3%	8.3%
1991	0.4%	3.5%	0.9%	6.6%
1992	0.6%	3.3%	1.2%	6.1%
1995	1.1%	4.7%	1.6%	7.2%

Source: L. Johnston, "University of Michigan Annual National Survey of Secondary School Students."
Lansing: University of Michigan News and Information Services, 11 December 1995.

Heroin and Junkie Musicians

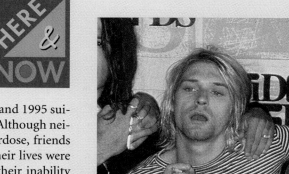

The most recent surge in heroin abuse has been particularly visible among popular musical artists. Especially notable were the 1994 and 1995 suicide deaths of Kurt Cobain and Shannon Hoon. Although neither rock star actually died from a narcotic overdose, friends and associates agree that the tragic endings to their lives were precipitated by severe addiction to heroin and their inability to escape drug dependence despite repeated attempts. Although the most visible victims, Cobain and Hoon were only two of a long list of rock and roll artists who died because of the allure of heroin and the life-shortening impact of its addiction. Other artistic notables who have succumb to this tragic dependence include Hole's Kristen Pfaff, Skinny Puppy's Dwayne Goettel, and the Replacements' Bob Stinson.

Source: J. Colapinto. "Rock and Roll Heroin." *Rolling Stone* (May 30, 1996): 15–20.

Kurt Cobain

1988 to 64,000 in 1994 (Colapinto 1996) and deaths from overdoses were up 80% from 1990, reaching 3500 in 1994 (Thompson 1995; Karch 1996b).

The reasons for these disturbing changes in heroin use patterns and attitude are not immediately apparent. It has been speculated that because antidrug efforts in the late 1980s and early 1990s targeted cocaine they inadvertently encouraged drug users to replace cocaine with heroin. Another possible reason for increased heroin use is that many drug dealers previously selling cocaine switched to heroin due to greater profits ("Heroin '96" 1996; Treaster and Holloway 1991), making heroin even more readily available. Whatever the reasons, it has become imperative to educate all populations about the dangers of this potent drug and reverse the present trend of escalating use and complacency about its dangers.

Stages of Dependence Initially, the effects of heroin are often unpleasant, especially after the

first injection. It is not uncommon to experience nausea and vomiting or to feel sick after administration; gradually, however, the euphoria overwhelms the aversive effects (Goldstein 1994). There are two major stages in the development of a psychological dependence on heroin or other opioid narcotics.

1. In the rewarding stage, euphoria and positive effects occur in at least 50% of users. These positive feelings and sensations increase with continued administration and encourage use (see page 240, "Here and Now").

2. Eventually, the heroin or narcotic user must take the drug to avoid withdrawal symptoms that start about 6 to 12 hours after the last dose. At this stage, it is said that "the monkey is on his back." This stage is psychological dependence. If one grain of heroin (about 65 milligrams) is taken over a two-week period on a daily basis, the user becomes physically dependent on the drug.

A Heroin Addict in Seattle

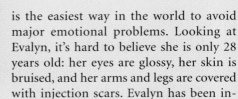

Seattle is one of several large metropolitan areas where the trend for using heroin by young people is particularly disturbing. Evalyn (not her real name) is a 28-year-old female from a suburban, middle-class family who claims to have started using heroin at the age of 13 after running away from an abusive father. She claims that the drug helped relieve her depression and described her first experience as "marvelous and so exciting." For Evalyn, heroin helps her to sleep, dream, escape, and experience oblivion. She claims heroin is the easiest way in the world to avoid major emotional problems. Looking at Evalyn, it's hard to believe she is only 28 years old: her eyes are glossy, her skin is bruised, and her arms and legs are covered with injection scars. Evalyn has been injecting into her foot because more accessible veins have already been used so much for heroin injections that they have collapsed. When asked if she will ever quit or seek treatment for her heroin addiction, she responds that she will "someday," but now she is scared to . . .   ■

Source: E. Weiss. "Seattle Scene Represents Nation's Rising Heroin Use." *All Things Considered,* National Public Radio (January 2, 1995).

Methods of Administration Many heroin users start by sniffing the powder or injecting it into a muscle (intramuscular) or under the skin ("skin popping"). Because of today's increased purity and decreased cost, more heroin users are administering their drug by smoking and snorting (Leland 1996).

Most established heroin addicts still prefer to **"mainline"** the drug (intravenous injection) ("Heroin '96" 1996). The injection device can be made from an eyedropper bulb, part of a syringe, and a hypodermic needle. "Mainlining" drugs causes the thin-walled veins to become scarred, and if done frequently, the veins will collapse. Once a vein is collapsed, it can no longer be used to introduce the drug into the blood. Addicts become expert in locating new veins to use: in the feet, the legs, the neck, even the temples. When addicts do not want "needle tracks" (scars) to show, they inject under the tongue or in the groin ("Opioids" 1996).

> **"mainline"**
> to inject a drug of abuse intravenously

Heroin Addicts and AIDS As noted already, because needle sharing is a common occurrence in populations of heavy heroin users, the transmission of deadly communicable diseases, such as acquired immune deficiency syndrome (AIDS), is a major problem (see Chapter 17). Over 50% of IV heroin users have been exposed to the AIDS virus. Fear of contracting this deadly disease has contributed to the increase of administering this drug by smoking and snorting (Bowersox 1995); however, many heroin users who start by smoking and snorting eventually progress to IV administration due to its more intense effects (Leland 1996).

Withdrawal Symptoms After the effects of the heroin wear off, the addict usually has only a few hours in which to find the next dose before severe withdrawal symptoms begin. A single "shot" of heroin only lasts four to six hours. It is enough to help addicts "get straight" or relieve the severe withdrawal symptoms called "dope sickness" but is not enough to give a desired "high" (Bearak 1992). Withdrawal symptoms start with a runny nose, tears, and minor stomach cramps. The addict may feel as if he or she is coming down with a bad cold ("Opioids" 1996). Between 12 and 48 hours after the last dose, the addict loses all of his or her appetite, vomits, has diarrhea and abdominal cramps, feels alternating chills and fever, and develops goose pimples all over (going "cold turkey"). Between two and four days later, the addict continues to experience some of the symptoms just described, as well as aching bones and

Table 10.4   **Symptoms of Withdrawal from Heroin, Morphine, and Methadone**

Symptoms	Time in Hours		
	Heroin	Morphine	Methadone
Craving for drugs; anxiety	4	6	24–48
Yawning, perspiration, runny nose, tears	8	14	34–48
Pupil dilation, goose bumps, muscle twitches, aching bones and muscles, hot and cold flashes, loss of appetite	12	16	48–72
Increased intensity of preceding symptoms, insomnia, raised blood pressure, fever, faster pulse, nausea	18–24	24–36	≥72
Increased intensity of preceding symptoms, curled-up position, vomiting, diarrhea, increased blood sugar, foot kicking ("kicking the habit")	26–36	36–48	—

muscles and powerful muscle spasms that cause violent kicking motions ("kicking the habit"). After four to five days, symptoms start to subside, and the person may get his or her appetite back (Way and Way 1992). However, attempts to move on in life will be challenging because compulsion to keep using the drug remains strong.

The severity of the withdrawal varies according to the purity and strength of the drug used and to the personality of the user. The symptoms of withdrawal from heroin, morphine, and methadone are summarized in Table 10.4. Withdrawal symptoms from opioids such as morphine, codeine, meperidine, and others are similar, although the time frame and intensity vary (O'Brien 1995).

Treatment of Heroin and Other Narcotic Dependence

The ideal result of treatment for dependency on heroin or other narcotics is to help the addict live a normal, productive, and satisfying life without drugs. In reality, relatively few heroin users become absolutely "clean" from drug use; thus, therapeutic compromise is often necessary (Millstein 1992). In the real world, treatment of heroin dependency is considered successful if the addict (1) stops using heroin, (2) no longer associates with dealers or users of heroin, (3) avoids dangerous activities often associated with heroin use (such as needle sharing, injecting unknown drugs, and frequenting shooting galleries), (4) improves employment status, (5) refrains from criminal activity, and (6) is able to enjoy normal family and social relationships (McLellan et al. 1993). For many heroin addicts, these goals can be achieved by substituting a long-lasting synthetic narcotic, such as methadone, in place of the short-acting heroin (Best et al. 1996). The substitute narcotic is

A heroin addict mainlining his drug.

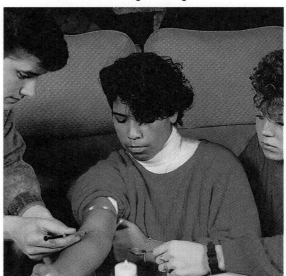

made available to heroin-dependent people from drug treatment centers under the direction of trained medical personnel. The dispensing of the substitute narcotic is tightly regulated by governmental agencies. The rationale for the substitution is that a long-acting drug, such as methadone, can conveniently be taken once a day to prevent the unpleasant withdrawal symptoms that occur within four hours after each heroin use (see Table 10.4). Although the substitute narcotic may also have abuse potential and be scheduled by the DEA (see Table 10.2), it is given to the addict in its oral form; thus its onset of action is too slow to cause a

rush like that associated with heroin use, so its abuse potential is substantially less. In addition, the cost to society is dramatically reduced; according to one study, an untreated heroin addict costs the community $21,000 for six months, but the cost of methadone maintenance for a person dependent on heroin is only $1750 for the same period (Grinspoon 1995).

Currently, methadone is approved by the FDA for "opiate maintenance therapy" in the treatment of heroin (or other narcotic) dependency (Grinspoon 1995). Proper use of methadone has been shown to effectively decrease illicit use of narcotics

FINDING a BALANCE Recovery through Journal Writing—A Way to Counter Life Stress and Drug Abuse

If it weren't for Kurt Cobain, Tom could be the poster child for Generation X. Although his experiences are unique, his plight is a familiar one—trying to make sense of a crazy world and understand just exactly how to fit in it. Looking back over the past five years, Tom's road has not been an easy one. Five years ago, no one, including Tom, would have predicted that he would one day be a heroin addict. How did it all begin? At some point in high school Tom began to feel isolated, he explained, feeling as if he didn't fit in with the rest of the crowd. Once regarded as a promising honor student by his teachers and considered very attractive by his peers, Tom's soul began to drift at the end of the tenth grade in a direction toward reckless abandon.

As with most exposures to drugs, there is never only one influencing factor. In Tom's case, several issues came into play: the writings of Thomas Wolfe, Timothy Leary, and Jack Keroac; constant tension with his parents (which he describes as serious codependency); the death of a close friend; and curiosity tempered with feelings of immortality. First Tom experimented with alcohol, then pot, followed by LSD with a little coke thrown in. By the time Tom was 16, the path of his life had changed dramatically and drugs were a daily habit. In November 1994, he

took the plunge into heroin. It began when he went to a party. A friend whom he had met there mentioned that he knew a guy who dealt heroin.

I was at a pretty low point in my life. I was going against the norm, and it seemed like this was the most extreme way to do it. So I snorted it twice and was ready to go with it. I didn't know all the repercussions, and I wasn't fully aware of the grasp, but soon there was no way out.

I loved the feeling, like a warm breeze throughout your body, and I thought, "This is great!" On Christmas day, after not having used in a couple of days, I broke out in a hot-cold sweat. I could never get comfortable. I had these flu-like feelings and I knew what it was. Once you feel it, you say, I'm never gonna feel this again. It's what keeps an addict an addict. So I went almost a whole year without missing more than a day.

Tom will tell you quite frankly that using a drug like heroin suppresses any natural emotions or feelings that one should have in the course of a day. Withdrawal is all the more haunting because the feelings that have been suppressed come back, begging to be dealt with. Recovery is pure hell. Says Tom, "When you're hooked on using it, you know you don't want to be. You want to quit and get some meds. At first you're an emotional basket case. Once you're OK, you want to go back and get high again. It's powerfully baffling."

Equally baffling is the behavior one undertakes to acquire the dope. On the way back from a Grate-

and other undesirable behavior related to drug dependence (Grinspoon 1995; Swan 1994). Another drug called LAAM (1-alpha-acetyl-methadol) has been clinically tested and approved to treat narcotic addiction (Goldstein 1995). LAAM is a very long-acting narcotic and is more convenient because it requires only three administrations per week to block heroin withdrawal symptoms (Best et al. 1996). A third narcotic, buprenorphine, which is currently used as an analgesic, also is being tested in the treatment of narcotic dependence. Its minimal potential for dependence makes this drug a desirable substitute for heroin (Swan 1993; Best et al. 1996). See Table 10.5 for a comparison of these three drugs.

Some people, including professionals involved in drug abuse therapy, view heroin or narcotic addiction as a "failure of the will" and see methadone treatment as substituting one addiction for another (Goldstein 1994). As a result, unrealistic treatment expectations are sometimes imposed on heroin addicts, leading to high failure rates. For example, many methadone treatment programs may distribute inadequate methadone doses to maintain heroin or narcotic abstinence; alternatively, narcotic-dependent patients may be told

---

ful Dead concert in Albany, New York, Tom convinced the guys in his van to pull off into a less than desirable neighborhood so he could get a quick fix. The trip to the projects nearly cost him his life. Several hours later he was found unconscious by a policeman in the front seat of his van, with his belt around his bicep and a needle still in his arm.

Just as it was a friend who introduced Tom to heroin, it was a friend who, after getting out of jail, had a heart-to-heart talk with Tom that made him realize a recovery program offered his only chance for getting his life back together and recovering his soul. With financial help from his parents and grandparents, he flew to Minneapolis and checked into the Hazelden Drug and Alcohol Addiction Treatment Center for a month-long program of heroin addiction treatment. One of the characteristics of an addict is deception, and Tom was a master of it. "Everyone there thought I was doing so well. I was the star leader, yet the whole time I was on the phone getting some dope set up for me at home. I guess I wasn't ready to make the change," he admitted with a sense of honest disappointment in his voice.

Tom is ready now. Two weeks ago he started taking naltrexone, an opiate blocker, and his outlook on life has changed dramatically. In Tom's words, it demolishes the problem before it even begins. He no longer has to choose between heroin and a normal life—naltrexone has made that choice for him. Its use has allowed him to move on with his life.

If Tom's black cloud has a silver lining, perhaps it can be found in the writing process of people like Jack Keroac and Thomas Wolfe. Writing can be a very cathartic expression of one's feelings; in fact, journal writing is considered one of the most effective ways to get in touch with the soul. As a coping technique, it is employed by many therapists to begin the soul-searching process that ultimately allows us to come face to face with our fears and fully embrace our shadow side. Today, the pen is the sword that brings justice to our demons, such as heroin.

Journal writing not only allows us to release our thoughts and feelings safely, but the process of journaling also provides a glimpse into our behaviors and patterns of thoughts and feelings that lead to these behaviors, and hence become responsible for their continuation. Although not sufficient as a solo treatment, journaling is certainly regarded as a stepping-stone toward wholeness.

> I do a lot of writing now—everyday. I do a lot of creative writing and I draw a lot. I also correspond with a lot of people who used to be in my life, those people whom I shut out years ago while using heroin. I'm learning to make amends.

For Tom, every day is a struggle, yet every day is also an inspiration. ■

Source: Brian Luke Seaward

Table 10.5 Comparison of Narcotic Substitutes Used in Opiate Maintenance therapy

Properties	Methadone	LAAM	Buprenophine
Administration	Oral	Oral	Oral or sublingual
Frequency of doses	Daily	Three times per week	Daily
Other uses	Analgesic	None	Analgesic
Physical dependence	Yes	Yes	Little
Causes positive subjective effects	Yes	Some	Yes
Abuse potential	Yes	Limited	Limited

Source: N. Swan. "Two NIDA-Tested Heroin Treatment Medications Move Toward FDA Approval." *NIDA Notes* (March–April 1993): 45.

their methadone will be terminated within six months regardless of their progress in the program. Such ill-advised policies often drive clients back to their heroin habits and demonstrate that many professionals who treat heroin and narcotic dependency do not understand that methadone is not a cure for heroin addiction, but is a means to achieve a healthier, more normal lifestyle (Millstein 1992; Swan 1994a).

It also is essential to understand that even proper use of methadone does not guarantee resolution of heroin or narcotic addiction. To maximize the possibility of successful treatment, the clients must also receive regular counseling sessions to help modify the drug-seeking behavior as well as receive on-site professional care, including job training, career development, education, general medical care, and family counseling. These supplemental services dramatically improve the success rate of narcotic dependence treatment (McLellan et al. 1993; Grinspoon 1995a).

◢ Other Narcotics

A large number of nonheroin narcotics are used for medical purposes. However, many are also distributed in the "streets," such as morphine, methadone, codeine, hydromorphone (Dilaudid), meperidine (Demerol), and other synthetics. A few of the most commonly abused opioids will be discussed briefly in the following sections. Except where noted, they are all Schedule II drugs.

Morphine

As noted earlier, morphine is the standard by which other narcotic analgesic agents are measured. It has been used to relieve pain since it was first isolated in 1803. Morphine has about half the analgesic potency of heroin but 12 times the potency of codeine.

Morphine is commonly used to relieve moderate to intense pain that cannot be controlled by less potent and less dangerous narcotics. Because of its potential for serious side effects, morphine is generally used in a hospital setting where emergency care can be rendered, if necessary. Most pain can be relieved by morphine if high enough doses are used (Reisine and Pasternak 1995); however, morphine is most effective against continuous dull pain.

The side effects that occur when using therapeutic doses of morphine include drowsiness, changes in mood, and inability to think straight. In addition, therapeutic doses depress respiratory activity; thus, morphine decreases the rate and depth of breathing and produces irregular breathing patterns. Like the other narcotics, it can create an array of seemingly unrelated effects throughout the body, including nausea and vomiting, constipation, blurred vision, constricted pupils, and flushed skin.

The initial response to morphine is varied. In normal people who are not suffering pain, the first exposure can be unpleasant, with nausea and vomiting being the prominent reactions. However, continual use often leads to a euphoric response and encourages dependence. When injected subcutaneously, the effects of heroin and morphine are almost identical; this situation occurs because heroin is rapidly metabolized in the body into morphine. After intravenous administration, the onset of heroin's effects is more rapid and more intense than those of morphine because heroin is more lipid-soluble and enters the brain faster. Because heroin is easier to manufacture and is more potent, it is more popular in illicit trade than morphine. Even so, morphine also has substantial abuse potential and is classified as a Schedule II substance (McEvoy 1993).

Tolerance to the effects of morphine can develop very quickly if the drug is used continuously. For example, an addict who is repeatedly administering the morphine to get a "kick" or maintain a "high" must constantly increase the dose. Such users can build up to incredible doses. One addict reported using 5 grams of morphine daily; the normal analgesic dose of morphine is 50 to 80 *milligrams* per day (Jaffe and Martin 1990). Such high doses are lethal in a person without tolerance to narcotics.

Methadone

Methadone was first synthesized in Germany in 1943, when natural opiate analgesics were not available because opium could not be obtained from the Far East during World War II. Methadone was first called *Dolophine,* after Adolph Hitler; one company still uses that trade name. (On the "street," methadone pills are often called "dollies.") As previously described, methadone is often substituted for heroin in the treatment of narcotic-dependent people. It is an effective analgesic, equal to morphine if injected and more active if taken orally.

The physiological effects of methadone are the same as those of morphine and heroin. As a narcotic, methadone produces psychological dependence, tolerance, and then physical dependence if repeated doses are taken. It is effective for about 24 to 36 hours; therefore, the addict must take methadone daily to avoid narcotic withdrawal. It is often considered as addictive as heroin if injected; consequently, because methadone is soluble in water, it is formulated with insoluble, inert ingredients to prevent it from being injected by narcotic addicts.

Among methadone's most useful properties are cross-tolerance with other narcotic drugs and a less intense withdrawal response. If it reaches a sufficiently high level in the blood, methadone blocks heroin euphoria. In addition, withdrawal symptoms of patients physically dependent on heroin or morphine and the postaddiction craving can be suppressed by oral administration of methadone. The effective dose for methadone maintenance is 50–100 milligrams per day to treat severe withdrawal symptoms (Karch 1996b).

The value of substituting methadone for heroin lies in its longer action. Because addicts no longer need heroin to prevent withdrawal, they often can be persuaded to leave their undesirable associates, drug sources, and dangerous lifestyles. The potential side effects from methadone are the same as those from morphine and heroin, including constipation and sedation; yet if properly used, methadone is a safe drug.

When injecting methadone, some people feel the same kind of euphoria that can be obtained from heroin. Methadone addicts receiving maintenance treatment sometimes become euphoric if the dose is increased too rapidly. There are cases of people who injected crushed methadone pills and developed serious lung conditions from particles that lodged in the tissue, creating a condition somewhat like emphysema. The number of deaths from methadone overdose has been higher than those from heroin in some major cities like New York. Many of these deaths involved young children who took the methadone brought home by parents in maintenance programs or teenagers who tried to shoot up with "street" methadone or methadone in combination with other drugs. Methadone overdoses can be reversed by the antagonist naloxone if the person is found in time.

Fentanyl

Fentanyl (Sublimaze) is a very potent narcotic analgesic (200 times more potent than morphine) that is often administered intravenously for general anesthesia. It is also used in transdermal systems (patches on the skin) in the treatment of chronic pain (Duragesic); occasionally reports surface of individuals abusing a fentanyl patch by licking, swallowing or even smoking it (Marquardt and Tharratt 1994). Fentanyl is not a natural opiate compound, but is readily synthesized and can be modified into drugs that retain potent narcotic properties.

It is estimated that some 100 different active forms of fentanyl could be synthesized; up to now, about ten derivatives have appeared on the "street." They are considered to be "designer" drugs (see Chapter 3); because of their great potency and ease of production, they have sometimes been used to replace heroin on the "street." Fentanyl-type drugs can appear in the same forms and colors as heroin, so there is nothing to alert users that they have been sold a heroin substitute (Henderson 1988). Due to their powerful effects, these drugs are especially dangerous, and incredibly small doses can cause fatal respiratory depression in an unsuspecting heroin user (Greenhouse 1992). (One "designer" fentanyl, 3-methyl fentanyl, is 6000 times more potent than heroin.) During the past decade, more than 100 deaths have been reported in the United States due to overdoses from fentanyl-related drugs. Most have occurred in California and New York (Karch 1996b). Because these drugs are sometimes very difficult to detect in the blood due to the small quantities used, there is no reliable information regarding the extent of fentanyl abuse.

Hydromorphone

Hydromorphone (Dilaudid) is prepared from morphine and used as an analgesic and cough suppressant. It is a stronger analgesic than morphine and is used to treat moderate to severe pain. Nausea, vomiting, constipation, and euphoria may be less marked with hydromorphone than with morphine (Karch 1996b). On the "street," it is taken in tablet form or injected.

Meperidine

Meperidine (Demerol) is a synthetic drug that frequently is used as an analgesic for treatment of moderate pain; it can be taken in tablet form or injected. Meperidine is about one-tenth as powerful as morphine, and its use can lead to dependence. This drug is sometimes given too freely by some physicians because tolerance develops, requiring larger doses to maintain its therapeutic action. With continual use, it causes physical dependence.

Meperidine addicts may use large daily doses (3 to 4 grams per day). In 1994, this drug was responsible for 36 overdose deaths in the United States (Karch 1996b).

MPTP, a "Designer" Tragedy Attempts to synthesize illicit *designer* versions of meperidine by street chemists have proved tragic for some unsuspecting drug addicts. In 1976, a young drug addict with elementary laboratory skills attempted to make a meperidine-like drug by using shortcuts in the chemical synthesis. Three days after self-administering his untested drug product, the drug user developed a severe case of tremors and motor problems identical to Parkinson's disease, a neurological disorder generally occurring in the elderly. Even more surprising to attending neurologists was that this young drug addict improved dramatically after treatment with levodopa, a drug that is very effective in treating traditional Parkinson's disease. After 18 months of treatment, the despondent addict committed suicide. An autopsy revealed he had severe brain damage that was almost identical to that occurring in classical Parkinsonian patients (Davies et al. 1979). It was concluded that a by-product resulting from the sloppy synthesis of the meperidine-like designer narcotic was responsible for the irreversible brain damage.

This hypothesis was confirmed by a separate and independent event on the West Coast in 1981 when a cluster of relatively young heroin addicts (aged 22–42) in the San Francisco area also developed symptoms of Parkinson's disease. All of these patients had consumed a new "synthetic heroin," obtained on the streets, that was produced by attempting to synthesize meperidine-like drugs (Langston et al. 1983). Common to both incidents was the presence of the compound MPTP, which was a contaminant resulting from the careless synthesis. MPTP is metabolized to a very reactive molecule in the brain that selectively destroys neurons containing the transmitter dopamine in the motor regions of the basal ganglia (see Chapter 6). Similar neuronal damage occurs in classical Parkinson's disease over the course of 50–70 years, whereas ingestion of MPTP dramatically accelerates the degeneration to a matter of hours (Goldstein 1995). As tragic as the MPTP incident was, it was heralded as an important scientific breakthrough: MPTP is now used by researchers as a tool to study why Parkinson's disease occurs and how to treat it effectively.

Codeine

Codeine is a naturally occurring constituent of opium and the most frequently prescribed of the narcotic analgesics. It is used principally as a treatment for minor to moderate pain and as a cough suppressant. Maximum pain relief from codeine occurs with 30 to 50 milligrams. Usually, when prescribed for pain, codeine is combined with either a salicylate (such as aspirin) or acetaminophen (Tylenol). Aspirin-like drugs and opioid narcotics interact in a synergistic fashion to give an analgesic equivalence greater than what can be achieved by aspirin or codeine alone.

Although not especially powerful, codeine may still be abused. Codeine-containing cough syrup is currently classified as a Schedule V drug. Because the abuse potential is considered minor, the FDA has ruled that codeine cough products can be sold without a prescription; however, the pharmacist is required to keep them behind the counter and must be asked in order to obtain codeine-containing cough medications. In spite of the FDA ruling, about 50% of the states have more restrictive regulations and require that codeine-containing cough products be available only by prescription.

Although codeine dependence is possible, it is not very common; most people that abuse codeine develop narcotic dependence previously with one of the more potent opioids. In general, large quantities of codeine are needed to satisfy a narcotic addiction; therefore, it is not commonly marketed on the "street."

Pentazocine

Pentazocine (Talwin) was first developed in the 1960s in an effort to market an effective analgesic with low abuse potential. When taken orally, its analgesic effect is slightly greater than that of codeine. Its effects on respiration and sedation are similar to those of the other opioids, but it does not prevent withdrawal symptoms in a narcotic addict. In fact, pentazocine will precipitate withdrawal symptoms if given to a person on methadone maintenance who needs an analgesic

(Reisine and Pasternak 1995). Pentazocine is not commonly abused because its effects can be unpleasant, resulting in dysphoria. It is classified as a Schedule IV drug.

Propoxyphene

Propoxyphene (Darvon, Dolene) is structurally related to methadone, but it is a much weaker analgesic, about half as potent as codeine. Like codeine, propoxyphene is frequently given in combination with aspirin or acetaminophen. Although it was once an extremely popular analgesic, the use of propoxyphene has declined as questions about its potency have been raised. Some research suggests this narcotic is no more effective in relieving pain than aspirin (Reisine and Pasternak 1995). To a large extent, new, more effective non-narcotic analgesics have replaced propoxyphene. In very high doses, it can cause delusions, hallucinations, and convulsions. Alone, propoxyphene causes little respiratory depression; however, when combined with alcohol or other CNS depressants, this drug can depress respiration.

◢ Narcotic-Related Drugs

Although not classified as narcotics, the following drugs are either structurally similar to narcotics (dextromethorphan) or are used to treat narcotic withdrawal (clonidine) or overdose (naloxone).

Dextromethorphan

Dextromethorphan is a synthetic used in cough remedies and can be purchased without prescription. Although its molecular structure resembles that of codeine, this drug does not have analgesic action nor does it cause typical narcotic dependence. However, there have been scattered reports across the country of cough medicine abuse with dextromethorphan, especially by high school and college students. It is claimed that high doses of this drug can cause mild hallucinations and stimulation (Karch 1996a) like PCP.

The following is an account of a 21-year-old male who consumed a high dose (approximately

360 milligrams) of dextromethorphan from a common cough medicine:

> When the dextromethorphan peaked, the most I can remember is laying on my bed thinking "Wow, that's odd, how I can still move my legs even though they aren't attached to my body!" That was way cool and didn't bother me a bit. I was totally convinced my body was separated into two parts, but I was amazed I could control them both. (From the web site— www.frognet.net/dxm/dxmexper.html)

Dextromethorphan is sometimes mixed with drugs such as alcohol, amphetamines, and cocaine to give unusual psychoactive interactions. As of 1996, the DEA had taken no steps to restrict the use of dextromethorphan in OTC products.

Clonidine

Clonidine (Catapres) was discovered in the late 1970s. It is not a narcotic analgesic and has no direct effect on the opioid receptors; instead, it stimulates receptors for noradrenaline, and its principal use is as an oral antihypertensive. Clonidine is mentioned here because it is a nonaddictive, noneuphoriagenic prescription medication with demonstrated efficacy in relieving some of the physical effects of opiate withdrawal (such as vomiting and diarrhea). However, clonidine does not alter narcotic craving or generalized aches associated with withdrawal (O'Brien 1995). The dosing regimen is typically a 7- to 14-day inpatient treatment for opiate withdrawal. Length of treatment can be reduced to 7 days for withdrawal from heroin and short-acting opiates; the 14-day treatment is needed for the longer-acting methadone-type opiates. Because tolerance to clonidine may develop, opiates are discontinued abruptly at the start of treatment. In this way, the peak intensity of withdrawal will occur while clonidine is still maximally effective (McEvoy 1993).

One of the most important advantages of clonidine over other treatments for opiate withdrawal detoxification is that it shortens the time for withdrawal to 14 days compared with several weeks or months using standard procedures, such as methadone treatment. The potential disadvantage of taking clonidine is that it can cause serious side effects of its own, the most serious being sig-

nificantly lowered blood pressure, which can cause fainting and blacking out (Hoffman and Lefkowitz 1995). Overall, its lack of abuse potential makes clonidine particularly useful in treating narcotic dependence.

Naloxone

Naloxone is a relatively pure narcotic antagonist. The drug attaches to opiate receptors in the brain and throughout the body and does not activate them, but rather prevents narcotic drugs, such as heroin and morphine, from having an effect. By itself, naloxone does not cause much change, but it potently blocks or reverses the effects of all narcotics. Because of its antagonistic properties, naloxone is a useful antidote in the treatment of narcotic overdoses; thus, administration of naloxone reverses life-threatening, narcotic-induced effects on breathing and the cardiovascular system. However, if not used carefully, this antagonist will also block the analgesic action of the narcotics and initiate severe withdrawals in narcotic-dependent people (Reisine and Pasternak 1995).

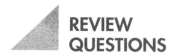

REVIEW QUESTIONS

1. What effects of narcotics cause them to have abuse potential?

2. Why is the clinical use of heroin illegal in the United States, but the use of morphine is not?

3. What are the principal clinical uses of the opioid narcotics?

4. What is the relationship between endorphin systems and the opioid narcotics?

5. Why has there recently been an increase in heroin abuse in the United States?

6. What are the principal withdrawal effects when heroin use is stopped in addicts?

7. How does "methadone maintenance" work for the treatment of narcotic dependence? Explain a possible drawback to this approach.

EXERCISES FOR THE WEB

Exercise 1: Narcotics Anonymous

Narcotics Anonymous is an international, community-based association of recovering drug addicts. Started in 1947, the NA movement is one of the world's oldest and largest of its type, boasting nearly twenty thousand weekly meetings in seventy countries. This web site hopes to explain what Narcotics Anonymous is and what its recovery program offers to drug addicts. The site describes the organization of NA services at the local, national, and international levels. The way in which Narcotics Anonymous cooperates with others

concerned about drug abuse in their countries and communities is explained. Finally, the site provides information on NA's membership and indicators of the success of Narcotics Anonymous.

Exercise 2: Opium in Hong Kong

An in-depth history of the Opium War in Hong Kong is revealed on this web page. Links to reports on Hong Kong found in the *New York Times, Washington Post, Reuters,* and *Time* are also accessible.

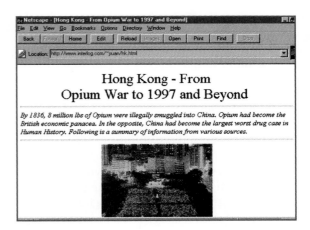

8. What are "shooting galleries," and why are they so important in the spread of AIDS?

9. What have been the consequences of "designer" narcotics?

10. How does morphine compare with heroin?

 KEY TERMS

analgesics   speedballing
opioid   "mainline"
antitussives

 SUMMARY

The term *narcotic* refers to naturally occurring substances derived from the opium poppy and their synthetic substitutes. These drugs are referred to as the opioid (or opiate) narcotics because of their association with opium. For the most part, the opioid narcotics possess abuse potential, but they also have important clinical value and are used to relieve all kinds of pain (they are analgesic), suppress coughing (they are antitussive), and stop diarrhea.

2 The principal side effects of the opioid narcotics, besides their abuse potential, include drowsiness, respiratory depression, nausea and vomiting, constipation, inability to urinate, and sometimes a drop in blood pressure. These side effects can be annoying or even life-threatening, so caution is required when using these drugs.

3 Heroin is the most likely of the opioid narcotics to be severely abused; it is easily prepared from opium and has a rapid, intense effect.

4 When narcotics such as heroin are first used by people not experiencing pain, the drugs can cause unpleasant, dysphoric sensations. However, euphoria gradually overcomes the aversive effects. The positive feelings increase with narcotic use, leading to psychological dependence. After psychological dependence, physical dependence occurs with frequent daily use, which reinforces the narcotic abuse. If the user stops taking the drug after physical dependence has occurred, severe withdrawal symptoms result.

5 Tolerance to narcotics can occur rapidly with intense use of these drugs. This tolerance can result in the use of incredibly large doses of narcotics that would be fatal to a nontolerant person.

6 Methadone and LAAM are frequently used to help narcotic addicts stop using heroin or one of the other, more addicting drugs. Oral methadone relieves the withdrawal symptoms that would result from discontinuing narcotics. Methadone can also cause psychological and physical dependence, but it is less addicting than heroin and easier to control. Another long-acting narcotic, buprenorphine, is also being used in narcotic maintenance programs.

7 Fentanyl is a very potent synthetic opioid narcotic. It is easily synthesized and can be converted into other fentanyl-like drugs that are as much as 3000 to 6000 times more potent than heroin itself. Detection and regulation of these fentanyl derivatives by law enforcement agencies are very difficult. The fentanyl-type drugs are being used as heroin substitutes and have already killed many narcotic addicts because of their unexpected potency.

8 Attempts to create designer narcotics have led to the synthesis of very potent fentanyl-like drugs that are responsible for a number of overdose deaths. In addition, attempts to synthesize a meperidine (Demerol) designer drug resulted in the inadvertent creation of MPTP, a very reactive compound that causes dramatic Parkinson's disease in its users.

REFERENCES

Abel, E. L. *Marijuana: The First Twelve Thousand Years.* New York: Plenum, 1980.

Austin, G. A. *Perspective on the History of Psychoactive Substance Use.* NIDA Research Issues no. 24. Washington, DC: U.S. Department of Health, Education, and Welfare, 1978.

Bearak, B. "Junkies Playing Roulette with Needles." *Salt Lake Tribune* (29 November 1992): A-4.

Best, S., A. Oliveto, and T. Kosten. "Opioid Addiction, Recent Advances in Detoxification and Maintenance Therapy." *CNS Drugs* 6 (October 1996): 301–14.

Bourne, P. G., ed. *Acute Drug Emergencies: A Treatment Manual.* New York: Academic, 1976.

Bowersox, J. A. "Heroin Update: Smoking, Injecting Cause Similar Effects, Usage Patterns May Be Shifting." *NIDA Notes* 10 (July/August 1995): 8–9.

Brecher, E. M. *Licit and Illicit Drugs.* Boston: Little, Brown, 1972.

Colapinto, J. "Rock and Roll Heroin." *Rolling Stone* (May 30, 1996): 15–20, 58–60.

Darke, S., and W. Hall. "Levels and Correlates of Polydrug Use Among Heroin Users and Regular Amphetamine Users." *Drug and Alcohol Dependence* 39 (1995): 231–5.

Davies, G., A. Williams, S. Markey, M. Ebert, E. Caine, C. Reickert, and I. Kopin. "Chronic Parkinsonism Secondary to Intravenous Injection of Meperidine Analogues." *Psychiatry Research* 1 (1979): 249–54.

DiChiara, G., and A. North. "Neurobiology of Opiate Abuse." *Trends in Pharmacological Sciences* 13 (May 1992): 185–93.

Drug Abuse Warning Network (DAWN). "Annual Medical Examiner Data, 1990." In *Data from the Drug Abuse Warning Network.* ADAMHA DHHS Publication no. 91–1880. Washington, DC: U.S. Department of Health and Human Services, 1991.

Facts and Comparisons Drug Newsletter, Update 14 (March 1995): 21.

Golding, A. "Two Hundred Years of Drug Abuse." *Journal of the Royal Society of Medicine* 86 (May 1993): 282–6.

Goldstein, A. In *Addiction from Biology to Drug Policy,* 137–54. New York: Freeman, 1994.

Goldstein, F. "Pharmacological Aspects of Substance Abuse." In *Remington's Pharmaceutical Sciences,* 19th ed., edited by A. R. Genaro. Easton, PA: Mack, 1995: 780–794.

Greenhouse, C. "NIDA Lays Plans for Quicker Response to Drug Crises." *NIDA Notes* 7 (January–February 1992): 20.

Grinspoon, L. "Psychotherapy for Methadone Patients." *Harvard Mental Health Letter* 12 (October 1995a): 7.

Grinspoon, L. "Treatment of Drug Abuse and Addiction—Part II." *Harvard Medical Letter* 12 (October 1995b): 1–4.

Hall, W., J. Bell, and J. Carless. "Crime and Drug Use Among Applicants for Methadone Maintenance." *Drug and Alcohol Dependence* 31 (1993): 123–9.

Henderson, G. "Designer Drugs: Past History and Future Prospects." *Journal of Forensic Sciences* 33 (1988): 569–75.

"Heroin '96: What Americans Need to Know." *Prevention Pipeline* 8 (November/December, 1996) 20.

Hoffman, B., and R. Lefkowitz. "Catecholamines, Sympathomimetic Drugs, and Adrenergic Receptor Antagonists." In *The Pharmacological Basis of Therapeutics,* 9th ed., edited by J. Hardman and L. Limbird, 1673–96. New York: McGraw-Hill, 1995.

Jaffe, J., and M. Martin. "Opioid Analgesics and Antagonists." In *The Pharmacological Basis of Therapeutics,* 8th ed., edited by A. Gilman, T. Rall, A. Nies, and P. Taylor. New York: Pergamon, 1990: 522–573.

Johnston, L. "University of Michigan Annual National Survey of Secondary School Students." Lansing: University of Michigan News and Information Services, 9 April 1993. Available from author at 412 Maynard Ave., Ann Arbor, MI.

Karch, S. "Hallucinogens." In *The Pathology of Drug Abuse,* 241–80. New York: CRC, 1996a.

Karch, S. "Narcotics." In *The Pathology of Drug Abuse,* 281–408. New York: CRC, 1996b.

Kennedy, D. "Flirting with Disaster." *Entertainment Weekly* (August 9, 1996): 18–26.

Kreek, M. "Multiple Drug Abuse Patterns and Medical Consequences." In *Psychopharmacology: The Third Generation of Progress,* edited by Herbert Meltzer, 1597–1604. New York: Raven Press, 1987.

"LAAM—A Long-Acting Methadone for Treatment of Heroin Addiction." *Medical Letter* 36 (10 June 1994): 52.

Langston, J., P. Ballard, J. Tetrud, and I. Irwin. "Chronic Parkinsonism in Humans due to a Product of Meperidine-Analogue Synthesis." *Science* 219 (1983): 979–980.

Leland, J. "The Fear of Heroin Is Shooting Up." *Newsweek* (August 26, 1996): 55–6.

Maas, P. "The Menace of China White." *Parade Magazine* (September 18, 1994): 4.

Marquardt, K., and R. S. Tharratt. "Inhalation Abuse of Fentanyl Patch." *Clinical Toxicology* 32 (1994): 75–8.

"Mary." *Rolling Stone* 30 (1996): 42–3.

Maurer, D., and V. Vogel. *Narcotics and Narcotic Addiction,* 3rd ed. Springfield, IL: Thomas, 1967.

McEvoy, G., ed. "Opiate Agonists." In *American Hospital Formulary Service Drug Information.* Bethesda, MD: American Society of Hospital Pharmacists, 1993.

McLellen, T., O. Arndt, D. Metzger, G. Woody, and C. O'Brian. "The Effects of Psychosocial Services in Substance Abuse Treatment." *Journal of the American Medical Association* 269 (21 April 1993): 1953–59.

Meddis, S. "USA's Illegal Drug Bill: $40 Billion." *USA Today* (20 June 1991): 1-A.

Millstein, R. "Methadone Revisited," *NIDA Notes* 7 (July–August 1992): 3–4.

Newsweek (August 26, 1996): 54.

Nowak, R. "Cops and Doctors: Drug Busts Hamper Pain Therapy." *Journal of NIH Research* 4 (May 1992): 27–29.

O'Brien, C. "Drug Addiction and Drug Abuse." In *The Pharmacological Basis of Therapeutics,* 9th ed., edited by J. Hardman and L. Limbird, 557–77. New York: McGraw-Hill, 1995.

"Opioids." *Medical Letter* 38 (May 10, 1996).

Pfefferbaum, B., and C. Hagberg. "Pharmacological Management of Pain in Children." *Journal of the American Academy of Child and Adolescent Psychiatry* 32 (1993): 235–42.

Reisine, T., and G. Pasternak. "Opioid Analgesics and Antagonists." In *The Pharmacological Basis of Therapeutics,* 9th ed., edited by J. Hardman and L. Limbird, 521–555. New York: McGraw-Hill, 1995.

Scott, J. M. *The White Poppy: A History of Opium.* New York: Funk & Wagnalls, 1969.

Shoemer, K. "Rockers, Models and the New Allure of Heroin." *Newsweek* (August 26, 1996): 50–53.

Sterne, A. E. "A Life of Opium Addiction." *Journal of Inebriety* 29 (Autumn 1907): 203–9.

Swan, N. "Two NIDA-Tested Heroin Treatment Medications Move Toward FDA Approval." *NIDA Notes* (March–April 1993): 45.

Swan, N. "Research Demonstrates Long-Term Benefits of Methadone Treatment." *NIDA Notes* 9 (1994a): 1, 4–5.

Swan, N. "Treatment Practitioners Learn About LAAM." *NIDA Notes* 9 (February–March 1994b): 5.

Thompson, C. "Deadly, Super-Pure Heroin Spreading." *Salt Lake Tribune* 250 (June 22, 1995): A-13.

Treaster, J. "Heroin Use Rises as Crack Wanes." *New York Times* (18 June 1991).

Treaster, J., and L. Holloway. "Potent New Blend of Heroin Ends 8 Very Different Lives." *New York Times* 143 (1994): 1, 13.

Way, W., and E. Way. "Opioid Analgesics and Antagonists." In *Basic and Clinical Pharmacology,* 5th ed., edited by B. Katzung, 420–36. Norwalk, CT: Appleton & Lange, 1992.

Weiss, E. "Seattle Scene Represents Nation's Rising Heroin Use." *All Things Considered,* National Public Radio (January 2, 1995).

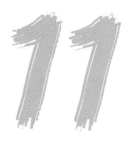

Stimulants

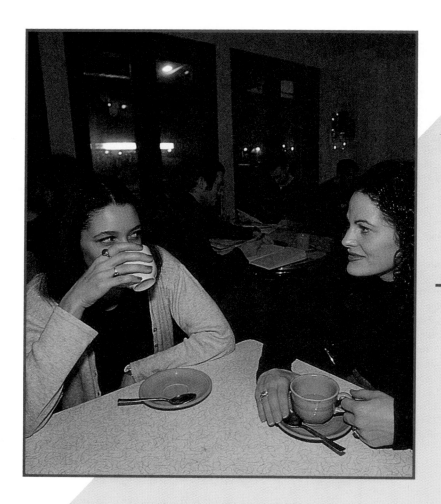

On completing this chapter
you will be able to: ▶

- The first therapeutic use of amphetamines was in inhalers to treat nasal congestion.
- Ritalin is a type of amphetamine used to treat hyperactive (attention deficit disorder) children.
- The most common FDA-approved use of amphetamines is as a diet aid to treat obesity.
- The number of deaths due to methamphetamine overdoses tripled from 1991 to 1994.

- "Ecstasy" is a "designer" drug that is chemically and pharmacologically related to amphetamines.
- The original Coca-Cola was a cocaine-containing tonic developed in the late 1800s.
- In the early 1980s, cocaine was viewed as a relatively harmless, glamorous substance by the media and some medical experts in this country.
- Smoking "freebased," or "crack," cocaine is more dangerous and more addicting

than other forms of administration.
- Many people who abuse cocaine have underlying mental illness.
- Caffeine is the most frequently used stimulant in the world.
- OTC decongestant drugs usually contain mild CNS stimulants.
- Herbal stimulants promoted as "natural highs" contain CNS stimulants that can be lethal.

- Explain how amphetamines work.
- Identify the FDA-approved uses for amphetamines.
- Recognize the major side effects of amphetamines on brain and cardiovascular functions.
- Identify the terms *speed, ice,* and *run* as they relate to amphetamine use.
- Explain what "designer" amphetamines are.
- Identify the three cocaine eras.

- Trace the changes in attitude toward cocaine abuse that occurred in the 1980s and explain why they occurred.
- Compare the effects of cocaine to those of amphetamines.
- Identify the four principal means of administering cocaine and their relative potencies.
- Distinguish the properties of "crack" that make it unique from other cocaine forms.
- Identify the different stages of cocaine withdrawal.

- Discuss the different approaches to treating cocaine dependence.
- Identify and compare the major sources of the caffeinelike xanthine drugs.
- List the principal physiological effects of caffeine.
- Compare caffeine dependence and withdrawal to that associated with the major stimulants.
- Understand the possible consequences of using herbal stimulants.

253

Stimulants are substances that cause the user to feel pleasant effects, such as a sense of increased energy, and a state of euphoria, or "high." This effect is illustrated in the following statement by a 24-year-old college student interviewed by Dr. Peter Venturelli:

> I've done cocaine three times. The first time was in college with some friends. I was drunk and nothing happened. . . . The second time, I felt like a million bucks. I could drink like a fish.

The user may also feel restless and talkative and have trouble sleeping. High doses used over the long term can produce personality changes or even dangerous behavior. Many users self-medicate psychological conditions (for example, depression) with stimulants. Because the initial effects of stimulants are so pleasant, these drugs are frequently abused, leading to dependence.

In this chapter, you will learn about two principal classifications of stimulant drugs. Major stimulants, including amphetamines and cocaine, are addressed first, given their prominent role in current drug abuse problems in the United States. The chapter concludes with a review of minor stimulants-in particular, caffeine. The stimulant properties of OTC sympathomimetics and "herbal highs" are also discussed.

(Because nicotine has unique stimulant properties, it is covered in Chapter 12, "Tobacco.")

Major Stimulants

All major stimulants cause increased alertness, excitation, and euphoria; thus, these drugs are referred to as **"uppers."** The major stimulants are classified as either Schedule I ("designer" amphetamines) or Schedule II (amphetamine and cocaine) controlled substances because of their abuse potential. Toxic effects of the major stimulants account for almost half of all drug-related unexplained sudden deaths in the United States (Goldstein 1994). Although these drugs have properties in common, they also have unique features that distinguish

"uppers"
CNS stimulants

them from one another. The similarities and differences of the major stimulants are discussed in the following sections.

Amphetamines

Amphetamines are potent CNS stimulants capable of causing dependence due to their euphorigenic properties and ability to eliminate fatigue. Despite their addicting effects, amphetamines can be legally prescribed by physicians. Consequently, amphetamine abuse occurs in people who acquire their drugs by both legitimate and illicit means.

The History of Amphetamines The first amphetamine was synthesized by the German pharmacologist L. Edeleano in 1887, but it was not until 1910 that this and several related compounds were tested in laboratory animals. Another 17 years passed before Gordon Alles, a researcher looking for a more potent substitute for ephedrine (used as a decongestant at the time), self-administered amphetamine and gave a firsthand account of its effects. Alles found that when inhaled or taken orally, amphetamine dramatically reduced fatigue, increased alertness, and caused a sense of confident euphoria (Grinspoon and Bakalar 1978).

Because of Alles's impressive findings, Benzedrine (amphetamine) inhalers became available in 1932 as a nonprescription medication in drugstores across America. The Benzedrine inhaler, marketed for nasal congestion, was widely abused for its stimulant action but continued to be available over the counter until 1949. Because of a loophole in a law that was passed later, not until 1971 were all potent amphetamine-like compounds in nasal inhalers withdrawn from the market (Grinspoon and Bakalar 1978).

Because of the lack of restrictions during this early period, amphetamines were sold for a variety of different ailments, including obesity, alcoholism, bed wetting, depression, schizophrenia, morphine and codeine addiction, heart block, head injuries, seasickness, persistent hiccups, and caffeine mania. Today, most of these uses are no longer approved as legitimate therapeutics but would be considered forms of drug abuse.

World War II provided a setting in which both the legal and "black market" use of amphetamines flourished (Grinspoon and Bakalar 1978). Because of their stimulating effects, amphetamines were widely used in World War II to counteract fatigue. For example, the German, Japanese, and British made extensive use of these drugs in the early 1940s. By the end of World War II, large quantities of amphetamines were readily available without prescription in seven different types of nasal inhalers.

In spite of warnings about these drugs' addicting properties and serious side effects, the U.S. armed forces issued amphetamines on a regular basis during the Korean War. Korean veterans going back to college used amphetamine tablets to stay awake and cram for examinations, and other students quickly adopted the practice. Amphetamine use became widespread among truck drivers making long hauls; in fact, it is believed that among the earliest distribution systems for illicit amphetamines were truck stops along major U.S. highways. High achievers under continuous pressure in the fields of entertainment, business, and industry often relied on amphetamines to counteract fatigue. Homemakers used them for weight control and to combat boredom from unfulfilled lives. At the height of the U.S. epidemic in 1967, some 31 million prescriptions were written for **anorexiants** (diet pills) alone.

anorexiants
drugs that suppress the appetite for food

Today a variety of related drugs and mixtures exist, including amphetamine substances such as dextroamphetamine (Dexedrine), methamphetamine (Desoxyn), and amphetamine itself. Generally, if doses are adjusted, the psychological effects of these various drugs are similar, so they will be discussed as a group. Other drugs with similar pharmacological properties are phenmetrazine (Preludin), and methylphenidate (Ritalin). Common slang terms for the amphetamines include *speed, crystal, meth, bennies, dexies, uppers, pep pills, diet pills, jolly beans, copilots, hearts, footballs, white crosses,* and *ice.*

How Amphetamines Work Amphetamines are synthetic chemicals that are similar to natural neurotransmitters such as norepinephrine (nora-drenaline), dopamine, and the stress hormone epinephrine (adrenaline). The amphetamines exert their pharmacological effect by increasing the release and blocking the metabolism of these catecholamine substances as well as serotonin (see Chapter 6), both in the brain and nerves associated with the sympathetic nervous system. Because amphetamines cause release of norepinephrine from sympathetic nerves, they are classified as *sympathomimetic* drugs. The amphetamines generally cause an arousal or activating response (also called the "fight-or-flight response") that is similar to the normal reaction to emergency situations or crises.

Amphetamines also cause alertness so that the individual becomes aroused, hypersensitive to stimuli, and feels "turned on." These effects occur even without external sensory input. This activation may be a very pleasant experience in itself, but a continual high level of activation may convert to anxiety, severe apprehension, or panic.

Amphetamines have potent effects on dopamine in the reward (pleasure) center of the brain (see Chapter 6). This action probably causes the "flash," or sudden feeling of intense pleasure that occurs when amphetamine is taken intravenously. Some users describe the sensation as a "whole body orgasm," and many associate intravenous methamphetamine use with sexual feelings. The actual effect of these drugs on sexual behavior is quite variable.

What Amphetamines Can Do A curious condition commonly reported with heavy amphetamine use is **behavioral stereotypy,** or getting "hung up." This term refers to a simple activity that is done repeatedly. An individual who is "hung up" will get caught in a repetitious thought or act for hours. For example, he or she may take objects apart, like radios or clocks, and carefully categorize all the parts, or sit in a tub and bathe all day, persistently sing a note, repeat a phrase of music, or repeatedly clean the same object. This phenomenon seems to be peculiar to potent stimulants such as the amphetamines and cocaine. Similar patterns of repetitive behavior also

behavioral stereotypy
meaningless repetition of a single activity

occur in psychotic conditions, which suggests that the intense use of stimulants such as amphetamines or cocaine alters the brain in a manner like that causing psychotic mental disorders (American Psychiatric Association 1994).

Chronic use of high doses of amphetamines causes dramatic decreases in the brain content of the neurotransmitters dopamine and serotonin that persist for months, even after drug use is stopped (Gygi et al. 1996). These decreases have been shown to reflect the death of CNS neurons that release these transmitters. It is not clear why this neuronal change occurs or how it affects behavior.

Approved Uses   Until 1970, amphetamines were prescribed for a large number of conditions, including depression, fatigue, and long-term weight reduction. In 1970, the FDA, acting on the recommendation of the National Academy of Sciences, restricted the legal use of amphetamines to three medical conditions: (1) narcolepsy, (2) hyperkinetic (attention deficit disorder) behavior, and (3) short-term weight reduction programs (Goldstein 1995).

Narcolepsy   Amphetamine treatment of **narcolepsy** is not widespread because this condition is a relatively rare disorder. The term *narcolepsy* comes from the Greek words for "numbness" and "seizure." A person who has narcolepsy falls asleep as frequently as 50 times a day if he or she stays in one position for very long. Taking low doses of amphetamines helps keep narcoleptic people alert.

> **narcolepsy**
> a condition causing spontaneous and uncontrolled sleeping episodes

Hyperkinetic Behavior   This common behavioral problem in children and adolescents involves an abnormally high level of physical activity (**hyperkinesis**), an inability to focus attention, and frequent disruptive behavior. About 4 out of every 100 grade-school children and 40% of schoolchildren referred to mental health clinics because of behavioral disturbances are hyperactive. The

> **hyperkinesis**
> excessive movement

drug commonly used to treat hyperkinetic (attention deficit disorder) children is the amphetamine-related methylphenidate or Ritalin (discussed later in this chapter).

Weight Reduction   By far the most common use of amphetamines is for the treatment of obesity. Amphetamines and chemically similar compounds are used as anorexiants to help such people control appetite. Amphetamines are thought to act by affecting the appetite center in the hypothalamus of the brain and decreasing food intake. The FDA has approved short-term use of amphetamines for weight loss programs, but has warned against their potential for abuse. Many experts feel that the euphoric effect of amphetamines is the primary motivation for their continued use in weight reduction programs. It is possible that many obese people have a need for gratification that can be satisfied by an amphetamine-like drug. If the drug is taken away, these individuals return to food to satisfy their need and sometimes experience "rebound," causing them to gain back more weight than they lost.

Side Effects of Therapeutic Doses   The two principal side effects of therapeutic doses of amphetamines include (1) abuse potential, which has already been discussed at length, and (2) cardiovascular toxicities. Many of these effects are due to the amphetamine-induced release of epinephrine from the adrenal glands and norepinephrine from the nerves associated with the sympathetic nervous system. The effects include increased heart rate, elevated blood pressure, and damage to vessels, especially small veins and arteries (Max 1991). In users with a history of heart attack, coronary arrhythmia, or hypertension, amphetamine toxicity can be severe or even fatal.

Current Misuse   Because amphetamine drugs can be readily and inexpensively synthesized in makeshift laboratories for illicit sales, can be administered by several routes, and cause a more sustained effect, these drugs are more popular than cocaine in many parts of the United States (Chavez 1996). Surveys suggest that there was a decline in the abuse of amphetamines in the late

1980s and early 1990s in parallel with the trend in cocaine abuse (Johnston 1996). However, in 1993 the declines were replaced by an alarming rise in the number of adolescents that abused amphetamines compared with 1992 (approximately 10%). Particularly troubling has been the dramatic rise in deaths (151 to 433) and visits to emergency rooms (4,900 to 17,400) that were caused by methamphetamines from 1991 to 1994 (Chavez 1996). The recent surge in the abuse of high doses of methamphetamine and its frightening social impact caused the U.S. Attorney General, Janet Reno, to propose a "National Methamphetamine Strategy" in 1996; it included plans to deal with methamphetamine-related criminal activity, violence, and law enforcement problems (Reno 1996).

Because of the potential for serious side effects, U.S. medical associations have asked all physicians to be more careful about prescribing amphetamines. In fact, presently, use is recommended only for narcolepsy and some cases of hyperactivity in children (Hoffman and Lefkowitz 1995). In spite of FDA approval, most medical associations do not recommend the use of amphetamines for weight loss. Probably less than 1% of all prescriptions now written are for amphetamines, compared with 8% in 1970.

Amphetamine abusers commonly administer a dose of 10 to 30 milligrams. Besides the positive effects of this dose-the "high"-it can cause hyperactive, nervous, or jittery feelings that encourage the use of a depressant such as a benzodiazepine, barbiturate, or alcohol to relieve the discomfort of being "wired" (Hoffman and Lefkowitz 1995).

A potent and commonly abused form of amphetamine is **speed,** an illegal methamphetamine available as a white crystalline powder for injection. The profit for the speed manufacturer is substantial enough to make illicit production financially attractive. The cost ranges from $50 to $150 per gram (Reno 1996). Methamphetamine is relatively easy to synthesize even by individuals without expertise in chemistry. Such people, referred to as "cook-

speed

an injectable methamphetemine used by drug addicts

ers," produce methamphetamine batches by using cookbook-style recipes (often obtained in jail or over the Internet). At least two predominant methods used for making methamphetamine result in highly variable products from clandestine laboratory to laboratory (Irvine and Chin 1991). The most popular recipe uses common OTC ingredients-ephedrine, pseudoephedrine, and phenylpropanolamine-as precursor material for the methamphetamine. To discourage the illicit manufacture of this potent stimulant, the Comprehensive Methamphetamine Control Act was passed in October 1996. This law increases penalties for trafficking in methamphetamine and in the **precursor chemicals** used to create this drug, and gives the government authority to regulate and seize these substances (Schwartz 1996).

precursor chemicals

chemicals used to produce a drug

Due to the ease of production and the ready availability of chemicals used to prepare methamphetamine, a constant supply of this drug has remained on the market. Currently, the wholesale trafficking of this stimulant is dominated by international polydrug trafficking organizations; in particular, Mexico-based groups have produced unprecedented quantities of high-purity methamphetamine that have saturated illicit markets in the western United States (Reno 1996; Johnson 1996).

Today, so-called meth or speed labs are frequently raided by law enforcement agencies across the country as local drug entrepreneurs try to grab a share of the profits. In 1995, the DEA shut down almost 300 illegal methamphetamine labs, most of which were in the western United States (Reno 1996); these statistics do not include the activities of local and state drug enforcement officials. The laboratory operators are usually well armed, and the facilities frequently booby-trapped with explosives. Not surprisingly, these operations pose a serious threat to their neighbors (Reno 1996).

Patterns of High-Dose Use Amphetamines can be taken orally, intravenously, or by smoking. The intensity and duration of effects vary according to the mode of administration. The "speed freak" uses chronic, high doses of amphetamines intravenously. Another approach to administering amphetamines is smoking **ice,** which can cause effects as potent, but perhaps more prolonged and erratic, than intravenous doses . The cycle or pattern of use often starts with several days of repeated administrations, usually of "speed," gradually increasing in amount and frequency. This pattern of intense stimulant use is called a **run.** Some users inject several thousand milligrams in a single day (Goldstein 1995) and the run can continue for as long as 15 days (Reno 1996). Initially, the user may feel energetic, talkative, enthusiastic, happy, confident, and powerful, and may initiate and complete highly ambitious tasks. He or she will be unable to sleep and will usually eat very little. His or her pupils will be dilated, mouth dry, and body temperature elevated, a condition known as **hyperpyrexia.**

> **ice**
> a smokable form of methamphetamine

> **run**
> intense use of a stimulant, cosisting of multiple administrations over a period of days

> **hyperpyrexia**
> elevated body temperature

After the first day or so, unpleasant symptoms become prominent as the dosage is increased. Symptoms commonly reported at this stage are teeth grinding, disorganized patterns of thought and behavior, stereotypy, irritability, self-consciousness, suspiciousness, and fear. Hallucinations and delusions can occur that are similar to a paranoid psychosis and indistinguishable from schizophrenia (American Psychiatric Association 1994; Flaum and Schultz 1996). The person is likely to show aggressive and antisocial behavior for no apparent reason. Severe chest pains, abdominal discomfort that mimics appendicitis, and fainting from overdosage are sometimes reported. "Cocaine bugs" represent one bizarre effect of high doses of potent stimulants such as amphetamines: The user experiences strange feelings, like insects crawling under the skin. The range of physical and mental symptoms from low to high doses is summarized in Table 11.1.

Toward the end of the run, the adverse symptoms dominate. When the drug is discontinued because the supply is exhausted or the symptoms become too unpleasant, an extreme crash can occur, followed by prolonged sleep, sometimes lasting several days. On awakening, the person is lethargic, hungry, and often severely depressed. The amphetamine user may overcome these effects by smoking ice or injecting speed, thereby initiating a new cycle. Barbiturates, benzodiazepines, and opiate narcotics are sometimes used to ease the "crash" or to terminate an unpleasant run (see Chapter 7). As one user described it:

> Speed is a rush-everything seems very clear intellectually. Alcohol doesn't seem to affect you. You sweat like you're working out, chain-smoke cigarettes, solve the world's problems, clean your kitchen floor, and write a letter you have to burn in the morning. That's in the first 45 minutes. Coming down is rough though, especially with cheap speed like white cross.
>
> *From the files of Peter Venturelli, interview with a 42-year-old female, 1995*

Continued use of massive doses of amphetamine often leads to considerable weight loss, sores in the skin, nonhealing ulcers, liver disease, hypertensive disorders, cerebral hemorrhage (stroke), heart attack, kidney damage, and seizures (Hall and Hando 1993). For some of these effects, it is impossible to tell whether they are caused by the drug, poor eating habits, or other factors associated with the lifestyle of people who inject methamphetamine.

Speed freaks are generally unpopular with the rest of the drug-taking community, especially "acid-heads" (addicts who use LSD), because of the aggressive, unpredictable behavior associated with use of potent stimulants. In general, drug abusers who take high doses of these agents, such as amphetamines or cocaine, are more likely to be involved in violent crimes than those who abuse other drugs (Miller and Kozel 1991). Consequently, these individuals may live together in "flash houses" that are solely occupied by chronic amphetamine or stimulant addicts. Heavy users

Table 11.1   **Summary of the Effects of Amphetamines on the Body and Mind**

	Body	Mind
Low Dose	Increased heartbeat	Decreased fatigue
	Increased blood pressure	Increased confidence
	Decreased appetite	Increased feeling of alertness
	Increased breathing rate	Restlessness, talkativeness
	Inability to sleep	Increased irritability
	Sweating	Fearfulness, apprehension
	Dry mouth	Distrust of people
	Muscle twitching	Behavioral stereotypy
	Convulsions	Hallucinations
	Fever	Psychosis
	Chest pain	
	Irregular heartbeat	
High Dose	Death due to overdose	

are generally unable to hold steady jobs because of their drug habits and often have a parasitic relationship with the rest of the illicit drug-using community.

Although claims have been made that amphetamines do not cause physical dependence, it is almost certain that the depression (sometimes suicidal), lethargy, and abnormal sleep patterns occurring after high chronic doses are part of withdrawal (Goldstein 1995). This type of rebound effect is opposite to that experienced with withdrawal from CNS depressants (see Chapter 7). Withdrawal from depressants cause severe and toxic overstimulation, even to the point of convulsions.

Amphetamine Combinations Amphetamines are frequently used in conjunction with a variety of other drugs, such as barbiturates, benzodiazepines, alcohol, and heroin (Hall and Hando 1993). Amphetamines intensify, prolong, or otherwise alter the effects of

speedballs

a combination of amphetamine or cocaine with an opioid narcotic, often heroin

LSD, and the two drugs are sometimes combined. The majority of speed users have also had experience with a variety of psychedelic and other drugs. In addition, people dependent on opiate narcotics frequently use amphetamines or cocaine. These combinations are called **speedballs.**

"Designer" Amphetamines Underground chemists can synthesize drugs that mimic the psychoactive effects of amphetamines. Although the production of such drugs diminished in the early 1990s, a recent surge in use by American teens has resulted in an approximate 5% annual use rate in high students (Johnston 1996). These substances have become known as *desinger drugs* see (Chapter 4).

Designer amphetamines sometimes differ from the parent compound by only a single element. These "synthetic spinoffs" pose a significant abuse problem because often several different designer amphetamines can be made from the parent compound and still retain the abuse potential of the original substance.

For many years the production and distribution of designer amphetamines were not illegal, even though they were synthesized from controlled substances. In the mid-1980s, however, the DEA actively pursued policies to curb their production and sale. Consequently, many designer amphetamines were outlawed under the Substance Analogue Enforcement Act (1986), which makes illegal any substance that is similar in structure or psychological effect to any substance already scheduled, if it is manufactured, possessed, or sold with the intention that it be consumed by humans (Beck 1990).

The principal types of designer amphetamines are

▲ Derivatives from amphetamine and methamphetamine that retain the CNS stimulatory effects, such as methcathinone ("CAT").

▲ Derivatives from amphetamine and methamphetamine that have prominent hallucinogenic effects besides their CNS stimulatory action, such as MDMA (Ecstasy).

Because the basic amphetamine molecule can be easily synthesized and readily modified, new amphetamine-like drugs continue to appear on the streets. Although these designer amphetamines are thought of as new drugs when they first appear, in fact, most were originally synthesized from the 1940s to the 1960s by pharmaceutical companies trying to find new decongestant and anorexiant drugs to compete with the other amphetamines. Some of these compounds were found to be too toxic to be marketed but have been rediscovered by "street chemists" and are being sold to unsuspecting victims trying to experience a new sensation. See Table 11.2 for a list of these designer amphetamines.

Some designer drugs of abuse that are chemically related to amphetamine include DOM (STP), methcathinone (Called "CAT" or "bathtub speed"), MDA, and MDMA (or methylenedioxymethamphetamine, called "Ecstasy," "X," "E," "XTC," or "Adam"). All of these drugs are currently classified as Schedule I agents.

MDMA (Ecstasy) Among the designer amphetamines, MDMA continues to be the most popular. It gained widespread popularity in the United States throughout the 1980s, and its use peaked in 1987 despite its classification as a Schedule I drug in 1985 by the DEA. At the height of its use, 39% of the undergraduates at Stanford University reported to have used MDMA at least once (Randall 1992a). In the late 1980s and early 1990s, use of MDMA declined in this country, but about this time it was "reformulated": this reformulation was not in a pharmacological sense but in a cultural context.

The "rave" scene in England provided a new showcase for MDMA or Ecstasy (Randall 1992a). Partygoers attired in "Cat in the Hat" hats and psychedelic jumpsuits paid $20 to dance all night to heavy electronically generated sound mixed with computer-generated video and laser light shows.

Table 11.2 "Designer" Amphetamines

Amphetamine Derivative	Properties
Methcathinone ("CAT")	Properties like those of methamphetamine and cocaine
Methylenedioxy**methamphetamine** (MDMA, "Ecstasy")	Stimulant and hallucinogen
Methylenedioxy**amphetamine** (MDA)	More powerful stimulant and less powerful hallucinogen than MDMA
4-Methylaminorex	CNS stimulant like amphetamine
N, N-Dimethyl**amphetamine**	One-fifth potency of amphetamine
4-Thiomethyl-2, 5-dimethoxy**amphetamine**	Hallucinogen
Para-methometh**amphetamine**	Weak stimulant

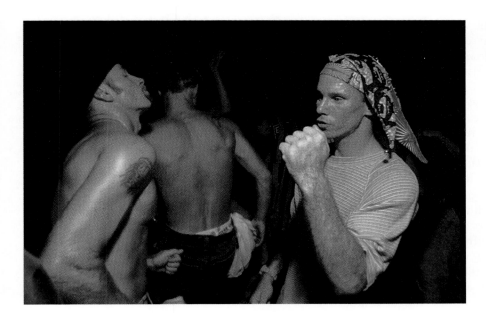

Dancers at a "rave" often consume Ecstasy for sensory enhancement.

For another $20, an Ecstasy tablet could be purchased for the sensory enhancement caused by the drug (Randall 1992b). It is estimated that as many as 31% of English youth in range of 16-25 years old have used Ecstasy (Grob et al. 1996). The British "rave" counterculture and its generous use of Ecstasy was exported to the United States in the early 1990s, with its high-tech music and video trappings being encouraged by low-tech laboratories that illegally manufactured the drug in this country. Some have compared the "rave" culture of the 1990s and its use of MDMA to the acid-test parties of the 1960s and their use of LSD and amphetamines (Randall 1992a). The following is an account by a young college woman who first used Ecstasy at a rave party when 22 years of age:

> I'd tried other drugs such as LSD and speed, but [Ecstasy] was different. I can't describe the exact feeling except that I was in . . . a euphoric state of mind, a mystical trance. My friends and I couldn't stop hugging and saying how much we loved each other . . . . Things went downhill from there . . . one day I swallowed [a large dose] . . . I was scared stiff. I blacked out, but woke the next morning very hot and with my body in spasms. Eventually I ended up in a psychiatric hospital . . . It was the most frightening experience of my life. (From N. Saunders. "E Is

for Ecstasy". Internet address: http://www.hyper-real.com/drugs/)

The patent for MDMA was first issued in 1914 to E. Merck in Darmstadt, Germany, for use as an appetite suppressant (Grob et al. 1996). No pharmaceutical company has ever manufactured MDMA for public marketing, and the FDA has never approved it for therapy (Beck 1990). MDMA was first found by the DEA on the streets in 1972 in a drug sample bought in Chicago (Beck 1990). The DEA earnestly began gathering data on MDMA abuse a decade later, which led to its classification as a Schedule I substance in 1985 despite the very vocal opposition by a number of psychiatrists who had been using MDMA since the late 1970s to facilitate communication, acceptance, and fear reduction in their patients (Beck 1990). MDMA and related designer amphetamines are somewhat unique from other amphetamines in that, besides causing excitation, they have prominent hallucinogenic effects, as well (see Chapter 13). These drugs have been characterized as combining the properties of amphetamine and LSD (Shifano and Magni 1996). The psychedelic effects of MDMA are likely caused by release of the neurotransmitter serotonin. After using hallucinogenic amphetamines, the mind is often flooded with a variety of irrelevant and incoherent thoughts and exaggerated sensory experiences and is more receptive to suggestion.

MDMA is often viewed as a "smooth amphetamine" and does not appear to cause the severe depression, or "crash," often associated with frequent high dosing of the more traditional amphetamines. Most users tend to be predominantly positive when describing their initial MDMA experiences (Taylor 1994). They claim the drug causes a dramatic drop in defense mechanisms or fear responses, while feeling an increased empathy for others. Combined with its stimulant effects, this action often increases intimate communication and association with others (Beck 1990; Goldstein 1995). However, many users do experience adverse effects, such as loss of appetite, grinding of teeth, muscle aches and stiffness, sweating, and a rapid heartbeat. In addition, fatigue can be experienced for hours or even days after use. In high doses, MDMA can cause paranoid psychosis, panic attacks, and seizures (Shifano and Magni 1996). Despite these side effects, there are few reports of severe toxicity or death in the United States from using MDMA (Taylor 1994): in contrast, at least 15 young people in England were killed in the early 1990s because of this designer amphetamine. In every case a recreational dose of this drug had been taken by the victim at a "rave" where crowds were packed together and dancing vigorously (Randall 1992a). In these fatal cases, the victims collapsed unconscious while dancing and started to convulse. The combination of rapidly rising body temperature (up to 110 °F), racing pulse, and plummeting blood pressure resulted in death from 2 to 60 hours after hospital admission. The lethality of MDMA under these conditions appears to be related to its ability to elevate body temperature and cause dehydration. Thus, mixed with the crowd, hot environment of a "rave" and extreme physical exertion while dancing, the drug causes a deadly episode of hyperthermia (Taylor 1994).

Methylphenidate: A Special Amphetamine

Methylphenidate (Ritalin) is related to the amphetamines but is a relatively mild CNS stimulant that has been used to alleviate depression. Research now casts doubt on its effectiveness for treating depression, but it is effective in treatment of narcolepsy (a sleep disorder). As explained previously, methylphenidate has also been found to aid in calming children suffering from attention deficit disorder and is currently the drug of choice for this purpose. The potency of methylphenidate lies between that of caffeine and amphetamine. Although it is not used much on the street by hardcore drug addicts, there have been reports of use by high school and college students because of claims that it helps them to "study better," "party harder," and experience a buzz (Hinkle and Winckler 1996). High doses of Ritalin can cause tremors, seizures, and strokes. Methylphenidate has been classified as a Schedule II drug, like the other prescribed amphetamines.

Cocaine

Over the last 10 to 15 years, cocaine abuse has become one of the greatest drug concerns in the U.S. society. In the so-called war against drugs, cocaine eradication is considered to be a top priority. The tremendous attention recently directed at cocaine reflects the fact that from 1978 to 1987 the United States experienced the largest cocaine epidemic in history. Antisocial and criminal activities related to the effects of this potent stimulant have become highly visible and widely publicized (Grinspoon 1993).

As recently as the early 1980s, cocaine use was not believed to cause dependency because it did not cause gross withdrawal effects, as do alcohol and narcotics (Goldstein 1994). In fact, a 1982 article in *Scientific American* stated that cocaine was "no more habit forming than potato chips" (Van Dyck and Byck 1982). This perception has clearly been proven false: cocaine is so highly addictive that it is readily self-administered not only by humans but by laboratory animals as well (Fischman and Johanson 1996). Surveys suggest that 1.4 million Americans are current cocaine users (NIDA 1995).

There is no better substance than cocaine to illustrate the "love-hate" relationship that people can have with drugs. Many lessons can be learned by understanding the impact of cocaine and the social struggles that have ensued as people have tried to determine their proper relationship with this substance.

The History of Cocaine Use

Cocaine has been used as a stimulant for thousands of years. Its history can be classified into three eras, based on geographical, social, and therapeutic considerations. Learning about these eras can help us understand current attitudes about cocaine.

The First Cocaine Era

The first cocaine era was characterized by an almost harmonious use of this stimulant by South American Indians living in the regions of the Andean Mountains and dates back to about 2500 B.C. in Peru. It is believed that the stimulant properties of cocaine played a major role in the advancement of this isolated civilization, providing its people with the energy and motivation to realize dramatic social and architectural achievements while being able to endure tremendous hardships in barren, inhospitable environments. The *Erythroxylon coca* shrub (cocaine found in the leaves) was held in religious reverence by these people until the time of the Spanish Conquistadors (Golding 1993).

The first written description of coca chewing in the New World was by explorer Amerigo Vespucci in 1499:

> They were very brutish in appearance and behavior, and their cheeks bulged with the leaves of a certain green herb which they chewed like cattle, so that they could hardly speak. Each had around his neck two dried gourds, one full of that herb in their mouth, the other filled with a white flour like powdered chalk. . . . [This was lime, which was mixed with the coca to enhance its effects.] When I asked . . . why they carried these leaves in their mouth, which they did not eat, . . . they replied it prevents them from feeling hungry, and gives them great vigor and strength. (Aldrich and Barker 1976, 3)

When the Spanish conqueror Francisco Pizarro invaded Peru in the sixteenth century, he found coca to be the center of the Incan social and religious systems. According to legend, the coca plant was divine.

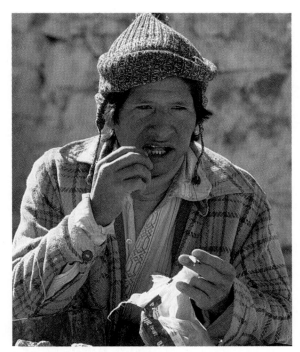

An Andean chews coca leaves.

It is ironic that there are no indications that these early South American civilizations had any significant social problems with cocaine, considering the difficulty it has caused contemporary civilizations. The ancient Indians appeared to be able to live harmoniously with this drug and even take advantage of its unique pharmacological properties to advance their societies. There are three possible explanations for their positive experiences with coca:

1. The Andean Indians maintained control of the use of cocaine. For the Incas, coca could only be used by the conquering aristocracy, chiefs, royalty, and other designated honorables (Aldrich and Barker 1976).

2. These Indians used the unpurified form of cocaine in the coca plant, while later civilizations purified the drug and thus dramatically increased its potency and the likelihood of abuse.

3. Chewing the coca leaf was a slow, sustained form of administering the drug; therefore, the

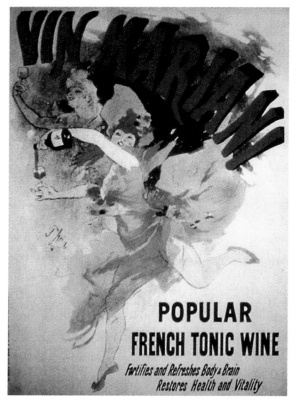

The "refreshing" element in Vin Mariani was coca extract.

effect was much less potent than snorting, intravenous injection, or smoking-techniques most often used today.

The Second Cocaine Era

A second major cocaine era began in the nineteenth century. During this period, scientific techniques were used to elucidate the pharmacology of cocaine and identify its dangerous effects. It was also during this era that the threat of cocaine to society-both its members and institutions-was first recognized (DiChiara 1993). At about this time, scientists in North America and Europe began experimenting with a purified, white, powdered extract made from the coca plant.

In the last half of the nineteenth century, Corsican chemist Angelo Mariani removed the active ingredients from the coca leaf and identified cocaine. This purified cocaine was added into cough

drops and into a special Bordeaux wine called *Vin Mariani*. The Pope gave Mariani a medal in appreciation for the fine work he had done. The cocaine extract was publicized as a magical drug that would free the body from fatigue, lift the spirits, and cause a sense of well-being, and the cocaine-laced wine became widely endorsed throughout the civilized world (Fischman and Johanson 1996). Included in a long list of luminaries who advocated this product for an array of ailments were the Czar and Czarist of Russia; the Prince and Princess of Wales; the Kings of Sweden, Norway, and Cambodia; commanders of the French and English armies; President McKinley of the United States; H. G. Wells; August Bartholdi (sculptor of the Statue of Liberty); and some 8000 physicians.

The astounding success of this wine attracted imitators, all making outlandish claims. One of these cocaine tonics was a nonalcoholic beverage named Coca-Cola, which was made from African kola nuts and advertised as the "intellectual beverage and temperature drink"; it contained 4-12 milligrams per bottle of the stimulant (DiChiara 1993). By 1906 Coca-Cola no longer contained detectable amounts of cocaine, but caffeine had been substituted in its place.

In 1884, the esteemed Sigmund Freud published his findings on cocaine in a report called "Uber Coca." Freud recommended this "magical drug" for an assortment of medical problems, including depression, hysteria, nervous exhaustion, digestive disorders, hypochondria, "all diseases which involve degenerations of tissue," and drug addiction.

In response to a request by Freud, a young Viennese physician, Karl Koller, studied the ability of cocaine to cause numbing effects. He discovered that it was an effective local anesthetic that could be applied to the surface of the eye and permit painless minor surgery to be conducted. This discovery of the first local anesthetic had tremendous worldwide impact. Orders for the new local anesthetic, cocaine, overwhelmed pharmaceutical companies.

Soon after the initial jubilation over the virtues of cocaine came the sober realization that with its benefits came severe disadvantages. As more people used cocaine, particularly in tonics and patent medicines, the CNS side effects and abuse liability became painfully evident. By the turn of the century, cocaine was being processed from the coca plant and purified routinely by drug companies. People began to snort or inject the purified form of this popular powder, which increased both its effects and its dangers. The controversy over cocaine exploded before the American public in newspapers and magazines.

As medical and police reports of cocaine abuse and toxicities escalated, public opinion demanded that cocaine be banned. In 1914, the Harrison Act incorrectly classified both cocaine and coca as narcotic substances (cocaine is a stimulant) and outlawed their uncontrolled use.

Although prohibited in patent and nonprescription medicines, prescribed medicinal use of cocaine continued into the 1920s. Medicinal texts included descriptions of therapeutic uses for cocaine to treat fatigue, vomiting, seasickness, melancholia, and gastritis. However, they also included lengthy warnings about excessive cocaine use, "the most insidious of all drug habits" (Aldrich and Barker 1976).

Little of medical or social significance occurred for the next few decades (Fischman and Johanson 1996). The medicinal use of cocaine was replaced mostly by the amphetamines during World War II because cocaine could not be supplied from South America. (Cocaine is not easily synthesized, so even today, the supply of cocaine, both legal and illegal, continues to come from the Andean countries of South America.) During this period, cocaine continued to be employed for its local anesthetic action, was available on the "black market," and was used recreationally by musicians, entertainers, and the wealthy. Because of the limited supply, the cost of cocaine was prohibitive for most would-be consumers. Cocaine abuse problems remained of minor concern until the 1980s.

The Third Cocaine Era

With the 1980s came the third major era of cocaine use. This era started much like the second in that the public and even the medical community were naive and misinformed about the drug. Cocaine was viewed as a glamorous substance and portrayed by the media as the drug of celebrities. Its use by prominent actors, athletes, musicians, and other members of

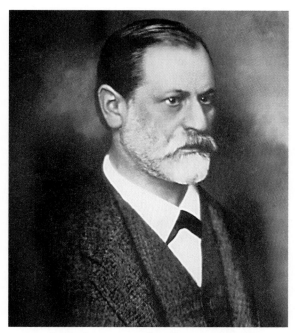

Sigmund Freud was an early advocate of cocaine, which he referred to as a "cure-all."

a fast-paced, elite society was common knowledge. By 1982, over 20 million Americans had tried cocaine in one form or another, compared with only 5 million in 1974 (Green 1985).

The following is an example of a report from a Los Angeles television station in the early 1980s, which was typical of the misleading information being released to the public:

> Cocaine may actually be no more harmful to your health than smoking cigarettes or drinking alcohol; at least that's according to a six-year study of cocaine use [described in *Scientific American*]. It concludes that the drug is relatively safe and, if not taken in large amounts, it is not addictive. (Byck 1987).

With such visibility, an association with prestige and glamour, and what amounted to an indirect endorsement by medical experts, the stage was set for another epidemic of cocaine use. Initially, the high cost of this imported substance limited its use. With increased demand came increased supply, and prices tumbled from an unaffordable

$100 per "fix" to an affordable $10. The epidemic began.

By the mid-1980s, cocaine permeated all elements of society. No group of people or part of the country was immune from its effects. Many tragic stories were told of athletes, entertainers, corporate executives, politicians, fathers and mothers, high school students, and even children using and abusing cocaine. It was no longer the drug of the laborer or even the rich and famous. It was everybody's drug and everybody's problem (Golding 1993). As one user recounts:

> I think I was an addict. I immediately fell in love with cocaine. I noticed right away it was a drug that you had power with, and I wanted more and more.

> *From the files of Peter Venturelli, interview*
> *with a 22-year-old male, 1995*

Cocaine Production Because cocaine is derived from the coca plant, which is imported from the Andean countries, America's problems with this drug have had a profound effect on several South American countries. With the dramatic rise in U.S. cocaine demand in the early 1980s, coca production in South America increased in tandem. The coca crop is by far the most profitable agricultural venture in some of these countries. In addition, this crop is easily cultivated and easily maintained (the coca plant is a perennial and remains productive for decades), and can be harvested several times a year (on average, two to four). The coca harvest has brought many jobs and some prosperity to these struggling economies. According to *National Geographic,* coca exports bring between $500 million and $1 billion to Bolivia annually. In U.S. terms, this figure is a relatively small amount, but for a poor country such as Bolivia, this money can mean the difference between life and death for many impoverished families (Boucher 1991).

In spite of U.S. efforts, coca production increased from 1994 to 1995 in Colombia, Peru, and Bolivia. The profits (1 kilogram of cocaine brings farmers $1000), combined with the traditional view held by the people in Latin American countries that coca is a desirable substance, have made it difficult to persuade farmers to change crops just to satisfy the demanding gringos (Haven 1996).

In conjunction with local governments, the United States has attempted to destroy coca crops directly by burning, cutting, spraying herbicides, and even the introduction of coca-eating caterpillars (Boucher 1991). The result has been that thousands of coca field workers are jobless and frustrated (Associated Press 1996).

Cocaine Processing Cocaine is one of several active ingredients from the leaves of *Erythroxylon coca* (its primary source). The leaves are harvested two or three times per year and used to produce coca paste, which contains up to 80% cocaine. The paste is processed in clandestine labs to form a pure, white hydrochloride salt powder. Often purified cocaine is

> **adulterated**
> comtaminating substances are mixed in to dilute the drugs

adulterated (or "cut") before it is sold on the "streets" with substances such as powdered sugar, talc, arsenic, lidocaine, strychnine, and methamphetamine. Adverse responses to administering street cocaine are sometimes caused by the additives, not the cocaine itself. The resultant purity of the cut material ranges from 10% to 85%.

Cocaine is often sold in the form of little pellets, called "rocks," or as flakes or powder. If it is in pellet form, it must be crushed before used. Such exotic names as Peruvian rock and Bolivian flake are bandied about to convince the buyer that the "stash" is high grade. Other street names used for cocaine include *blow, snow, flake, C, coke, toot, white lady, girl, cadillac, nose candy, gold dust,* and *stardust.*

Current Attitudes and Patterns of Abuse

Given contemporary medical advances, we have greater understanding of the effects of cocaine and toxicities and dependence it produces. The reasons for abusing cocaine are better understood as well. For example, it is clear that as many as 30% of chronic cocaine users are self-medicating psychiatric disorders such as depression, attention deficit disorders, or anxiety (Grinspoon 1993). Such

Figure 11.1

Trends in cocaine and crack use by high school seniors, 1975–1996. These data represent the percentages of high school seniors surveyed who reported using cocaine during the year.

Note: Crack cocaine did not become widely available until 1986.

Source: L. Johnson. "University of Michigan Annual National Surveys of Secondary Students." Lansing: University of Michigan, 1996.

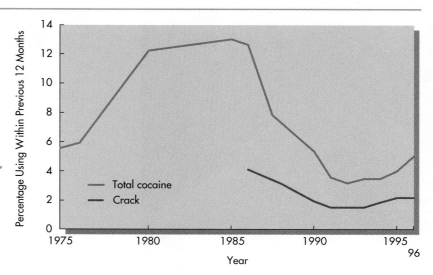

knowledge helps in identifying and administering effective treatment. The hope is that society will never again be fooled into thinking that cocaine abuse is glamorous or an acceptable form of entertainment.

Attempts are being made to use this understanding (some recently acquired, some merely relearned) to educate people about the true nature of cocaine. Such education was likely responsible for trends of declining cocaine use observed from 1987 to 1991 (see Figure 11.1). Decreases occurred in virtually every age group evaluated during this period. Surveys during this time revealed that, in general, cocaine use became less acceptable; these changes in attitude almost certainly contributed to the dramatic reduction in use (Johnston 1994). However, since 1992, the cocaine abuse has rebounded, especially in young populations (Figure 11.1) (Johnston 1996). Although it is not clear why the declines ceased, some experts have speculated that attitudes about cocaine use are again changing and eventually may lead to a new era of cocaine problems (Johnston 1996).

It is important to note that in general even when the total number of cocaine users was declining, the number of heavy users actually increased, resulting in a stable pattern of total cocaine consumption over the past decade (Hudgins et al. 1995). As a consequence, more people

are consuming larger quantities, which often leads to severe toxicity requiring emergency care.

Cocaine Administration Cocaine can be administered orally, inhaled into the nasal passages, injected intravenously, or smoked. The form of administration is important in determining the intensity of cocaine's effects, its abuse liability, and the likelihood of toxicity (Fischman and Johanson 1996).

Oral administration of cocaine produces the least potent effects; most of the drug is destroyed in the gut or liver before it reaches the brain. The result is a slower onset of action with a milder, more sustained stimulation. This form is least likely to cause health problems and dependence (Grinspoon 1993). South American Indians still take cocaine orally to increase their strength and for relief from fatigue. Administration usually involves prolonged chewing of the coca leaf, resulting in the consumption of about 20-400 milligrams of the drug (DiChiara 1993). Oral use of cocaine is not common in the United States.

"Snorting" involves inhaling cocaine hydrochloride powder into the nostrils, where deposits form in the lining of the nasal chambers and approximately 100 milligrams of the drug passes through the mucosal tissues into the bloodstream (DiChiara 1993). Substantial CNS stimulation

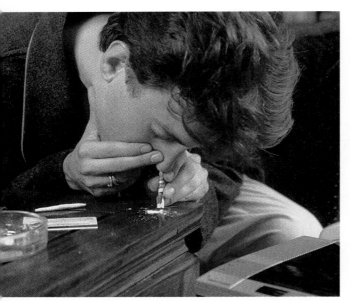

Snorting cocaine causes substantial stimulation often followed by a rebound depression.

occurs in several minutes, persists for 30 to 40 minutes, and then subsides. The effects occur more rapidly and are shorter-lasting and more intense than those achieved with oral administration, as more of the drug enters the brain more quickly. Because concentrations of cocaine in the body are higher after snorting than after oral ingestion, the side effects are more severe. One of the most common consequences of snorting cocaine is rebound depression, or "crash," which is of little consequence after oral consumption. As a general rule, the intensity of the depression correlates with the intensity of the euphoria (Goldstein 1995).

According to studies performed by the National Institute on Drug Abuse, about 10% to 15% of those who try intranasal (snorting) cocaine go on to heavier forms of dosing, such as intravenous (IV) administrations. Intravenous administration of cocaine is a relatively recent phenomenon because the hypodermic needle was not widely available until the late 1800s. This form of administration has contributed to many of the cocaine problems that appeared at the turn of the century. IV administration allows large amounts of cocaine to be introduced very rapidly into the body and causes severe side effects and

dependence. Within seconds after injection, cocaine users experience an incredible state of euphoria. The "high" is intense but short-lived; within 15 to 20 minutes, the user experiences dysphoria and is heading for a "crash." To prevent these unpleasant rebound effects, cocaine is readministered every 10 to 30 minutes. Readministration continues as long as there is drug available.

This binge activity resembles that seen in the methamphetamine "run." When the cocaine supply is exhausted, the binge is over (Goldstein 1994). Several days of abstinence may separate these episodes; the average cocaine addict binges once to several times a week, with each binge lasting 4 to 24 hours. Cocaine addicts claim that all thoughts turn toward cocaine during binges; everything else loses significance. This pattern of intense use is how some people blow all of their money on cocaine, as the following scenario illustrates:

> I'm working hard for my old man and I'm even selling [cocaine] at work a little bit, but now I'm starting to get to the point where you know the whole thing is one big lie. I didn't even know what the truth was anymore. I just started lying to everybody about things. I was making this kind of money, . . . but I got so f-addicted to this stuff, you don't even know you're lying anymore. And I started doing so much of it that I started losing money and I started losing other people's as well. I had to lie to those people, and I started screwing those people just so I could get my next fix.

From the files of Peter Venturelli, interview with a 22-year-old-male, 1995

Freebasing is a method of reducing impurities in cocaine and preparing the drug for smoking. It produces a type of cocaine that is more powerful than normal cocaine hydrochloride. One way to "freebase" is to treat the cocaine hydrochloride with a liquid base such as sodium carbonate or ammonium hydroxide. The cocaine dissolves, along with many of the impurities commonly found in it (such as amphetamines, licodaine, sugars, and others). A solvent, such as petroleum or

freebasing
coversion of cocaine into its alkaline form for smoking

ethyl ether, is added to the liquid to extract the cocaine. The solvent containing the cocaine floats to the top and is drawn off with an eyedropper; it is placed in an evaporation dish to dry, and crystalized cocaine residue is then crushed into a fine powder, which can be smoked in a special glass pipe.

The effects of smoked cocaine are as intense or greater than those achieved through intravenous administration (Fischman and Johanson 1996). The onset is very rapid, the euphoria is dramatic, the depression is severe, the side effects are dangerous, and the chances of dependence are high (Grinspoon 1993). The reason for these intense reactions to inhaling cocaine into the lungs is that the drug passes rapidly through the lining of the lungs and into the many blood vessels present; it is then carried almost directly to the brain.

Freebasing became popular in the United States in the 1980s due to the fear of diseases such as AIDS and hepatitis that are transmitted by sharing contaminated hypodermic needles. But freebasing involves other dangers. Because the volatile solvents required for freebasing are very explosive, careless people have been seriously burned or killed during processing (Siegel 1985). "Street" synonyms used for freebased cocaine include *baseball, bumping, white tornado, world series,* and *snowtoke.*

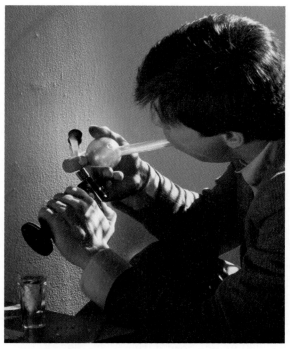

"Freebasing" paraphernalia. A water pipe is often used to smoke freebased cocaine, or "crack." Cocaine administered by smoking is very potent and fast acting; the effect lasts for 10 to 15 minutes, after which depression occurs. This is the most addicting form of cocaine.

"Crack" Between 1985 and 1986, a special type of freebased cocaine known as **crack** or *rock* appeared on the streets (Goldstein 1994). By 1988, approximately 7% of the young adult population had tried crack; as of 1992 the use of crack had fallen substantially to 1.5%, but rebounded to 2.1% by 1996. This rebound is thought to reflect a lack of perceived risk from this drug (Johnston 1996). Crack is inexpensive and can be smoked without the dangerous explosive solvents mentioned earlier in the discussion of freebasing. It is made by taking powdered cocaine hydrochloride and adding sodium bicarbonate (baking soda) and water. The paste that forms removes impurities as well as the hydrochloride from the cocaine.

> **crack**
>
> already processed and inexpensive "freebased" cocaine, ready for smoking

The substance is then dried into hard pieces called *rocks,* which may contain as much as 90% pure cocaine. Other slang terms for crack include *base, black rock, gravel, Roxanne,* and *space basing.*

Like freebased cocaine, crack is usually smoked in a glass water pipe. When the fumes are absorbed into the lungs, they act rapidly, reaching the brain within 8 to 10 seconds. An intense "rush" or "high" results, and later a powerful state of depression, or "crash," occurs. The high may last only 3 to 5 minutes, and the depression may persist from 10 to 40 minutes or longer in some cases. As soon as crack is smoked, the nervous system is greatly stimulated by the release of dopamine, which seems to be involved in the rush. Cocaine prevents resupply of this neurotransmitter, which may trigger the crash.

Because of the abrupt and intense release of dopamine, smoked crack is viewed as a drug with tremendous potential for addiction (Grinspoon 1993) and is considered by users to be more enjoyable than cocaine administered intravenously (Fischman and Johanson 1996). In fact, some people with serious cardiovascular disease continue their use of crack despite knowledge of the serious risk for heart attacks and strokes (Fischman and Foltin 1992). Crack and cocaine marketing and use are often associated with criminal activity. For example, nearly 30% of the homicide victims in New York City have cocaine in their bodies (Swan 1995).

In general, crack use is more common among African-American and Hispanic populations than among white Americans. However, the difference in prevalence does not appear to be racially related, but rather due to socioeconomic circumstances (Lillie-Blanton et al. 1993). Of special concern is the use of crack among women during pregnancy. Children born under these circumstances have been referred to as **crack babies;** their population is estimated to include as many as 900,000 infants born during 1989-1992 (Knight-Ridder News Service 1992). Even though the effects of crack on fetal development are not fully understood, many clinicians and researchers have predicted that these crack babies will impose an enormous social

> **crack babies**
> ———
> infants born to women who use crack cocaine during pregnancy

burden. However other experts have expressed concern that the impact of cocaine on the fetus is grossly overstated and suggested that behavioral problems seen in these children are more a consequence of social environment than direct pharmacological effects (Fischman and Johanson 1996). Clearly, more studies will be required to determine the full impact of using this drug during pregnancy.

It is not coincidental that the popularity of crack use paralleled the AIDS epidemic in the mid-1980s. Because crack administration does not require injection, theoretically the risk of contracting the HIV virus from contaminated needles is avoided. Even so, incidence of HIV infection in crack users is still very high, because crack smokers also use cocaine intravenously and 30% to 40% of the IV users are HIV-positive (Des Jarlais

1992)-see Chapter 16. Another reason for the high incidence of HIV infections (as well as other venereal diseases, such as syphilis and gonorrhea) among crack users is the dangerous sexual behavior in which these people participate. Crack is commonly used as payment for sex, not to mention that users are much less inclined to be cautious about their sexual activities while under the influence of this drug (Des Jarlais 1992).

Major Pharmacological Effects of Cocaine Cocaine has profound effects on several vital systems in the body. With the assistance of modern technology, the mechanisms whereby cocaine alters body functions have become better understood today. Such knowledge will hopefully lead to better treatment of cocaine dependence.

Most of the pharmacological effects of cocaine use stem from enhanced activity of catecholamine (dopamine, noradrenaline, adrenaline) and serotonin transmitters. It is believed that the principal action of the drug is to block the reuptake of these substances following their release from neurons. The consequence of such action is to prolong the activity of these transmitter substances at their receptors and substantially increase their effects. The summation of cocaine's effects on these four transmitters causes CNS stimulation (Woolverton and Johnston 1992). The increase of noradrenaline activity following cocaine administration increases the effects of the sympathetic nervous system and alters cardiovascular activity (see discussion later).

Central Nervous System Because cocaine has stimulant properties, it has antidepressant effects as well. In fact, some users self-administer cocaine to relieve severe depression or the negative symptoms of schizophrenia (Seibyl et al. 1992; Mendelson and Mello 1996), but in general its short-term action and abuse liability make cocaine unsatisfactory for the treatment of depression disorders. The effects of stimulation appear to increase both physical and mental performance while masking fatigue. High doses of cocaine cause euphoria (based on the form of administration) and enhance the sense of strength, energy, and performance. Because of these positive effects, cocaine has intense reinforcing properties, which encourage continual use and dependence (Woolverton and Johnston 1992).

The feeling of exhilaration and confidence caused by cocaine can easily transform into irritable restlessness and confused hyperactivity (Grinspoon 1993). In addition, high chronic doses alter personality, frequently causing psychotic behavior that resembles paranoid schizophrenia (American Psychiatric Association 1994; Fischman and Johanson 1996). For example, in an interview with Dr. Peter Venturelli, a 17-year-old-female explained that a cocaine-abusing friend " . . . was so coked up that he carved the word 'pain' in his arm and poured coke on it. He thought it symbolized something." In some urban hospitals as many as 38% of the patients admitted for psychiatric reasons abuse cocaine (Galanter et al. 1992). In addition, cocaine use heightens the risk of suicide (Ehrman 1992), major trauma, and violent crimes (Brookoff et al. 1993). In many ways, the CNS effects of cocaine are like those of amphetamines, although perhaps with a more rapid onset, a more intense high due partially to the manner in which the drugs are administered), and a shorter duration of action (Goldstein 1995).

Besides dependence, other notable CNS toxicities that can be caused by cocaine use include headaches, temporary loss of consciousness, seizures, and death (Benowitz 1992). Some of these effects may arise from the increased body temperature caused by this drug (Grinspoon 1993).

Cardiovascular System Cocaine can initiate pronounced changes in the cardiovascular system by enhancing the sympathetic nervous system, increasing the levels of adrenaline, and causing vasoconstriction (Grinspoon 1993). The initial effects of cocaine are to increase heart rate and elevate blood pressure. At the same time that the heart is being stimulated and working harder, the vasoconstriction effects deprive the cardiac muscle of needed blood (Fischman and Johanson 1996). Such a combination can cause severe heart arrhythmia (an irregular contraction pattern) or heart attack. Other degenerative processes have also been described in the hearts and blood vessels of chronic cocaine users (Fischman and Johanson 1996). In addition, the vasoconstrictive action of

this sympathomimetic can damage other tissues, prompting a stroke, lung damage in those who smoke cocaine, destruction of nasal cartilage in those who snort the drug, and injury to the gastrointestinal tract (Goldstein 1995).

Local Anesthetic Effect Cocaine was the first local anesthetic used routinely in modern-day medicine. There is speculation that the ancient Andes Indians of South America used cocaine-filled saliva from chewing coca leaves as a local anesthetic for surgical procedures (Aldrich and Barker 1976). However, this assumption is contested by others (Byck 1987). Even so, cocaine is still a preferred local anesthetic for minor pharyngeal (back part of the mouth and upper throat area) surgery due to its good vasoconstriction (reduces bleeding) and topical, local numbing effects. Although relatively safe when applied topically, significant amounts of cocaine can enter the bloodstream and, in sensitive people, cause CNS stimulation, toxic psychosis, or even on rare occasions, death (*Medical Letter* 1996).

Cocaine Withdrawal

Considerable debate has arisen as to whether cocaine withdrawal actually happens and, if so, what it involves. With the most recent cocaine epidemic and the high incidence of intense, chronic use, it has become apparent that nervous systems do become tolerant to cocaine and that, during abstinence, withdrawal symptoms occur (Goldstein 1995). In fact, because of CNS dependence, the use of cocaine is less likely to be stopped voluntarily than is the use of other illicit drugs (Schwartz et al. 1991). Certainly, if the withdrawal experience is adverse enough, a user will be encouraged to resume the cocaine habit.

The intensity of cocaine withdrawal is proportional to the duration and intensity of use. The physical withdrawal symptoms are relatively minor compared with those caused by long-term use of CNS depressants and by themselves are not considered to be life-threatening (Woolverton and Johnston 1992). Short-term withdrawal symptoms include depression (chronic cocaine users are 60 times more likely to commit suicide than nonusers), sleep abnormalities, craving for the drug, agitation, and anhedonia (inability to experience pleasure). Long-term withdrawal effects include a return to normal pleasures, accompanied by mood swings and occasional craving triggered by cues in the surroundings (Grinspoon 1993; Mendelson and Mello 1996).

Of particular importance to treatment of the chronic cocaine users is that abstinence after bingeing appears to follow three unique stages, each of which must be dealt with in a different manner if relapse is to be prevented. These phases are classified as: phase 1, or "crash" (occurs nine hours to four days after drug use is stopped); phase 2, or withdrawal (one to ten weeks); and finally, phase 3, or extinction (indefinite). The basic features of these phases are outlined in Table 11.3 (Gawin 1992).

Treatment of Cocaine Dependence Cocaine dependency is classified as a psychiatric disorder by the American Psychiatric Association (1994). Treatment of this condition has improved as experience working with these patients has increased. Even so, success rates vary for different programs. From 30% to 90% of the patients who persist in outpatient treatment programs are considered to be "successfully treated" (Gawin 1991). The problem with such assessments is that they do not take into account patients who drop out of programs. Also, no clear-cut criteria for qualifying success have been established. For example, is success considered to be abstaining from cocaine for one year, two years, five years, or forever?

No one treatment technique has been found to be significantly superior to others or universally effective (Mendelson and Mello 1996); consequently, substantial disagreement exists as to what is the best strategy for treating cocaine dependency, and there is a major ongoing effort by federal agencies and scientists to find effective therapy for cocaine addiction (Leshner 1996). Most treatments are directed at relieving craving (Kleber 1992). Major differences in treatment approaches include (1) whether outpatient or inpatient status is appropriate, (2) which drugs and what dosages should be used to treat patients during the various stages of abstinence, and (3) what length of time the patient should be isolated from cocaine-accessible environments. It is important to treat each individual patient according to his or her unique needs. Some factors that need

Table 11.3   **Cocaine Abstinence Phases**

	Phase 1: "Crash"	Phase 2: Withdrawal	Phase 3: Extinction
Time since last binge	24–48 hours	1–10 weeks	Indefinite
Features	*Initial* Agitation, depression, anorexia, suicidal thoughts *Middle* Fatigue, no craving, insomnia *Late* Extreme fatigue, no craving, exhaustion	*Initial* Mood swings, sleep returns, some craving, little anxiety *Middle and late* Anhedonia, anxiety, intense craving, obsessed with drug seeking	Normal pleasure, mood swings, occasional craving, cues trigger craving

Source: Gawin (1991).

to be considered when formulating a therapeutic approach include the following:

Why did the patient begin using cocaine, and why has dependency occurred?

What is the severity of abuse?

How has the cocaine been administered?

What is the psychiatric status of the patient; are there underlying or coexisting mental disorders, such as depression or attention deficit disorder?

What other drugs are being abused along with the cocaine?

What is the patient's motivation for eliminating cocaine dependence?

What sort of support system (family, friends, co-workers, and so on) will sustain the patient in the abstinence effort?

Outpatient Versus Inpatient Approaches The decision as to whether to treat a patient dependent on cocaine as an outpatient or inpatient is based on a number of issues. For example, inpatient techniques allow greater control than outpatient treatment; thus, the environment can be better regulated, the training of the patient can be more closely supervised, and his or her responses to treatment can be more closely monitored. In contrast, the advantages of the outpatient approach are that supportive family and friends are better able to encourage the patient, the surroundings are more comfortable, and natural, potential problems that might occur when the patient re-

turns to a normal lifestyle are more likely to be identified; in addition, such treatment is less expensive.

Cocaine-dependent patients should be matched to the most appropriate strategy based on their personalities, psychiatric status, and the conditions of their addiction (Mendelson and Mello 1996). For instance, a cocaine addict who lives in the ghetto, comes from a home with other drug-dependent family members, and has little support probably would do better in the tightly controlled inpatient environment. However, a highly motivated cocaine addict who comes from a supportive home and a neighborhood that is relatively free of drug problems would probably do better on an outpatient basis.

Therapeutic Drug Treatment Several drugs have been used to treat cocaine abstinence, although none has been found to be universally effective (Leshner 1996). Table 11.4 lists those that have been used in each of the three principal phases of cocaine abstinence. Besides relieving acute problems of anxiety, agitation, and psychosis, drugs can also diminish cocaine craving; this effect is achieved by giving drugs such as bromocryptine or L-dopa that stimulate the dopamine transmitter system or the narcotic, buprenorphine. As mentioned, the pleasant aspects of cocaine likely relate to its ability to increase the activity of dopamine in the limbic system. When cocaine is no longer available, the dopamine system becomes less active, causing depression and anhedonia, which results in tremendous craving for cocaine. The intent of these cocaine substitutes is to stimu-

Table 11.4 Medications Used in Treatment of Cocaine Abstinence at Various Phases

Phase	Drug	Drug Group (Rationale)
1. Crash	Benzodiazepines	Depressants (relieve anxiety)
2. Withdrawal	Bromocryptine, L-dopa	Dopamine agonist (relieve craving))
3. Extinction	Desipramine, imipramine	Antidepressant (relieve depression and craving)

Source: J. Mendelson and N. Mello. "Management of Cocaine Abuse and Dependence." *New England Journal of Medicine* 334 (1996): 965-72.

Recovery Through Using Humor

To see the twinkle in her eyes and the genuine smile that graces her face, you would never know that Donna was a cocaine addict—an addiction that nearly killed her. The twinkle and smile reveal what the mask of cocaine hid for years. Her story goes like this.

Donna was a self-described overachiever. By the age of 19, she had earned a bachelor's degree in nursing. By the age of 20, she had received her master's degree. Perhaps it was an attempt to please her parents. Perhaps it was an attempt to fill a void. Nevertheless, whatever Donna did, she excelled at. The road to success was not without its potholes, however. During her junior year in college, Donna began to take speed, which then led to alcohol, which in turn led to cocaine-a downward spiral toward death.

"Back when I was in school, you could get a doctor's prescription for amphetamines. A lot of people took these to lose weight. I took them so I could stay up late and study." As Donna describes it, speed can bring you up, and alcohol can bring you down. Soon she found herself becoming dependent on both substances to achieve a false sense of balance in her life. At age 23, Donna was married and her professional career in nursing was skyrocketing. Alcohol became a constant friend, soon to be joined by cocaine as her drug of choice for what she calls the last three years of her 11-year addiction history.

"Where did I get the cocaine?" she asks with a giggle. "I got it from several of the physicians whom I worked with. You know, one out of every five cocaine addicts is a white-collar professional. We're not all street bums," she explained. "The first time I used cocaine, I loved it. But what it was doing was filling a void. Cocaine was a magic bullet. It took me away from my childhood pain [you could call this an abandonment issue]. It also ruined my life. I knew eventually I was going to die."

Ironically, even as a psychiatric nurse who worked with the chronically mentally ill, Donna managed to hide her addiction problem from her professional colleagues. "As a rule, health care professionals who are addicts tend to be overachievers. Even on a bad day, we still look pretty good. It never occurred to anyone that I had a drug problem. Everyone loved me and cared for me. My friends and colleagues were enablers. They thought I was depressed because I was going through a divorce at the time, so they helped me by covering for me and doing some of my work. It kept me sick longer."

Donna put up a good front, but eventually the habit began to take its toll. Having spent over $250,000 in a three-year period, looking run-down

---

late dopamine activity and relieve the cravings. Although this approach sometimes works initially, it is temporary. In the third phase of cocaine abstinence, antidepressants such as desipramine are effective for many cocaine-dependent patients in relieving underlying mood problems and occasional cravings.

The beneficial effects of these drugs are variable and not well studied. There is some debate over their use. Drugs are, at best, only adjuncts in the treatment of cocaine dependence; they are never long-term solutions by themselves (Carrol 1994). Successful treatment of cocaine abuse re-

quires intensive counseling; strong support systems from family, friends, and co-workers; and a highly motivated patient (See "Recovering Through Humor" above). It is important to realize that a complete "cure" from cocaine dependence is possible: ex-addicts cannot return to cocaine and control its use (Kleber 1992). The following is an example of the constant battle of one cocaine addict who is attempting to break the habit:

> I had several years of sobriety [from cocaine use] until recently when I relapsed on crack . . . I don't know if I am addicted to crack. I still want

and depressed (she lost 30 pounds, slimming down to 90 pounds), and with the quality of her work performance suffering dramatically, the signs and symptoms of addictions became more visible. A friend began to see through the lies and deceptions and one day called her on the carpet. Sensing that Donna was suicidal and ready to die, her friend called Donna's parents in a successful attempt to get her some help. Almost by force, Donna entered a 30-day treatment program, the day after she quit her job.

It was a very long road to recovery. From the month-long treatment program, she entered a halfway house for three months (a humbling experience, she admits) and then continued as an outpatient for the next nine months. She also underwent psychoanalysis treatment and attended Alcoholics Anonymous and Cocaine Anonymous meetings, which she still attends regularly even years later. There is a spiritual (not religious) approach to any 12-step program. As Donna explains, "In AA, you are allowed to discover God through a new understanding-a loving, accepting God, unlike the fire and damnation God I grew up with."

Humor, it is said, is a gift from God. By far it provides one of the most effective means to deal with stress. The word *silly* is derived from the word *selig*, meaning "blessed." *Humor* comes to use from the word *fluid* or *moisture*. "Humor is about having a fluid spirit," explains Donna, as she should know because humor therapy has become her calling.

"It was my sister who taught me the importance of silliness. It was my grandmother who gave me strength, hope, and inspiration." This special alchemy turned to gold in the course of Donna's recovery. "This may sound silly," she said, "but in treatment, we did meditation and visualization. Three times a wizard came to me with a message either on a scroll or in a crystal ball. The message was one word-humor. It was then I knew I needed to pursue the issue of laughter as a means to cope. I needed to learn to lighten up. so I studied with Annette Goodheart, M.D., Steve Allen, Jr., M.D., and Bernie Siegel, M.D." With a natural talent to speak in front of a crowd, Donna's future was cast in mirth. Today she is considered an expert in the field of humor therapy, traveling extensively throughout the international community to share the benefits of humor and laughter, and she doesn't preach theory. For Donna, it is her saving grace in the treatment of her addiction.

I have come to discover that the degree [to which] you are willing to experience your sorrow is proportional to that which you will experience your joy. Joy and sorrow are wired on the same neural pathway.

The twinkle in her eyes, the smile on her face, and the laugh in her voice say it all. ◼

the drug, perhaps to cover the sadness and make me feel happy again . . . I love the excitement I felt with the drug . . . My focus is one-tracked . . . I need help but I don't know if I want it. (From America Online, Dewey CBS 1996)

Recovery from Cocaine Dependence Although numerous therapeutic approaches exist for treating cocaine addiction, successful recovery is not likely unless the individual is substantially benefited by giving up the drug. Research has shown that treatment is most likely to succeed in patients who are middle-class, employed, and married; for example, 85% of addicted medical professionals recover from cocaine addiction. These people can usually be convinced that they have too much to lose in their personal and professional lives by continuing their cocaine habit. In contrast, a severely dependent crack addict who has no job, family, home, or hope for the future isn't likely to be persuaded that abstinence from cocaine would be advantageous, so therapy usually is not successful (Grinspoon 1993).

Polydrug Use by Cocaine Abusers Treatment of most cocaine abusers is complicated by the fact that they are polydrug (multiple drug) users. It is unusual to find a person who only abuses cocaine. For example, it has been reported that 60% to 90% of cocaine abusers also use alcohol (Fischman and Johanson 1996). In general, the more severe the alcoholism, the greater the severity of the cocaine dependence. For most cases, alcoholism develops after the cocaine abuse pattern (Carrol et al. 1993) because the alcohol is used to relieve some of the unpleasant cocaine effects, such as anxiety, insomnia, and mood disturbances (Sands and Ciraulo 1992). This drug combination is a particularly dangerous one for several reasons:

1. The presence of both cocaine and alcohol (ethanol) in the liver results in the formation of a unique chemical product called *cocaethylene,* which is created in the reaction of ethanol with a cocaine metabolite. Cocaethylene is often found in high levels in the blood of victims of fatal drug overdoses and appears to enhance the euphoria as well as the cardiovascular toxicity of cocaine (Fischman and Johanson 1996).

2. Both cocaine and alcohol can damage the liver; thus their toxic effects on the liver are summed when the drugs are used in combination (Sands and Ciraulo 1992).

3. The likelihood of damaging a fetus is enhanced when both drugs are used together during pregnancy (Sands and Ciraulo 1992).

4. Cardiovascular stress is substantially enhanced in the presence of both drugs; thus, people with underlying coronary artery disease are 18 times more likely to suffer sudden death from cardiovascular factors when using this combination (Sands and Ciraulo 1992).

As with amphetamines, cocaine abusers also frequently coadminister narcotics, such as heroin; this combination is called a speedball and has been associated with an especially high risk for HIV infection (Mendelson and Mello 1996). Cocaine users often combine their drug with other depressants, such as benzodiazepines, or marijuana (Sands and Ciraulo 1992) to help reduce the severity of the crash after their cocaine binges. Codependence on cocaine and a CNS depressant can complicate treatment but must be considered.

Cocaine and Pregnancy One of the consequences of widespread cocaine abuse is that literally thousands of babies are born each year in the United States having been exposed to cocaine in the womb. Cocaine use during pregnancy is highest in poor, inner-city regions; estimates of its prevalence range from 3% to 50% according to the metropolitan area (Mayes 1992). It is likely that in the United States more than $1 billion is spent annually for maternal care of cocaine-using women during their pregnancies. The majority of these **cocaine babies** are abandoned by their mothers and left to the welfare system for care.

> **cocaine babies**
> children exposed to cocaine while in the womb

It is not clear exactly what types of direct effects cocaine has on the developing fetus. It is known that cocaine use during pregnancy can cause vasoconstriction of placental vessels, thus interfering with oxygen and nutrient exchange between mother and child, or contraction of the uterine muscles, resulting in trauma or premature birth. Current data also suggest that infants exposed to cocaine during pregnancy are more likely to suffer a small head (microencephaly), premature delivery, reduced birthweight (Coles et al. 1992), and increased irritability and subtle learning and cognitive deficits (Fischman and Johanson 1996). Some controversial early studies have suggested that cocaine use during pregnancy can also cause permanent malformation of the brain, strokes, SIDS (sudden infant death syndrome), permanent learning deficits, and behavioral disorders. However, these studies have been criticized because (1) the pregnant populations examined were not well defined and properly matched, (2) use of other drugs (such as alcohol) with cocaine during pregnancy was often ignored, and (3) the effects of poor nutrition, poor living conditions, and a traumatic lifestyle were not considered when analyzing the results. Due to these problems, much of the earlier work examining prenatal effects of cocaine is flawed and the conclusions are questionable (Grinspoon 1993; Fischman and Johanson 1996). Unfortunately, because of the dubious findings of these studies, the popular press has predicted a devastating long-term outcome for the

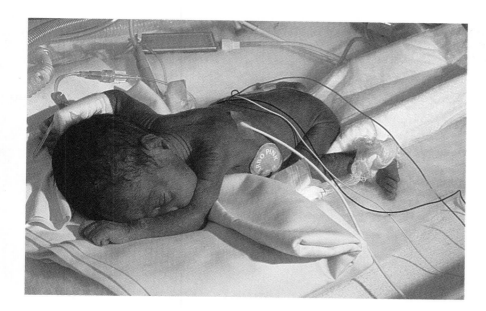

Infants born to crack-using mothers are often premature.

"cocaine babies" without reliable scientific proof. Consequently, these children are often difficult to place in adopting families. Because of this social rejection, the predictions of behavioral and social problems may come true for reasons unrelated to prenatal exposure to cocaine (Mathias 1992).

◢ Minor Stimulants

Minor stimulants enjoy widespread use in the United States because of the mild lift in mood provided by their consumption. The most popular of these routinely consumed agents are methylxanthines (commonly called *xanthines*), such as caffeine, which are consumed in beverages made from plants and herbs. Other minor stimulants are contained in OTC medications, such as cold and hay fever products; these will be mentioned briefly in this Chapter but discussed at greater length in Chapter 15. Because of their frequent use, some dependence on these drugs can occur; however, serious dysfunction due to dependence is infrequent. Consequently, abuse of xanthines such as caffeine is not viewed as a major health problem (Heishman and Henningfield 1992).

Caffeinlike Drugs (Xanthines) Caffeine is the world's most frequently used stimulant and perhaps its most popular drug (Heishman and Henningfield 1992). Beverages and foods containing caffeine are consumed by almost all adults and children living in the United States today (see Table 11.5). In this country, the average daily intake of caffeine is 4 milligrams/kilogram (280 milligrams per 70-kilogram man or the equivalent of approximately 3 cups of coffee), with 3% of the population consuming 600 milligrams or more per day (Heishman and Henningfield 1992). The most common sources of caffeine include coffee beans, tea plants, kola nuts, maté leaves, guaraná paste, and yoco bark.

Although the consumption of caffeine-containing drinks can be found throughout history, the active stimulant caffeine was discovered by German and French scientists in the early 1820s. Caffeine was described as a substance with alkaloid (basic) properties that was extracted from green coffee beans and referred to as *kaffebase* by Ferdinand Runge in 1820 (Gilbert 1984). In the course of the next 40 to 60 years, caffeine was identified in several other genera of plants, which were used as sources for common beverages. These included tea leaves (originally the drug was

Table 11.5 **Caffeine Content of Beverages and Chocolate**

Beverage	Caffeine Content (mg)/cup	Amount
Brewed coffee	90–125	5 oz
Instant coffee	35–164	5 oz
Decaffeinated coffee	1–6	5 oz
Tea	25–125	5 oz
Cocoa	5–25	5 oz
Coca-Cola	45	12 oz
Pepsi-Cola	38	12 oz
Mountain Dew	54	12 oz
Chocolate bar	1–35	1 oz.

called *thein*); guaraná paste (originally the drug was called *guaranin*); Paraguay tea, or maté; and kola nuts. Certainly, the popularity of these beverages over the centuries attests to the fact that most consumers find the stimulant effects of this drug desirable.

The Chemical Nature of Caffeine Caffeine belongs to a group of drugs that have similar chemical structures and are known as the **xanthines**. Besides caffeine, other xanthines are theobromine (means "divine leaf"), discovered in cacao beans (used to make chocolate) in 1842, and theophylline (means "divine food"), isolated from tea leaves in 1888. These three agents have unique pharmacological properties (which are discussed later), with caffeine being the most potent CNS stimulant.

xanthines

the family of drugs that include caffeine

Beverages Containing Caffeine To understand the unique role that caffeine plays in U.S. society, it is useful to gain perspective on its most common sources: unfermented beverages.

Coffee Coffee is derived from the beans of several species of *coffea* plants. The *coffea arabica* plant grows as a shrub or small tree and reaches 4 to 6 meters in height when growing wild. Coffee beans are primarily cultivated in South America and East Africa and constitute the major cash crop for exportation in several underdeveloped countries.

The name *coffee* was likely derived from the Arabian word *kahwa;* some argue it was named after the Ethiopian prince *Kaffa,* the suggested site of origin for the coffee tree. From Ethiopia, the coffee tree was carried to Arabia and cultivated (Kihlman 1977); it became an important element in Arrabial civilization and is mentioned in writings dating back to A.D. 900.

Coffee probably reached Europe through Turkey and was likely used initially as a medicine. By the middle of the seventeenth century, coffeehouses had sprung up in England and France- places to relax, talk, and learn the news. These coffeehouses turned into the famous "penny universities" of the early eighteenth century, where for a penny a cup, you could listen to some of the great literary and political figures of the day.

Coffee was originally consumed in the Americas by English colonists, although tea was initially preferred. Tea was replaced by coffee following the Revolutionary War. Because tea had become a symbol of English repression, the switch to coffee was more a political statement than a change in taste. The popularity of coffee grew as U.S. boundaries moved west. In fact, daily coffee use continued to increase until it peaked in 1986, when annual coffee consumption averaged 10 pounds per person. Although concerns about the side effects associated with caffeine use have since caused some decline in coffee consumption, this beverage still plays a major role in the lifestyles of most Americans (Sawynok and Yaksh 1993).

Tea Tea is made from the *Camellia sinensis* plant, which is native to China and parts of India, Burma, Thailand, Laos, and Vietnam. As mentioned, tea contains two xanthines: caffeine and theophylline. As with coffee, the earliest use of tea is not known.

Although apocryphal versions of the origin of tea credit Emperor Shen Nung in 2737 B.C., the first reliable account of the use of tea as a medicinal plant is from an early Chinese manuscript written around A.D. 350. The popular use of tea slowly grew. The Dutch brought the first tea to Europe in 1610, where it was accepted rather slowly; however, with time, it was adopted by the British as a favorite beverage and became an integral part of their daily activities. In fact, the tea trade constituted one of the major elements of the English economy. Tea revenues made it possible for England to colonize India and also helped to bring on the Opium Wars in the 1800s, which benefited British colonialism (see chapter 10).

The British were constantly at odds with the Dutch as they attempted to monopolize the tea trade. Even so, the Dutch introduced the first tea into America at New Amsterdam around 1650. Later, the British gained exclusive rights to sell tea to the American colonies. Because of the high taxes levied by the British government on tea being shipped to America, tea became a symbol of British rule.

Soft Drinks The second most common source of caffeine is soft drinks. In general, the caffeine content per 12-ounce serving ranges from 30 to 60 milligrams (see Table 11.5). Soft drinks account for most of the caffeine consumed by U.S. children and teenagers, and for many people, a can of cola has replaced the usual cup of coffee.

Social Consequences of Consuming Caffeine-Based Beverages It is impossible to accurately assess the social impact of consuming beverages containing caffeine, but certainly the subtle (and sometimes not so subtle) stimulant effects of the caffeine present in these drinks have had some social influence. These beverages have become integrated into social customs and ceremonies and recognized as traditional drinks.

Today, drinks containing caffeine are consumed by many people with ritualistic devotion the first thing in the morning, following every meal, and at frequent interludes throughout the day known as "coffee breaks" or "tea times." The immense popularity of these products is certainly a consequence of the stimulant actions of caffeine. Both the dependence on the "jump-start" effect of caffeine and the avoidance of unpleasant withdrawal consequences in the frequent user assure the continual popularity of these products.

These effects are illustrated by the following comments from college students (from Internet http://www.thejack.nau.edu/0913/lige2.html/,1996):

> Tina (freshman, psychology major): "I get headaches if I do not have my . . . Coca-Cola. The tension builds up in my head and I feel nauseous . . . As soon as I drink Coke, it goes away. I'm definitely addicted."

> Eric (senior, geology major): "I wake up and feel like I could fall asleep walking down the street. That's how I tell I need [coffee]."

> Jesse (senior, biology major): "I have worked at a coffeehouse for two years. I see customers come in dragging their feet . . . Once [customers] get it, though, they go 'Now I can get through my day.' Some people are more . . . on the edge if they don't get it [coffee]."

Other Natural Caffeine Sources Although coffee and tea are two of the most common sources of natural caffeine in the United States, other caffeine-containing beverages and food are popular in different parts of the world. Some of the most common include guaraná from Brazil, maté from Argentina, Southern Brazil, and Paraguay; and kola nuts from West Africa, West Indies, and South America (Kihlman 1977).

Chocolate Although chocolate contains small amounts of caffeine (see Table 11.5), the principal stimulant in chocolate is the alkaloid theobromine, named after the cocoa tree, *Theobroma cacao*. (*Theobroma* is an Aztec word meaning "fruit of the gods.") The Aztecs thought very highly of the fruit and seed pods from the cacoa tree, and they used the beans as a medium of exchange in bartering. The Mayan Indians adopted the food and made a warm drink from the beans that they called *chocolatl* (meaning "warm drink"). The original chocolate drink was a very thick concoction that had to be eaten with a spoon. It was unsweetened because the Mayans apparently did not know about sugar cane.

Hernando Cortés, the conqueror of Mexico, took some chocolate cakes back to Spain with him in 1528, but the method of preparing them remained a secret for nearly 100 years. It was not until 1828 that the Dutch worked out a process to remove much of the fat from the kernels to make a chocolate powder that was the forerunner of the cocoa we know today. The cocoa fat, or *cocoa butter* as it is called, was later mixed with sugar and pressed into bars. In 1847, the first chocolate bars appeared on the market. By 1876, the Swiss had developed milk chocolate, which is highly popular in today's confectionaires.

OTC Drugs Containing Caffeine Although the consumption of beverages is by far the most common source of xanthines, a number of popular OTC products contain significant quantities of caffeine. For example, many OTC analgesic products contain approximately 30 milligrams of caffeine per tablet (Anacin). Higher doses of 100 to 200 milligrams per tablet are included in stay-awake (No-Doz, Caffedrine) and "picker-upper" (Vivarin) products (PDR 1997). The addition of caffeine to these OTC medications is highly controversial and has been criticized by clinicians who are unconvinced of caffeine's benefits. Some critics believe that the presence of caffeine in these OTC medicines is nothing more than a psychological gimmick to entice customers through mild euphoric effects provided by this stimulant.

Despite this criticism, accumulating evidence indicates that caffeine has some analgesic (pain-relieving) properties of its own (Sawynok and Yaksh 1993). Recent studies suggest that 130 milligrams, but not 65 milligrams, of caffeine is superior to a placebo in relieving nonmigraine headaches. In addition, the presence of caffeine has been shown to enhance aspirin-medicated relief from surgical pain (such as tooth extraction). Based on such findings, more clinicians are recommending the use of caffeine in the management of some types of headaches and minor to moderate pains (Sawynok and Yaksh 1993).

Physiological Effects of the Xanthines The xanthines significantly influence several important body functions. Although the effects of these drugs are generally viewed as minor and short-term (Goldstein 1994), when used in high doses or by people who have severe medical problems, these drugs can be dangerous. The following sections summarize the responses of the major systems to xanthines.

CNS Effects Among the common xanthines, caffeine has the most potent effect on the CNS, followed by theophylline; theobromine has relatively little influence. Although the CNS responses of users can vary considerably, in general, 100 to 200 milligrams of caffeine enhances alertness, causes arousal, and diminishes fatigue (Heishman and Hennington 1992). Caffeine is often used to block drowsiness and facilitate mental activity, such as when cramming for exams into the early hours of the morning. In addition, caffeine stimulates the formation of thoughts but does not improve learning ability in the wide-awake student. The effects of caffeine are most pronounced in unstimulated, drowsy consumers (Goldstein 1994). The CNS effects of caffeine also diminish the sense of boredom (Nehlig et al. 1992). Thus, people engaged in dull, repetitive tasks, such as assembly-line work, or nonstimulating and laborious exercises, such as listening to a boring professor, often consume caffeine beverages to help compensate for the tedium. Most certainly, xanthine drinks are popular because they cause these effects on brain activity.

Adverse CNS effects usually occur with doses greater than 300 milligrams per day. Some of these include insomnia, an increase in tension, anxiety, and initiation of muscle twitches. Doses over 500 milligrams can be dysphoric (unpleasant) and can cause panic sensations, chills, nausea, and clumsiness. Extremely high doses of caffeine, from 5 to 10 grams, frequently result in seizures, respiratory failure, and death (Heishman and Henningfield 1992).

Cardiovascular and Respiratory Effects Drugs that stimulate the brain usually stimulate the cardiovascular system as well. The response of the heart and blood vessels to xanthines is dependent on dose and previous experience with these mild stimulants. Tolerance to the cardiovascular effects occurs with frequent use (Heishman and Hennington 1992). With low doses (100 to 200 milligrams), heart activity can either increase, decrease, or do nothing; at higher doses (over 500 milligrams), the rate of contraction of the heart increases. Xanthines usually cause minor vasodilation in most of the body. In contrast, the cerebral blood vessels are vasoconstricted by the action of caffeine. In fact, cerebral vasoconstriction likely accounts for this drug's effectiveness in relieving some minor vascular headaches caused by vasodilation of the cerebral vessels.

Among the xanthines, theophylline has the greatest effect on the respiratory system, causing air passages to open and facilitate breathing. Because of this effect, tea has often been recommended to relieve breathing difficulties, and theophylline is frequently used to treat asthma-related respiratory problems.

Other Effects The methylxanthines have noteworthy, albeit mild, effects on other systems in the body. They cause a minor increase in the secretion of digestive juices in the stomach, which can be significant to individuals suffering from stomach ailments such as ulcers. These drugs also increase urine formation (as any heavy tea drinker undoubtedly knows).

Caffeine Intoxication Consuming occasional low doses of the xanthines (equivalent of two to three cups of coffee per day) is relatively safe for most users (Heishman and Hennington 1992; Margen 1994). However, frequent use of high doses causes psychological as

caffeinism
symptoms caused by taking high chronic doses of caffeine

well as physical problems called **caffeinism.** This condition is found in about 10% of the adults who consume coffee (Heishman and Hennington 1992).

The CNS components of caffeine intoxication are recognized as a "psychoactive substance-induced psychiatric disorder" in *DSM-IV* (American Psychiatric Association 1994) criteria established by the American Psychiatric Association. The essential features of this disorder are restlessness, nervousness, excitement, insomnia, flushed face, diuresis, muscle twitching, rambling thoughts and speech, and stomach complaints. These symptoms can occur in some people following a dose as low as 250 milligrams per day. Caffeine doses in excess of 1 gram per day may cause muscle twitching, rambling thoughts and speech, heart arrhythmias, and motor agitation. With higher doses, ringing in the ears and flashes of light can occur.

Some researchers suggest consuming large quantities of caffeine is associated with cancers of the bladder, ovaries, colon, and kidneys. These claims have not been reliably substantiated (Margen 1994; Gurin 1994).

One problem with many such studies is that they assess the effect of coffee consumption on cancers rather than the effect of caffeine itself. Because coffee contains so many different chemicals, it is impossible to determine specifically the effect of caffeine in such research (Gurin 1994). Other reports claim that caffeine promotes cyst formation in female breasts. Although these conclusions also have been challenged, many clinicians advise patients with mammilary cysts to avoid caffeine (Margen 1994). Finally, some reports indicate that very high doses of caffeine given to pregnant laboratory animals can cause stillbirths or offspring with low birthweights or limb deformities. Recent studies found that moderate consumption of caffeine (less than 300 milligrams per day) did not significantly affect human fetal development (Mills 1993); however, intake of more than 300 milligrams per day during pregnancy has been associated with an increase in spontaneous fetal loss (*Facts and Comparisons Drug Newsletter* 1994). Mothers are usually advised to avoid or at least reduce caffeine use during pregnancy (Margen 1994).

Table 11.6   Caffeine Withdrawal Syndrome

Symptom	Duration
Headache	Several days to 1 week
Decreased alertness	2 days
Decreased vigor	2 days
Fatigue and lethargy	2 days
Nervousness	2 days

Source: Based on S. Holtzman. "Caffeine as a Model Drug of Abuse." *Trends in Pharmacological Sciences* 11 (1990): 355-6.

Based on the information available, no strong evidence exists to suggest that moderate use of caffeine leads to disease (Margen 1994). There are, however, implications that people with existing severe medical problems-such as psychiatric disorders (such as severe anxiety, panic attacks, and schizophrenia), cardiovascular disease, and possibly breast cysts-are at greater risk when consuming caffeine. Realistically, other elements-such as alcohol and fat consumption and smoking-are much more likely to cause serious health problems (Gurin 1994).

Caffeine Dependence Caffeine causes limited dependence, which is relatively minor compared with that of the potent stimulants; thus, the abuse potential of caffeine is also much lower and dependence is less likely to interfere with normal daily routines (Heishman and Henningfield 1992). However, caffeine is so readily available and socially accepted (almost expected) that the high quantity of consumption has produced many modestly dependent users (Holtzman 1990). The degree of physical dependence on caffeine is highly variable, but related to dose, and is also considerably lower than that with the major stimulants. A recent study reported that caffeine doses as low as 100 milligrams per day can cause significant withdrawal effects, such as headaches, fatigue, mood changes, muscle pain, flulike symptoms, and nausea in some people (Holtzman 1990).

With typical caffeine withdrawal, these effects can persist for several days (see Table 11.6). Although these symptoms are unpleasant, they usually are not severe enough to prevent most people from giving up their coffee or cola drinks, if desired. It is noteworthy that two-thirds of those patients who are treated for caffeinism relapse into their caffeine-consuming habits (Heishman and Henningfield 1992).

Variability in Responses Caffeine is eventually absorbed entirely from the gastrointestinal tract after oral consumption. In most users, 90% of the drug reaches the bloodstream within 20 minutes and is distributed into the brain and throughout the body very quickly (Sawynok and Yaksh 1993). The rate of absorption of caffeine from the stomach and intestines differs from person to person by as much as sixfold. Such wide variations in the rate at which caffeine enters the blood from the stomach likely account for much of the variability in responses to this drug (Nehlig et al. 1992).

OTC Sympathomimetics

Although often overlooked, the sympathomimetic decongestant drugs included in OTC products such as cold, allergy, and diet aid medications have stimulant properties like those of caffeine (Appelt 1993). For most people, the CNS impact of these drugs is minor, but for those people who are very sensitive to these drugs, they can cause jitters and interfere with sleep. For such individuals, OTC products containing the sympathomimetics should be avoided prior to bedtime.

The common OTC sympathomimetics are shown in Table 11.7 and include ephedrine and phenylpropanolamine. In the past, these two OTC agents were packaged to look like amphetamines (called "look-alike drugs") and legally sold on the "street," usually to children or high school students. Although much less potent than amphetamines (though they can be used as precursor chemicals to make methamphetamine), these minor stimulants can be abused and have caused deaths. Attempts to regulate look-alike drugs re-

| Table 11.7 | Common OTC Sympathomimetics |

Drug	OTC Product (form)
Phenylpropanolamine	Decongestant, diet aid (oral)
Ephedrine	Decongestant (oral, nasal spray or drops)
Levodesoxyephedrine	Decongestant (nasal inhalant)
Naphazoline	Decongestant (nasal spray or drops)
Oxymetazoline	Decongestant (nasal spray or drops)
Phenylephrine	Decongestant (oral, nasal spray or drops, eye drops)
Psuedoephedrine	Decongestant (oral)
Tetrahydozoline	Decongestant (eye drops)
Xylometazoline	Decongestant (nasal spray or drops)

Source: Based on B. Bryant and T. Lombardi. "Cold and Allergy Products." In *Handbook of Nonprescription Drugs,* 10th ed., edited by T. Covington. Washington, DC: American Pharmaceutical Association, 1993.

sulted in passage of the federal and state Imitation Controlled Substances Acts. These statutes prohibit the packaging of OTC sympathomimetics to appear like amphetamines.

These laws have not resolved the problem, however. Other products called "act-alikes" have been created. Although the packaging of the act-alike does not resemble that of amphetamine capsules, these minor stimulants are promoted on the street as "harmless speed" and "OTC uppers." It is likely that use of such products will lead to the abuse of more potent stimulants (Brown 1991).

Herbal Stimulants

Some OTC sympathomimetics are also found in herbal stimulants sold by mail and in novelty stores, beauty salons, and health food stores (Lane 1996). These pills are sold under names such as "Cloud 9," "Ultimate Xphoria, "Herbal Ecstasy," and contain stimulants such as ephedrine, ephedra, or ma huang (*Pharmacy Times* 1996). These products are particularly promoted to high school and college students as *natural highs* to be used as diet aids or energy boosters. Excessive use of these products can cause seizures, heart attacks, and strokes (see "Finding a Balance," page 284). In fact, more than 15 deaths and 400 cases of severe reactions have been reported in the United States from excessive use of these products (*Pharmacy Times* 1996). The FDA recently issued a warning about the dangers of these products, but has not been able to remove herbal stimulants from the market because of a 1994 federal law that prohibits such action until the FDA conclusively proves the dangers of these substances (*Pharmacy Times* 1996). Even though federal agencies are barred from action, states such of Ohio and Texas have successfully restricted the marketing of ephedrine-containing pills (Lane 1996).

Herbal Ecstasy and Natural Problems

The heart is considered to be the most important organ in the body, and not just because it pumps blood to every cell tissue. The heart is deemed significant because of its symbolic meaning as well. It represents the core of our existence. The heart signifies both love and courage. In fact, the word *courage* means "big heart." When anything goes wrong with the heart, we feel it physically, emotionally, and spiritually. Changes in feelings are not uncommon with drug use; it is one reason why they are taken-to alter feelings, enhance mood, and reach a state of ecstasy.

Ecstasy. The word brings thoughts and feelings of euphoria and bliss. It used to bring those thoughts to Johnny but not anymore. Johnny was a cautious drug user, or so he thought. Reading up on the drug Ecstasy, he opted for the herbal choice. This way, he thought, he couldn't lose.

> I was told it was safe. I wanted a good experience. I had friends who took the regular stuff and it was laced with heroin. That's not for me. So I got some herbal Ecstasy and, boom, I was in heaven. Every cell in my body was alive and in pleasure.

Herbal Ecstasy contains large concentrations of caffeine, ephedra, and other stimulants, enough to send the nervous and hormonal systems out of balance. This sense of being on the edge explains much of its appeal. Johnny's first experience was titillating. So much so, in fact, that he had to do it again. But this time the dynamics changed. Something was different. Within minutes of ingesting his stash, Johnny felt the same rush as with his first time, but it came with an incredible pain in his chest. A friend who was with him jokingly said, "Don't worry, you're having a heart attack." It was no joke. The rapid succession of ventricular contractions peaked at a tumultuous level, then stopped. Johnny laid on the floor virtually unconscious. At the age of 23, he almost became one more statistic. Rushed to the hospital emergency room, his heart attack proved to be less than fatal.

Mindy Green is a research assistant at the Herb Research Center (HRC) in Boulder, Colorado. She and her colleagues field phone calls (approximately 60,000 per year) on a host of topics relating to the use of herbs. Cases like Johnny's that make the news send a flood of phone calls to the HRC office about the use of herbal Ecstasy.

"It's a tragic situation. Several deaths have been attributed to herbal Ecstasy," Mindy explains. "It's unfortunate that these kids are being told this is a safe alternative to street drugs. My belief is the responsible use of herbs does not include recreational use of them."

The experience has made Johnny sad, ambivalent, and a bit scared. The damage to his heart will remain for life, a condition that he is now slowly learning to accept. Acceptance is a process, as Johnny has learned. In describing his feelings about the experience, he recites the serenity prayer: "God, give me the serenity to accept the things I cannot change, the courage to change the things I can, and the wisdom to know the difference." ∎

REVIEW QUESTIONS

1. Should the FDA continue to approve amphetamines for the treatment of obesity? Why?

2. How are methamphetamine and Ecstasy similar, and how do they differ?

3. What are the dangers of designer drugs in general, and of designer amphetamines in particular?

4. What have past experiences taught us about cocaine? Do you think we have finally learned our lesson concerning this drug?

5. Why does the method of cocaine administration make a difference in how a user is affected

EXERCISES FOR THE WEB

Exercise 1: Cocaine

Cocaine Anonymous is a fellowship of men and women who share their experience, strength and hope with each other so that they may solve their common problem and help others to recover from their addiction. The only requirement for membership is a desire to stop using cocaine and all other mind-altering substances. There are no dues or fees for membership; the organization is fully self-supported through contributions. CA is not allied with any sect, denomination, political party, organization, or institution. They do not wish to engage in any controversy, and they neither endorse nor oppose any causes. This fellowship's primary purpose is to stay free from cocaine and all other mind-altering substances, and to help others achieve the same freedom.

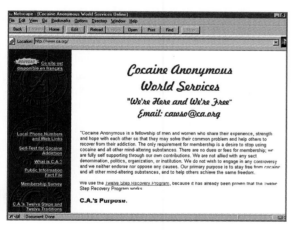

Exercise 2: Inhalants

Inhalant use among youth has risen dramatically over the past 10 years. The Wisconsin Prevention Resource Center provides information on alcohol and other drug use. This article, entitled "Prevention Strategies to Reduce Inhalant Use and Abuse" offers a detailed perspective on how to reduce inhalant use.

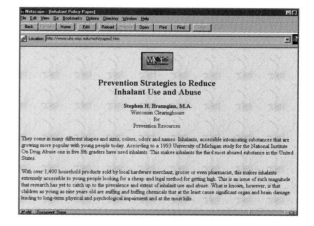

---

by this drug? Use examples to substantiate your conclusions.

6. Why do people use crack cocaine, and what are the major toxicities caused by use of high doses of this stimulant?

7. How is cocaine dependence treated? What are the rationales for the treatments?

8. How does caffeine compare with cocaine and amphetamine as a CNS stimulant?

9. Because of caffeine's potential for abuse, do you think the FDA should control it more tightly? Defend your answer.

10. Do you feel that herbal stimulants should be available OTC? Explain your answer.

KEY TERMS

"uppers"
anorexiants
behavioral stereotypy
narcolepsy
hyperpyrexia
speed
precursor chemicals
ice
run
speedball
hyperkinesis
adulterated
freebasing
crack
crack babies
cocaine babies
xanthines
caffeinism

SUMMARY

1 Amphetamines, originally developed as decongestants, are potent stimulants. Some amphetamines have been approved by the FDA (a) as diet aids to treat obesity, (b) treatment for narcolepsy, and (c) treatment for hyperkinetic problems (attention deficit disorder) in children.

2 In therapeutic doses, amphetamines can cause agitation, anxiety, and panic due to their effects on the brain; in addition, they can cause an irregular heartbeat, increased blood pressure, and heart attack or stroke. Intense, high-dose abuse of these drugs can cause severe psychotic behavior, stereotypy, and seizures as well as the severe cardiovascular side effects just mentioned.

3 *Speed* refers to the use of intravenous methamphetamine. *Ice* is smoked methamphetamine. A *run* is a pattern of intense, multiple dosing over a period of days that can cause serious neurological, psychiatric, and cardiovascular consequences.

4 "Designer" amphetamines are chemical modifications of original amphetamines. Some designer amphetamines, such as "Ecstasy," retain abuse potential and are often marketed "on the street" under exotic and alluring names.

5 In the late 1970s and early 1980s, cocaine was commonly viewed by the U.S. public as a relatively safe drug with glamorous connotations. By the mid-1980s, however, it was apparent that cocaine was a very addicting drug with dangerous side effects.

6 The CNS and cardiovascular effects of both amphetamines and cocaine are similar. However, cocaine's effects tend to occur more rapidly, be more intense, and wear off more quickly than those of amphetamines.

7 The intensity of the cocaine effect and the likelihood of dependence occurring are directly related to the means of administration. Going from least to most intense effect, the modes of cocaine administration include chewing, "snorting," injecting, and smoking (or "freebasing").

8 "Crack" is cocaine that has been converted into its "freebase" form and is intended for smoking.

9 Cocaine withdrawal goes through three main stages: (a) the "crash," the initial abstinence phase consisting of depression, agitation, suicidal thoughts, and fatigue; (b) withdrawal, including mood swings, craving, anhedonia, and obsession with drug seeking; and (c) extinction, when normal pleasure returns and cues trigger craving and mood swings.

10 Treatment of cocaine dependence is highly individualistic and has variable success. The principal strategies include both inpatient and outpatient programs. Drug therapy often is used to relieve short-term cocaine craving and to alleviate mood problems and long-term craving. Psychological counseling and support therapy are essential components of treatment.

11 Caffeine is the most frequently consumed stimulant in the world. It is classified as a xanthine (methylxanthine) and is found in a number of beverages. It is also included in some OTC medicines such as analgesics and "stay-awake" products. Caffeine causes minor stimulation of cardiovascular activity, kidney function (it is a diuretic), and gastric secretion.

12 Dependence on caffeine can occur in people who regularly consume large doses. Withdrawal can cause headaches, agitation, and tremors. Although unpleasant, withdrawal from caffeine dependence is much less severe than that from amphetamine and cocaine dependence.

REFERENCES

Aldrich, M., and R. Barker. *Cocaine: Chemical, Biological, Social and Treatment Aspects,* edited by S. J. Mule. Cleveland, OH: CRC, 1976: 3–10.

American Psychiatric Association. "Substance-Related Disorders." In *Diagnostic and Statistical Manual,* 4th ed. *[DSM-IV],* A. Francis, chairperson, 175–272. Washington, DC: American Psychiatric Association, 1994.

Appelt, G. "Weight Control Products." In *Handbook of Nonprescription Drugs,* 10th ed., edited by T. Covington, 339–49. Washington, DC: American Pharmaceutical Association, 1993.

Associated Press, "Colombia Closes Narcotic Labs." *Boston Globe* (July 6, 1996): 6.

Beck, J. "The Public Health Implications of MDMA Use." In *Ecstacy,* edited by S. Peroutka, 77–103. Norwell, MA: Kluwar, 1990.

Benowitz, N. "How Toxic Is Cocaine?" In *1992 Cocaine: Scientific and Social Dimensions,* edited by Ciba, 125–48. Ciba Foundation Symposium 166. New York: Wiley, 1992.

Boucher, D. "Cocaine and the Coca Plant." *BioScience* 41 (1991): 72–6.

Brookoff, D., E. Campbell, and L. Shaw. "The Underreporting of Cocaine-Related Trauma." *American Journal of Public Health* 83 (1993): 369–71.

Brown, E., J. Prager, H. Lee, and R. Ramsey. "CNS Complications of Cocaine Abuse: Prevalence, Pathophysiology, and Neuroradiology. *American Journal of Radiology* 159 (July 1992): 137–47.

Brown, M. *Guide to Fight Substance Abuse.* Nashville, TN: International Broadcast Services, 1991.

Bryant, B., and T. Lombardi. "Cold and Allergy Products." In *Handbook of Nonprescription Drugs,* 10th ed., edited by T. Covington. Washington, DC: American Pharmaceutical Association, 1993: 89–115.

Byck, R. "Cocaine Use and Research: Three Histories." In *Cocaine: Chemical and Behavioral Aspects,* edited by S. Fisher, London: Oxford University Press, 1987: 3–17.

Carroll, K., B. Rounsaville, and K. Bryant. "Alcoholism in Treatment-Seeking Cocaine Abusers: Clinical and Prognostic Significance." *Journal in Studies of Alcohol 54* (1993): 199–208.

Carroll, K., B. Rounsaville, L. Gordon, C. Nich, P. Jatlow, R. Bisighini, and F. Gawin. "Psychotherapy and Pharmacotherapy for Ambulatory Cocaine Abusers." *Archives of General Psychiatry* 51 (1994): 177–87.

Chavez, N. "Methamphetamine Abuse Increases." *SAMSHA News* 4 (Winter/Spring, 1996): 29.

Coles, C., K. Platzman, I. Smith, M. James, and A. Falek. "Effects of Cocaine and Alcohol Use in Pregnancy on Neonatal Growth and Neurobehavioral Status." *Neurotoxicology and Teratology* 14 (1992): 22–33.

Des Jarlais. "AIDS and HIV Infections in Cocaine Users." In *Cocaine: Scientific and Social Dimensions,* edited by Ciba, 181–95. Ciba Foundations Symposium 166. New York: Wiley, 1992.

DiChiara, G. "Cocaine: Scientific and Social Dimensions. *Trends in Neurological Sciences* 16 (1993): 39.

Ehrman, J. "Cocaine Heightens Risk for Suicides." *ADAMHA News* 18 (May–June 1992): 17.

Facts and Comparisons Drug Newsletter. "Fetal Loss Associated with Caffeine." 13 (March 1994): 22.

Fischman, M., and R. Foltin. "Self-Administration of Cocaine by Humans: A Laboratory Perspective." In *Cocaine: Scientific and Social Dimensions,* edited by Ciba, 165–80. New York: Wiley, 1992.

Fischman, M., and C. Johanson. "Cocaine." In *Pharmacological Aspects of Drug Dependence: Towards an Integrated Neurobehavior. Approach Handbook of Experimental Pharmacology.* 159–195. edited by C. Schuster and M. Kuhar. 1996.

Flaum, M. and S. Schultz,, "When Does Amphetamine-Induced Psychosis Become Schizophrenia." *American Psychiatry* 153 (1996): 812–15.

Galanter, M., S. Egelko, G. DeLeon, C. Rohrs, and H. Franco. "Crack/Cocaine Abusers in the General Hospital: Assessment and Initiation of Care. *American Journal of Psychiatry* 149 (1992): 810–5.

Gawin, F. "Cocaine Addiction: Psychology and Neurophysiology." *Science* 251 (1991): 1580–6.

Gawin, F., and H. Kleber. "Evolving Conceptualizations of Cocaine Dependence." *Yale Journal of Biology and Medicine* 61 (1988): 123–36.

Gilbert, R. "Caffeine Consumption." In *The Methylxanthine Beverages and Foods: Chemistry, Consumption, and Health Effects.* New York: Liss, 1984.

Golding, A. "Two Hundred Years of Drug Abuse." *Journal of the Royal Society of Medicine* 86 (May 1993): 282–6.

Goldstein, A., In *Addiction from Biology to Drug Abuse,* 179–89. New York: Freeman 1994.

Goldstein, F. "Pharmacological Aspects of Substance Abuse." In *Remington's Pharmaceutical Sciences,* 19th ed., edited by A. R. Genaro. Easton, PA: Mack, 1995: 780–794.

Green, E. "Cocaine, Glamorous Status Symbol of the 'Jet Set,' Is Fast Becoming Many Students' Drug of Choice." *Chronicle of Higher Education* 13 (November 1985): 1, 34.

Greenhouse, C. "Designer Drugs at a Glance." *NIDA Notes* 7 (January–February 1992): 20–2.

Grinspoon, L. "Update on Cocaine." Parts 1 & 2. *Harvard Mental Health Letter* 10 (August–September 1993): 1–4.

Grinspoon, L., and J. Bakalar. "The Amphetamines: Medical Use and Health Hazards." In *Amphetamines Use, Misuse and Abuse,* edited by D. Smith. Boston, MA: Hall, 1978: 18–33.

Grob, C., R. Poland, L. Chang, and T. Ernst. "Psychobiological Effects of 3.4-Methylenedioxymethamphetamine in Humans: Methodological Considerations and Preliminary Observations." *Behavioral Brain Research* 73 (1996): 103–7.

Gurin, J. "Coffee and Health." *Consumer Reports* (October 1994): 650–1.

Gygi, M., S. Gygi, M. Johnson, D. Wilkins, J. Gibb, and G. R. Hanson. "Mechanisms for Tolerance to Methamphetamine Effects." *Neuropharmacology* 35 (1996): 751–757.

Hall, W., and J. Hando. "Illicit Amphetamine Use Is a Public Health Problem in Australia." *Medical Journal of Australia* 159 (1993): 643–4.

Haven, P. "Cocaine Still Colombia's Most Lucrative Cash Crop." *Salt Lake Tribune* 251 (March 24, 1996): A8.

Heishman, S., and J. Henningfield. "Stimulus Functions of Caffeine in Humans: Relation to Dependence Potential." *Neuroscience and Behavior* Review 16 (1992): 273–87.

Hinkle, J., and S. Winckler. "Vitamin R: The Expansion of Ritalin Abuse." *PRN (Pharmacy Recovery Network) A PhA* 4 (April–June, 1996): 1.

Hoffman, B., and R. Lefkowitz. "Catecholamines, Sympathomimetics Drugs, and Adrenergic Receptor Antagonists." In *The Pharmacological Basis of Therapeutics.* 9th ed., edited by J. Hardman and L. Limbird, 199–248. New York: McGraw-Hill 1995).

Holtzman, S. "Caffeine as a Model Drug of Abuse." *Trends in Pharmacological Sciences* 11 (1990): 355–6.

Hudgins, R., J. McCusker, and A. Stoddard. "Cocaine Use and Risky Injection and Sexual Behaviors." *Drug and Alcohol Dependence* 37 (1995): 7–14.

Irvine, G., and L. Chin. "The Environmental Impact and Adverse Health Effects of the Clandestine Manufacture of Methamphetamine." In *Methamphetamine Abuse: Epidemiologic Issues and Implications,* 33–42. NIDA Research Monograph Series 15. Washington, DC: U.S. Government Printing Office, 1991.

. "Drug Addiction and Drug Abuse." In *The Pharmacologic Basis of Therapeutics,* 8th ed., edited by A. Gilman, T. Rall, A. Nies, and P. Taylor, 522–73. New York: Pergamon, 1990.

Johnson, K. "Feds Draw a Battle-line on Drugs, Methamphetamine Use Spreads East to Midwest." *USA Today* (27 September 1996): 3A.

Johnston, L. *University of Michigan Annual National Surveys of Secondary Students.* Lansing: University of Michigan, 1996. Available from author at 412 Maynard, Ann Arbor, MI.

Johnston, L. *Univeristy of Michigan Annual National Surveys of Secondary Students.* Lansing: University of Michigan, 1994. Available from author at 412 Maynard Ave., Ann Arbor, MI.

Kihlman, B. *Caffeine and Chromosomes.* Amsterdam: Elsevier, 1977.

Kleber, H. "Treatment of Cocaine Abuse: Pharmacotherapy." In *Cocaine Scientific and Social Dimensions,* edited by Ciba, 195–206. Ciba Foundation Symposium 166. New York: Wiley, 1992.

Knight-Ridder News Service. "Experts Call War on Drugs a $32 Billion Stalemate." *Salt Lake Tribune* 244 (21 September 1992): A-2.

Lane, E. "On 'Cloud 9'? Loose Regulation of Ephedrine Raises Some Questions." *Ogden Standard-Examiner* (April 21, 1996): 5E.

Leshner, A. "Molecular Mechanisms of Cocaine Addiction." *New England Journal of Medicine.* 335 (1996): 128–9.

Lillie-Blanton, M., J. Anthony, and C. Schuster. "Probing the Meaning of Racial/Ethnic Group Comparisons in Crack Cocaine Smoking." *Journal of the American Medical Association* 269 (1993): 993–7.

Margen, S. "Caffeine: Grounds for Concern." *U.C. Berkeley Wellness Letter* 10 (March 1994): 4.

Mathias, R. 'Crack Babies' Not a Lost Generation, Researchers Say." *NIDA Notes* 7 (January–February 1992): 16.

Max, B. "This and That: The Ethnopharmacology of Simple Phenethylamines and the Questions of Cocaine and the Human Heart." *Trends in Pharmacological Sciences* 12 (1991): 329–33.

Mayes, L., R. Granger, M. Bornstein, and B. Zucker. "The Problem of Prenatal Cocaine Exposure." *Journal of the American Medical Association* 15 (1992): 406–8.

Medical Letter. "Acute Reaction to Drugs of Abuse." 38 (1996): 43.

Mendelson, J. and N. Mello. "Management of Cocaine Abuse and Dependence." *New England Journal of Medicine* 334 (1996): 965–72.

Miller, M., and N. Kozel. "Introduction and Overview." In *Methamphetamine Abuse: Epidemiologic Issues and Implications,* 1–5. NIDA Research Monograph Series 115.

Washington, DC: U.S. Government Printing Office, 1991.

Mills, J., et al. "Moderate Caffeine Use and the Risk of Spontaneous Abortion and Intrauterine Growth Retardation." *Journal of the American Medical Association* 269 (1993): 593–602.

National Institute on Drug Abuse (NIDA). "The Facts About Cocaine Abuse and Treatment." *NIDA Notes* (September/October 1995)

Nehlig, A., J. Daval, and G. Debry. "Caffeine and the Central Nervous System: Mechanisms of Action, Biochemical, Metabolic and Psychostimulant Effects." *Brain Research Review* 17 (1992): 139–70.

Pagliaro, L., L. Jaglalsingh, and A. Pagliaro. "Cocaine Use and Depression." *Canadian Medical Association Journal* 147 (1992): 1636.

Pharmacy Times, "New York County Bans Herbal Stimulants.: 62 (1996): 8.

Physicians' Desk Reference, Medical Economics, Montvale, NJ, 51 edition (1997).

Randall, T. "Ecstasy-Fueled 'Rave' Parties Become Dances of Death for English Youths." 268 (1992a): 1505–6.

Randall, T. "Rave' Scene, Ecstasy Use, Leap Atlantic." *Journal of the American Medical Association* 268 (1992b): 1506.

Reno, J. (U.S. Attorney General). "National Methamphetamine Strategy" (message to the President of the United States). U.S. Department of Justice, Office of the Attorney General (April 1996).

Sands, B., and D. Ciraulo. "Cocaine Drug-Drug Interactions." *Journal of Clinical Psychopharmacology* 12 (1992): 49–55.

Sato, M. "A Lasting Vulnerability to Psychosis in Patients with Previous Methamphetamine Psychosis." *The Neurobiology of Drug and Alcohol Addiction. Annals of the New York Academy of Sciences* 654–28 June 1992): 160–70.

Sawynok, J., and T. Yaksh. "Caffeine as an Analgesic Adjuvant: A Review of Pharmacology and Mechanisms of Action." *Pharmacological Reviews* 45 (1993): 43–85.

Schwartz, R. "New Meth Law Protects OTC Market." *American Druggist* 213 (November 1996): 18.

Schwartz, R. M. Lyenberg, and N. Hoffman. "Crack Use by American Middle-Class Adolescent Polydrug Users." *Journal of Pediatrics* 118 (1991): 150–5.

Seibyl, J., L. Brenner, J. Drystal, R. Johnson, and D. Charney. "Mazindol and Cocaine Addiction in Schizophrenia." *Biological Psychiatry* 31 (1992): 1172–83.

Shifano, F., and G. Magni. "MCMA (Ecstasy) Abuse: Psychopathological Features and Craving for Chocolate: A Case Series." *Biological Psychiatry* 3 (1996): 763–767.

Seigel, R. K. "Treatment of Cocaine Abuse." *Journal of Psychoactive Drugs* 17 (1985): 52.

Swan, N. "31% of New York Murder Victims Had Cocaine in their Bodies." *NIDA Notes* 10 (March/April 1995): 4.

Taylor, J. "All-New MDMA FAQ." Internet (computer networking service), Usenet News, sci.med.pharmacy (27 May 1994).

Van Dyck, C., and R. Byck. "Cocaine." *Scientific American* 246 (1982): 128–41.

Woolverton, W., and K. Johnston. "Neurobiology of Cocaine Abuse." *Trends in Pharmacological Sciences* 13 (1992): 193–200.

12 Tobacco

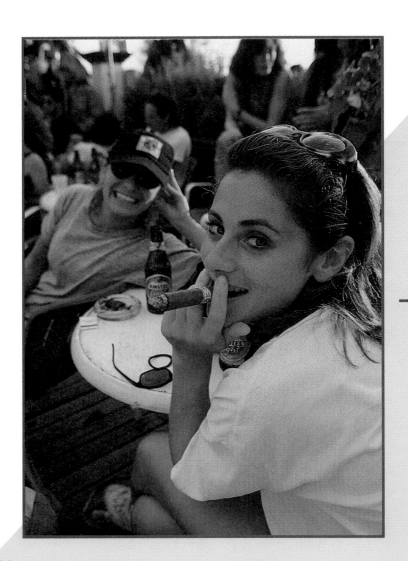

**On completing this chapter
you will be able to:** ▶

- Approximately 29% of the U.S. population age 12 and older smokes.
- In the United States, nicotine dependency resulting from cigarette smoking is the most common form of drug addiction. Addiction to nicotine causes more deaths and disease than all other addictions to licit and illicit drugs.
- Tar and nicotine levels in cigarettes have dropped considerably over the last 40 years.
- Native Americans used tobacco in every manner: smoked as cigars, cigarettes (wrapped in corn husks), and pipes; as a syrup to be swallowed or applied to the gums; chewed and snuffed; and administered rectally as a ceremonial enema.
- Tobacco inspired the first major drug controversy of global dimensions.
- In the 1600s, Turkey, Russia, and China imposed death penalties for smoking.
- People aged 26 to 34 have the highest rates of smoking.
- As educational levels increase, men are increasingly more likely to quit smoking than are women.
- Tobacco farming is the sixth largest legal cash crop in the United States.
- The manufacturing cost for cigarettes (not counting the tobacco) is approximately three cents a pack.
- Since the first Surgeon General's report on smoking and health in 1964, nearly 10 million people in the United States have died from causes attributable to smoking.
- Research indicates that a connection exists between *prenatal* nicotine exposure and smoking in later life.
- The Camel cartoon character, Joe Camel, was as recognizable to 6-year-olds as the Mickey Mouse silhouette that denotes the Walt Disney Company.

Learning Objectives

- Assess the addictiveness of nicotine.
- Specify the percentage and number of people who smoke in the United States.
- Explain how the quality of leaf tobacco has changed since the mid-1950s.
- Describe the effect of nicotine on the nervous system.
- List five ways in which tobacco is absorbed.
- Specify three ways that cigarette smoking is a costly addiction.
- Identify the two types of smokeless tobacco products.
- Explain how cigarettes are responsible for chronic illnesses.
- Define the terms *mainstream smoke, sidestream smoke, passive smoking,* and *environmental tobacco smoke.*
- Give the approximate percentage of adolescents in the United States who have tried smoking.
- List the main methods for quitting smoking.
- Explain the association between cigarette smoking and the use of illicit drugs and alcohol.
- List the four primary aspects of tobacco control laws at the state level.

I'm 43 years old and have smoked cigarettes most of my life. I began around age 11, sneaking cigarettes with my friends. I tried to quit and actually did quit for over six years. But, as soon as some major problem affected me, like right before my first divorce, I just started back up again. I know I have to quit sooner or later while my health is still intact. Smoking cigarettes is like begging for big-time health problems. You certainly don't get healthier with each puff inhaled! (From Venturelli's research files, 43-year-old male high school teacher, September 10, 1996)

Tobacco Use: Scope of the Problem

Cigarette smoking is the major, most preventable cause of disease and premature death in the United States. In surveys of such legitimate drugs as alcohol, nicotine, and caffeine, the number one killer drug continues to be cigarettes. They are responsible for approximately 1192 deaths every day and 435,000 annually, while alcohol kills approximately 100,000 annually (Aldrich 1995, 28). Another series of statistics shows that 180,000 die of coronary heart disease, 36,000 from stroke, 156,000 from cancer, and 60,000 from chronic pulmonary disease and other causes (Bartacchi et al. 1995, 49). Furthermore, 150,000 yearly cases of bronchitis and pneumonia result in young children whose parents smoke (*CBS Evening News* 1994).

A researcher at the University of Michigan, Dr. Lloyd D. Johnston, has said "[O]ne in four regular smokers will eventually die from tobacco use. I don't know any other product, including guns, that has that death rate" (Ryan 1994, 5). Indeed, nicotine dependency through cigarette smoking is not only the most common form of drug addiction, but also the one that causes more death and disease than all other addictions combined (USDHHS 1994). (See Figure 12.1.)

Figure 12.1

U.S. Deaths from Tobacco and Other Drugs Circa 1990
Almost three times as many Americans die from tobacco-related illnesses such as cardiovascular and respiratory diseases and cancer as die from alcohol-, cocaine-, and heroin-related problems combined.

Sources: Drug Abuse Warning Network, *Morbidity and Mortality Weekly Report,* U.S. Vital Statistics

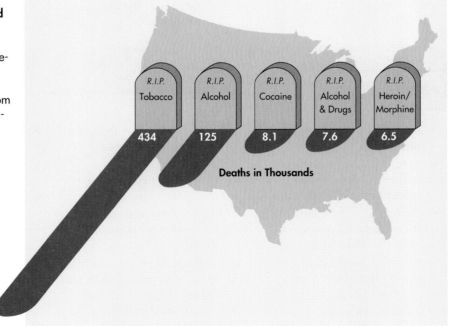

Current Tobacco Use

In 1993, 46 million adults aged 18 years and older (24 million men and 22 million women) in the United States were current smokers. Smoking among adults decreased dramatically from 42% of the population in 1965 to 25% in 1993. During this period, the percentage of smokers among the adult male population declined from 52% to 28%; the percentage of adult female smokers declined from 34% to 23% (CDC 1995); see Table 12.1. A more recent study conducted in 1995 showed that approximately 61 million Americans smoked cigarettes. This number represents a smoking rate of 29% among the U.S. population age 12 and older (SAMHSA 1996). An additional estimated 6.9 million Americans (3.3% of the population) used smokeless tobacco in 1995. Additional significant findings related to smoking include the following:

▲ More than 146 million people aged 12 years and older (71% of the population) have tried

smoking cigarettes; 64 million (31%) have smoked cigarettes within the past year; and almost 54 million (26%) have smoked cigarettes within the past month (NIDA 1995).

▲ People aged 26 to 34 have the highest rates of smoking.

▲ Almost 28 million males (30% of the population) and 26 million females (25%) have smoked cigarettes within the past month (NIDA 1995).

U.S. cigarette use by region is as follows: 32% of the population in the North Central region, 29% in the South region, 26% in the West region, and 28% in the Northeast region. The rate of smoking is estimated at 27% of the population in large metropolitan areas, 28% in small metropolitan areas, and 33% in nonmetropolitan areas (USDHHS 1996). Level of educational attainment was also correlated with tobacco usage. Thirty-seven percent of adults who did not complete high

Table 12.1   **Percent of Smoking Prevalence Among U.S. Adults, 1955–1993**
(18 Years of Age and Older)

Year	Population (millions)	Males	Females	Whites	Blacks
1955	—	56.9	28.4	—	—
1965	42.4	51.9	33.9	42.1	45.8
1966	42.6	52.5	33.9	42.4	45.9
1970	37.4	44.1	31.5	37.0	41.4
1974	37.1	43.1	32.1	36.4	44.0
1978	34.1	38.1	30.7	33.9	37.7
1979	33.5	37.5	29.9	33.3	36.9
1980	33.2	37.6	29.3	32.9	36.9
1983	32.1	35.1	29.5	31.8	35.9
1985	30.1	32.6	27.9	29.6	34.9
1987	28.8	31.2	26.5	28.5	32.9
1988	28.1	30.8	25.7	27.8	31.7
1990	25.5	28.4	22.8	25.6	26.2
1991	25.7	28.1	23.5	25.5	29.1
1992*	26.5	28.6	24.6	26.6	27.8
1993	25.0	27.7	22.5	24.9	26.1

(*) Estimates since 1992 incorporate people who have smoked at some point in their lives.

Source: Office on Smoking and Health, Centers for Disease Control and Prevention. Atlanta: U.S. Department of Health and Human Services, 1995.

school smoked cigarettes, while only 17% of college graduates smoked. The data also show that the average age of people who began daily cigarette use was 19.1 years in 1993, while the average age was 16.8 years in 1994. Thus daily cigarette use appears to be occurring at an earlier age (SAMHSA 1996, 99). (Additional information on the groups that use tobacco will follow later in this chapter.)

The History of Tobacco Use

Like alcohol, tobacco has a long history of use in this country. The tobacco plant was indigenous to the United States. In fact, tobacco was one of the New World's contributions to the rest of humanity. The word *tobacco* may have come from *tabaco,* which was a two-pronged tube used by the natives of Central America to take snuff. Columbus reported receiving tobacco leaves from the natives of San Salvador in 1492. However, the native peoples had been smoking the leaves for many centuries before Columbus arrived. Practically all of the natives from Paraguay to Quebec used tobacco. The Mayas regarded tobacco smoke as divine incense that would bring rain in the dry season. The oldest known representation of a smoker is a stone carving from a Mayan temple, which shows a priest puffing on a ceremonial pipe. The Aztecs used tobacco in folk medicine and religious ritual.

Indeed, Native Americans used tobacco in every manner known: smoked as cigars and cigarettes (wrapped in corn husks) and in pipes; as a syrup to be swallowed or applied to the gums; chewed and snuffed; and administered rectally as a ceremonial enema (Schultes 1978; Tobacco Institute 1982; O'Brien et al. 1992).

In the 1600s, Turkey, Russia, and China all imposed death penalties for smoking. In Turkey, smoking was introduced in the 1600s, spread in popularity, and instantly created two camps. On the one hand, poets praised tobacco as one of four elements of the world of pleasure: tobacco, opium, coffee, and wine. Priests, on the other hand, were violently opposed to this substance. They created the legend that tobacco grew from Mohammed's spittle, after he was bitten by a viper, sucked out the venom, and spat.

Murad (Amurath) IV, known as Murad the Cruel, who reigned during 1623–1640, executed many of his subjects caught smoking.

> Whenever the Sultan went on his travels or on a military expedition, his halting-laces were always distinguished by a terrible increase in the number of executions. Even on the battlefield, he was fond of surprising men in the act of smoking, . . . he would punish them by beheading, hanging, quartering, or crushing their hands and feet and leaving them helpless between the lines. . . . Nevertheless, in spite of all the horrors of this lust [smoking] that seemed to increase with age, the passion for smoking still persisted. . . . Even the fear of death was of no avail with the passionate devotees of the habit. (Corti 1931, 138–9).

The Romanov tsars publicly tortured smokers and exiled them to Siberia. The Chinese decapitated anyone caught dealing in tobacco with the "outer barbarians." Yet smoking continued to grow to epidemic proportions. Despite their opposition to anything foreign, the Chinese became the heaviest smokers in Asia, thus facilitating the later spread of opium smoking. Thus, no nation whose population has learned to use tobacco products has been successful in outlawing use or getting people to stop.

Snuffing first became fashionable in France during the reign of Louis XIII and spread throughout the European aristocracy. Snuffing was regarded as daintier and more elegant than constantly exhaling smoke. King Louis XIV, however, detested all forms of tobacco and would not permit its use in his presence. (He would have banned it, but he needed the tax revenue that tobacco brought in.) His sister-in-law, Charlotte of Orleans, was one of the few at court who agreed with him. As she wrote to her sister, "It is better to take no snuff at all than a little; for it is certain that he who takes a little will soon take much, and that is why they call it 'the enchanted herb,' for those who take it are so taken by it that they cannot go without it." Napoleon is said to have used seven pounds of snuff per month (Corti 1931).

Popularity in the Western World

When tobacco reached Europe, it was at first merely a curiosity, but its use spread rapidly. Europeans had no name for the process of inhaling smoke, so they called this "drinking" smoke. Perhaps the first European to inhale tobacco smoke was Rodrig de Jerez, a member of Columbus's crew. He had seen people smoking in Cuba and brought the habit to Portugal. When he smoked in Portugal, his friends, seeing smoke coming from his mouth, believed he was possessed by the devil! As a result, he was placed in jail for several years (Heimann 1960; O'Brien et al. 1992).

In 1559, the French ambassador to Portugal, Jean Nicot, grew interested in this novel plant and sent one as a gift to Catherine de Medici, Queen of France. The plant was named *Nicotiana tabacum* after him.

The next several hundred years saw a remarkable increase in the use of tobacco. Portuguese sailors smoked it and left tobacco seeds scattered around the world. Over the next 150 years, the Portuguese introduced tobacco to trade with India, Brazil, Japan, China, Arabia, and Africa. Many large tobacco plantations around the world were started by the Portuguese at this time.

An early Christian religious leader, Bishop Bartolome de las Casas (1474–1566), reported that Spanish settlers in Hispaniola (Haiti) smoked rolled tobacco leaves in cigar form like the natives. When the bishop asked about this disgusting habit, the settlers replied that they found it impossible to give up.

As the use of tobacco spread, so did the controversy about whether it was bad or good. *Tobacco use inspired the first major drug controversy of global dimensions.* As a medicine, tobacco was at first almost universally accepted. Nicholas Monardes, in his description of New World plants (dated 1574), recommended tobacco as an infallible cure for 36 different maladies. It was described as a holy, healing herb—a special remedy sent by God to humans.

Opponents of tobacco use disputed its medical value. They pointed out that tobacco was used in the magic and religion of Native Americans. Tobacco was attacked as an evil plant, an invention of the devil. King James I of England was fanatically opposed to smoking. In an attempt to limit tobacco use, he raised the import tax on tobacco and also sold the right to collect the tax (Austin 1978; O'Brien et al. 1992).

Nevertheless, tobacco use increased. By 1614, the number of tobacco shops in London had mushroomed to over 7000, and demand for tobacco usually outstripped supply. Tobacco was literally worth its weight in silver, so to conserve it, users smoked it in pipes with very small bowls. Use of tobacco grew in other areas of the world as well.

In 1642, Pope Urban VIII issued a formal decree forbidding the use of tobacco in church under penalty of immediate excommunication. This decree was in response to the fact that priests and worshippers had been staining church floors with tobacco juice. One priest in Naples sneezed so hard after taking snuff that he vomited on the altar in full sight of the congregation. In response, Pope Innocent X issued another edict against tobacco use in 1650, but the clergy and the laity continued to take snuff and smoke. Finally, in 1725, Pope Benedict XIII, himself a smoker and "snuff-taker," annulled all previous edicts against tobacco (Austin 1978).

History of Tobacco Use in America

Tobacco played a significant role in the successful colonization of the United States (Langton 1991, 21). In 1610, John Rolfe was sent to Virginia to set up a tobacco industry. At first, the tobacco planted in Virginia was a native species, *Nicotiana rustica,* that was harsh and did not sell well. But in 1612, Rolfe managed to obtain some seeds of the Spanish tobacco species *Nicotiana tabacum,* and by 1613, the success of the tobacco industry and the Virginia colony was assured.

The history of tobacco smoking in the United States is rich in terms of the tremendous number of laws, rules, regulations, and customs that have arisen out of the habit of smoking. Many states have had laws prohibiting the use of tobacco by young people as well as women of any age. In the 1860s, for instance, it was illegal in Florida for anyone under the age of 21 to smoke cigarettes. A 20-year-old caught smoking could be taken to court and compelled to reveal his source (the cigarette "pusher"). In Pennsylvania, as in South Carolina, any child not informing on his or her cigarette supplier was a criminal.

Up to the turn of the century, chewing and snuffing were the most common ways of using tobacco in the United States. In 1897, half of all tobacco was prepared for chewing. Law required that spittoons be placed in all public buildings until 1945 ("Cigars" 1988).

Cigars became popular in the United States in the early 1800s. Cigar manufacturers fought the introduction of cigarettes for many years. They spread rumors that cigarettes contained opium, were made with tobacco from discarded cigar butts and with paper made by Chinese lepers, and so on. By about 1920, cigarette consumption started to exceed that of cigars. The introduction of the cigarette-rolling machine in 1883 had spurred cigarette consumption because they became cheaper than cigars. By 1885, a billion cigarettes a year were being produced. Americans consumed over 815 billion cigarettes in 1988, or about 5000 per person age 18 or older. More recent estimates show that the number of cigarettes manufactured in the United States rose from 667 billion in 1983 to 695 billion in 1991 to 702 billion from 1992 to 1993. Though domestic consumption has dropped, the increases result from foreign demand of U.S. tobacco leaf and U.S. cigarette manufacturers offering discounted cigarettes and lower prices on premium brands.

An example of a historical (early 1900s) spittoon that would have been placed in a public building

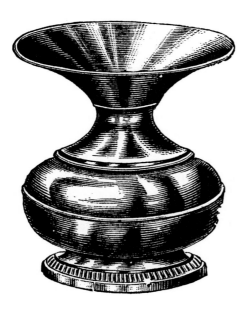

Tobacco Production

Tobacco farming is the sixth largest legal cash crop in the United States, ranking behind corn, soybeans, hay, wheat, and cotton (Foster et al. 1989, 121). North Carolina and Kentucky are the two leading growers of tobacco (O'Brien et al. 1992, 6).

While there are over 60 species of plants, ***Nicotiana tabacum*** is the primary species of tobacco cultivated in the United States. Its mature leaves are 1 to 2.5 feet long. The nicotine content ranges from 0.3% to 7%, depending on the variety, leaf position on the stalk (the higher the position, the more nicotine), and growing conditions. The flavor of tobacco comes from *nicotianin,* also called *tobacco camphor* (U.S. Surgeon General 1979; O'Brien et al. 1992, 1).

> ***nicotiana tabacum***
> primary species of tobacco cultivated in the United States

After harvesting and drying, tobacco leaves are shredded, blown clean of foreign matter and stems, remoisturized with glycerine or other chemical agents, and packed in huge wooden barrels called *hogsheads.* These barrels are placed in storehouses for one to two years to age, during which time the tobacco becomes darker and loses moisture, nicotine, and other volatile substances. When aging has been completed, moisture is again added and the tobacco is blended with other varieties.

There are many types of tobacco, with varying characteristics of harshness, mildness, and flavor. **Bright,** also called **flue-cured** or **Virginia,** is the most common type used in cigarettes. (Flue-cured tobacco is heated in curing sheds to speed the drying process.) Developed just before the Civil War, this technique made tobacco smoke more readily inhalable.

> **bright, flue-cured, or Virginia**
> the most common type of tobacco used in cigarettes

The amount of leaf tobacco in a cigarette has declined by roughly 25% since 1956. There are two reasons for this drop, not considering the introduction of filtertip cigarettes. (If a filtertip is the same size as a plain cigarette, it has about one-third less tobacco.) The first reason is the use of reconstituted sheets of tobacco. Parts of the tobacco leaves and stems that were discarded in earlier years are now ground up, combined with many other ingredients to control factors such as moisture, flavor, and color, and then rolled out as a flat, homogenized sheet of reconstituted tobacco. This sheet is shredded and mixed with regular leaf tobacco, thus reducing production costs. Nearly one-fourth of the tobacco in a cigarette comes from tobacco scraps made into reconstituted sheets.

A second technological advance has further reduced the amount of tobacco needed. This process, called **puffing,** is based on freeze-drying the tobacco and then blowing air or an inert gas, such as carbon dioxide, into it. The gas expands, or puffs up, the plant cells so they take up more space, are lighter, and can absorb additives better.

puffing
a method for reducing the amount of tobacco in cigarette production

Tobacco additives are not controlled by the Food and Drug Administration (FDA) or any other government agency. Additives may include extracts of tobacco, as well as nontobacco flavors such as licorice, cocoa, fruit, spices, and floral compositions. (Licorice was first used in tobacco as a preservative around 1830 and became appreciated only later as a sweetener.) Synthetic flavoring compounds also may be used.

In the 1870s, a "cigarette girl" could roll about four cigarettes per minute by hand. When James Duke leased and improved the first cigarette-rolling machine in 1883, he could make about 200 cigarettes per minute. This advance was the last link in the chain of development leading to the modern American blended cigarette. Today's machines make over 3600 uniform cigarettes per minute.

Tar and nicotine levels in cigarettes have dropped considerably over the last 40 years (Palfai and Jankiewicz 1991; Bartecchi et al. 1995). Most cigarettes today are low-tar and low-nicotine types. The filtertip, in which the filter is made of cellulose or in some cases charcoal, has also become common; over 90% of all cigarettes sold currently in the United States are filtertips (Stellman and Garfinkel 1986; *Tobacco Industry Profile* 1988). The filter does help remove some of the harmful substances in smoke, but most, such as carbon monoxide, pass through into the mouth and lungs. To date, 43 cancer-causing substances have been identified out of the 4700 substances used in cigarettes (Bartecchi et al. 1995, 49). Many are known carcinogens, whereas the health consequences of many more have not been adequately analyzed.

The manufacturing cost for cigarettes (not counting the tobacco) is about three cents a pack. Total cost varies with the manufacturer but usually does not exceed five to seven cents a pack. The total amount spent by American consumers is about $25 billion a year for all tobacco products, with over 90% of that for cigarettes. In 1986, the tax revenue on all cigarettes to the U.S. government was about $4 billion, with over $1.5 billion more in state taxes. In 1994, annual revenues for cigarette makers reached $48 billion (Brownlee et al. 1994).

Government Regulation In the early 1960s, attitudes toward tobacco use began to change in the United States (see "Fighting the Drug War," page 299). Prior to this time, tobacco was perceived as being devoid of any negative consequences. After years of study and hundreds of research reports about the effects of smoking, the Advisory Committee to the U.S. Surgeon General reported in 1964 that "cigarette smoking is causally related to lung cancer in men; the magnitude of the effects of cigarette smoking far outweighs all other factors." In 1965, Congress passed legislation setting up the National Clearinghouse for Smoking and Health. This organization has the responsibility of monitoring, compiling, and reviewing the world's medical literature on the health consequences of smoking.

Reports were published by this clearinghouse in 1967, 1968, and 1969. The statistical evidence presented in 1969 made it difficult for Congress to avoid warning the public that smoking was dangerous to their health. Since November 1, 1970, all cigarette packages and cartons have had to carry this label: "Warning: The Surgeon General Has Determined That Cigarette Smoking Is Dangerous to Your Health." In 1984, Congress enacted legislation requiring cigarette advertisements and packages to post four distinct warnings (see Figure 12.2), which are to be rotated every three months.

Figure 12.2

Warnings on cigarette labels. Four warnings must be rotated on cigarette packages. The messages are based on the reports of the U.S. Surgeon General on *The Health Consequences of Smoking* (1985) and went into effect on October 12, 1985.

> SURGEON GENERAL'S WARNING: Quitting Smoking Now Greatly Reduces Serious Risks to Your Health.

> SURGEON GENERAL'S WARNING: Smoking Causes Lung Cancer, Heart Disease, Emphysema, and May Complicate Pregnancy.

> SURGEON GENERAL'S WARNING: Smoking by Pregnant Women May Result in Fetal Injury, Premature Birth, and Low Birth Weight.

> SURGEON GENERAL'S WARNING: Cigarette Smoke Contains Carbon Monoxide.

Further pressure on Congress prompted laws to be passed that prohibited advertising tobacco on radio and television after January 2, 1971. The intent was to limit the media's ability to make smoking seem glamorous and sophisticated. The loss in revenue to radio and television was enormous.

The 1979 publication *Smoking and Health: A Report of the Surgeon General* gave what was then up-to-date information on research about the effects of tobacco on cardiovascular disease, bronchopulmonary disease, cancer, peptic ulcer, and pregnancy. It also emphasized the increase in smoking by women and girls over the past 15 years. The 1981 U.S. Surgeon General's report, *The Changing Cigarette,* gave further information, and the 1985 report, *The Health Consequences of Smoking,* gave research findings showing the relationship of smoking, cancer, and chronic lung disease in the workplace.

As this edition goes to press, subject to final congressional approval is the news that the to-bacco companies—RJR Nabisco, Philip Morris, Brown & Williamson and Lorillard—reached a decision with attorneys general in nearly 40 states to have the tobacco companies pay out $368.5 billion over the next twenty-five years for compensations to states for health care costs of smokers in treatment. Further, the agreement also calls for paying lawsuits to smokers, finance health research and promote education programs targeted to youth who are potentially contemplating smoking or are current cigarette smokers. The agreement also stipulates that Joe Camel and the Marlboro Man will no longer be used in advertising whether they be billboard advertising, T-shirt giveaways, and other methods of promoting particular brands of cigarettes. Finally all cigarette manufacturers will be held liable to additional penalties if the number of teenage smokers does not decline by half within the next seven years. To date, this is the most sweeping government-initiated action taken against tobacco manufacturers (Smolowe, 30 June 1997, 24–29).

Since 1985, numerous other reports on smoking and health by the U.S. Surgeon General have been issued; they invariably repeat the assertions about the devastating effects of cigarette smoking (Bartecchi et al. 1995). For a historical summation of the developments between cigarette consumption and efforts to diminish cigarette use, see Table 12.2.

Pharmacology of Nicotine

In 1828, nicotine was separated out as a component of tobacco. **Nicotine** is a colorless, highly volatile liquid alkaloid. It has no therapeutic application or action, and it is considered a volatile and powerful poison. Usually inhaled, "tobacco smoke is an aerosol, a colloid system consisting of a liquid dispersed in a gaseous medium, as in a fog or disinfectant spray" (Palfai and Jankiewicz 1991, 348). When smoked, tobacco enters the lungs as a water-soluble liquid contained in the watery portion of the mucous membranes. When chewed, nicotine is extracted from chewing or absorbing finely

nicotine
a colorless, highly volatile liquid alkaloid

FIGHTING THE DRUG WAR

For decades, cigarette smoking was portrayed as something glamorous, sexy, cool . . . especially in advertisements paid for by tobacco companies. In the 1960s, the Marlboro Man galloped across American TV screens, offering the subliminal promise that men who smoked Marlboros could be equally macho. For women who smoked, the message was that they could attract men like him.

By the end of the 1970s, when people first began to realize that smoking might not be the healthiest habit, the positive images from advertisements were so deeply ingrained in their psyches, and the addictions so deeply ingrained in their brains, that most people couldn't—or didn't want to—give up their butts.

Even in the late 1980s and early 1990s, when it was widely accepted that smoking cigarettes, or using tobacco in other forms, could actually kill you, Joe Camel was splattered across billboards and magazine ads, drawing in the youth of America with his "be cool" message. Unfortunately, the messages worked. In the mid-1990s, roughly 25% of people living in the United States used tobacco. Approximately 90% of new smokers every year are younger than 18. Though technically it is illegal for those under 18 to buy cigarettes, it is nearly impossible to enforce this law. Cigarettes are just too accessible, and the allure is too strong.

In the summer of 1996, President Bill Clinton moved boldly toward curbing the power of the tobacco companies, as part of a larger effort to stop smoking among teenagers, and signed an Executive Order that subjected tobacco to regulation by the FDA. For its part, the FDA—under the rigorous leadership of Dr. David Kessler—declared cigarettes to be "the delivery system for an addictive drug, nicotine."

The FDA's conclusion was supported by an Italian study, led by Gaetano di Chiara, whose results were published in the summer of 1996. Di Chiara's team conducted research on rats that had been injected with a small dose of nicotine—about the same amount that a smoker receives from a single drag on a cigarette. The researchers then monitored the biochemical changes that occurred in the *nucleus accumbens,* an area of the brain that appears to control the process of addiction. They found that levels of dopamine, a powerful brain chemical, increased dramatically in the outermost shell of the nucleus accumbens, which in turn has numerous connections to the *amygdala,* one of the brain's most important emotional centers. This finding was important because Di Chiara's group had determined earlier that a virtually identical pattern of biochemical activity accompanies injections of cocaine, amphetamines, and morphine.

Will President Clinton's order stick after the departure of the FDA's crusading Dr. Kessler? If it does, cigarette sales would require a photo I.D. that includes proof of age; magazines read by large numbers of teens would be allowed to run only black-and-white, all-text tobacco ads; billboards promoting tobacco products would be banned within 1000 feet of schools or playgrounds; cigarette machine placement would be sharply restricted; and tobacco companies would not be allowed to sponsor sporting events or include tobacco-related logos on products such as hats, T-shirts, and gym bags.

Whether those measures will be sufficient to prevent future generations from causing their own lives to go up in smoke remains to be seen. ∎

ground tobacco leaves in the mouth. **Tobacco chewing** involves the absorption of nicotine through the mucous lining of the mouth; **snuff dipping,** another method of administration, involves placing a pinch of tobacco

> **tobacco chewing**
> the absorption of nicotine through the mucous lining of the mouth

between the gums and the cheek.

The amount of tobacco absorbed varies according to five factors: (1) the exact composition of the tobacco used (Doweiko 1996); (2) how densely the tobacco is packed in the cigarette

> **snuff dipping**
> placing a pinch of tabacco between the gums and the cheek

Table 12.2 Significant Developments Related to Smoking and Health 1964–1995

1964	▲ *Smoking and Health: Report of the Advisory Committee to the Surgeon General,* the first major U.S. report on smoking and health, is published. It concludes that cigarette smoking is a cause of lung cancer in men and a suspected cause in women, and identifies many other causal relationships and smoking-disease associations. The report calls for "appropriate" remedial action.
	▲ The National Interagency Council on Smoking and Health, the first national antismoking coalition, is formed.
	▲ Cigarette manufacturers establish a voluntary Cigarette Advertising Code for television and radio.
	▲ The American Medical Association (AMA) officially calls smoking "a serious health hazard."
	▲ The State Mutual Life Assurance Company becomes the first company to offer life insurance to nonsmokers at discounted rates.
1965	▲ Congress passes the Federal Cigarette Labeling and Advertising Act, requiring the following health warning on all cigarette packages: "Caution: Cigarette Smoking May Be Hazardous to Your Health."
	▲ Public Health Service (PHS) establishes the National Clearinghouse for Smoking and Health.
1966	▲ A health warning label appears on all cigarette packages.
1967	▲ A report of the Surgeon General concludes that smoking is the principal cause of lung cancer.
	▲ The Federal Communications Commission (FCC) rules that the Fairness Doctrine applies to cigarette advertising. Stations broadcasting cigarette commercials must donate air time to antismoking messages.
	▲ The Federal Trade Commission (FTC) releases the first report on tar and nicotine yield in cigarette brands.
1968	▲ Action on Smoking and Health is formed to serve as a legal action arm for the antismoking community.
1969	▲ The National Association of Broadcasters (NAB) endorses phasing-out cigarette ads on television and radio.
1970	▲ The Public Health Cigarette Smoking Act of 1969 is enacted, banning cigarette advertising on television and radio and requiring a stronger health warning on cigarette packages: "Warning: The Surgeon General Has Determined That Cigarette Smoking Is Dangerous to Your Health."
	▲ The World Health Organization (WHO) takes a public position against cigarette smoking.
1971	▲ The Surgeon General proposes a government ban on smoking in public places.
	▲ Cigarette advertising ends on radio and television. Fairness Doctrine antismoking messages also end.
	▲ Cigarette manufacturers' voluntary agreement to list tar and nicotine yield in all advertising becomes effective.
1972	▲ A report of the Surgeon General identifies involuntary smoking as a health risk.
	▲ Under a consent order with the FTC, six major cigarette companies agree to include a "clear and conspicuous" health warning in all cigarette advertisements.
1973	▲ Congress enacts the Little Cigar Act of 1973, banning little cigar ads from television and radio.
	▲ The Civil Aeronautics Board requires "no smoking" sections on all commercial airline flights.
	▲ Arizona becomes the first state to restrict smoking in a number of public places and the first to do so explicitly because environmental tobacco smoke exposure is a public hazard.
1975	▲ Cigarettes are discontinued in K-rations and C-rations to soldiers and sailors.

1977	▲ The American Cancer Society (ACS) sponsors the first national "Great American Smokeout." ▲ Doctors Ought to Care is formed to provide a focal point for physicians' antismoking advocacy, especially through counteradvertising.
1978	▲ The National Clearinghouse for Smoking and Health is renamed the Office on Smoking and Health. ▲ Utah enacts the first state law banning tobacco advertisements on any billboard, streetcar sign, streetcar, or bus.
1979	▲ Minneapolis and St. Paul become the first cities to ban the distribution of free cigarette samples.
1980	▲ A report of the Surgeon General highlights health consequences of smoking to women. ▲ PHS announces "Health Objectives for the Nation," which include a goal to reduce smoking to below 25% of adults by 1990. ▲ The FTC begins testing cigarettes for carbon monoxide yields.
1981	▲ A report of the Surgeon General focuses on "The Changing Cigarette." It concludes that no cigarette or level of tobacco consumption is safe.
1982	▲ A report of the Surgeon General focuses exclusively on smoking and cancer. ▲ Congress temporarily doubles the federal excise tax on cigarettes to 16 cents per pack, to take effect from January 1, 1983, to October 1, 1985. It marks the first such increase since 1951. ▲ ACS, American Lung Association (ALA), and American Heart Association (AHA) form a tripartite Coalition on Smoking OR Health, primarily to coordinate federal legislative activities related to smoking control. ▲ The National Cancer Institute (NCI) reorganizes its smoking research program, as the Smoking, Tobacco and Cancer Program, to focus on smoking behavior research and interventions.
1983	▲ A report of the Surgeon General focuses exclusively on smoking and cardiovascular disease. ▲ San Francisco passes a law to include smoking restrictions in private workplaces.
1984	▲ A report of the Surgeon General focuses exclusively on smoking and chronic obstructive lung disease. ▲ Congress enacts the Comprehensive Smoking Education Act, requiring rotational health warnings on cigarette packages and advertisements. ▲ The FDA approves nicotine polacrilex gum as a "new drug." ▲ The Surgeon General announces his goal of a smoke-free society by 2000.
1985	▲ A report of the Surgeon General covers smoking and occupational exposures. ▲ Minnesota enacts the first state legislation to earmark a portion of the state cigarette excise tax to support antismoking programs. ▲ STAT (Stop Teenage Addiction to Tobacco) is formed to focus on teenage tobacco use.
1986	▲ A report of the Surgeon General focuses exclusively on the health consequences of involuntary smoking. ▲ A special report of the Surgeon General documents the health consequences of using smokeless tobacco. ▲ Congress enacts the Comprehensive Smokeless Tobacco Health Education Act of 1986. It requires rotation of three health warnings on smokeless tobacco packages and advertisements and bans smokeless tobacco advertising on broadcast media. ▲ Congress extends permanently the 16 cents per pack federal excise tax on cigarettes. ▲ Californians for Nonsmokers' Rights goes national, becoming Americans for Nonsmokers' Rights. It was originally formed as California GASP (Group Against Smoking Pollution) in 1976. ▲ Minnesota enacts the first state law to ban free distribution of smokeless tobacco samples. ▲ Congress imposes a federal excise tax on smokeless tobacco products.

Table 12.2 (continued)

1987	▲ The Department of Health and Human Services (DHHS) establishes a smoke-free environment in its facilities, affecting 120,000 DHHS employees nationwide. ▲ The Minnesota Sports Commission votes to ban tobacco advertising in the Metrodome Sports Stadium effective in 1992, the first such action in the United States.
1988	▲ A report of the Surgeon General concentrates exclusively on nicotine addiction. ▲ A congressionally mandated smoking ban takes effect on domestic airline flights scheduled for two hours or less. Northwest Airlines voluntarily bans smoking on all flights in North America. ▲ ALA sponsors the first annual "Non-Dependence Day." ▲ California voters pass a referendum raising the state cigarette excise tax by 25 cents per pack, the largest cigarette excise tax increase in U.S. history. Revenues earmarked for public health purposes.
1989	▲ A report of the Surgeon General marks the twenty-fifth anniversary of the first Smoking and Health report; it focuses on progress since the first report.
1990	▲ The Environmental Protection Agency (EPA) issues a draft risk assessment on environmental tobacco smoke (ETS). ▲ The Office of the Inspector General (OIG), DHHS, issues a report concluding that laws curtailing minors' access to tobacco are ignored. It proposes a minors' access to tobacco model law for states. ▲ The airline smoking ban goes into effect, banning smoking on all scheduled domestic flights of six hours or less. ▲ The Secretary of the DHHS denounces "Uptown" cigarettes, a brand to be targeted to blacks— the manufacturer cancels its plans to market the cigarettes.
1991	▲ The National Institute for Occupational Safety and Health (OSH), part of the Centers for Disease Control and Prevention (CDC), issues a bulletin recommending that ETS be reduced to the lowest feasible concentration in the workplace. ▲ The NCI and the ACS join together in the American Stop Smoking Intervention Study (ASSIST), funding 17 states over a period of seven years at a cost of $165 million. ▲ The federal cigarette excise tax increases to 20 cents.
1992	▲ The first federal legislation is enacted to require states to adopt and enforce restrictions on tobacco sales to minors. Penalties are to be imposed on state substance abuse funding without proper enforcement. ▲ OIG, DHHS, issues a report documenting the widespread use of smokeless tobacco, particularly among young athletes. ▲ A transdermal nicotine patch is introduced. ▲ The Joint Commission on Accreditation of Healthcare Organizations (JCAHO) requires hospitals to be smoke-free as of January 1994 to maintain accreditation. ▲ The FTC takes its first enforcement action under the Smokeless Tobacco Act, alleging that the Pinkerton Tobacco Company's Red Man brand name appeared illegally during a televised event. ▲ The World Bank establishes a formal policy on tobacco, including discontinuing loans or investments for tobacco agriculture in developing countries.
1993	▲ The EPA releases final risk assessment of ETS, classifying it as a "Group A" carcinogen. ▲ Representatives of the tobacco industry file a suit against the EPA related to the findings of its ETS risk assessment. ▲ The OSH provides tobacco control resources to the remainder of states not funded under project ASSIST. ▲ The FDA prohibits over-the-counter smoking-deterrent products because they have not been shown to be effective.

1993 (cont.)	▲ The U.S. Postal Service eliminates smoking in all of its facilities. ▲ The federal cigarette excise tax increases to 24 cents. ▲ Congress enacts a smoke-free policy for Women, Infants and Children (WIC) clinics. ▲ The Office of the U.S. Trade Representative and DHHS meet to discuss tobacco trade issues, creating the Task Force on Tobacco Exports to review the government's activities involving tobacco trade. ▲ Congress enacts legislation requiring all American cigarettes to contain at least 75% American-grown tobacco and requiring a tariff on imported tobacco to help finance the federal tobacco crop subsidy program. ▲ A working group of 16 state Attorneys General releases recommendations for implementing smoke-free policies in fast-food restaurants.
1994	▲ A report of the Surgeon General focuses on tobacco use among youth. ▲ Congress enacts the Pro-Children Act of 1994, requiring all federally funded children's services to become smoke-free. ▲ Occupational Safety and Health Administration (OSHA) announces proposed regulations to prohibit smoking in the workplace, except in separately ventilated smoking rooms. ▲ The six major domestic cigarette manufacturers testify before the U.S. House Subcommittee on Health and the Environment that they do not manipulate the nicotine levels in cigarettes. ▲ FDA Commissioner Kessler testifies that cigarettes may qualify as drug delivery systems, bringing them within the jurisdiction of the FDA. ▲ Mississippi becomes the first state to sue the tobacco industry to recover Medicaid costs for tobacco-related illnesses. ▲ The Department of Defense (DOD) bans smoking in all of its workplaces. ▲ The Robert Wood Johnson Foundation and the AMA launch the Smokeless States grant program to fund local initiatives for tobacco control and prevention.
1995	▲ *The Journal of the American Medical Association* publishes articles on documents from the Brown and Williamson Tobacco Corporation, indicating the industry's early knowledge of the harmful effects of tobacco use and the addictive nature of nicotine. ▲ The Philip Morris Company recalls its cigarette brands due to the presence of contaminants. The CDC investigates reports of possible health effects. ▲ FDA Commissioner Kessler declares tobacco use to be a pediatric disease. ▲ The Department of Justice reaches a settlement with Philip Morris to remove tobacco advertisements from the line of sight of TV cameras in sports stadiums to ensure compliance with the federal ban on tobacco ads on TV. ▲ The FTC reports that the cigarette industry spent $6 billion on advertising and promotions in 1993.

Source: Centers for Disease Control and Prevention (CDC). "Smoking and Health Information—Significant Developments Related to Smoking and Health 1964–1995." Atlanta: U.S. Department of Health and Human Services, 1995.

(Doweiko 1996, 172) and the length of the cigarette smoked; (3) whether a filter is used and the characteristics of the filter; (4) the volume of smoke inhaled; and (5) the number of cigarettes smoked throughout the day.

◢ Physiological Effects

In large doses, nicotine is highly toxic. It has been used as an insecticide, and at higher concentration levels, it has the same effects as a poison. The symptoms of nicotine poisoning include sweating, vomiting, mental confusion, diminished pulse rate, and breathing difficulty. Respiratory failure from the paralysis of muscles usually brings on death.

Nicotine is the substance in tobacco that causes dependence because of how it is metabolized and the effects it produces. Many regular users smoke about 20 to 30 cigarettes per day, or one every 30 to 40 minutes.

Nicotine is a curious drug because it first stimulates and then depresses the nervous system. The stimulus effect is due to release of norepinephrine and the fact that nicotine mimics the action of acetylcholine. Nicotine thus stimulates cholinergic receptors (nicotinic type) first but is not removed from the receptors very rapidly; the next effect is depression, caused by blocked nerve activity. Nicotine increases the respiration rate at low dose levels because it stimulates the receptors in the carotid artery (in the neck) that monitor the brain's need for oxygen. It stimulates the cardiovascular system by releasing epinephrine, which increases coronary blood flow, heart rate, and blood pressure. The effect is to raise the oxygen requirements of the heart muscle but not the oxygen supply. This action may trigger heart attacks in susceptible people (Armitrage et al. 1985; USDHHS/CDC 1993, 857).

Initially, nicotine stimulates salivary and bronchial secretions, then inhibits them. The excess saliva associated with smoking is caused by the irritating smoke, not the nicotine itself (Taylor 1980; Benowitz 1988).

Nicotine and perhaps other substances in tobacco smoke tend to inhibit hunger contractions in the stomach for up to one hour. At the same time, this substance causes a slight increase in blood sugar and deadens the taste buds. These factors may explain the decreased feelings of hunger experienced by many smokers. Smokers have often reported that they gain weight after they stop smoking and that their appetite increases. In addition, when someone who smokes one or more packs a day quits, there may be a decrease in heart rate (two to three beats per minute) and up to a 10% decrease in basal metabolic rate. The body is being stressed less, so it converts more food into fat.

Nicotine and other products in smoke, such as carbon monoxide, produce still other effects. Up to 10% of all the hemoglobin in smokers may be in the form of carboxyhemoglobin. This type of hemoglobin cannot carry oxygen, so up to 10% of the smoker's blood is effectively out of circulation as far as normal oxygen–carbon dioxide exchange is concerned. This situation could easily cause a smoker to become breathless following exertion. It is a factor in heart attacks and in the lower birth-weight and survival rate of infants born to women who smoke during pregnancy (discussed later in this chapter).

Addictive Characteristics of Nicotine

Nicotine produces an intense effect on the central nervous system, and both inhaled tobacco smoke and mouth absorption of smokeless tobacco are akin to taking an intravenous injection of nicotine. Cigarette tobacco contains between 1.5% and 3% nicotine, with each cigarette containing between 29 to 30 milligrams of the drug (Fort 1969, 154–5; Sullivan 1991). (In 1980, an average cigarette contained less than 1 milligram of nicotine.) Although tolerance to nicotine builds up rapidly, the fatal dose for adults is 60 milligrams—a cigar contains between 15 and 40 milligrams. It is virtually impossible to overdose, even though nicotine is a poison in large quantities because a smoker feels the effects before any lethal amount can accumulate in the body (Schelling 1992, 431).

Clove Cigarettes

Indonesian **clove cigarettes** were first used by young Americans in the 1980s. In 1980, 12 million clove cigarettes were sold in this country; by 1984, sales had increased to 150 million. The popularity of clove cigarettes has recently begun to diminish, however.

The aroma of clove cigarettes masks the neg-

> **clove cigarettes**
> Indonesian aromatic-type cigarettes with more tobacco, tar, nicotine, and carbon monoxide than standard cigarettes in the U.S.

eugenol

the organic chemical in clove cigarettes that delivers the aroma when inhaled

ative physical effects of nicotine. As a result, adolescent and adult smokers often assume that these cigarettes are safer than tobacco cigarettes. The truth is that **eugenol,** the organic chemical that gives clove its aroma, anesthetizes the back of the throat, reducing the apparent harshness of the smoke and allowing deeper inhalation. Further, these cigarettes consist of more than 60% tobacco and possess a greater amount of tar, nicotine, and carbon monoxide than regular cigarettes manufactured in the United States. Users have reported excessive wheezing, fluid retention in the lungs, and bloody phlegm after smoking clove cigarettes.

◢ Cigarette Smoking: A Costly Addiction

Every day 3,000 young people become regular smokers. Every day 6,000 teens under age 18 smoke their first cigarette. Every day more than 1,000 adults die prematurely as a result of an adolescent decision. (USDHHS 1996, 2).

The inevitability of cigarette addiction is undisputable. More than 24 billion packages of cigarettes are purchased annually in the United States, and approximately 400,000 deaths are attributed to cigarette smoking. Studies have shown that 70% of current smokers want to quit but cannot. Cigarette smoking is so addictive that 83% of smokers smoke every day; in contrast, only 10% of illicit drug users are daily users. Furthermore, 85% of people who try an illicit drug quit using that substance, but only 63% of people who try cigarettes quit smoking (USDHHS 1994).

In 1993, smoking-attributable costs for medical care reached $50 billion. These costs include hospital, physician, and nursing home expenditures, prescription drugs, and home health care expenditures. Each of the approximately 24 billion packages of cigarettes sold in 1993 amounted to $2.06 spent on medical care attributable to smok-

ing. Of this $2.06, approximately $0.89 was paid through public sources. Thus, it costs the American taxpayer $0.89 for medical care expenses for each pack of cigarettes smoked by others, regardless of whether he or she smokes!

Mortality Rates

About 10 million people in the United States have died from causes attributed to smoking (including heart disease, emphysema, and other respiratory diseases) since the first Surgeon General's report on smoking and health was issued in 1964 (USDHHS 1995). Nearly 19% of all preventable causes of death in the United States can be attributed to tobacco use (Bartecchi et al. 1995).

Although the past 25 years has been marked by a steady decline in cigarette consumption (see Table 12.1), the risk of premature death is significantly higher (about 70%) for cigarette smokers than for nonsmokers. Cigarette smoking results in more than 5 million total years of potential life being lost annually (USDHHS 1995).

According to the U.S. Surgeon General, estimates of premature deaths associated with cigarette smoking range from 400,000 to 418,000 per year (USDHHS 1995), including 134,000 deaths from heart disease, 120,000 deaths from lung cancer [87% of all lung cancer deaths are attributable to smoking ("Facts About Smoking"), 31,000 deaths from other forms of cancer, 65,000 deaths from chronic lung disease, 23,000 deaths from stroke, and about 82,000 deaths from other diagnoses (see Figure 12.3).

A 35-year-old male who smokes two packs a day has a life expectancy that is 8.1 years shorter than his nonsmoking counterpart (U.S. Surgeon General 1985; Callahan 1987; USDHHS/CDC 1993, 863). The death rate increases with the amount smoked: A two-pack-a-day smoker has a mortality rate twice as high as a nonsmoker. Overall mortality rates are greater for those who smoke longer; death rates are directly proportional.

Various cigarettes have different tar and nicotine contents; the effects they produce—and thus the mortality rate—vary as well. Smokers of low-tar and -nicotine cigarettes have a mortality ratio

Figure 12.3

(A) 418,000 Deaths Attributable to Cigarette Smoking, United States, 1990

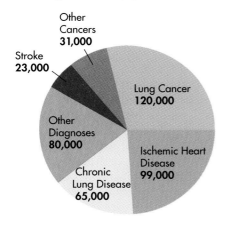

Source: CDC SAMMEC *MMWR* 42 (1993): 645–9.

(B) Comparative Causes of Annual Deaths in the United States

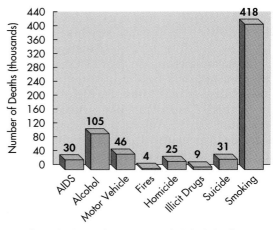

Note: All mortality data are for 1990, except alcohol, which is for 1987.

Sources: HIV/AIDS Surveillance Report; National Safety Council Accident Facts; Monthly Vital Statistics Report; SAMMEC; Alcohol-Related Death Index.

50% greater than that of nonsmokers but 15% to 20% less than that of cigarette smokers as a group (U.S. Surgeon General 1981; DeAngelis 1989).

Overall mortality ratios decline the longer ex-smokers abstain from smoking. People who stop smoking before age 50 reduce their risk of dying over the next 15 years by 50%. The mortality rate for ex-smokers is related to the *number* of cigarettes they used to smoke per day and the *age* at which they started to smoke. The mortality rate for cigar smokers is somewhat higher than that for nonsmokers and is related to the number of cigars smoked daily. The mortality rate for pipe smokers is slightly greater than that for nonsmokers.

Chronic Illness

Not only do cigarette smokers tend to die at an earlier age than nonsmokers, but they also have a higher probability of contracting certain diseases (Schuckit 1984; American Cancer Society 1990; USDHHS 1995). Following the U.S. Surgeon Gen-

eral's report in 1964, the National Center for Health Statistics began collecting information on smoking. These findings have been helpful in assessing the relationships between tobacco use and illnesses, disability, and other health indicators. Among other things, the center found that men and women currently smoking cigarettes have more chronic health problems than people who never smoked. A dose–response relationship also exists between the number of cigarettes smoked per day and particular illnesses. For instance, men who smoke two packs of cigarettes a day have a four times higher rate of chronic bronchitis and/or **emphysema** than do nonsmokers. The rate for women smoking two or more packs a day is nearly ten times higher.

emphysema

a common type of lung disease often resulting from smoking

Other indicators of sickness studied were workdays lost, days spent in bed because of illness, and days of limited activity resulting from chronic disease. Male smokers had a 33% excess and female smokers a 45% excess of workdays lost compared with nonsmokers. Male former smokers had a 41% excess and female former smokers a 43% excess of workdays lost. The U.S. Office of Technology Assessment (now disbanded) had estimated that cigarettes cost Americans $68 billion annually in tobacco-related health care costs and lost productivity (American Cancer Society 1996). This amount represents a tremendous financial and productivity loss for the nation.

Data on disability and illness show continued high risk among former smokers. The most likely reason for this relationship is that smokers quit because of a smoking-related illness that has already severely damaged the cardiovascular system or lungs.

Cardiovascular Disease Overwhelming evidence shows that cigarette smoking increases the risk of cardiovascular disease (Callahan 1987; Fiore et al. 1989; Bartecchi et al. 1995, 44). Cigarettes caused almost 180,000 deaths from cardiovascular disease in the United States in 1990 (Bartecchi et al. 1995, 49). Data collected for the United States, the United Kingdom, Canada, and other countries show that smoking is a major risk factor for heart attack. The probability of heart attack is related to the amount smoked, which has a synergistic relationship to other risk factors, such as obesity.

Smoking cigarettes is a major risk factor for arteriosclerotic disease and for death from arteriosclerotic aneurysm of the aorta (Palfai and Jankiewicz 1991). (An *aneurysm* is a weakened area in a blood vessel that forms a blood-filled sac and may rupture.) Smokers have a higher incidence of atherosclerosis of the coronary arteries that supply blood to the heart (the arteries become blocked with fat deposits), and the effect is dose-related. Both the carbon monoxide and the nicotine in cigarette smoke can precipitate angina attacks (painful spasms in the chest when the heart muscle does not get the blood supply it needs).

Smokers of low-tar and -nicotine cigarettes have less risk of coronary heart disease, but their risk still exceeds that of nonsmokers. The risk goes down if the person quits; after about 10 years, the risk of coronary disease in ex-smokers approaches

that in nonsmokers. Women who smoke and use oral contraceptives have a significantly higher risk of death or disability from stroke, heart attack, and other cardiovascular diseases than nonsmokers, whether on or off "the pill."

Cancer Lung cancer is the leading cause of cancer death in the United States, claiming 127,000 victims a year (American Cancer Society 1996). There were an estimated 521,000 deaths from all types of cancer in 1995, of which 120,000 were from lung cancer (American Cancer Society 1996, 7). Lung cancer is the most common type in men and in women. Lung cancer in women has increased dramatically—up fourfold in 25 years. Lung cancer mortality rates for women are increasing more rapidly than for men. Women who smoke die sooner, just as male smokers do; a direct relationship has been found between smoking and lung cancer in both genders.

Approximately 82% of lung cancer cases in men and 75% in women are caused by cigarette smoking. Less than 10% of nonsmokers get lung cancer. What's more, 85% to 90% of all deaths from lung cancer are smoking-related (American Cancer Society 1996).

The risk of lung cancer increases with the following factors:

▲ Amount smoked, as measured by the number of cigarettes smoked per day

▲ Duration of smoking

▲ Age at which the person started smoking

▲ Degree of inhalation

▲ Tar and nicotine content of the cigarettes

Use of filter cigarettes and of lower-tar and -nicotine cigarettes decreases the lung cancer mortality rate, but it is still significantly higher than that for nonsmokers. If a smoker quits, the lung cancer mortality rate goes down but will not approach the nonsmoker rate until 10 years of abstinence.

Pipe and cigar smokers are more likely to contract lung cancer than nonsmokers but less likely to do so than habitual cigarette smokers. Common types of cancers among cigar and pipe smokers include cancers of the mouth, larynx, and esophagus.

Person with tobacco-related illness

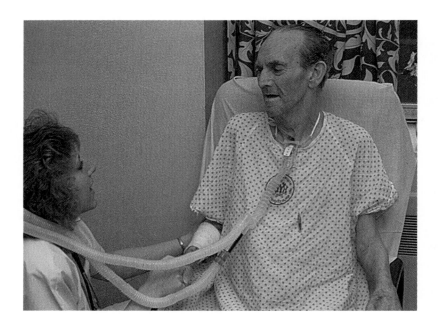

Exposure to certain air pollutants in the environment or in industry—especially the asbestos, uranium, nickel, and chemical industries—acts synergistically with cigarette smoking to increase lung cancer mortality rates far above what would be the rate for each separately without smoking.

Heavy smoking can severely damage the lungs and cause emphysema.

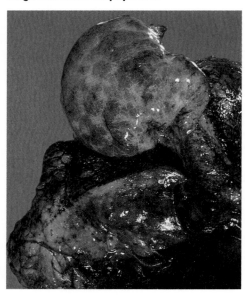

Cancer of the larynx is significantly higher in smokers compared with nonsmokers and is related to the amount smoked. A compounding effect has also been shown to exist between smoking and alcohol consumption and between exposure to asbestos and smoking, increasing the likelihood of getting cancer of the larynx. The risk of laryngeal cancer goes down if the person stops smoking; as with lung cancer, however, this form of cancer does not reach the level for nonsmokers for nearly 10 years.

A causal relationship also exists between smoking and cancers of the oral cavity, esophagus, urinary bladder, pancreas, and kidneys.

Bronchopulmonary Disease Cigarette smoking is the leading cause of bronchopulmonary disease, which includes a host of lung ailments (Bartecchi et al. 1995, 49). Cigarette smokers have higher death rates from pulmonary emphysema and chronic bronchitis and more frequently have impaired pulmonary function and other symptoms of pulmonary disease than nonsmokers (American Cancer Society 1997).

Respiratory infections are more prevalent and more severe among cigarette smokers—particularly heavy smokers—than among nonsmokers. The risk of developing or dying from bronchopulmonary disease among pipe or cigar smokers is higher than that for nonsmokers but less than for cigarette smokers. Ex-smokers have lower death rates from bronchopulmonary disease than do continuing smokers.

The cause of lung damage may be impaired immune system activity in lung tissue, genetic factors, and deficiencies in certain substances in the tissues. People with a low amount of an enzyme called *alpha-1-antitrypsin* are known to be more likely to develop emphysema. Smoking is especially dangerous for such people.

As mentioned, smokers are more prone to develop bronchopulmonary disease in the presence of air pollutants, such as sulfur oxides and asbestos, than are nonsmokers. Coal dust, cotton dust, and chlorine exert additive effects with cigarette smoking in damaging the lungs. Likewise, exposure to fumes and dust—especially talc and carbon black in the rubber industry and uranium and gold dust in the mining industry—act synergistically with cigarette smoking in the development of bronchopulmonary disease.

It is now understood how cigarette smoking causes one of the most common lung diseases, emphysema. Smoking produces inflammation of the lung tissue and increases the protein elastase in the tissue. Elastin, a structural material in the lungs, is broken down by elastase enzyme. In the long run, the lung tissue is damaged extensively, causing emphysema (U.S. Surgeon General 1984; USDHHS 1995).

Effects on the Fetus

Women who are younger than 23 years of age make up the fastest-growing segment of smokers in the United States (Bartecchi et al. 1995, 49). This trend is unfortunate because cigarette smoking during pregnancy has a significantly harmful effect on the development of the fetus, the survival of the newborn infant, and the continued development of the child (see the Here and Now box). Adverse effects on pregnancy range from increased risk for spontaneous abortion to impaired fetal growth, stillbirth, premature birth, and neonatal death. Babies born to mothers who smoke have a lower average body weight and length and have a smaller head circumference (Bartecchi et al. 1995,

49). The amount a woman smokes will impact the size of the child she bears. If a smoking woman gives up this habit for the entire duration of the pregnancy, her child will probably be of normal size and strength.

The below-average weight of babies born to smokers is caused by carbon monoxide and nicotine (Cook et al. 1990). Carbon monoxide reduces the oxygen-carrying capacity of the fetus's blood, just as it does the mother's. Fetal growth is retarded because the tissue becomes starved for oxygen. Inhaled nicotine enters the mother's blood from her lungs and rapidly constricts the blood flow to the placenta, reducing available oxygen and nutrients until the effect of the nicotine has worn off. In addition, nicotine crosses the blood–placenta barrier to the fetal bloodstream. It has the same effects on the fetus's nervous system and blood circulation as on the mother's. However, the fetus cannot metabolize nicotine efficiently, so the effects last longer for the child than for the mother.

One known carcinogen in tobacco smoke, *benzo(a)pyrene,* crosses the placenta and enters the fetal blood. Experiments with pregnant mice exposed to benzo(a)pyrene showed that their offspring had a markedly higher incidence of cancer. The impact of smoking during pregnancy on the incidence of cancer in infants is not known. In addition, if the father smokes but the mother does not, the infant may still be affected by secondhand smoke.

Infants born to mothers who smoke have a reduced probability of survival. They are more likely to die from **sudden infant death syndrome (SIDS)** and other causes related to their retarded growth. Long-term effects may be observed in physical growth, mental development, and behavioral characteristics of those babies who survive the first four weeks of life. It appears that children of mothers who smoke do not catch up with children of nonsmoking mothers in various stages of development, at least up to age 11. Smoking during pregnancy may also cause hyperkinesis in children.

sudden infant death syndrome (SIDS)
unexpected and unexplainable death that occurs while infants are sleeping

Pregnant Smoking Mothers and Their Daughters

HERE & NOW

A recent study by Dr. Denise Kandel of Columbia University suggests a strong relationship between prenatal exposure to smoking and the exposed female child's likelihood to smoke later in life. Prior to this study, prenatal exposure to smoking had been linked to "impairments in memory, learning, cognition, and perception in the growing child." In addition, this study suggests that exposed female children are "four times as likely to begin smoking during adolescence and to continue smoking than daughters of women who did not smoke during pregnancy."

An article describing this work noted, "The study suggests that nicotine, which crosses the placental barrier, may affect the female fetus during an important period of development so as to predispose the brain to the addictive influence of nicotine more than a decade later" (Mathias 1995). Prenatal smoking, however, had no strong effect on the smoking of male children; the researchers did not find any strong evidence to explain this result, calling this odd relationship "speculative."

The disturbing recent trend in female adolescent smoking is illustrated in Figure 12.4. This trend had previously been linked to a number of factors, but Dr. Kandel's work was the first to document this possible connection between prenatal nicotine exposure and smoking later in life.

The researchers worked to ensure that later smoking was a result of prenatal—not postnatal—smoking by the mother. They found that "regardless of the amount or duration of current or past maternal smoking, the strongest correlation between maternal smoking and a daughter's smoking occurred when the mother smoked during pregnancy."

Dr. Kandel plans to continue her research and probe into other aspects of prenatal exposure to nicotine by following the participants in her study for another six years. ■

Source: R. Mathias. "Daughters of Mothers Who Smoked During Pregnancy Are More Likely to Smoke, Study Says." *NIDA Notes* 10.5 (September/October 1995): II, 14.

Figure 12.4
Trends in Adolescent Girls' Current Use of Cigarettes

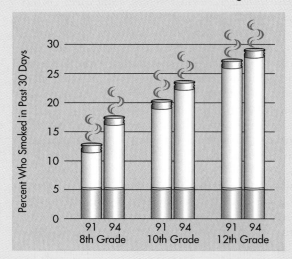

According to NIDA's *Monitoring the Future* study, the percentage of adolescent girls who smoke cigarettes has increased in the last four years. Although smoking among adolescent girls has been linked to many different factors, Dr. Kandel's study is the first to document a possible link between prenatal exposure to nicotine and an adolescent girl's tendency to smoke cigarettes.

Source: NIDA's Monitoring the Future Studies, 1991–94

Tobacco Use Without Smoking

Although it is customary to associate the effects of tobacco use with smoking, in fact millions of nonsmokers experience tobacco effects through their use of smokeless tobacco products.

Although a resurgence has occurred in the use of all forms of smokeless tobacco, plug, leaf, and snuff, the greatest cause for concern centers on the increased use of **"dipping snuff."** Dipping snuff, which is highly addictive, exposes the body to levels of nicotine equal to those obtained with cigarettes. **Chewing tobacco** and **snuff** are two types of smokeless tobacco products that are commonly referred to as "spit tobacco."

dipping snuff

Placing a pinch of smokeless tobacco between the gums and the cheek

chewing tabacco

tobacco leaves shredded and twisted into strands for chewing purposes

Both types consist of tobacco leaves that are shredded and twisted into strands and then either chewed or placed in the cheek between the lower lip and gum. In this process, nicotine, along with a number of carcinogens, is absorbed through the oral tissue. In **snuffing,** tobacco is "snorted" instead of being chewed or placed in the cheek.

snuffing

snorting chewing tobacco nasally

Smokeless tobacco contains powerful chemicals, including nicotine, nitrosamines, polycyclic aromatic hydrocarbons, and dozens of other carcinogens, that can injure tissues in the mouth and throat (see "Here and Now"' page 312). The findings have been made regarding smokeless tobacco:

1. About 5 million U.S. adults use smokeless tobacco.

2. In 1986, the U.S. Surgeon General concluded that smokeless tobacco is not a safe substitute for smoking cigarettes because of three reasons: it can cause cancer, it can produce a number of noncancerous oral conditions, and it can lead to nicotine addiction and dependence.

3. Oral cancer occurs several times more frequently among snuff dippers than among nontobacco users. (See the Case in Point box.)

4. The risk of cancer of the cheek and gum may reach nearly 50% among long-term snuff users.

5. The use of smokeless tobacco is increasing among male adolescents and young male adults.

6. According to the U.S. Department of Agriculture, U.S. output of moist snuff has risen 83% since 1981, when it reached 30 million pounds, to an estimated 55 million pounds in 1994.

7. The Centers for Disease Control and Prevention's 1994 Youth Risk Behavior Survey reported that 20% of male high-school students used smokeless tobacco.

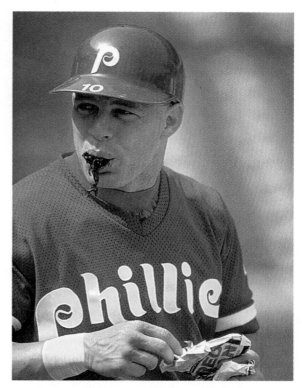

Despite the well-known health hazards of tobacco products, athletes, such as this baseball player, often use smokeless tobacco.

The increasing popularity of snuff tobacco (see Figure 12.5) is due to more effective and persistent advertising campaigns depicting famous athletes using such products. Some experts also believe that the increasing popularity of this tobacco product relates to its ability to satisfy the addiction to nicotine where smoking is prohibited (as it is in increasingly smoke-free environments). Thus, snuffing in place of smoking is perceived as an alternative to smoke-free environments.

The prevalence of smokeless tobacco use was highest among individuals with the lowest levels of education. The prevalence was 1.4% among those with more than 16 years of schooling and 4.6% among those with less than 12 years of schooling. In addition, use in the United States varied substantially by region: 4.6% in the South, 2.8% in the Midwest, 2.1% in the West, and 1.3% in the Northwest. Smokeless tobacco use was far more prevalent in the rural areas than in urban areas.

Think Twice About "Chewing"

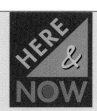

Dear Readers:

What follows is an edited version of an article by Susan Miller Degnan, a newspaper reporter for the *Miami Herald.* It was sent to me [Ann Landers] by an 84-year-old fan in Harlingen, Texas, who urged me to "keep up the good work." I hope you will be as moved by it as I was. Here it is:

There may never have been a quieter time in the 117-year history of the Philadelphia Phillies than when Rick Bender, a longtime sandlot ballplayer, walked into their clubhouse in early March with the U.S. Surgeon General.

Bender's face—what was left of it—jolted the Phillies so much that when they took the field that day, not a single cheek was filled with tobacco."

"Put it this way," said Bender, 31, a beekeeper in Montana, "I have a face you will never forget.

Half a jaw. Partial tongue. Cavernous neck. Three remaining teeth. And scars he can't help but cut when he shaves the few hairs that still grow after radiation treatments. It took four operations to halt the mouth cancer doctors attributed to Bender's daily use of two cans of finely ground tobacco snuff, also known as dip, which he packed between his lower lip and gum.

"He scared me out of the chimney," said pitcher Terry Mulholland, who dipped for 17 years. "I thought, 'I'm 30 years old. It's time to grow up.'"

If major league baseball had its way, it would sever the growth at its roots. Smoking, dipping, and chewing tobacco neither promote physical health nor portray a wholesome image for young people who idolize athletes.

Mulholland quit dipping, but his teammates couldn't last. By the ninth inning, cheeks were bulging.

Smokeless tobacco has been linked to baseball since the game's rules were roughed out in 1845. It was as easy to spit on the baseball field as on the corn field. Still is. A 1988 study funded by the National Cancer Institute found that 40 percent of pro players dip or chew, a figure that dwarfs use in other sports.

Dipping half a tin of snuff daily is like inhaling 30 to 40 cigarettes. The nicotine is so addictive that it has been compared to heroin.

Along with alcohol and cigars, Babe Ruth chewed vigorously and dipped. He even snorted snuff and was advised to stop because of impacted nasal passages. Ruth continued to do it all and died of throat cancer in 1948. He was 53.

"A tobacco ban in baseball?" Pirates manager Jim Leyland responded with a cigar dangling from his mouth. "It's ridiculous, a total invasion of privacy. We have a lot of other things we should be paying attention to rather than telling some poor SOB he can't put chew in his mouth."

And now this is Ann talking: I hope every baseball player who uses smokeless tobacco will take this seriously. Youngsters look up to you and think everything you do is cool. Do you want to be responsible for some kid ending up like Rick Bender? Please think about it.

Other adverse medical reactions can result from an addiction to smokeless tobacco as illustrated by the following: In April 1997, Mets baseball pitcher Pete Harnisch was removed from a weekend start because he was not "mentally" prepared to pitch (The Associated Press, 8 April 1997). Harnisch was placed on a 15-day disabled list by the New York Mets after having quit cold turkey his 13-year addiction to smokeless tobacco products on March 19.

After quitting, the major symptoms he experienced were night sweats, shakes, raw nerves, edginess, sleep deprivation, and shaking that lasted the day prior to his medical removal from pitching. Harnisch's physician said that his symptoms were common of tobacco withdrawal. ■

Source: Susan Miller Degnan, *Miami Herald,* 9 October 1993: Living Section.

Figure 12.5

Per Capita Consumption of Tobacco Products, 1981–1991

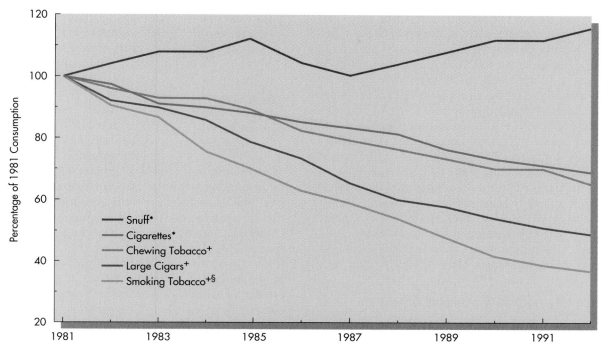

Notes: (*) Per person 18 and over. (+) Per male 18 and over. (§) Smoking tobacco = pipe, roll-your-own, and small cigars.

Source: U.S. Department of Agriculture. *Tobacco Situation and Outlook Report.* U.S. Department of Agriculture, Economic Research Service, TS-223, 1993.

Among adults, there were approximately equal numbers of snuff and chewing tobacco users. Daily use was more prevalent for snuff users than for users of chewing tobacco. The type of smokeless product varied considerably by age. Generally, younger users (18–44 years old) were more likely to take snuff, while older users (45 years and older) were more likely to choose chewing tobacco. Many smokeless tobacco users also smoked cigarettes. Among current users, 22.9% were also current smokers and 33.3% were former users.

Unlike cigarette consumption, which has been steadily declining, consumption of moist snuff has increased markedly for many years; indeed, it is the only product whose use is increasing. Consumption of moist snuff in the United States tripled between 1972 and 1991. In addition, increased restrictions on cigarette smoking in public places and the workplace have motivated some smokers to switch to moist snuff.

Significant changes in the demographics have been noted among smokeless tobacco users since 1970. Although black men of all ages and older white men (45 years and older) have decreased their use of smokeless tobacco, use among white men aged 18–44 years has increased nearly fivefold (Giovino et al. 1994). Smokeless tobacco use among older women (45 years and older) also decreased markedly, although use among black women remains high.

How safe are smokeless tobacco products compared with cigarettes? A study conducted by the University of Southern California found that taking one pinch of snuff has effects equivalent to those derived from smoking three or four cigarettes. The likelihood of getting oral cancer increases significantly for anyone who uses smokeless tobacco daily for 3.5 years or longer (Perry 1990, 20–23; USDHHS 1995) (see "Here and Now," page 312). Other evidence has shown that continued use of smokeless products can cause cancer of the pharynx and esophagus. The incidence of developing these cancers is related to the duration of use and the type of product used because "long-term snuff users have a 50% greater risk of developing oral cancer than nonusers" ("Smokeless Tobacco" 1990). Other, less serious effects of using smokeless tobacco include severe inflammation of gum tissue, tooth decay, and receding gums and tooth loss ("Smokeless Tobacco" 1990; Giovino et al. 1994).

In response to these developments, Congress enacted the Comprehensive Smokeless Tobacco Health Education Act of 1986. It requires rotation of three health warnings on smokeless tobacco packages and advertisements and bans smokeless tobacco advertising on broadcasting media (see Table 12.2).

Secondhand and Sidestream Smoke

Cigarette smoke drawn through the mouthpiece and inhaled directly from a cigarette is classified as **mainstream smoke** (MS). **Sidestream smoke** (SS), or second-hand smoke, refers to the smoke that comes directly from the lighted tip of a cigarette between puffs. **Passive smoking** (PS) refers to nonsmokers' inhalation of tobacco smoke. In addition, the term **environmental tobacco smoke** (ETS) is used to refer to the mixture of predominantly sidestream smoke and exhaled mainstream smoke that is inhaled by the passive smoker (USDHHS 1994).

Studies of smoking and its effects have directed increased attention to sidestream smoke because the burning tobacco smoke that pollutes the air is breathed in by smokers and nonsmokers alike. This type of smoke contains much higher concentrations of some irritating and hazardous substances—such as carbon monoxide, nicotine,

> **mainstream smoke**
> the smoke drawn directly through the mouthpiece of a cigarette
>
> **sidestream smoke**
> smoke released into the air from a lighted cigarette

> **passive smoking**
> nonsmoker's inhalation of tobacco smoke
>
> **environmental tobacco smoke**
> the mixture of predominantly sidestream smoke and exhaled mainstream smoke that is inhaled by the passive smoker

and ammonia—than inhaled mainstream smoke. Because it contains more particles of smaller diameter, sidestream smoke is therefore more likely to be deposited deep in the lungs (Bartecchi et al. 1995).

A U.S. news telecast reported that secondhand smoke kills 50,000 nonsmokers yearly (*CBS Evening News* 1994). If several people smoke in an enclosed area, the carbon monoxide (CO) level may exceed the safe limit recommended by the Environmental Protection Agency (EPA). Under conditions of heavy smoking and poor ventilation, high concentrations of CO can occur from sidestream smoke. CO gas is not removed by most standard air filtration systems. It can be diluted only by increasing ventilation with fresh air containing low levels of CO. Formation of CO can be reduced by increasing the amount of oxygen available during the burning of the tobacco. This goal can be achieved by using perforated cigarette paper and perforated filtertips. Regular and small cigars produce more CO than cigarettes because the tobacco leaf wrapper reduces the amount of oxygen available at the burning zone. The levels of CO created by smokers may cause nonsmokers with coronary disease to have angina attacks.

◢ Who Smokes?

Given what we know today about the effects of smoking, it's hard to understand why people smoke. Lifetime users are understandably addicted; quitting is hard. Following are some statistics that describe who is smoking:

1. In 1994, an estimated 60 million Americans were current smokers. This number gives a smoking rate of 29% for the population age 12 and older.

2. Current smokers are more likely to be heavy drinkers and illicit drug users. Among smok-

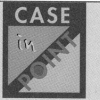

Youth and Smoking

By age 18, nearly two-thirds of adolescents in the United States have tried smoking. The overall national prevalence of current smoking (that is, individuals who have smoked within the last 30 days) for persons aged 12–18 years was estimated at 16% in 1989 (USDHHS 1994). Among high school seniors, the prevalence of past-month smoking was 28% in 1992.

The following sociodemographic findings relate to adolescent smoking (also see Figure 12.6 regarding the effects of various influences on the likelihood of smoking for 11–19-year-olds):

▲ Youths aged 12–16 years who are current smokers are almost twice as likely to be home without a parent or other adult for ten or more hours per week than teens who never smoked.

▲ Teens who smoke are more likely to be socially distant from their parents or guardians.

▲ High school seniors growing up on a farm or in the country are more likely to smoke than those growing up in large cities.

▲ As the likelihood of having smoked in the past month increases, the quality of school performance decreases. Other factors that are fre-

quently linked to such youth include increased consumption of other licit and illicit drugs, school truancy, dysfunctional families, crime-related behavior, and unprotected sex.

▲ Four-year college/university-bound seniors are less likely to smoke than high school seniors not planning to further their education at a college or university.

▲ Males planning to enter the armed forces after high school are more likely to be past-month smokers.

▲ Seniors who are less religiously inclined are more likely to be smokers.

▲ Male students who left school before graduating are more than twice as likely to report smoking the past week. Female students who dropped out are less likely to smoke than male dropouts (33% versus 52%).

▲ White dropouts are more likely to smoke than black dropouts (46% versus 17%).

▲ Tobacco use among adolescence is associated with a range of health-compromising behaviors, including being involved in fights, carrying weapons, engaging in higher-risk sexual behavior, and using alcohol and other drugs. ■

ers, the rate of heavy alcohol use (five or more drinks on five or more days in the past month) was 14% and the rate of current illicit drug use was 13%. Among nonsmokers, only 3% were heavy drinkers and 3% were illicit drug users. (More detail about smoking and licit and illicit drug use will be discussed in the section, "Tobacco as a Gateway Drug.")

3. Approximately 4.5 million youths aged 12–17 were current smokers in 1995; the rate of smoking among this group was 20%—up from 18.9% in 1994. The current rate of smoking was highest in the 18–25-year-old age group (35%) and the 26–34-year-old

group (32%). The smoking rate was 28% among adults age 35. (See the Case in Point box, "Youth and Smoking," for greater detail.)

4. In regards to smoking and racial and/or ethnic ancestry, no significant differences in smoking rates were found. With smokeless tobacco, however, use was more prevalent among whites (3.9%) than among blacks (1.3%) or Hispanics (1.2%). In considering gender, adult men had somewhat higher rates of smoking than adult women, but smoking rates for 12–17-year-olds showed no differences between males and females (USDHHS 1996).

Figure 12.6

The Effects of Various Influences on the Likelihood of Smoking (11- to 19-year-olds)

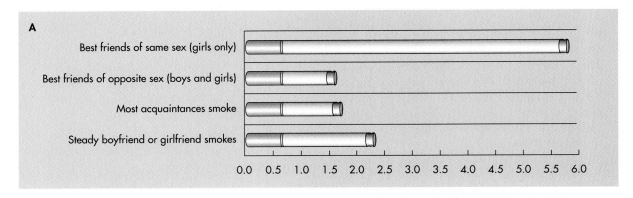

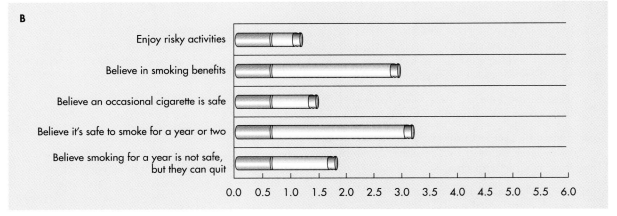

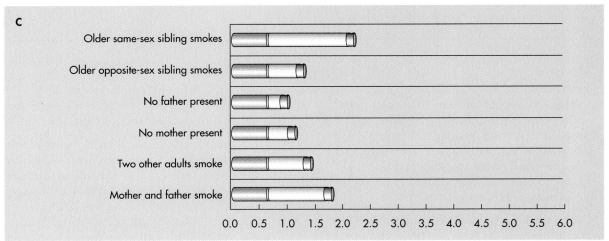

The figures show the odds that a teenager with a particular characteristic is a current smoker. The odds are based on a comparison to a hypothetical 15-year-old white non-Hispanic teen with no family members or friends who smoke, who thinks an occasional cigarette is dangerous, and that smoking offers no benefits. The likelihood of smoking for this hypothetical teen is 1.85%. The first box shows that a female teen whose best friends smoke is nearly six times as likely as the baseline teen to smoke.

Source: Attitudes and Practices Survey (TAPS). Atlanta, GA: Centers for Disease Control, 1995.

5. Similar and other findings are shown in Table 12.3, which describes past-month use of cigarettes by age groups, race/ethnicity, and sex for the period 1985–1995. Since 1985, cigarette use has been steadily declining, except for 1994 and 1995, when the percentages remained relatively stable. Whites have the highest past-month smoking rate (29.7%), while blacks have the second highest rate (28.1%), and Hispanics have the third highest rate (24.7%) (SAMHSA 1996). In addition, past-month use of cigarettes is higher for males (31.0%) than for females (26.8%).

6. Level of educational attainment was correlated with tobacco usage. While national health surveys have found that gender, educa-

tion, and race and ethnicity strongly affect the likelihood of smoking, researchers believe that educational achievement levels are better predictors of smoking than gender (Pierce et al. 1989). Approximately 38% of adults who had not completed high school were current smokers, while only 16% of college graduates smoked (SAMHSA 1996).

Reasons for Smoking

Nicotine dependency through cigarette smoking is not only the most common form of drug addiction, but the one that causes more deaths and disease than all other addictions combined (USDHHS 1994, 34). Tobacco use continues

---

Table 12.3 Past-Month Use of Cigarettes, by Age Group, Race/Ethnicity, and Sex: 1985–1995

Demographic Characteristics	1985	1988	1990	1991	1992	1993	1994	1995
Total	38.7†	35.3†	32.6	33.0*	31.9	29.6	28.6	28.8
Age Group								
12–17	29.4*	22.7	22.4	20.9	18.4	18.5	18.9	20.2
18–25	47.4†	45.6†	40.9	41.7	41.5	37.9	34.6	35.3
26–34	45.7†	42.1*	42.4*	37.3	38.2	34.2	32.4	34.7
≥35	35.5*	32.4	28.9	31.6	30.0	28.2	27.9	27.2
Race/Ethnicity								
White	38.9†	35.2*	33.6	33.5	32.8	30.3	29.4	29.7
Black	38.0†	34.2	29.9	31.2	29.8	26.2	28.4	28.1
Hispanic	40.0†	35.6†	28.5	33.6†	29.2	29.0	25.8	24.7
Other	—	—	25.7	28.0	25.4	27.6	20.5	23.5
Sex								
Male	43.4†	39.5†	36.0*	35.2	34.1	32.2	31.5	31.0
Female	34.5†	31.4*	29.4	31.1*	30.0	27.3	26.0	26.8

Note: The population distributions for the 1993, 1994, and 1995 NHSDAs are post-stratified to population projections of totals based on the 1990 decennial census. NHSDAs from 1985 through 1992 used projections based on the 1980 census. The change from one census base to another has little effect on estimated percentages reporting drug use, but may have significant effect on estimates of number of drug users in some subpopulation groups.
Estimates for 1985 through 1993 may differ from estimates for these survey years that were published in other NHSDA reports. The estimates shown here for 1985 through 1993 have been adjusted to improve their comparability with estimates based on the new version of the NHSDA instrument that was fielded in 1994 and subsequent NHSDAs.
Because of the methodology used to adjust the 1985 through 1993 estimates, some logical inconsistency may exist between estimates for a given drug within the same survey year. For example, some adjusted estimates of past-year use may appear to be greater than adjusted lifetime estimates. These inconsistencies tend to be small, rare, and not statistically significant.
(*) Difference between estimate and 1995 estimate is statistically significant at the 0.05 level.
(†) Difference between estimate and 1995 estimate is statistically significant at the 0.01 level.
(—) Low precision; no estimate reported.
Source: Substance Abuse and Mental Health Services Administration (SAMHSA), Office of Applied Studies, National Household Survey on Drug Abuse (NHSDA).

despite the fact that, since the 1960s, medical research and government assessments have clearly proved that smoking leads to premature death.

If you were to ask tobacco users why they smoke, their answers would be quite similar:

1. It's relaxing.

2. It decreases the unpleasant effects of tension, anxiety, and anger.

3. It satisfies the craving.

4. It's a habit.

5. I do it for the stimulation, increased energy, and arousal.

6. I like manipulating objects that have become satisfying habits (the cigarette, pipe, and so on).

In addition,

7. Female high school students (34%) smoke to lose weight (Rovner 1991; Wentz 1993, 127).

8. Nicotine functions as a mild tranquilizer moderating anxious or aggressive moods (Krough 1992).

9. Parents and/or siblings smoke (Rovner 1991; Wentz 1993, 127).

10. A close friend or boyfriend/girlfriend smokes (USDHHS 1994, 137).

Tobacco use fosters dependence for a number of reasons:

1. The habit can be rapidly and frequently reinforced by inhaling tobacco smoke (about 10 reinforcements per cigarette, or 200 with one pack).

2. The rapid metabolism and clearance of nicotine allows frequent and repeated use, which is encouraged by the rapid onset of withdrawal symptoms.

3. Smoking has complex pharmacological effects, both central and peripheral, that may satisfy a variety of the smoker's needs.

4. Some groups offer psychological and social rewards for use, especially the peer groups of young people.

5. Smoking patterns can be generalized; that is, the smoker becomes conditioned to continue smoking with other activities. For example, some smokers feel the need to smoke after a meal, when driving, and so on.

6. Smoking is reinforced by both pharmacological effects and ritual.

7. There is no marked performance impairment; in fact, smoking enhances performance in some cases. (Nicotine produces a state of alertness, prevents deterioration of reaction time, and improves learning.)

These reasons may not only explain why people continue to smoke, but also reveal why it is hard for them to stop. For example, only some 10% to 15% of current alcohol drinkers are considered problem drinkers, but approximately 85% to 90% of cigarette smokers consider themselves to be addicted to nicotine (USDHHS 1994).

Smokers appear to regulate their intake of nicotine. For example, the smoker of a low-nicotine cigarette is likely to smoke more and inhale more deeply. The average one-pack-a-day smoker is estimated to self-administer 7500 pulses (one pulse per inhalation) of nicotine to specific nicotinic receptors in the brain per year. This rate greatly surpasses the stimulation rate of any other known form of substance abuse. A habit that is reinforced as frequently and easily as smoking is very hard to break.

Other factors responsible for creating the addiction to nicotine are:

1. Cigarettes are relatively inexpensive; a pack-a-day habit costs less than an hour's work at the federal minimum wage level.

2. Cigarettes are readily available.

3. No equipment other than a lighter or match is needed.

4. Cigarettes are portable and easy to store.

5. Cigarettes are legal for individuals over age 18.

6. Other rewarding behaviors can occur while smoking (for example, drinking, socializing, and eating).

An incident that happened as Synanon, a treatment program for heroin addicts, illustrates how powerfully addictive the smoking habit is. Synanon policy dictates that addicts cannot use any drugs while being rehabilitated. In 1970,

Synanon decided to ban cigarettes because of their cost and because they seemed to serve as a crutch for people getting off other drugs. About 100 people left and chose possible readdiction to hard drugs rather than stay at Synanon without cigarettes. Residents of Synanon noted that the withdrawal symptoms for tobacco lasted much longer than those for other drugs, and they believed it was easier to quit heroin than cigarettes!

Relapse or Readdiction

Whenever I go back to smoking after having stopped for several months, I would always convince myself that I could easily stop again and that my health would be fine if I only had one to three cigarettes per day. Now that I think back, I realize that I am probably a life-addicted person. I'm a lifer! Don't let anyone kid you: Nicotine is really a "hardcore" drug, and it's horribly addictive.

From Venturelli's research files, interview with a 53-year-old male, May 18, 1991

Relapse or readdiction to tobacco can result if the ex-smoker does not use smoking cessation aids after overcoming nicotine withdrawal symptoms during the first few weeks of abstinence. Various internal and external stimuli may serve as triggers for craving or withdrawal symptoms. Stressful situations—such as an argument with a spouse, encounters with friends who smoke, and various types of social events—may prompt a response similar to withdrawal. This reaction sets the stage for readdiction.

The Motivation Not to Smoke

When habitual smokers stop smoking on their own, without the use of smoking cessation aids, they may experience a variety of unpleasant withdrawal effects, including craving for tobacco, irritability, restlessness, sleep disturbances, gastrointestinal disturbances, anxiety, and impaired concentration, judgment, and psychomotor performance (see "Finding a Balnce," page 321). The intensity of withdrawal effects may be mild, moderate, or severe; it is not always correlated with the amount smoked. One interview revealed the following:

Quitting is very hard once you're addicted to nicotine. In a London subway, I once saw a sign that said, "Addiction to nicotine is worse than addiction to heroin." At the time I first read this sign, I thought it was a complete exaggeration. But now, eight years later, I am convinced it's true.

From Venturelli's research files, interview with a 53-year-old male, May 18, 1991

The onset of nicotine withdrawal symptoms may occur within hours or days after quitting and may persist from a few days to several months. Frustration over these symptoms leads many people to start smoking again (Cook et al. 1990; Schelling 1992). As the same interviewee stated:

Whenever I quit smoking, I go through weeks of anguish and craving for just one more cigarette. Yeah, quitting is really tough, especially during the first few days. The desire to smoke is very strong at first. But then slowly, ever so so slowly, the craving begins to fade. After three months, the worst is over. Yet, even after a year, you can suddenly think of how great it would be to have just one cigarette.

Research shows that smoking cessation should be a gradual process, as this type of withdrawal eliminates the severe symptoms of craving for nicotine. According to the National Institute on Drug Abuse (NIDA), "rates of relapse are highest in the first few weeks and months and diminish considerably after three months" (NIDA 1995). (See Figure 12.7.) The optimal treatment for smoking cessation will also include behavioral therapies (NIDA 1995). Behavioral modification treatments report 33% long-term abstinence with 50% recidivism. "Studies have shown that pharmacological treatment combined with psychological treatment, including psychological support and skill training to overcome high-risk situations, result in some of the highest long-term abstinence rates" (NIDA 1995).

In 1993, an estimated 48 million adults were former smokers. Successful cessation was higher among men (52%), whites (52%), and people living at or above the poverty level (52%), and increased proportionally with age. In terms of

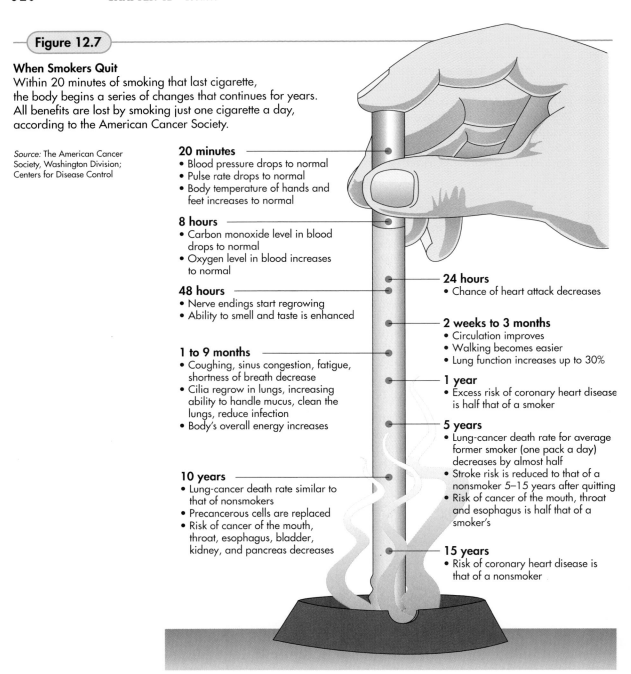

Figure 12.7

When Smokers Quit
Within 20 minutes of smoking that last cigarette,
the body begins a series of changes that continues for years.
All benefits are lost by smoking just one cigarette a day,
according to the American Cancer Society.

Source: The American Cancer
Society, Washington Division;
Centers for Disease Control

20 minutes
• Blood pressure drops to normal
• Pulse rate drops to normal
• Body temperature of hands and
  feet increases to normal

8 hours
• Carbon monoxide level in blood
  drops to normal
• Oxygen level in blood increases
  to normal

48 hours
• Nerve endings start regrowing
• Ability to smell and taste is enhanced

1 to 9 months
• Coughing, sinus congestion, fatigue,
  shortness of breath decrease
• Cilia regrow in lungs, increasing
  ability to handle mucus, clean the
  lungs, reduce infection
• Body's overall energy increases

10 years
• Lung-cancer death rate similar to
  that of nonsmokers
• Precancerous cells are replaced
• Risk of cancer of the mouth,
  throat, esophagus, bladder,
  kidney, and pancreas decreases

24 hours
• Chance of heart attack decreases

2 weeks to 3 months
• Circulation improves
• Walking becomes easier
• Lung function increases up to 30%

1 year
• Excess risk of coronary heart disease
  is half that of a smoker

5 years
• Lung-cancer death rate for average
  former smoker (one pack a day)
  decreases by almost half
• Stroke risk is reduced to that of a
  nonsmoker 5–15 years after quitting
• Risk of cancer of the mouth, throat
  and esophagus is half that of a
  smoker's

15 years
• Risk of coronary heart disease is
  that of a nonsmoker

education levels, the prevalence of cessation was lowest among persons with 9–11 years of education (Massachusetts Medical Society 1994).

When relapse rates for heroin users, cigarette smokers, and alcoholics were plotted in a graph, the curves indicating the relapse percentages over a one-year period were virtually identical. These data were taken from people who sought treatment, however. Heroin users and alcoholics who quit drugs on their own have much higher success rates.

Each year, approximately 17 million people try to quit their smoking habit for at least a day during the American Cancer Society's Great

Early Nicotine Addiction and Cessation

The state of Virginia is cigarette territory, and it's fair to say that Richmond is filled with a cloudy air of acceptance with the behavior of smoking, especially for teenagers. High schools are typically filled with hormones, rebellious tempers, and peer pressure. It was the latter factor that influenced Claire, a native of Richmond, to start smoking at age 15. In an effort to make friends with a girl who was popular in school and, in turn, become more popular herself, Claire lit her first cigarette. After a few coughs, she took to it immediately. Knowing that her parents wouldn't approve, she kept her secret from them as best she could. "I would open my bedroom window and blow the smoke outside, and then spray myself with perfume," she says. "Looking back now, I'm sure they knew. How could they not?"

In high school, Claire would smoke about two packs a week. Today, at age 36, she smokes about that many cigarettes per day, although she typically lights up, then walks around, and comes back to find that half the cigarette has turned to ashes. For the first time since she first started to inhale, Claire is now thinking of quitting. She quit once before, she admits with a slight laugh—for about four hours. "It was so hard." She explains, "You know it's not good, you know it's not healthy, but let's face it, it's addictive. There is a certain fear in letting go, a fear of the unknown." When asked about the allegations that cigarette companies covertly added more addictive chemicals to their products, a trace of anger can be heard in her voice. "God, it would have been so much easier to quit if that wasn't the case, but I have got to tell you, no one made me start smoking."

Today there are tremendous social pressures to limit smoking, particularly in public buildings such as airports. Claire, who hates to fly, found herself recently on a plane headed to California to attend a family wedding. With a layover in Dallas, she thought she would have time for a cigarette, but she soon discovered that she would have to pass through airport security to light up outside. Being short on time, she resorted to an old high school behavior and lit up in the women's room, unfazed by the airport regulations. Any thoughts about quitting smoking quickly surrendered to her fear of flying. Fear is a common emotion in Claire's life, and one often associated with the behavior of lighting up. Recently, however, her desire to quit smoking has grown much stronger.

The first step in modifying behavior is the initiation of a desire to change, followed by a conscious decision to make a change. Next, the individual actually follows through with a new behavior via a substitution. The final step is evaluating the entire process to see what gains, if any, have been made. Health behaviorists know that no successful attempt to change a behavior such as cigarette smoking can begin until there is a desire to do so. As is often the case, the embers of desire are often extinguished by the flooding waters of fear. In Claire's case, however, the feelings of fear are ebbing with the passing of each day. Desire to change is in the air.

Adding to this desire is a different kind of pressure, coming from her three boys. "School drills it into them about the dangers of cigarette smoking and drug abuse, and this [message] comes home on a regular basis." Her eldest son (age 10) often challenges her by saying, "If you quit smoking, I'll start working out." As she reflects on the impact that her behavior might have on the boys, her desire to quit grows even stronger.

"I think about it every day. I think about it every morning when I get up, and every night when I go to bed, and several times in between." A number of factors have pulled Claire toward this way of thinking—most importantly, the effect that this behavior might have on the health of her three children. She wants her kids to be physically active, and hopes that they take up sports when they become older. She fears that her smoking habit may impair their health and performance, something she doesn't want. Claire has thought about both hypnosis and nicotine patches. "I only know of one person who has had success with hypnosis, but several people who have tried the patch with great success."

The seeds of behavioral change have been planted. Although no specific goal has been set nor a specific date selected, Claire is confident that one day she will no longer have the urge to light up a cigarette.

American Smokeout. Of these quitters, more than 4 million still abstain from smoking after three months. Nearly 90% of those who have tried to quit attempt to do so on their own by either stopping "cold turkey" or using other methods that will be discussed later in this chapter.

Alternative Activities for Successfully Quitting

The American Cancer Society has developed a list of alternative activities that the new ex-smoker might try as aids to get through the withdrawal period. When the craving for a cigarette arises, the smoker may engage in these behaviors:

▲ Nibble on fruit, celery, or carrots.

▲ Chew gum or spices such as ginger, cinnamon bark, or cloves.

▲ Use replacements in conjunction with quitting smoking, such as the nicotine patch or nicotine gum. (Such cessation smoking aids will be discussed in greater detail in the next section.)

▲ Perform moderately strenuous physical activity, such as bicycling, jogging, or swimming (if the person's heart and lungs are not too badly damaged from smoking).

▲ Spend as much time as possible in places where smoking is prohibited, such as movie theaters, libraries, and other smoke-free environments.

▲ Use mouthwash after each meal.

▲ Associate with nonsmokers for long periods of time.

We add two tips from personal experience (Venturelli):

▲ Chew or slowly dissolve sugarless minted candy during the entire day.

▲ Get rid of the drug paraphernalia, such as ashtrays and lighters. (The seriousness of the ex-smoker's intentions can often be gauged by how willing the individual is to give up an expensive ashtray, cigarette box, or engraved lighter.)

Smoking Cessation Aids

At the end of World War II, three-quarters of young men smoked; the fraction is now less than a third and going down. (Schelling 1992)

The number of cigarette-smoking adults dropped from 42% of the population in 1965 to 25% in 1993 (American Cancer Society). There is no one "right" way to quit this habit. Successful cessation may include one or a combination of methods, including using step-by-step manuals, attending self-help classes or counseling, or using nicotine replacement therapy. A number of stop smoking aids are currently available, such as those discussed below.

Nicotine Gum Besides self-help books, acupuncture, "cold turkey" techniques, hypnosis, and self-help with behavioral modification (for further details on these methods, see Table 12.4), Nicorette, a nicotine chewing gum, is now available without a prescription. The purpose of this gum is to lessen the craving desire for nicotine by substituting the gum for a cigarette so that small amounts of nicotine can be absorbed in the mouth's lining and into the bloodstream (Ricks 1996, B1; Krough 1992; American Cancer Society).

Nicotine Patches The 24-hour transdermal nicotine patch was introduced to the public in January 1992. Popularly known as the "nicotine patch" or

A transdermal patch, an example of a recent popular remedy for quitting smoking.

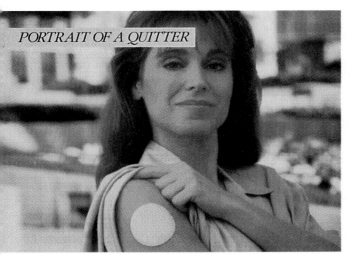

PORTRAIT OF A QUITTER

Table 12.4	**Kicking the Habit** To wean oneself from cigarettes means denying the central nervous system a substance that induces pleasure. There are a variety of methods to break the habit, but experts say wanting to break the habit is half the battle.

Method	Description	Duration	Pros/Cons
Acupuncture Cost: About $200 but depends on program.	Needles are placed primarily in the scalp and ears to stimulate production of enkephalins, the chemical messengers found at nerve endings. These chemicals have a morphine-like effect on the brain and theoretically override desire for nicotine.	From one month to six weeks. Patients come in once a week for a treatment. Relaxation tapes also are used.	Some people have an aversion to needles. But if patients can stomach it, the technique is 80% successful, practitioners say.
Cold turkey Cost: None	The oldest method of breaking the smoking habit involves giving up cigarettes altogether.	Can take a week for some people, months for others. The time it takes to break the habit depends on how often the smoker "sneaks" a cigarette.	Because of a lack of supervision, there is often a tremendous desire to smoke, and each cigarette enhances the desire for nicotine. The technique can be 100% successful for individuals. There have been no studies conducted on this method versus medically supervised techniques.
Hypnosis Cost: $50 to $100 per session.	The smoker is hypnotized to enhance the power of suggestion.	Some people need just a single session, while others need more.	National studies have not established the effectiveness of hypnosis. Smokers who have tried the technique often turn to medically supervised nicotine patch or nicotine gum programs.
Nicotine gum Cost: $36.99 for 96 pieces of gum.	Smokers chew gum laced with nicotine to replace the substance found in cigarettes. The gum is often offered as part of behavioral modification programs.	From 10 to 12 pieces of the prescription gum are recommended per day, with a maximum of 30. Each piece is chewed for 30 minutes. The program lasts 3–6 months.	There have been complaints about the taste and texture of the gum, which some say is like cardboard. The effectiveness rate is 40% to 50%.
Nicotine patch Cost: $56.99 for a two-week supply.	Smokers receive decreasing doses of nicotine from a patch that adheres to the body. A different patch is worn daily and is rotated to different parts of the body to prevent skin irritation.	Generally involves a six-week program in which patches with decreasing amounts of nicotine are worn.	The patch has to be worn faithfully. Some people will forget to put on a patch; others on occasion sneak a cigarette, defeating the purpose because the amount of nicotine is increased in the body. National studies place the overall effectiveness at 60%.
Self-help with behavioral modification Cost: $10 refundable deposit for a four-week program on how to quit.	The American Medical Association and the American Cancer Society offer a "How to Quit" program of audio- and video tapes. The program focuses on four areas: How to Keep My Mouth Busy; How to Keep My Hands Busy; Calm My Nerves; and Focus My Concentration.	A four-week program.	The success of the program depends largely on the smoker's desire to quit. It is endorsed by the AMA and the ACS because it changes the smoker's need to have a cigarette. AMA studies show that the program is more effective than behavior modification alone.

Source: D. Ricks. "What a Drag: How Nicotine Gets Its Hammerlock on Users." *Salt Lake Tribune* 251 (21 March 1996): B1, B8.

A 1994 study by the University of Iowa showed that: (1) Two methods—hypnosis and acupuncture—worked well. Thirty-six percent of smokers using hypnosis and 30% who underwent acupuncture quit for approximately three months; (2) Sixteen percent of smokers using nicotine gum were not smoking three months later; (3) Smokers who were told verbally to quit without any other assistance had a 7% success rate after three months; and (4) The best smoking cessation aid was the nicotine patch, with a 60% success rate.

"the patch," it is marketed under the brand names Nicoderm and Habitrol.

The patch, which is directly applied and worn on the skin, releases a continuous flow of small doses of nicotine to quell the desire for cigarette-provided nicotine. The method of delivering nicotine to the skin reduces the withdrawal symptoms as the smoker attempts to quit. The prescription requirement for purchasing the nicotine patch was recently removed, and it is now sold as an over-the-counter drug.

Figure 12.8

Cigarette Marketing Expenditures

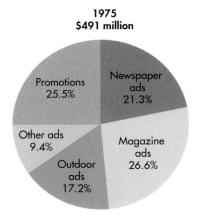

1975
$491 million

- Promotions 25.5%
- Newspaper ads 21.3%
- Other ads 9.4%
- Magazine ads 26.6%
- Outdoor ads 17.2%

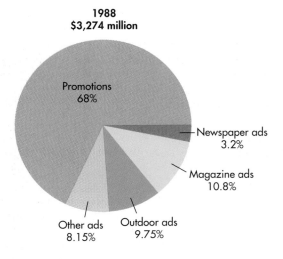

1988
$3,274 million

- Promotions 68%
- Newspaper ads 3.2%
- Magazine ads 10.8%
- Outdoor ads 9.75%
- Other ads 8.15%

Source: C. E. Bartecchi, T. D. MacKenzie, and R. W. Shrier. "The Global Tobacco Epidemic." *Scientific American* (May 1995): 49.

◢ Social Issues: Looking to the Future

If smoking is so unhealthy and everyone knows it, why is it so pervasive? In the following section, we will examine how expenditures by the tobacco industry promote the use of this drug.

Economic Interests

The tobacco industry spends approximately $4 billion each year on advertising (USDHHS 1994, 160), making cigarettes the second most promoted consumer product. In fact, when the total spent on print and billboard advertising is taken into account, the tobacco industry spends approximately $40 annually on every smoker in the United States.

In 1990, $435 billion was spent on outdoor advertising and transit posters for cigarettes (see Figure 12.8). Some 10% to 12% of the revenues generated by the tobacco industry went for advertising and promotional expenditures. Approximately $3 billion was spent for promotional activities, while an all-time low of $887 million was spent on advertising. Since 1971, print advertising expenditures have steadily declined (a 14% drop in magazine advertising and a 7% drop in newspaper advertising), primarily because of government bans (discussed earlier in the chapter).

The advertising campaigns invariably portray smokers as sexy, healthy, and adventurous, enjoying recreation and close relationships with lovers and friends. These themes are especially appealing to youth (Altman et al. 1987; USDHHS 1994). The *Journal of the American Medical Association* has reported that the "Joe Camel" cartoon character is as recognizable to 6-year-olds as the Mickey Mouse silhouette that denotes the Walt Disney Company. In fact, the character is even familiar to many 3-year-olds and is generally more identifiable to children than to adults, according to the research (see Figure 12.9).

As the consumption of cigarettes has declined in the United States, new markets abroad have expanded. Western nations like the United States and Canada have been fairly successful in broadcasting that the use of tobacco is hazardous to your health. In 1989, Canada introduced a ban on all tobacco advertising, sponsorship, and indirect advertising of Canadian origin (USDHHS 1994). Per capita consumption in primarily nonindustrialized Third World countries has steadily increased with the availability of tobacco produced in the United States.

American-brand cigarettes hold prestige for middle- and lower-class groups in many foreign societies. In India, for example, along with English cigarettes, U.S. cigarettes are considered superior in quality and are a status symbol for those who can afford to purchase such luxury items.

In some countries, such as China, approximately 90% of the male population smokes. Such nations represent an incredibly appealing market to U.S. cigarette manufacturers. Given the shrinking markets in the United States and most other modern industrialized nations, U.S. manufacturers feel compelled to look overseas for new revenues. They have found lucrative markets in many Third World nations. Tobacco sales are becoming stronger in certain foreign markets while becoming weaker in others.

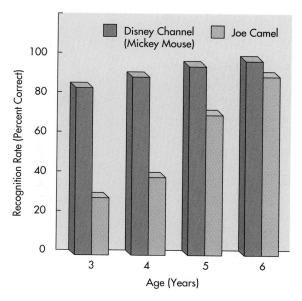

Figure 12.9

Recognition of Logos by Children

Tobacco as a Gateway Drug

Just recently, conclusive research findings have indicated that tobacco is more of a serious **gateway drug** than previously expected. For example, nearly all heroin addicts initially began using gateway drugs such as alcohol and/or tobacco products. (Granted, most people who drink alcohol and use tobacco do not become heroin addicts!)

> **gateway drugs**
>
> drugs whose use leads to the use of other drugs; alcohol, cigarettes, and marijuana are considered gateway drugs

Biochemical evidence proving that the use of gateway drugs leads to the abuse of others is weak.

> **patterns of behavior**
>
> consistent and related behaviors that occur together, such as marijuana use and euphoria, alcohol abuse, and intoxication

However, some findings are quite interesting. "The decisions to use tobacco or other gateway drugs set up **patterns of behavior** that make it easier for a user to go on to other

drugs" ("Non-Smoking Youth" 1991). In other words, smokers have developed the behavioral patterns that may lead them to experiment and use other licit and illicit drugs.

Research indicates that cigarette smokers are more likely to use alcohol, marijuana, and cocaine than are nonsmokers (Giovino et al. 1995, 55). Figure 12.10 shows a strong association between cigarette smoking and the use of illicit drugs and alcohol by 12- to 17-year-old smokers. "[I]n the 12- through 17-year-old group (Figure 12.10) . . . those who smoked daily were approximately 14 times more likely to have binged on alcohol, 114 times more likely to have used marijuana at least 11 times, and 32 times more likely to have used cocaine at least 11 times than those who had not smoked" (USDHHS 1994, 36). Other studies have shown similar relationships between cigarette smoking and the prevalence of other drug use. In addition, more smokable preparations are now available for various drugs such as cocaine (crack), methamphetamine (ice), phencyclidine (PCP),

Figure 12.10

Use of Illicit Drugs and Alcohol by 12- to 17-Year-Old Smokers and Nonsmokers, 1995

Source: Substance Abuse and Mental Health Services Administration (SAMHSA), Office of Applied Studies (OAS). *Preliminary Estimates from the 1995 National Household Survey on Drug Abuse,* Advance Report 18. Rockville, MD: NCADI, August 1996.

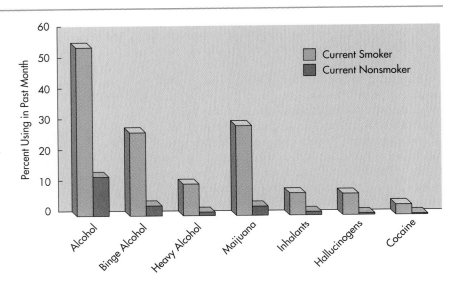

and heroin (USDHHS 1988, 38; USDHHS 1995). As smokers who become polydrug users report that tobacco is one of the first drugs they used, it is apparent that cigarette smoking skills can easily be transferred to other smokable drugs and may facilitate the process of experimenting with these drugs.

Smoking Prohibition Versus Smokers' Rights

In response to the percentage of the U.S. population that has effectively banned smoking from certain public facilities, people who desire to continue smoking have formed action groups to press their right to smoke. These groups have largely been organized by several tobacco companies. Through mailing lists, newsletters, and slick magazine promotions, the groups advocate and report on the following issues:

▲ How the rights of smokers have been eroded in public and private places

▲ How to write to members of Congress, and other political leaders, urging them to uphold smokers' rights

▲ How to lobby effectively for smoking in the workplace

▲ How the harmful effects of second-hand smoke have been exaggerated or remain unproven

▲ How people who enjoy smoking have won major battles, preserving their right to smoke

Although some modest gains have been made by these groups, the trend to restrict and ban cigarette smoking continues to be very strong. Antismoking groups have been highly successful in their own efforts.

Restrictions on the sale of cigarettes and tobacco products remain very strong. For example, an eight-state survey revealed that three-fourths of people (77%–86%) believed that stronger enforcement of minors' access laws would keep teens away from smoking. Most respondents (69%–77%) also believed that banning all cigarette machines would be an effective measure in achieving this goal (CDC 1996). Another recent national survey funded by the Robert Wood Johnson Foundation found that adults in the United States overwhelmingly support specific actions to make tobacco less accessible to minors. For example, 94% support ID verification by vendors selling to anyone appearing under-age, and 78% support keeping all tobacco products (including cigarette lighters!) behind counters to prevent shoplifting by minors.

In the recent past, efforts to reduce tobacco use focused on individual smoking cessation. This approach has resulted in only limited success. More recently, tobacco-use prevention and reduction efforts have relied on a public health or environmental approach. The environmental approach includes changing public policies regarding tobacco use. Today, prevention efforts focus on regulating the sale and use of tobacco and increasing taxes on tobacco products.

Smoke-Free Indoor Air The four primary aspects of tobacco control laws in each state are smoke-free indoor air, youth access to tobacco products, advertising of tobacco products, and excise taxes on tobacco products.

As of July 1995, 47 states required some variation of smoke-free indoor air. Forty-one states have laws restricting smoking in state government work sites. In contrast, only 21 state laws restrict smoking in private workplaces. Thirty-one states have laws that regulate smoking in restaurants, and some have laws that regulate smoking in other locations, such as day-care centers, hospitals, public transportation facilities, grocery stores, and enclosed arenas.

Youth Access to Tobacco A total of 32 states have enacted laws that prohibit the purchase, possession, or use of tobacco products by minors. Although no state has completely banned the sale of tobacco products through vending machines, none allows such sales to minors. In fact, 32 states have created additional restrictions intended to reduce youth access to vending machines. Twelve states ban the placement of vending machines in areas accessible to young persons and allow their placement only in bars, liquor stores, adult clubs, and other adult-oriented establishments.

Licensing Thirty-three state laws require some form of retail licensure for the sale of tobacco products.

Advertising Only nine states have laws restricting the advertising of tobacco products.

Taxing Cigarettes All states tax cigarettes. The average tax is 31.5 cents per pack, but ranges from 2.5 cents per pack in Virginia to 75 cents per pack in Michigan. In all states, the tax is a fixed amount, not a percentage of the price per pack. In addition, smokeless tobacco products are taxed in 42 states. Thus, statewide enforcement, preemptive legislation (legislation prohibiting any local jurisdiction from enacting reductions that are more stringent than the state law or restrictions that may vary from state law), court decisions, and federal legislation all influence and control the impact of state tobacco control legislation (CDC 1995).

In short, the willingness of nonsmokers to speak up as firmly as necessary against smoking and exposure to second-hand smoke has inspired restrictive legislation against tobacco use, which in turn affects smoking habits. As stated above, a complete network of laws defines, controls, and restricts smoking—from purchasing tobacco to the consumption of cigarettes or other types of tobacco products, such as smokeless and pipe tobacco, cigars, and the like.

Several organized groups of nonsmokers have made quite an impact, including Action on Smoking and Health (ASH), the Group Against Smokers' Pollution (GASP), the American Lung Association, the American Cancer Society, and medical and dental associations. These groups have been instrumental in passing legislation restricting or banning smoking in public places; banning cigarette commercials on television; and prohibiting smoking on commercial aircraft, interstate buses, and in some restaurants, elevators, indoor theaters, libraries, art galleries, and museums.

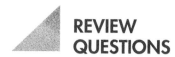

REVIEW QUESTIONS

1. If smoking is the most preventable cause of disease and premature death in the United States, why do people continue to smoke?

2. How effective are the health warning labels on cigarette packages? Interview two or three smokers about these warning labels.

3. List and define the diseases that cigarette smokers are most likely to contract.

4. What effects do cigarettes have on the fetus?

EXERCISES FOR THE WEB

Exercise 1:
Smoking From All Sides

The "Smoking From All Sides" web page is an attempt to discuss smoking in an unbiased fashion. Additional links to check out include "Health Aspects," "Tobacco History," "Pro-Smoking Documents," and "Smoking Glamour."

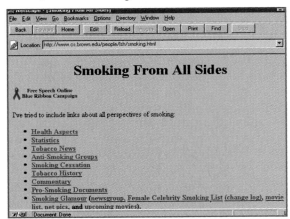

Exercise 2:
Nicotine and Tobacco Web Page

The "Nicotine and Tobacco" web page discusses issues related to smoking, tobacco and health. Startling statistics on the number of people a year who die from tobacco use is one such issue.

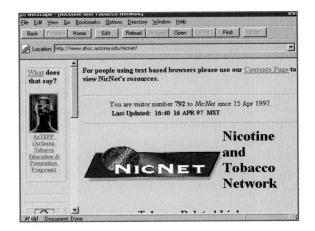

5. Why is smokeless tobacco perceived as safer than other forms of tobacco?

6. Who is more likely to smoke, and why?

7. Why do people who smoke become dependent on tobacco?

8. As tobacco markets in the United States have shrunk, what has happened abroad?

9. Why has the use of snuff dramatically increased since 1987?

10. Assess the major methods for quitting smoking. Which methods are most likely to succeed?

11. How is smoking related to the use of alcohol and illicit drug use?

12. Do you think smokers should have the right to smoke in public places? Explain.

KEY TERMS

Nicotiana tabacum
bright, flue-cured, or Virginia
puffing
nicotine
tobacco chewing
snuff dipping
eugenol
emphysema
sudden infant death syndrome (SIDS)
dipping snuff
chewing tobacco
snuff
snuffing
mainstream smoke
sidestream smoke
passive smoking

environmental tobacco smoke
gateway drug
patterns of behavior

SUMMARY

1 Nicotine is by far one of the most addictive drugs.

2 Approximately 29% of the U.S. population age 12 and older smokes; an additional 6.9 million Americans are users of smokeless tobacco.

3 The quality of leaf tobacco has changed throughout the years of production. Since 1956, the amount of leaf tobacco in a cigarette has declined by approximately 25%. Most cigarettes today are low-tar and low-nicotine types, and 90% are filtertips.

4 Nicotine is the substance in tobacco that causes dependence. This drug initially stimulates and then depresses the nervous system.

5 The amount of tobacco absorbed varies according to five factors: (a) the exact composition of tobacco being used; (b) how densely the tobacco is packed in the cigarette and the length of the cigarette smoked; (c) whether a filter is used and the characteristics of the filter; (d) the volume of the smoke inhaled; and (e) the number of cigarettes smoked throughout the day.

6 Cigarette smoking is an addiction that is costly in three ways: (a) 400,000 deaths in the United States are attributed to cigarette smoking; (b) in 1993, smoking-attributable costs for medical care totaled $50 billion; and (c) the American taxpayer pays $0.89 in medical care expenses for each pack of cigarettes smoked by others.

7 *Chewing tobacco* and *snuff* are types of smokeless tobacco products that are commonly referred to as "spit tobacco." Both types consist of tobacco leaves that are shredded and twisted into strands and then either chewed or placed in the cheek between the lower lip and gum.

8 Research clearly shows that the tar and nicotine content of cigarettes affect mortality rates. Cigarette smokers tend to die at an earlier age than nonsmokers. They also have a greater probability of contracting various illnesses, including types of cancers, chronic bronchitis and emphysema, diseases of the cardiovascular system, and peptic ulcers. In addition, smoking has adverse effects on pregnancy and may harm the fetus.

9 Cigarette smoke is classified as either *mainstream smoke* (MS), the smoke drawn directly through the mouthpiece of the cigarette, or *sidestream smoke* (SS). *Passive smoking* refers to nonsmokers' inhalation of tobacco smoke. The term *environmental tobacco smoke* (ETS) is widely used to refer to the mixture of predominantly SS and exhaled MS that is inhaled by the passive smoker.

10 By age 18, approximately two-thirds of adolescents in the United States have tried smoking. Among high school seniors, the prevalence of past-month smoking is 28%.

11 The primary methods for quitting smoking are step-by-step manuals, acupuncture, "cold turkey" techniques, hypnosis, nicotine gum, nicotine patches, and self-help with behavioral modification.

12 Current smokers are more likely to be heavy drinkers and illicit drug users than nonsmokers.

13 The four primary aspects of tobacco-control laws in each state are smoke-free indoor air, youth access to tobacco products, advertising of tobacco products, and excise taxes on tobacco products.

REFERENCES

Aldrich, L. "Tobacco Tax Increases Would Reduce Smoking." In *Smoking*, edited by K. L. Swisher, 28–30. San Diego, CA: Greenhaven Press, 1995.

Associated Press, 8 April 1997. Available from a1/chew.html

Altman, D. G., M. D. Slater, C. L. Albright, and N. Maccoby. "How an Unhealthy Product Is Sold: Cigarette Advertising in Magazines, 1960–1985." *Journal of Communication* 37 (1987): 95–106.

American Cancer Society. *Cancer Facts and Figures.* Atlanta, GA: American Cancer Society, 1990.

American Cancer Society. "Questions About Smoking, Tobacco, and Health . . . and the Answers." Available from www.cancer.org/smoking.html.

American Cancer Society. "Tobacco Use." March 1997. Available from www.cancer.org/tobacco.html.

American Cancer Society. *Cancer: Facts and Figures—1996.* Atlanta, GA: American Cancer Society, 1996.

Armitrage, A. K., C. T. Dollery, C. F. George, T. H. Houseman, P. J. Lewis, and P. M. Turner. "Absorption and Metabolism of Nicotine from Cigarettes." *British Medical Journal* 4 (1985): 313–6.

Austin, G. A. *Perspectives on the History of Psychoactive Substance Use.* Washington, DC: National Institute on Drug Abuse, 1978.

Bartecchi, C. E., T. D. MacKenzie, and R. W. Shrier. "The Global Tobacco Epidemic." *Scientific American* (May 1995): 49.

Benowitz, N. L. "Pharmacological Aspects of Cigarette Smoking and Nicotine Addiction." *New England Journal of Medicine* 319 (1988): 1318–30.

"Beware Those Spicy Cigarettes." *Consumer Reports* 50 (1985): 641.

Brownlee, S., and S. V. Roberts with M. Cooper, E. Goode, K. Hetter, and A. Wright. "Should Cigarettes Be Outlawed?" *U.S. News and World Report* (18 April 1994): 32–36, 38, 43.

Callahan, M. "How Smoking Kills You." *Parade Magazine* 213 (December 1987): 209–11.

CBS Evening News (8 February 1994), New York, NY.

Centers for Disease Control (CDC). "The Surgeon General's 1989 Report on Reducing The Health Consequence of Smoking: 25 Years of Progress (Executive Summary)." *Morbidity and Mortality Weekly Report* 38, Supplement 5-2 (1989): 1.

Centers for Disease Control and Prevention (CDC). CDC Surveillance Summaries. *Morbidity and Mortality Weekly Report* 44 (November 3, 1995).

Centers for Disease Control and Prevention (CDC). *Tobacco Sales to Youth.* Atlanta, GA: Centers for Disease Control and Prevention, Substance Abuse and Mental Health Services Administration, June 1996.

"Cigars." *Encyclopedia Americana.* Danbury, CT: Grolier, 1988.

Cook, P. S., R. C. Petersen, and D. T. Moore. "Alcohol, Tobacco, and Other Drugs May Harm the Unborn." Rockville, MD: U.S. Department of Health and Human Services, 1990.

Corti, E. C. *A History of Smoking.* London: Harrap and Company, 1931.

DeAngelis, T. "Behavior Is Included in Report on Smoking." *APA Monitor* 20, no. 3 (1989): 1, 4.

Degnan, S. M., *Miami Herald* (9 October 1993): Living Section.

Doweiko, H. E. *Concepts of Chemical Dependence,* 3rd ed. Pacific Grove, CA: Brooks/Cole, 1996.

"Facts About Smoking" [mimeographed fact sheet]. South Bend, IN: American Lung Association of Northern Indiana.

Fiore, M. C., T. E. Novotny, J. P. Pierce, E. J. Hatziandreau, K. M. Patel, and R. M. Davis. "Trends in Cigarette Smoking in the U.S.—The Changing Influence of Gender and Race." *Journal of the American Medical Association* 261 (January 1989): 49–56.

Fort, J. *The Pleasure Seekers.* Indianapolis: Bobbs-Merrill, 1969.

Foster, C. D., N. R. Jacobs, and M. A. Siegel, eds. *Illegal Drugs and Alcohol—America's Anguish.* Wylie, TX: Information Plus, 1989.

Giovino, G. A., J. E. Henningfield, S. L. Tambour, L. G. Escobedo, and J. Slade. "Epidemiology of Tobacco Use and Dependence." *Epidemiologic Reviews* 17 (1995): 48–65.

Giovino, G. A., M. W. Schooley, B. P. Zhu, J. H. Chrismon, S. L. Tambour, and J. P. Peddicord. "Trends and Recent Patterns in Selected Tobacco-Use Behaviors. Surveillance Summary." *Mortality and Morbidity Weekly Report* 43 (SS-3) (1994): 1–43.

Grabowski, H., and S. M. Hall, eds. *Pharmacological Adjuncts in Smoking Cessation.* Washington, DC: U.S. Government Printing Office, 1985.

Heimann, R. K. *Tobacco and Americans.* New York: McGraw-Hill, 1960.

Henning, R. I., R. T. Jones, and P. Fischman. "The Titration Hypothesis Revisited: Nicotine Gum Reduces Smoking Intensity." In *Pharmacological Adjuncts in Smoking Cessation,* NIDA Research Monograph 53, edited by J. Grabowski and S. M. Hall, 27–41. Rockville, MD: National Institute on Drug Abuse, 1985.

Indiana Prevention Resource Center. *Factline on: Tobacco.* Bloomington, IN: Trustees of Indiana University or the Indiana Division of Mental Health, 1995.

Jaffe, J. H., and M. Kanzler. "Smoking as an Addictive Disorder." In *Cigarette Smoking as a Dependence Process,* Research Monograph 23, edited by N. A. Krasnegor, 4–23. Washington, DC: National Institute on Drug Abuse, U.S. Department of Health, Education, and Welfare, 1979.

Krasnegor, N. A. "Introduction." In *The Behavioral Aspects of Smoking,* Research Monograph 26, edited by N. A. Krasnegor, 1–6. Washington, DC: National Institute on Drug Abuse, Department of Health, Education, and Welfare, 1979.

Krough, David. "Smoking—Why Is It So Hard to Quit? Priorities of the American Council on Science and Health," New York, NY (Spring 1992): 29–32.

Langton, P. A. *Drug Use and the Alcohol Dilemma.* Boston: Allyn and Bacon, 1991.

Liska, Ken. *Drugs and the Human Body.* New York: Macmillan, 1990.

Massachusetts Medical Society. "Health Objectives for the Nation: Cigarette Smoking Among Adults—United States, 1993." *Morbidity and Mortality Weekly Report* 43 (1994): 925–930.

National Institute on Drug Abuse (NIDA). *Cigarette Smoking.* CAP 42. Rockville, MD: National Institute on Drug Abuse, January 1995.

"Non-Smoking Youth Better Resist Other Drugs." *Prevention Newsline* 4, no. 3 (Spring 1991): 5.

O'Brien, R., S. Cohen, G. Evans, and J. Fine. *The Encyclopedia of Drug Abuse,* 2nd ed. New York: Facts on File and Greenspring, 1992.

Office of Smoking and Health, U.S. Department of Health and Human Services (USDHHS). *Reducing the Health Consequences of Smoking: 25 Years of Progress: A Report of the Surgeon General.* DHHS pub. no. (CDC) 89-8411. Washington, DC: USDHHS, 1989.

Palfai, T., and H. Jankiewicz. *Drugs and Human Behavior.* Dubuque, IA: Brown, 1991.

Perry, S. "Recognizing Everyday Addicts." *Current Health* 2, no. 16 (May 1990): 20–3.

Pierce, J. J., et al. "Trends in Cigarette Smoking in the United States—Educational Differences Are Increasing." *Journal of the American Medical Association* 261 (6 January 1989): 23–32.

Pomerleau, O. F. "Behavioral Factors in the Establishment, Maintenance, and Cessation of Smoking." In *The Behavioral Aspects of Smoking,* Research Monograph 26, edited by N. A. Krasnegor, 47–67. Washington, DC: National Institute on Drug Abuse, U.S. Department of Health, Education, and Welfare, 1979.

Ricks, D. "What a Drag: How Nicotine Gets Its Hammerlock on Users." *Salt Lake Tribune* 251 (21 March 1996): B1, B8.

Rovner, S. "Up in Smoke: Why Do So Many Kids Ignore All the Evidence Condemning Cigarettes?" *Washington Post,* National Weekly Edition (16–22 December 1991): 20–21.

Ryan, B. E. "Whole Lotta Smokin' Goin' On: Tobacco and Health." *The Prevention Pipeline* 7 (1994): 4–7.

Schelling, T. C. "Addictive Drugs: The Cigarette Experience." *Science* (24 January 1992): 430–3.

Schultes, R. E. "Ethnopharmacological Significance of Psychotropic Drugs of Vegetal Origin." In *Principles of Psychopharmacology,* 2nd ed., edited by W. G. Clark and J. del Giudice, 41–70. New York: Academic Press, 1978.

"Smokeless Tobacco, Think Before You Chew." Leaflet. Chicago, IL: American Dental Association, 1990.

Smolowe, J. "Stepping on Big Tobacco." *Time* 149, 30 June 1997, 24–29.

Stellman, S. D., and L. Garfinkel. "Smoking Habits and Tar Levels in a New American Cancer Society Prospective Study of 1.2 Million Men and Women." *Journal of the National Cancer Institute* 76 (1986): 1057–63.

Substance Abuse and Mental Health Services Administration (SAMHSA), Office of Applied Studies (OAS). *Preliminary Estimates from the 1995 National Household Survey on Drug Abuse,* Advance Report 18. Rockville, MD: NCADI (National Clearinghouse for Alcohol and Drug Information), August 1996.

Sullivan, L. "Nicotine Dependence." In *Drug Abuse and Drug Abuse Research. Third Triennial Report to Congress,* DHHS Publication No. (ADM) 91-1704. U.S. Department of Health and Human Services, 1991.

Taylor, P. "Ganglionic Stimulating and Blocking Agents." In *The Pharmacological Basis of Therapeutics,* 6th ed., edited by A. G. Gilman, L. S. Goodman, and A. Gilman, 211–9. New York: Macmillan, 1980.

Tobacco Institute. *About Tobacco Smoke.* Washington, DC: Tobacco Institute, 1982.

U.S. Department of Health and Human Services (USDHHS). *The Health Consequences of Smoking: Nicotine Addiction: A Report of the Surgeon General, 1988,* DHHS Publication No. (CDC) 88-8406. U.S. Department of Health and Human Services, Public Health Service, Centers for Disease Control, Center for Health Promotion and Education, Office on Smoking and Health, 1988.

———. *Preventing Tobacco Use Among Young People: A Report of the Surgeon General.* Atlanta, GA: U.S. Department of Health and Human Services, Public Health Service, Centers for Disease Control and Prevention, National Center for Chronic Disease Prevention and Health Promotion, Office on Smoking and Health, 1994.

———. *Tobacco-Control Activities in the United States, 1992–1993: Biennial Report to Congress.* Atlanta, GA: U.S. Department of Health and Human Services, Public Health Service, Centers for Disease Control and Prevention, National Center for Chronic Disease Prevention and Health Promotion, Office on Smoking and Health, 1995.

U.S. Department of Health and Human Services (USDHHS) and Centers for Disease Control (CDC). "Current Trends: Mortality Trends for Selected Smoking-Related Cancers and Breast Cancer—United States 1950–1990." *Morbidity and Mortality Weekly Report* 12, no. 44 (12 November 1993): 863–6.

———. "Current Trends: Use of Smokeless Tobacco Among Adults—United States, 1991." *Morbidity and Mortality Weekly Report* 42, no. 14 (16 April 1993): 263–6.

———. *Cigarette Smokers—Related Mortality,* Atlanta, GA: U.S. Department of Health and Human Services

———. *CDC's Tobacco Use Prevention Program: Working Toward a Healthier Future,* Atlanta, GA: Office of Smoking and Health, 1996.

U.S. Surgeon General. *Smoking and Health: A Report of the Surgeon General.* Publication no. (PHS) 79-50066. Washington, DC: U.S. Department of Health, Education, and Welfare, 1979.

———. *The Changing Cigarette.* Publication no. (PHS) 81-51056. Washington, DC: U.S. Department of Health, Education, and Welfare, 1981.

———. *The Health Consequences of Smoking.* Washington, DC: 1984.

———. *The Health Consequences of Smoking: Cancer and Chronic Lung Disease in the Workplace.* Washington, DC: U.S. Government Printing Office, 1985.

Volle, R. L., and G. B. Koelle. "Ganglionic Stimulating and Blocking Agents." In *The Pharmacological Basis of Therapeutics,* 6th ed., edited by L. S. Goodman and A. Gilman, 565–74. New York: Macmillan, 1975.

Wentz, C. "Editorial: 22.2 Million American Women Just Don't Get It." *Journal of Women's Health* 3 (4 November 1993): 127–128.

13 Hallucinogens (Psychedelics)

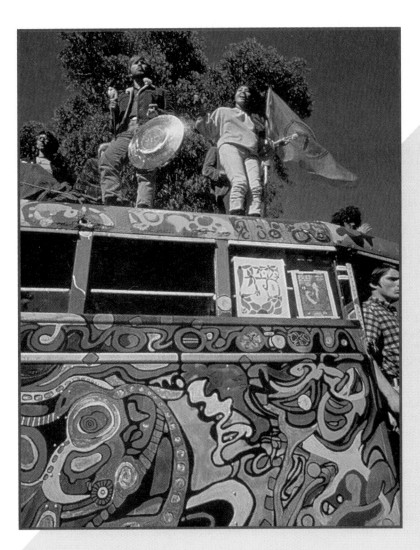

On completing this chapter
you will be able to:

- Many ancient mystics used hallucinogens as part of their religious ceremonies.
- Hallucinogens were abused by relatively few people in the United States until the social upheaval of the 1960s.
- The Native American Church in the United States can legally use the psychedelic mescaline as part of its religious ceremonies.
- Some hallucinogens—such as LSD, MDA, and Ecstasy—have been used by psychia-trists to assist in psychotherapy with certain patients.
- Hallucinogens such as LSD do not tend to cause physical dependence.
- The senses are grossly exaggerated and distorted under the influence of hallucinogens.
- For some users, hallucinogens can cause frightening, nightmarish experiences called "bad trips."
- PCP was originally developed as a general anesthetic.
- PCP is sometimes used as an additive in "street" hallucinogens.
- Intense use of PCP can cause psychotic episodes accompanied by tremendous strength, making management of users by medical or law enforcement personnel very dangerous.
- Inhalant drugs of abuse killed over 1000 adolescents in 1994.

- Identify the three principal types of hallucinogens and their four principal hallucinogenic effects.
- Explain why hallucinogens became so popular during the 1960s.
- Describe the nature of the sensory changes that occur due to the influence of hallucinogens.
- Outline how psychedelic, stimulant, and anticholinergic effects are expressed in the three principal types of hallucinogens.
- Describe the rationale for using hallucinogens in psychotherapy.
- Explain how the abuse liability of hallucinogens differs from that associated with other commonly abused drugs.
- Describe the effects that environment and personality have on the individual's response to hallucinogens.
- Discuss the occurrence of psychosis and "flashbacks" following LSD use.
- Identify the problems of purity with "street" LSD.
- Characterize how PCP differs from other hallucinogens.
- Identify the abused inhalants, who uses them, and the hazards they cause.

First time I tried [LSD], I was in college. I just saw tracers, no big visuals. Everything was enhanced or something. It made me jittery, but not tense. I could really drink.

From Venturelli's files, Joe, age 24, 1996

I was doing acid [LSD] on Thanksgiving. The turkey begged my Dad not to carve it. Another time my James Dean poster told me to kill myself and I wasn't worth living. So I tried.

From Venturelli's files, Val, age 17, 1996

These quotes from young adults illustrate the sensory and emotional distortions that can be caused by using **hallucinogens.** In this chapter we will begin with a brief historical review of the use of hallucinogens, tracing the trend in the United States from the 1960s to today. Next, the nature of hallucinogens and the effects they produce will be examined. The rest of the chapter addresses the various types of psychedelic agents: LSD types, phenylethylamines, anticholinergics, and other miscellaneous substances.

hallucinogens

substances that alter sensory processing in the brain, causing perceptual disturbances, changes in thought processing, and depresonalization

◢ The History of Hallucinogen Use

People have known and written about drug-related hallucinations for centuries. Throughout the ages, individuals who saw visions or experienced hallucinations were perceived as being holy or sacred, receiving divine messages, or possibly as being bewitched and controlled by the devil. There are many indications that medicine men, shamans, witches, oracles, and perhaps mystics and priests of various groups were familiar with drugs and herbs that caused such experiences and today are known as hallucinogens.

Prior to the 1960s, several psychedelic substances, such as mescaline from the peyote cactus, could be obtained from chemical supply houses with no restriction in the United States. Abuse of

hallucinogens did not become a major social problem in this country until this decade of racial struggles, the Vietnam War, and violent demonstrations. Many individuals frustrated with the hypocrisy of "the establishment" tried to "turn on and tune in" by using hallucinogens as pharmacological crutches.

Psychedelic drugs became especially popular when some medical professionals such as then-Harvard psychology professor, Timothy Leary, reported that these drugs allowed users to get in touch with themselves and achieve a peaceful inner serenity (Associated Press 1996). At the same time, it became well publicized that the natural psychedelics (such as mescaline and peyote) were and had been for many years used routinely by some religious organizations of Native Americans for enhancing spiritual experiences. This factor contributed to the mystical, supernatural aura associated with hallucinogenic agents and added to their enticement to a so-called dropout generation.

With widespread use of LSD, it was observed that this and similar drugs may induce a form of psychosis-like schizophrenia (American Psychiatric Association 1994). The term **psychotomimetic** was coined to describe these compounds; it means "psychosis mimicking" and is still used in medicine today. The basis for the designation is the effects of these drugs that induce mental states that impair an individual's ability to recognize and respond appropriately to reality.

psychotomimetic

substances that cause psychchosis-like syptoms

By the mid-1960s, federal regulatory agencies had become concerned with the misuse of hallucinogens and the potential emotional damage caused by these drugs. Access to hallucinogenic agents was restricted, and laws against their distribution were passed. Despite the problems associated with these psychedelics, some groups demanded that they be allowed to use these substances.

The Native American Church

The hallucinogen peyote plays a central role in the ceremonies of Native Americans who follow a reli-

Protests against the Vietnam War in the 1960s and 1970s demonstrated the social frustration which likely contributed to widespread use of LSD.

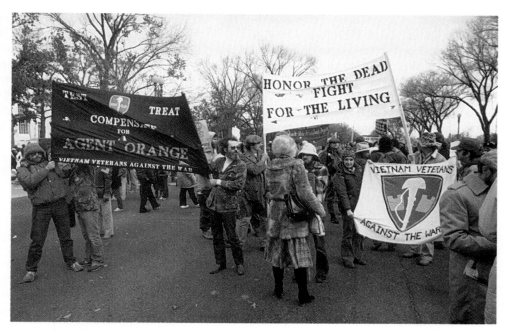

gion that is a combination of Christian doctrine and Native American religious rituals. Members of this Church are found as far north as Canada. They believe that God made a special gift of this sacramental plant to them so that they might commune more directly with Him. The first organized peyote church was the First-Born Church of Christ, incorporated in 1914 in Oklahoma. The Native American Church of the United States was chartered in 1918 and is the largest such group at present (approximately 100,000 to 200,000 members).

Because of the religious beliefs of the members of the Native American Church concerning the powers of peyote, when Congress legislated against its use in 1965, it allowed room for religious use of this psychedelic plant. The American Indian Religious Freedom Act of 1978 was an attempt by Congress to allow the members of the Native American Church access to peyote due to constitutional guarantees of religious freedom. Due to controversy inspired by the original piece of legislation, an amendment to the 1978 act was signed in 1994 that specifically protected the use of peyote in Native American Church ceremonies.

This amendment also prohibits use of peyote for nonreligious purposes (Becenti 1994).

Timothy Leary and the League of Spiritual Discovery

In 1966, three years after being fired by Harvard because of his controversial involvement with hallucinogens, Timothy Leary undertook a constitutional strategy intended to retain legitimate access to another hallucinogen, LSD. He began a religion called the League of Spiritual Discovery; LSD was the sacrament. This unorthodox religious orientation to the LSD experience was presented in a manual called *The Psychedelic Experience* (Leary et al. 1964), which was based on the *Tibetan Book of the Dead*. It became the "bible" of the psychedelic drug movement.

The movement grew, but most members used "street" LSD and did not follow Leary's directions. Leary believed that the hallucinogenic experience was only beneficial under proper control and guidance. But most members of this so-called religion merely used the organization as a front to gain access to an illegal drug. Federal authorities did not agree with Leary's *freedom of religion* interpretation and in 1969 convicted him for possession of marijuana and LSD and sentenced him to 20 years imprisonment (Stone 1991). Before being incarcerated, Leary escaped to Algeria and wandered for a couple of years before being extradited to the United States. He served several years in jail and was released in 1976.

Even in his later years, Leary continued to believe that U.S. citizens should be able to use hallucinogens without government regulation. He died in 1996 at the age of 75 years, revered by some but cursed by others (Letters 1996).

◢ Hallucinogen Use Today

Today, the use of hallucinogens (excluding marijuana) is primarily a young adult phenomenon (Johnston et al. 1996). Although the use rate has

not returned to that of the late 1960s and early 1970s (approximately 16%), the increase in high school seniors lifetime use from 9.2% in 1992 to 14.0% in 1996 is very disturbing (Table 13.1). Of particular concern is the 50% increase in LSD use during this time (Johnston 1996). It has been speculated that this increase reflects the ignorance of a new generation about the potential problems of the hallucinogens and a shift from using the widely publicized drugs of abuse such as cocaine and heroin (Johnston et al. 1996).

◢ The Nature of Hallucinogens

Agreement has not been reached on what constitutes a hallucinogenic agent (O'Brien 1996), for several reasons. First, a variety of seemingly unrelated drug groups can produce hallucinations, delusions, or sensory disturbances under certain conditions; for example, besides the traditional hallucinogens (such as LSD), anticholinergics, cocaine, amphetamines, and steroids can cause hallucinations.

What's more, responses to even the traditional hallucinogens can vary tremendously from person to person and from experience to experience. It is apparent that multiple mechanisms are involved in the actions of these drugs, which contributes to the array of responses that they can cause. These drugs most certainly influence the complex inner workings of the human mind and have been described as **psychedelic, psychotogenic,** or (as already mentioned) psychotomimetic. The features

psychedelic
substances that expand or heighten perception and consciousness

psychotogenic
substances that initiate psychotic behavior

of hallucinogens that distinguish them from other drug groups are their ability to alter perception, thought, and feeling in such a manner that does not normally occur except in dreams or during experiences of extreme religious exaltation (Jaffe 1990). We will examine these characteristics throughout this chapter.

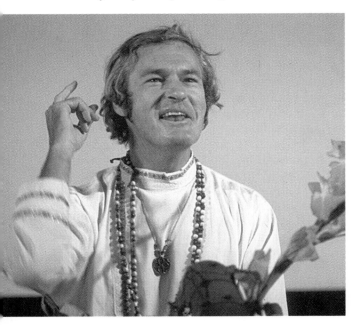

Timothy Leary attempted to legalize LSD in the 1960s.

Table 13.1   **Trends in the Use of Inhalants, LSD, and All Hallucinogens by Eighth-graders through Young Adults from 1992 to 1996.** For this survey, inhalants and marijuana were not considered as hallucinogens

	Used During Lifetime				Used During Year				Used During Month			
	1992	1994	1995	1996	1992	1994	1995	1996	1992	1994	1995	1996
Eighth-graders												
Inhalants	17.4%	19.9%	21.6%	21.2%	9.5%	11.7%	12.8%	12.2%	4.7%	5.6%	6.1%	5.8%
LSD	3.2	3.7	4.4	5.1	2.1	2.4	3.2	3.5	0.9	1.1	1.4	1.5
All hallucinogens	3.8	4.3	5.2	5.9	2.5	2.7	3.6	4.1	1.1	1.3	1.7	1.9
Tenth-graders												
Inhalants	16.6	18.0	19.0	19.3	7.5	9.1	9.6	9.5	2.7	3.6	3.5	3.3
LSD	5.8	7.2	8.4	9.4	4.0	5.2	6.5	6.9	1.6	2.0	3.0	2.4
All hallucinogens	6.4	8.1	9.3	10.5	4.3	5.8	7.5	7.8	1.8	2.4	3.3	2.8
Twelfth-graders												
Inhalants	16.6	17.7	17.4	16.6	6.2	7.7	8.0	7.6	2.3	2.7	3.2	2.5
LSD	8.6	10.5	11.7	12.6	5.6	6.9	8.4	8.8	2.0	2.6	4.0	2.5
All hallucinogens	9.2	11.4	12.7	14.0	5.9	7.6	9.3	10.1	2.1	3.1	4.4	3.5
Young adults												
Inhalants	13.9	13.2	N.A.	N.A.	3.1	2.1	N.A.	N.A.	1.1	0.5	N.A.	N.A.
LSD	13.8	13.8	N.A.	N.A.	4.3	4.0	N.A.	N.A.	1.1	1.1	N.A.	N.A.
All hallucinogens	15.9	15.4	N.A.	N.A.	5.1	4.9	N.A..	N.A.	1.6	1.4	N.A.	N.A.
Ecstasy	3.9	3.8	N.A.	N.A.	1.0	0.7	N.A.	N.A.	0.3	0.2	N.A.	N.A.

Note: N.A., not available.

Source: L. Johnston. University of Michigan News Release, December 19, 1996.

Sensory and Psychological Effects

In general, LSD is considered the prototype agent against which other hallucinogens are measured. Typical users experience several stages of sensory experiences; they can go through all stages during a single "trip" or more likely, they will only pass through some. These stages include (1) heightened, exaggerated senses, (2) loss of control, (3) self-reflection, and (4) loss of identity and a sense of cosmic merging.

The following illustrations of the stages of the LSD experience are based primarily on an account by Solomon Snyder (1974), a highly regarded neu-

roscientist (one of the principal discoverers of endorphins; see Chapter 6), who personally experienced the effects of LSD as a young resident in psychiatry.

Altered Senses In his encounter with LSD, Snyder used a moderate dose of 100 to 200 micrograms and observed few discernible effects for the first 30 minutes except some mild nausea. After this time had elapsed, objects took on a purplish tinge and appeared to be vaguely outlined. Colors, textures, and lines achieved a richness Snyder had never before experienced. Perception was so exaggerated that individual skin pores "stood out and clamored for recognition" (p. 42). Objects became distorted; when Snyder focused on his thumb, it began to swell, undulate, and then moved forward in a menacing fashion. Visions filled with distorted imagery occurred when his eyes were closed. The sense of time and distance changed dramatically; "a minute was like an hour, a week was like an eternity, a foot became a mile" (p. 43). The present seemed to drag on forever, and the concept of future lost its meaning. The exaggeration of perceptions and feelings gave the sense of more events occurring in a time period, giving the impression of time slowing.

An associated sensation described by Snyder is called **synesthesia,** a crossover phenomenon between senses. For example, sound takes on visual dimensions and vice versa, enabling you to see sounds and hear colors. These altered sensory experiences are described as a heightened sensory awareness and relate to the first component of the psychedelic state (O'Brien 1996).

> **synesthesia**
>
> a subjective sensation of image of a sense other than the one being stimulated, such as an auditory sensation caused by a visual stimulus

Loss of Control   The second feature of LSD also relates to altered sensory experiences and a loss of control (O'Brien 1996). The user cannot determine whether the psychedelic trip will be a pleasant, comfortable experience or a "bad trip," with recollections of hidden fears and suppressed anxieties that can precipitate neurotic or psychotic responses. The frightening reactions may persist a few minutes or several hours and be mildly agitating or extremely threatening. Some bad trips can include feelings of panic, confusion, suspiciousness, helplessness, and a total lack of control. The following scenario illustrates how terrifying a bad trip can be:

> I was having problems breathing [and] my throat was all screwed up. The things that entered my mind were that I was dead and people were saying good-bye, because they really meant it. I was witnessing my own funeral. I was think-

ing that I was going to wake either in the back seat of a cop car or in the hospital.

> *From the files of Peter Venturelli, interview with a 19-year-old male, 1995*

Replays of these frightening experiences can occur at a later time, even though the drug has not been taken again; such recurrences are referred to as **"flashbacks."**

It is not clear what determines the nature of the sensory response. Perhaps it relates to the state of anxiety and personality of the user or the nature of

> **"flashback"**
>
> the recurrences of earlier drug-induced sensory experiences in the absence of the drug

his or her surroundings. It is interesting that Timothy Leary tried to teach his "drug disciples" that "turning on correctly means to understand the many levels that are brought into focus; it takes years of discipline, training and discipleship" ("Celebration #1" 1966). He apparently felt that, with experience and training, you could control the sensory effects of the hallucinogens. This is an interesting possibility but has never been well demonstrated.

Self-Reflection   Snyder (1974) makes reference to the third component of the psychedelic response in his LSD experience. During the period when sensory effects predominate, self-reflection also occurs. While in this state, Snyder explains, the user "becomes aware of thoughts and feelings long hidden beneath the surface, forgotten and/or repressed" (p. 44). As a psychiatrist, Snyder claims that this new perspective can lead to valid insights that are useful psychotherapeutic exercises.

Some psychotherapists have used or advocated the use of psychedelics for this purpose since the 1950s, as described by Sigmund Freud, to "make conscious the unconscious" (Snyder 1974, 44). It should be noted that, while a case can be made for the psychotherapeutic use of this group of drugs, the Food and Drug Administration (FDA) has not approved any of these agents for psychiatric use. The psychedelics currently available are considered to be too unpredictable in their effects and possess substantial risks (Abraham et al. 1996).

Not only is their administration not considered to be significantly therapeutic, but their use is deemed a great enough risk that the principal hallucinogenic agents are scheduled as controlled substances (see Chapter 4).

Loss of Identity and Cosmic Merging The final features that set the psychedelics apart as unique drugs are described by Snyder (1974) as the "mystical-spiritual aspect of the drug experience." He claims, "It is indescribable. For how can anyone verbalize a merging of his being with the totality of the universe? How do you put into words the feeling that 'all is one,' 'I am of the all,' 'I am no longer.' One's skin ceases to be a boundary between self and others" (p. 45). Because consumption of hallucinogen-containing plants has often been part of religious ceremonies, it is likely that this sense of cosmic merging and union with all humankind correlates to the exhilaratingly spiritual experiences described by many religious mystics.

The loss of identity and personal boundaries caused by hallucinogens is not viewed as being so spiritually enticing by all. In particular, for individuals who have rigid, highly ordered personalities, the dissolution of a well-organized and -structured world is terrifying because the drug destroys the individual's emotional support. Such an individual finds that the loss of a separate identity can cause extreme panic and anxiety. During these drug-induced panic states, which in some ways are schizophrenic-like, people have committed suicide or homicide. These tragic reactions are part of the risk of using hallucinogenics and explains some of the FDA's hesitancy to legalize or authorize them for psychotherapeutic use.

Mechanisms of Action

As with most drugs, hallucinogens represent the proverbial "two-edged sword." These drugs may cause potentially useful psychiatric effects for many people. However, the variability in positive versus negative responses, coupled with lack of understanding as to what factors are responsible for the variables, have made these drugs dangerous and difficult to manage.

Some researchers have suggested that all hallucinogens act at a common central nervous system (CNS) site to exert their psychedelic effects. Although this hypothesis has not been totally disproven, there is little evidence to support it. The fact that so many different types of drugs can cause hallucinogenic effects suggests that multiple mechanisms are likely responsible for their actions.

The most predictable and typical psychedelic experiences are caused by LSD or similar agents. Consequently, these agents have been the primary focus of studies intended to elucidate the nature of hallucinogenic mechanisms. Although LSD has effects at several CNS sites, ranging from the spinal cord to the cortex of the brain, its effects on the neurotransmitter serotonin most likely account for its psychedelic properties (Abraham et al. 1996). That LSD and similar drugs alter serotonin activity has been proven; how they affect this transmitter is not so readily apparent.

Although many experts believe changes in serotonin activity are the basis for the psychedelic properties of most hallucinogens, a case can be made for the involvement of norepinephrine, dopamine, acetylcholine, and perhaps other transmitter systems as well (see Chapter 6). Only additional research will be able to sort out this complex but important issue.

◢ Types of Hallucinogenic Agents

Due to recent technological developments, understanding of hallucinogens has advanced; even so, the classification of these drugs remains somewhat arbitrary. Many agents produce some of the pharmacological effects of the traditional psychedelics, such as LSD and mescaline.

A second type of hallucinogen includes those agents that have amphetamine-like molecular structures (referred to as *phenylethylamines*) and possess some stimulant action; this group includes drugs such as DOM (dimethoxymethyl*amphetamine*), MDA (methylenedioxy*amphetamine*), and MDMA (methylenedioxy*methamphetamine*). These agents vary in their hallucinogen or stimulant properties. MDA is more like an amphetamine (stimulant), while MDMA is more like LSD (hallucinogen). In large doses, however, each of the phenylethylamines causes substantial CNS stimulation.

The third major group of hallucinogens is the anticholinergic drugs, which block some of the receptors for the neurotransmitter acetylcholine (see Chapter 6). Almost all drugs that antagonize these receptors cause hallucinations in high doses. Many of these potent anticholinergic hallucinogens are naturally occurring and have been known, used, and abused for millennia.

Traditional Hallucinogens: LSD Types

The LSD-like drugs are considered to be the prototypical hallucinogens and are used as the basis of comparison for other types of agents with psychedelic properties. Included in this group are LSD itself and some hallucinogens derived from plants, such as mescaline from the peyote cactus, psilocybin from mushrooms, dimethyltryptamine (DMT) from seeds, and myristicin from nutmeg. Because LSD is the principal hallucinogen, its origin, history, and properties will be discussed in detail, providing a basis for understanding the other psychedelic drugs.

Lysergic Acid Diethylamide (LSD)   LSD is a relatively new drug, but similar compounds have existed for a long time. For example, accounts from the Middle Ages tell about a strange affliction that caused women to abort and others to develop strange burning sensations in their extremities. Today, we call this condition **ergotism** and know that it is caused by eating grain contaminated by the ergot fungus. This fungus produces compounds related to LSD called the *ergot alkaloids* (Goldstein 1994). Besides the sensory effects, the ergot substances can also cause hallucinations, delirium, and psychosis.

In 1938, Albert Hofmann, a scientist for Sandoz Pharmaceutical Laboratories of Basel,

> **ergotism**
> poisoning by toxic substances from the ergot fungus Claviceps purpurea

Switzerland, worked on a series of ergot compounds in a search for active chemicals that might be of medical value (Schwartz 1995). Lysergic acid was similar in structure to a compound called *nikethamide,* a stimulant, and Hofmann tried to create slight chemical modifications that might merit further testing. The result of this effort was the production of lysergic acid diethylamide, or LSD. Hofmann's experience with this new compound gave insight to the effects of this drug and are detailed in "Case in Point," page 341.

Soon after LSD was discovered, the similarity of experiences with this agent to the symptoms of schizophrenia were noted, which prompted researchers to investigate correlations between the two. The hope was to use LSD as a tool for producing an artificial psychosis to aid in understanding the biochemistry of psychosis. Interest in this use of LSD has declined because it is not generally accepted that LSD effects differ from natural psychoses (Abraham et al. 1996).

The use of LSD in psychotherapy has also been tried in connection with the treatment of alcoholism, autism, paranoia, schizophrenia, and various other mental and emotional disorders. Therapeutic use of LSD has not increased to any great extent over the years because of its limited success, legal aspects, difficulty in obtaining the pure drug, adverse reactions to the drug ("bad trips" can occur under controlled as well as uncontrolled conditions), and rapid tolerance buildup in some patients.

Nonmedical interest in LSD and related drugs began to grow during the 1950s and peaked in the 1960s, when LSD was used by millions of young Americans for chemical escape. Occasionally a "bad trip" would cause a user to feel terror and panic; these experiences resulted in well-publicized accidental deaths due to jumping from building tops or running into the pathway of oncoming vehicles (U.S. Department of Justice 1991b).

As with other hallucinogens, the use of LSD by teenagers declined somewhat over the past two decades but began to rise again in the early 1990s. The reason for this rise is thought to relate to a decline in the perceived dangers of using LSD and an increase in peer approval (Johnston 1996). These changes in attitude may reflect the recent reduc-

Albert Hofmann's Discovery

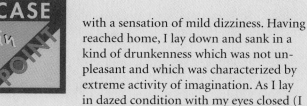

Following synthesis of the diethylamide derivative of lysergic acid in 1938, Hofmann noted nothing unusual about the product, so he stored it in a bottle on the laboratory shelf. In 1943, he checked over some of the synthetic compounds he had worked on and started making further tests of LSD. Most likely due to carelessness, a small amount must have entered his blood. Hofmann noted that

> Last Friday, April 16, 1943, I was forced to stop my work in the laboratory in the middle of the afternoon and to go home, as I was seized by a peculiar restlessness associated

with a sensation of mild dizziness. Having reached home, I lay down and sank in a kind of drunkenness which was not unpleasant and which was characterized by extreme activity of imagination. As I lay in dazed condition with my eyes closed (I experienced daylight as disagreeably bright), there surged upon me an uninterrupted stream of fantastic images of extraordinary plasticity and vividness and accompanied by an intense, kaleidoscope-like play of colors. This condition gradually passed off after about two hours.

Hofmann realized the experience was probably caused by the chemical he had been working with (Hofmann 1968). ■

---

tion in education concerning these drugs. Of high school seniors sampled in 1975, 11.3% had used LSD sometime during their life; that number declined to 8.7% in 1990 and rebounded to 11.7% in 1995 (Johnston 1995). Similar, but less dramatic, patterns were also observed in college and young adult populations (Johnston et al. 1996). LSD users are typically college or high school students, Caucasian, middle-class and risk-taking (Schwartz 1995).

Synthesis and Administration LSD is a complex molecule that requires about one week to be synthesized. Because of the sophisticated chemistry necessary for its production, LSD is not manufactured by local illicit laboratories. It appears that an illegal operation in San Francisco is the principal source of LSD for the United States and even much of the world. Because of LSD's potency, it has been difficult to locate the illicit LSD labs; small quantities of LSD are sufficient to satisfy the demand and can be easily transported without detection (Schwartz 1995).

The physical properties of LSD are not distinctive. In its purified form, LSD is colorless, odorless, and tasteless. It can be purchased in several forms, including tiny tablets (about one-tenth the size of

aspirins, called "microdots"), capsules, and occasionally even a liquid. The street names of LSD include *acid, blotter acid, microdot,* and *white lightning* (U.S. Department of Justice 1991b). Although LSD usually is taken by mouth, it is sometimes injected (Schwartz 1995).

LSD often is added to absorbent paper, such as blotter paper, that can be divided into small decorated squares. Each square is swallowed or chewed

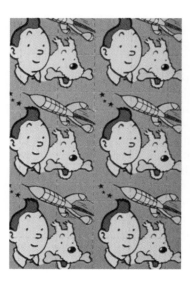

LSD blotter paper. Small amounts of LSD are added to decorated, absorbent paper. Each small square represents a single dose to be chewed or swallowed. The designs on the paper have no drug function.

and represents a single dose. One gram of LSD can provide 10,000 individual doses and be sold on the streets for $50,000 (Schwartz 1995).

Physiological Effects Like many hallucinogens, LSD is remarkably potent (Goldstein 1995). The typical dose today is 20–30 micrograms, compared with a typical dose of 150–300 micrograms in the 1960s. This difference in dose likely explains why today fewer users of LSD are experiencing severe side effects (U.S. Department of Justice 1991a). In monkeys, the lethal dose has been determined to be about 5 milligrams (mg) per kilogram (kg) of body weight.

When taken orally, LSD is readily absorbed and diffused into all tissues. It will pass through the placenta into the fetus and through the blood–brain barrier. The brain receives about 1% of the total dose.

Within the brain, LSD is particularly concentrated in the hypothalamus, the limbic system, and the auditory and visual reflex areas. Electrodes placed in the limbic system show an "electrical storm," or a massive increase in neural activity, which might correlate with the overwhelming flood of sensations and the phenomenon of synesthesia reported by the user (Goldstein 1995). LSD also activates the sympathetic nervous system; shortly after the drug is taken, body temperature, heart rate, and blood pressure rise, the person sweats, and the pupils of the eyes become dilated. Its effects on the parasympathetic nervous system cause an increase in salivation and nausea (Schwartz 1995). These systemic effects do not appear to be related to the hallucinogenic properties of the drug.

Pharmacokinetic experiments with LSD show that about half of the substance is cleared from the body within 3 hours, and more than 90% is excreted within 24 hours (Goldstein 1995). The effects of this hallucinogen can last 2–12 hours depending on the dose and previous experience with the drug (Schwartz 1995). Tolerance to the effects of LSD develops more rapidly and lasts longer than tolerance to other hallucinogens. Tolerance develops very quickly to repeated doses, probably because of a change in sensitivity of the target cells in the brain rather than a change in its metabolism. It wears off within a few days after the drug is discontinued. Because there are no with-drawal symptoms, a person does not become physically dependent, but some psychological dependency on LSD can occur (Mathias 1993).

Behavioral Effects Because LSD alters a number of systems in the brain, its behavioral effects are many and variable between individuals (Goldstein 1995). The following sections address common CNS responses to this drug.

Creativity and Insight. A question often raised by researchers interested in experimenting with LSD is, Does it help expand the mind, increasing insight creativity? This question is extremely difficult to answer because no one has ever determined the origin of insight and creativity. Moreover, each of us views these qualities differently.

Subjects under the influence of LSD often express the feeling of being more creative, but creative acts such as drawing and painting are hindered by the motor impairment caused by LSD. The products of artists under the influence of the drug usually prove to be inferior to those produced prior to the drug experience. Paintings done in LSD creativity studies have been described as reminiscent of "schizophrenic art."

In an often cited study, creativity, attitude, and anxiety tests on 24 college students found that LSD had no objective effect on creativity, although many of the subjects said they felt they were more creative (McGlothin et al. 1967). This paradox is noted in several studies of LSD use: The subjects feel they have more insight and provide better answers to life's problems, but they do not or cannot demonstrate this increase objectively. Overt behavior is not modified, and these new insights are short-lived unless they are reinforced by modified behavior.

In spite of these results, some researchers still contend that LSD can enhance the creative process. For example, Oscar Janigar, a psychiatrist at the University of California, Los Angeles, claims to have determined that LSD does not produce a tangible alteration in the way a painter paints; thus, it does not turn a poor painter into a good one. However, Janigar claims that LSD does alter the way the painter appraises the world and allows the artist to "plunge into areas where access was restricted by confines of perceptions" and consequently becomes more creative (Tucker 1987, 16).

Adverse Psychedelic Effects. It is important to remember that there is no typical pattern of response to LSD. The experience varies for each user as a function of the person's set, or expectations, and setting, or environment, during the experience. Two of the major negative responses are described as follows (Pahnke et al. 1970):

1. *The psychotic adverse reaction,* or *"freakout,"* is an intense, nightmarish experience. The subject may have complete loss of emotional control, and experience paranoid delusions, hallucinations, panic attacks, psychosis, and catatonic seizures. In rare instances, some of these reactions are prolonged, lasting days. In 1991, 4000 episodes were reported in U.S. emergency rooms due to adverse LSD reactions (Mathias 1993).

2. *The nonpsychotic adverse reaction* may involve varying degrees of tension, anxiety, fear, depression, and despair but not as intense a response as the "freakout." A person with deep psychological problems or a strong need to be in conscious control or one who takes the drug in an unfavorable setting is more likely to have an adverse reaction than a person with a well-integrated personality.

Severe LSD behavioral toxicity can be treated with tranquilizers or a benzodiazepine (Schwartz 1995).

Perceptual Effects. Because the brain's sensory processing is altered by a hallucinogenic dose of LSD, many kinds of unusual illusions can occur. Some users report seeing shifting geometrical patterns mixed with intense color perception; others observe the movement of stationary objects, such that a speck on the wall appears as a large blinking eye or an unfolding flower. Interpretation of sounds can also be scrambled; a dropped ashtray may become a gun fired at the user, for instance. In some cases, LSD alters perceptions to the extent that people feel they can walk on water or fly through the air. The sensation that the body is distorted and even coming apart is another common effect, especially for novice users. Thoughts of suicide and sometimes actual attempts can be caused by use of LSD as well (U.S. Department of Justice 1991b).

Many LSD users find their sense of time distorted, such that hours may be perceived as years or an eternity. As discussed earlier, users may also

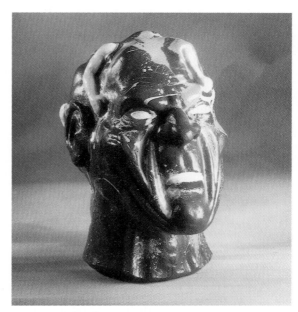

This piece of sculpture was done by a university student while under the influence of LSD.

have a distorted perception of their own knowledge or creativity; for instance, they may feel their ideas or work are especially unique, brilliant, or artistic. When analyzed by a person not on LSD, however, or explained after the "trip" is over, these ideas or creations are almost always quite ordinary.

In sum, LSD alters perception such that any sensation can be perceived in the extreme. An experience can be incredibly beautiful and uplifting. However, sometimes the experience can be very unpleasant, as described by one college student:

> Unfortunately, not all trips are good. I know one person who had a "bad trip," in which he felt little devils tearing him apart. One time he also remembered sitting in front of a glass of beer ready to drink it until the alcohol started to bubble and make air-popping noises. He's also had a few flashbacks that made him feel tranced and out of control. On one occasion, he said that objects were moving around the room and he had no power to stop them. He felt crazy for a while.
>
> *From the files of Peter Venturelli, interview with a 20-year-old male, 1995*

The "flashback" is an interesting but poorly understood phenomenon of LSD use. Although usually thought of as being adverse, sometimes flashbacks are pleasant and even referred to as "free trips" (Schwartz 1995). During a flashback, sensations caused by previous LSD use return, although the subject is not using the drug at the time.

There are three broad categories of negative LSD-related flashbacks:

1. *The "body trip"*—the recurrence of an unpleasant physical sensation

2. *The "bad mind trip"*—the recurrence of a distressing thought or emotion

3. *Altered visual perception*—the most frequent type of recurrence, consisting of seeing dots, flashes, trails of light, halos, false motion in the peripheral field, and other sensations (see "Case in Point" below for an example)

Flashbacks are most disturbing because they come on unexpectedly. Some have been reported as long as five years after use of LSD (Goldstein 1994); for most people, however, flashbacks usually subside within weeks or months after taking LSD (Schwartz 1995). The duration of a flashback is variable, lasting from a few minutes to several hours.

Although the precise mechanism of flashbacks is unknown, physical or psychological stresses and some drugs such as marijuana may trigger these experiences (Goldstein 1995). It has been proposed that flashbacks are an especially vivid form of memory that becomes seared into the subconscious mind due to the effects of LSD on the brain's transmitters. As one user describes it:

> It was like watching a video of my past, except it was intensified greatly and the colors were extreme. Faces and objects were melting and I got really scared and started to flip out.
>
> *From the files of Peter Venturelli, interview with a 19-year-old male, 1995*

Treatment consists of reassurance that the condition will go away and the use of a sedative like Valium if necessary, to treat the anxiety or panic that can accompany the flashback experience (Schwartz 1995).

Genetic Damage and Birth Defects Experiments conducted in the mid-1960s suggested that LSD could cause birth defects, based on the observation that, when LSD was added to a suspension of human white blood cells in a test tube, the chromosomes of these cells were damaged. From this finding, it was proposed that, when LSD was consumed by humans, it could cause damage to the chromosomes of the male sperm, female egg, or the cells of the developing infant. Such damage theoretically could result in congenital defects in offspring (Dishotsky et al. 1971).

Carefully controlled studies conducted after news of LSD's chromosomal effects were made public have not supported this hypothesis. Experiments have revealed that, in contrast to the test-tube findings, there is no chromosomal damage to white blood cells or any other cells when LSD is given to a human being (Dishotsky et al. 1971).

Studies have also shown that there are no carcinogenic or mutagenic effects from using LSD in experimental animals or humans, with the exception of the fruit fly. (LSD is a mutagen in fruit flies if given in doses that are equivalent to 100,000 times the hallucinogenic dose for humans.) Teratogenic effects occur in mice if LSD is given early in pregnancy. LSD may be teratogenic in rhesus monkeys if it is injected in doses (based on body weight) exceeding at least 100 times the usual hallucinogenic dose for humans. In other studies,

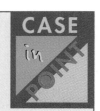

The "After Flash"

As a teenager John Doe took LSD approximately 30 times. Some 15 years later, he still sees grainy, photographic dots. He also sees "trails," blurred images associated with a moving object, such as a waving arm. "It's as if the lens of a camera were left open taking a time-lapse photograph." Doe also complains that the visual distortions also bring twinges of fear. "I have the feeling of coming on, a rush. It hits me in the gut, like going over the top of a hill. I take Valium, which stops it in its tracks" (Nadis 1990, 24). ■

women who took "street" LSD but not those given pure LSD had a higher rate of spontaneous abortions and births of malformed infants; this finding suggests that contaminants in adulterated LSD were responsible for the fetal effects and not the hallucinogen itself (Dishotsky et al. 1971).

Early Human Research In the 1950s, the U.S. government—specifically, the Central Intelligence Agency (CIA) and the army—became interested in reports of the effects of mind-altering drugs, including LSD. Unknown to the public at the time, these agencies conducted tests on humans to learn more about such compounds and determine their usefulness in conducting military and clandestine missions. These activities became public when a biochemist, Frank Olson, killed himself in 1953 after being given a drink laced with LSD. Olson had a severe psychotic reaction and was being treated for the condition when he jumped out of a tenth-story window. His family was told only that he had committed suicide. The connection to LSD was not uncovered until 1975. The court awarded Olson's family $750,000 in damages in 1976.

In 1976, the extent of these studies was revealed: nearly 585 soldiers and 900 civilians had been given LSD in poorly organized experiments in which participants were coerced into taking this drug or not told that they were being given it. Powerful hallucinogens such as LSD can cause se-rious psychological damage in some subjects, especially when they are unaware of what is happening.

The legal consequences of these LSD studies continued for years. As recently as 1987, a New York judge awarded $700,000 to the family of a mental patient who killed himself after having been given LSD without an explanation of the drug's nature. The judge said that there was a "conspiracy of silence" between the army, the Department of Justice, and the New York State Attorney General to conceal events surrounding the death of the subject, Harold Blauer.

Mescaline (Peyote)

Mescaline is one of approximately 30 psychoactive chemicals that have been isolated from the peyote cactus and used for centuries in the Americas. One of the first reports on the peyote plant was made by Francisco Hernandez of the court of King Philip II of Spain. King Philip was interested in reports from the earlier Cortés expedition about strange medicines the natives used and sent Hernandez to collect information about herbs and medicines. Hernandez worked on this project from 1570 to 1575 and reported the use of more than 1200 plant remedies, as well as the existence of many hallucinogenic plants. He was one of the first to record the eating of parts of the peyote cactus and the resulting visions and mental changes.

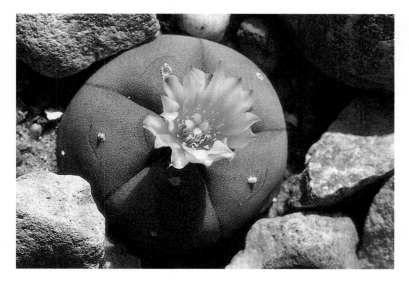

The peyote cactus contains a number of drugs; the best known is mescaline.

In the seventeenth century, Spanish Catholic priests asked their Indian converts to confess to the use of peyote, which they believed was used to conjure up demons. However, nothing stopped its use. By 1760, use of peyote had spread into what is now the United States.

Peyote has been confused with another plant, the mescal shrub, which produces dark red beans that contain an extremely toxic alkaloid called *cytisine*. This alkaloid may cause hallucinations, convulsions, and even death. In addition, a mescal liquor is made from the agave cactus. Partly because of misidentification with the toxic mescal beans, the U.S. government outlawed the use of both peyote and mescaline.

Mescaline is the most active drug in peyote; it induces intensified perception of colors and euphoria in the user. However, as Aldous Huxley said in *The Doors of Perception* (1954), his book about his experimentation with mescaline, "Along with the happily transfigured majority of mescaline takers there is a minority that finds in the drug only hell and purgatory." After Huxley related his experiences with mescaline, it was used by an increasing number of people.

Physiological Effects The average dose of mescaline that will cause hallucinations and other physiological effects is from 300 to 600 milligrams. It may take up to 20 peyote (mescal) buttons (ingested orally) to get 600 milligrams of mescaline.

Based on studies of animals, it is estimated that from 10 to 30 times the lowest dose that will cause behavioral effects in humans may be lethal. (About 200 milligrams is the lowest mind-altering dose.) Death in animals results from convulsions and respiratory arrest. Mescaline is perhaps 1000 to 3000 times less potent than LSD and 30 times less potent than another common hallucinogen, psilocybin (Mathias 1993), see later in this chapter.

Effects include dilation of the pupils (**mydriasis**), increase in body temperature, anxiety, visual hallucinations, and alteration of body image. The last effect is a type of hallucination in which parts of the body may seem to disappear or to become grossly distorted. Mescaline induces vomiting in many people and some muscular relaxation (sedation). Ap-

mydriasis

pupil dilation

parently, there are few after-effects or drug hangover feelings at low doses. Higher doses of mescaline slow the heart and respiratory rhythm, contract the intestines and the uterus, and cause headache, difficulty in coordination, dry skin with itching, and hypertension (high blood pressure).

Mescaline users report that they lose all awareness of time. As with LSD, the setting for the "trip" influences the user's reactions. Most mescaline users prefer natural settings, most likely due to the historical association of this drug with Native Americans and their nature-related spiritual experiences (often under the influence of this drug). The visual hallucinations achieved depend on the individual. Colors are at first intensified and may be followed by hallucinations of shades, movements, forms, and events. The senses of smell and taste are enhanced. Some people claim (as with LSD) that they can "hear" colors and "see" sounds, such as the wind. Synesthesia occurs naturally in a small percentage of cases.

At low to medium doses, an ecstatic state of euphoria is reported, often followed by a feeling of anxiety and less frequently by depression. Occasionally, users observe themselves as two people and experience the sensation that the mind and body are separate entities. A number of people have had cosmic experiences that are profound, almost religious, in which they discover a sense of unity with all creation. People who have this sensation often believe they have discovered the meaning of existence.

Mechanism of Action Within 30 to 120 minutes after ingestion, mescaline reaches a maximum concentration in the brain and may persist for up to nine or ten hours. Hallucinations may last up to two hours and are usually affected by the dose level. About half the dose is excreted unchanged after six hours and can be recovered in the urine for reuse (if peyote is in short supply). A slow tolerance builds up after repeated use, and there is cross-tolerance to LSD. As with LSD, mescaline intoxication can be alleviated or stopped by taking a dose of chlorpromazine (Thorazine, a tranquilizer) and to a lesser extent with diazepam (Valium). Like LSD, mescaline probably exerts much of its hallucinogenic effects by altering serotonin systems (Jaffe 1990).

Analysis of "street" samples of mescaline in a number of U.S. cities over the past decade shows that the chemical sold rarely is authentic. Regardless of color or appearance, these street drugs are usually other hallucinogens, such as LSD, DOM, or PCP. If a person decides to take hallucinogenic street drugs, "let the buyer beware." Not only is the actual content often different and potentially much more toxic than bargained for (they are frequently contaminated), but the dosage is usually unknown even if the drug is genuine.

Psilocybin The drug psilocybin has a long and colorful history. Its principal source is the *Psilocybe mexicana* mushroom of the "magic" variety (Goldstein 1994). It was first used by some of the early natives of Central America more than 2000 years ago. In Guatemala, statues of mushrooms that date back to 100 B.C. have been found. The Aztecs later used the mushrooms for ceremonial rites. When the Spaniards came into Mexico in the 1500s, the natives were calling the *Psilocybe mexicana* mushroom "God's flesh." Because of this seeming sacrilege, they were harshly treated by the Spanish priests.

Gordon Wasson identified the *Psilocybe mexicana* mushroom in 1955. The active ingredient was extracted in 1958 by Albert Hofmann, who also synthesized LSD. Doing research, Hofmann wanted to make certain he would feel the effects of the mushroom, so he ate 32 of them, weighing 2.4 grams (a medium dose by Indian standards) and then recorded his hallucinogenic reactions (Burger 1968).

Timothy Leary also tried some psilocybin mushrooms in Mexico in 1960; apparently the experience influenced him greatly. On his return to Harvard, he carried out a series of experiments using psilocybin with student groups. Leary was careless in experimental procedures and did some work in uncontrolled situations. His actions caused a major administrative upheaval, ending in his departure from Harvard.

One of Leary's questionable studies was the "Good Friday" experiment in which 20 theological students were given either a placebo or psilocybin in a double-blind study (that is, neither the researcher nor the subjects know who gets the placebo or the drug), after which all attended the same 2.5-hour Good Friday service. The experimental group reported mystical experiences whereas the control group did not (Pahnke and Richards 1966). Leary believed that the experience was of value and that, under proper control and guidance, the hallucinatory experience could be beneficial.

Psilocybin is not very common on the street. Generally, it is administered orally and is eaten either fresh or dried. Accidental poisonings are common for those who mistakenly consume poisonous mushrooms rather than the hallucinogenic variety.

The dried form of these mushrooms contains from 0.2% to 0.5% psilocybin. The hallucinogenic effects produced are quite similar to those of LSD, and there is a cross-tolerance between psilocybin, LSD, and mescaline. The effects caused by psilocybin vary with the dosage taken. Up to 4 milligrams will cause a pleasant experience, relaxation, and some body sensation. In some subjects, higher doses cause considerable perceptual and body image changes, accompanied by hallucinations, as illustrated in the following quote:

> The first time I shroomed, everything looked like it was made of plastic, like everything could

The psilocybe mushroom, source of psilocybin and psilocin.

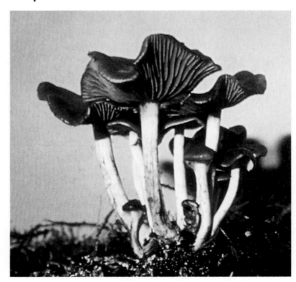

be folded up or something. Whatever somebody told me, I would believe it to be true. Like if I was drinking a beer and someone told me it was tequila, I would taste tequila.

From the files of Peter Venturelli, interview with a 20-year-old male, 1995

Psilocybin stimulates the autonomic nervous system, dilates the pupils, and increases the body temperature. There is some evidence that psilocybin is metabolized into psilocin, which is more potent and may be the principal active ingredient. Psilocin is found in mushrooms but in small amounts. Like the other hallucinogens, psilocybin apparently causes no physical dependence.

Dimethyltryptamine (DMT) DMT is a short-acting hallucinogen found in the seeds of certain leguminous trees native to the West Indies and parts of South America (Schultes 1978). It is also prepared synthetically in illicit laboratories. For centuries, the powdered seeds have been used as a snuff called *cohoba* in pipes and snuffing tubes. The Haitian natives claim that, under the influence of the drug, they can communicate with their gods. Its effects may last under one hour, which has earned it the nickname "the businessman's lunch break" drug.

DMT has no effect when taken orally; it is inhaled either as smoke from the burning plant or in vaporized form. DMT is sometimes added to pars-

Despite concerns and warnings about the dangers of using hallucinogens, some individuals are fascinated by what they view as the "mystical and spiritual" powers of such substances. For example, Mark Plotkin claims that the course of his life was completely changed in 1974 while enrolled at Harvard. He attended a lecture by Professor Richard Evans Schultes, an expert in ethnobotany. Schultes had lived in the Amazon for 13 years (1941–1953), where he studied medicinal plants. He was a leading authority on Amazonian botany, medicinal plants, cocoa, Mexican mushrooms, and hallucinogens. He imparted to his students a sense of the beauty, value, and wonder of the rainforest ecosystem and the tribal natives whose lives were so closely integrated with it. After the seminar, Mark decided he was going to spend the rest of his life studying ethnobotany in South America.

Several years later Mark had an opportunity to visit the Amazon region. Mark didn't go to the Amazon to study hallucinogens. His interests specifically lay in the medicinal plants thought to be useful for various chronic diseases, such as diabetes, cancer, and arthritis. However, Mark earned the trust of the indigenous people and in the course of his research was introduced to local hallucinogenic plants used by the Amazonian Indians to "commune with the spirit world." Mark's first exposure to the hallucinogens occurred one night in 1987. He described his experience:

When I turned back to the shaman, he was pointing a tube at me. With equal parts anxiety, excitement, fear, and anticipation, I placed the tube's bowl in my right nostril. The shaman held the other end between his lips and blew, starting off slowly and finishing with a mighty blast. The force seemed to propel the drug from the shaman's tube directly into my bloodstream and then into my very soul. . . .

Although my heart pounded painfully in my chest, a subtle sense of exhilaration accompanied the pain that wracked my body, . . . At the edge of my field of vision, tiny figures began to appear. By now my senses had been severally altered. My hearing was especially acute; I felt as if I could hear everything in the shabono [hut]. My field of vision had been greatly expanded: it was as if I were looking at the world through a wide-angle lens. At the edge of my field of

ley leaves or flakes, tobacco, or marijuana to induce its hallucinogenic effect. The usual dose is 60 to 150 milligrams. In structure and action, it is similar to psilocybin although not as powerful. Like the other hallucinogens discussed, DMT does not cause physical dependence.

Nutmeg High doses of nutmeg can be quite intoxicating, causing symptoms such as drowsiness, stupor, delirium, and sleep. Prison inmates have known about this drug for years, so in most prisons, use of spices such as nutmeg is restricted.

Nutmeg contains 5% to 15% myristica oil, which is responsible for the physical effects. Myris-

ticin (about 4%), which is structurally similar to mescaline, and elemicin are probably the most potent psychoactive ingredients in nutmeg. Myristicin blocks release of serotonin from brain neurons. Some scientists believe that it can be converted in the body to MDMA (a close relative of MDA, discussed later), which also affects the central nervous system. Mace, the exterior covering of the nutmeg seed, also contains the hallucinogenic compound myristicin.

Two tablespoons of nutmeg (about 14 grams) taken orally cause a rather unpleasant "trip" with a dreamlike stage; rapid heartbeat, dry mouth, and thirst are experienced as well. Agitation,

---

vision, the little figures [hekura—spirits of the forest] began to dance. . . . I felt that once again, I was slipping through a crack in the wall, moving from what we in the West perceive as reality into a different world—one that is an integral part of the Indian's reality. . . . Such an experience almost inevitably leaves you with more questions than answers. But it opens your mind and forces you to ask what is real and what isn't, what we know and what we have yet to learn."

Years later, under the tutelage of yet a different shaman, Mark waited for an appropriate moment to ask his mentor about the mystery of hallucinogens, specifically one referred to as Brunfelsia. "Grandfather, what if I wanted to take the potion?" he said.

"Awah," the shaman said, "No, this is a very dangerous plant. Many apprentices have taken it, and some have lost their minds. Some did not survive. If you take it, you will die."

Despite warnings about the psychiatric dangers of the hallucinogens, Mark remains convinced that the use of drugs such as LSD should be approached with "reverence" because he believes they can help the user explore new realms of consciousness and

spiritual dimensions usually not accessible. However, even Mark has come to appreciate that experimenting with mind-altering hallucinogens is risky and can prove to be extremely damaging, if not deadly. Part of Mark's teaching today is that hallucinogens are not meant to be used to escape reality, as they are by people who abuse them. And as the shaman indicated, the dangers of such use can be fatal. Mark sees a yearning in today's American culture, a quest for all things spiritual. As stress arises in our lives, so too does the hunger for a closer spiritual connection. But as Mark can attest, this moment is not the time to experiment with mind-altering hallucinogens. The consequences will prove damaging, if not deadly.

Following in the footsteps of his mentor Schultes, Mark currently lectures on the topic of ethnobotany and is involved with many projects to help save the rainforests around the world, which house thousands of plants with important medicinal purposes.

You can read more about Mark Plotkin and his research in his autobiographical missive, Tales of a Shaman's Apprentice: An Ethnobotanist Searches for New Medicines in the Amazon Rain Forest (Penguin Book 1993).

apprehension, and a sense of impending doom may last about 12 hours, with a sense of unreality persisting for several days (Claus et al. 1970).

Phenylethylamine Hallucinogens

The phenylethylamine drugs are chemically related to amphetamines. Phenylethylamines have varying degrees of hallucinogenic and CNS stimulant effects, which are likely related to their ability to release serotonin and dopamine, respectively. Consequently, the phenylethylamines that predominantly release serotonin are dominated by their hallucinogenic action and are LSD-like, while those more inclined to release dopamine are dominated by their stimulant effects and are cocaine-like.

Dimethoxymethylamphetamine (DOM or STP)

The basic structure of DOM is amphetamine. Nonetheless, it is a fairly powerful hallucinogen that seems to work through mechanisms similar to those of mescaline and LSD. In fact, the effects of DOM are similar to those caused by a combination of amphetamine and LSD, with the hallucinogenic effects of the drug overpowering the amphetaminelike physiological effects.

Designer" Amphetamines "Designer" amphetamines were discussed in Chapter 11 but are presented again here due to their hallucinogenic effects. Their hybrid actions as psychedelic stimulants not only make them a particularly fascinating topic for research but also provide a unique experience described by drug abusers as a "smooth amphetamine." This characterization likely accounts for the popularity of the designer amphetamines.

3,4-Methylenedioxyamphetamine (MDA) MDA, first synthesized in 1910, is structurally related to both mescaline and amphetamine. Early research found that MDA is an anorexiant (causing loss of appetite) as well as a mood elevator in some persons. Further research has shown that the mode of action of MDA is similar to that of amphetamine. It causes additional release of the neurotransmitters serotonin, dopamine, and norepinephrine.

MDA has been used as an adjunct to psychotherapy. In one study, eight volunteers who had previously experienced the effects of LSD under clinical conditions were given 150 milligrams of MDA. Effects of the drug were noted between 40 and 60 minutes following ingestion by all eight subjects. The subjective effects following administration peaked at the end of 90 minutes and persisted for approximately 8 hours. None of the subjects experienced hallucinations, perceptual distortion, or closed-eye imagery, but they reported that the feelings the drug induced had some relationship to those previously experienced with LSD. The subjects found that both drugs induced an intensification of feelings, increased perceptions of self-insight, and heightened empathy with others during the experience. Most of the subjects also felt an increased sense of aesthetic enjoyment at some point during the intoxication. Seven of the eight subjects said they perceived music as "three-dimensional" (Naranjo et al. 1967).

On the "street," MDA has been called the "love drug" because of its effects on the sense of touch and the attitudes of the users. Users often report experiencing a sense of well-being (likely a stimulant effect) and heightened tactile sensations (like a hallucinogenic effect) and thus increased pleasure through sex and expressions of affection. Those under the influence of MDA frequently focus on interpersonal relationships and demonstrate an overwhelming desire or need to be with or talk to people. Some users say they have a very pleasant "body high"—more sensual than cerebral, and more emphatic than introverted.

The unpleasant side effects most often reported are nausea, periodic tensing of muscles in the neck, tightening of the jaw and grinding of the teeth, and dilation of the pupils. "Street" doses of MDA range from 100 to 150 milligrams. Serious convulsions and death have resulted from larger doses, but in these cases, the quantity of MDA was not accurately measured. Ingestion of 500 milligrams of pure MDA has been shown to cause death. The only adverse reaction to moderate doses seems to be marked physical exhaustion, lasting as long as two days (Marquardt et al. 1978).

An unpleasant MDA experience should be treated the same as a "bad trip" with any hallucinogen. The person should be "talked down"

FIGHTING THE DRUG WAR

Ecstasy, an amphetamine with hallucinogenic properties, was *the* "designer drug" of the late 1980s and early 1990s. It remained legal until 1985, when the FDA determined that it could be seriously harmful and outlawed its use. Since then, the Ecstasy market has followed the typical designer drug scenario—limited access created higher demand, prompting the development of drugs that produced similar effects but could not be declared illegal.

Enter "Herbal Ecstasy," a stimulant derived from the Chinese herb *ma huang,* or ephedra. It is, in many ways, the brainchild of Scan Shayan, the 20-year-old chief executive officer of Global World Media, and some of his friends, who were eager to cash in on what they saw as a great market opportunity. Quoted in *Newsweek* in mid-1996, Shayan said, "We thought, God, if we could come up with an alternative product like [Ecstasy] that was safe, legal and natural, there would be a huge market for it." He met a group of herbalists who had been experimenting with mildly psychoactive herbs, and worked with them to develop Herbal Ecstasy.

Although Herbal Ecstasy does not have the hallucinogenic properties of its illegal predecessor, it carries the same cachet. It is marketed as a way to increase energy, heighten sexual sensation, and raise cosmic consciousness. Thanks to a 1994 law limiting the federal government's power to regulate herbs, vitamins, and diet pills, the FDA has only limited control over the production, distribution, and use of this product. Just because it's legal and natural, however, it doesn't mean that Herbal Ecstacy is safe.

Herbal Ecstasy, and other "herbal supplements" like it, first came under fire in mid-1996, after a 20-year-old college student died from the combined effects of ephedrine, pseudoephedrine, phenylpropanolamine, and caffeine—the active ingredients in Ultimate Xphoria, the herbal supplement he and his friends took while on spring break in Florida. Since then, the FDA and other critics have claimed that ephedra and ephedra-based substances can cause hypertension, palpitations, nerve damage, muscle damage, psychosis, stroke, memory loss, and, in some cases, seizures and death.

Many natural food stores that sold these ephedra-based supplements no longer carry them because these stimulants have no therapeutic value. Furthermore, many herbalists and members of the National Nutritional Foods Association (NNFA) have distanced themselves from these products, claiming they are not a legitimate part of the natural products industry. They remain available in some natural products stores and by mail, however, and they are marketed on the Internet.

In light of the acknowledged danger of these substances, and the FDA's lack of power to control them, some states, —including Florida, California, and New York, —have begun to work toward prohibiting the sale of certain ma huang products. A battle is also raging within the American Health Products Association between those who support the continued sale of ephedra-based products and those who do not.

Regardless of whether the FDA will ultimately be able to exert control over the distribution of these substances or whether it will remain in the hands of the natural products industry, it is clear that something must be done to protect the public health. As the director of the Utah Natural Products Alliance, Loren Israelsen said, ". . . the industry had better establish ground rules for itself and have the guts to enforce them."

Sources: Cowley, G. "Herbal Warning" *Newsweek* (May 6, 1996). p 61.
Mergentime, K. "Ephedra-Linked Death Sparks FDA Backlash" *Natural Foods Merchandiser* (June 1996).
Creative Loafine [Online]. October 1995.

(reassured) in a friendly and supportive manner. Usually, the use of other drugs is not needed, although medical attention may be necessary. Under the Comprehensive Drug Abuse Prevention and Control Act of 1970 (see Appendix A), MDA is classified as a Schedule I substance; illegal possession is a serious offense.

Methylenedioxymethamphetamine (MDMA)

MDMA is a modification of MDA, but is thought to have more psychedelic but less stimulant (for example, euphoria) activity than its predecessor. MDMA is also structurally similar to mescaline. This drug has become known as "Ecstasy," "XTC" and "Adam" (U.S. Department of Justice 1991b). (Ecstasy was also discussed in Chapter 11.)

MDMA was synthesized in 1912, but it only became widely used in the 1980s (Shulgin 1990). This "designer" amphetamine can be produced easily; the reaction can literally be set up in a "cookie jar" using a coffee filter. The synthesis is often done sloppily by illicit labs and causes contaminants in the final product (Randall 1992a). The unusual psychological effects it produces are part of the reason for its popularity. The drug produces euphoria, increased sensitivity to touch, and lowered inhibitions. Many users claim it intensifies emotional feelings without sensory distortion and that it increases empathy and awareness both of the user's body and of the aesthetics of the surroundings (Creighton et al. 1991; Taylor 1994). Some consider MDMA to be an aphrodisiac. Because MDMA lowers defense mechanisms and reduces inhibitions, it has even been used during psychoanalysis (Creighton et al. 1991; Grob et al. 1992).

In the 1980s, MDMA was popularized by articles in *Newsweek* (Adler 1985), *Time* (Toufexis 1985), and other magazines, which have mentioned the euphoric effects, potential therapeutic value, and lack of serious side effects, MDMA is still popular with college-age students and young adults (Johnston et al. 1996). Because of its effect to enhance sensations, MDMA has been used as part of a countercultural "rave" scene, including high-tech music and laser light shows. Observers report that MDMA-linked "rave" parties are reminiscent of the "acid parties" of the 1960s and 1970s (Randall 1992b; Iwersen and Schmoldt 1996).

Because of the widespread abuse of MDMA, the DEA prohibited its use by placing it on Schedule I in 1985 (Greenhouse 1992). At the time of the ban, it was estimated that up to 200 physicians were using the drug in psychotherapy (Greer and Tolbert 1990) and an estimated 30,000 doses a month were being taken for recreational purposes (*American Medical News* 1985).

MDMA is usually taken orally, but it is sometimes snorted or even occasionally smoked (Taylor 1994). After the "high" starts, it may persist for minutes or even an hour, depending on the person, the purity of the drug, and the environment in which it is taken. When "coming down" from an MDMA-induced high, people will often take small oral doses known as "boosters" to get high again. If they take too many boosters, they become very fatigued the next day. The average dose is about 75–150 milligrams; a number of cases of toxic effects have been reported at higher doses (Randall 1992a).

There is disagreement as to the possible harmful side effects of MDMA. Use of high doses can cause psychosis and paranoia (Iwersen and Schmoldt 1996). Some negative physiological responses caused by recreational doses include dilated pupils, dry mouth and throat, clenching of teeth (in 76% of users), muscle aches and stiffness (in 28% of users), fatigue (in 80% of users), insomnia (in 38% of users), agitation, and anxiety. Some of these reactions can be intense and unpredictable. Under some conditions, death can be caused by *hyperthermia* (elevated body temperature), instability of the autonomic nervous system, and kidney failure (Iwersen and Schmoldt 1996; Greenhouse 1992).

Several studies have demonstrated long-term damage to serotonin neurons in the brain following a single high dose of both MDMA and MDA (O'Brien 1996). Although the behavioral significance of this damage in humans is not clear, at the present time caution using this drug is warranted.

Anticholinergic Hallucinogens

The anticholinergic hallucinogens include naturally occurring alkaloid (bitter organic base) substances that are present in plants and herbs found around the world. These drugs are often mentioned in folklore and in early literature as being added to "potions." They are thought to have killed the Roman Emperor Claudius and to have poisoned Hamlet's father. Historically, they have been the favorite drugs used to eliminate inconvenient people (Marken et al. 1996). Hallucinogens affecting the cholinergic neurons also have been used by South American Indians for religious ceremonies (Schultes and Hofmann 1980) and were probably used in witchcraft to give the illusion of flying, to prepare sacrificial victims, and even to give some types of marijuana ("superpot") its kick.

The potato family of plants (Solanaceae) contain most of these mind-altering drugs. Three potent anticholinergic compounds are commonly found in these plants: (1) scopolamine, or hyoscine; (2) hyoscyamine; and (3) atropine. Scopolamine may produce excitement, hallucinations, and delirium even at therapeutic doses: with atropine, doses bordering on toxic levels are usually required to obtain these effects (Schultes and Hofmann 1973). All these active alkaloid drugs block some acetylcholine receptors (see Chapter 6).

The alkaloid drugs can be used as ingredients in cold symptom remedies because they have a drying effect and block production of mucus in the nose and throat. They also prevent salivation, so that the mouth becomes uncommonly dry and perspiration may stop. Atropine may increase the heart rate by 100% and cause the pupils to dilate markedly, causing inability to focus on nearby objects. Other annoying side effects of these anticholinergic drugs include constipation and difficulty in urinating. These inconveniences tend to discourage excessive abuse of these drugs for their hallucinogenic properties. Usually people who abuse these anticholinergic compounds are receiving the drugs by prescription (Marken et al. 1996).

Anticholinergics can cause drowsiness by affecting the sleep centers of the brain. At large doses, a condition occurs that is similar to a psychosis, characterized by delirium, loss of attention, mental confusion, and sleepiness (Carlini 1993). Hallucinations may also occur at higher doses. At very high doses, paralysis of the respiratory system may cause death.

Although hundreds of plant species naturally contain anticholinergic substances and consequently can cause psychedelic experiences, only a few of the principal plants will be mentioned here.

Atropa Belladonna: **The Deadly Nightshade Plant** Knowledge of this plant is very old, and its use as a drug is reported in early folklore. The name of the genus, *Atropa,* is the origin for the drug name *atropine,* and indicates the reverence the Greeks had for the plant. Atropos was one of the three Fates in Greek mythology, whose duty it was to cut the thread of life when the time came. This plant has been used for thousands of years by assassins and murderers. In *Tales of the Arabian Nights,* unsuspecting potentates were poisoned with atropine from the deadly nightshade or one of its relatives. Fourteen berries of the deadly nightshade contain enough drug to cause death.

The species name, *belladonna,* means "beautiful woman." The early Roman and Egyptian women knew that girls with large pupils were considered attractive and friendly. To create this condition, they would put a few drops of an extract of this plant into their eyes, causing the pupils to dilate (Marken et al. 1996). Belladonna has also had a reputation as a love potion.

Mandragora Officinarum: **The Mandrake** The mandrake contains several active psychedelic alkaloids: hyoscyamine, scopolamine, atropine, and mandragorine. Mandrake has been used as a love potion for centuries but has also been known for its toxic properties. In ancient folk medicine, mandrake was used to treat many ailments in spite of its side effects. It was recommended as a sedative, to relieve nervous conditions, and to relieve pain (Schultes and Hofmann 1980).

The root of the mandrake is forked and, viewed with a little imagination, may resemble the human body. Because of this resemblance, it has been credited with human attributes, which gave rise to many superstitions in the Middle Ages about its magical powers. Shakespeare referred to this plant in *Romeo and Juliet.* In her farewell speech, Juliet says, "And shrieks like mandrakes torn out of the earth, that living mortals hearing them run mad."

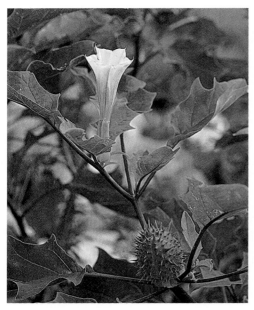

Datura stramonium, or jimsonweed, a
common plant that contains the hallucinogenic
drug scopolamine.

Hyoscyamus Niger: **Henbane** Henbane is a
plant that contains both hyoscyamine and scopolamine. In A.D. 60, Pliny the Elder spoke of henbane: "For this is certainly known, that if one takes
it in drink more than four leaves, it will put him
beside himself" (Jones 1956). Henbane was also
used in the orgies, or *bacchanalias,* of the ancient
world.

Although rarely used today, henbane has been
given medicinally since early times. It was frequently used to cause sleep, although hallucinations often occurred if given in excess. It was likely
included in witches' brews and deadly concoctions
during the Dark Ages (Schultes and Hofmann
1980).

Datura Stramonium: **Jimsonweed** The *Datura*
genus of the Solanaceae family (see earlier discussion) includes a large number of related plants
found worldwide. The principal active drug in this
group is scopolamine; there are also several less
active alkaloids.

Throughout history, these plants have been
used as hallucinogens by many societies. They are
mentioned in early Sanskrit and Chinese writings

and were revered by the Buddhists. There is also
some indication that the priestess (oracle) at the
ancient Greek temple of Apollo at Delphi was
under the influence of this type of plant when she
made prophecies (Schultes 1970). Prior to the supposed divine possession, she appeared to have
chewed leaves of the sacred laurel. A mystic vapor
was also reported to have risen from a fissure in
the ground. The sacred laurel may have been one
of the *Datura* species, and the vapors may have
come from burning these plants.

Jimsonweed gets its name from an incident
that took place in seventeenth-century Jamestown. British soldiers ate
this weed while trying to
capture Nathaniel Bacon,
who had made seditious remarks about the king. The
effect of the hallucinogen
was said to be " . . . a very pleasant comedy; for
they turn'd fools upon it for several days" (Beverly
1947, 139). Although still abused occasionally by
adventuresome young people, the anticholinergic
side effects of jimsonweed are so unpleasant that it
rarely becomes a long-term problem.

> **jimsonweed**
> a potent hallu-
> cinogenic plant

Other Hallucinogens

Technically, any drug that alters perceptions,
thoughts, and feelings in a manner that is not normally experienced but in dreams can be classified
as a hallucinogen. Because the brain's sensory
input is complex and involves several neurotransmitter systems, drugs with many diverse effects
can cause hallucinations (Jaffe 1990).

Three agents that do not conveniently fit into
the principal categories of hallucinogens will be
discussed in the following sections.

Phencyclidine (PCP) PCP is considered by many
experts as the most dangerous of the hallucinogens (U.S. Department of Justice 1991b). PCP was
developed in the late 1950s as an intravenous
anesthetic. Although it was found to be effective, it
had serious side effects that caused it to be discontinued for human use. Sometimes when people
were recovering from PCP anesthesia, they experienced delirium and manic states of excitation lasting 18 hours (Jaffe 1990). PCP is currently a

Schedule II drug, legitimately available only as an anesthetic for animals. It has been banned from veterinary practice since 1985 because of its high theft rate. Most, if not all, PCP used in the United States today is produced illegally (U.S. Department of Justice 1991b).

"Street" PCP is mainly synthesized from readily available chemical precursors in clandestine laboratories. Within 24 hours, "cooks" (the makers of street PCP) can set up a lab, make several gallons of the drug, and destroy the lab before the police can locate them. Liquid PCP is then poured into containers and ready for shipment (Sanchez 1988).

PCP first appeared on the street drug scene in 1967 as the *"PeaCe Pill."* In 1968, it reappeared in New York as a substance called "hog." By 1969, PCP was found under a variety of guises. It was sold as "angel dust" and sprinkled on parsley for smoking. It has sold on the streets under at least 50 different slang names, including *loveboat, lovely, key to street E, greed, wacky weed, supergrass, rocket fuel, elephant tranquilizer, snorts, cyclone, cadillac, earth, killer weed, embalming fluid,* and *flying saucers* (U.S. Department of Justice 1991b; Gorelick and Balster 1995).

In the late 1960s, PCP began to find its way into a variety of street drugs sold as psychedelics. By 1970, authorities observed that phencyclidine was used widely as a main ingredient in psychedelic preparations. It is still frequently substituted for and sold as LSD, mescaline, marijuana, and cocaine (Goldstein 1995).

One difficulty in estimating the effects or use patterns of PCP is caused by variance in drug purity. Also, there are about 30 **analogs** of PCP, some of which have appeared on the street. PCP has so many other street names that people may not know they are using it or they may have been deceived when buying what they thought was LSD or mescaline. Users may not question the identity of the substances unless they have a bad reaction.

analogs
drugs with similar structures

PCP is available as a pure, white crystalline powder, as tablets, or as capsules. However, because it is usually manufactured in makeshift laboratories, it is frequently discolored by contaminants from a tan to brown with a consistency ranging from powder to a gummy mass (U.S. Department of Justice 1991b). PCP can be taken orally, smoked, sniffed, or injected (American Psychiatric Association 1994). In the late 1960s through the early 1970s, PCP was mostly taken orally, but it is now commonly snorted or applied to dark brown cigarettes, leafy materials such as parsley, mint, oregano, marijuana, or tobacco and smoked (U.S. Department of Justice 1991b). By smoking PCP, the experienced user is better able to limit his or her dosage to a desired level. After smoking, the subjective effects appear within 1 to 5 minutes and peak within the next 5 to 30 minutes. The "high" lasts about 4 to 6 hours, followed by a 6- to 24-hour "comedown."

In the 1979 national drug survey performed by the National Institute on Drug Abuse, about 7% of the U.S. high school seniors had used PCP in a 12-month period; however, in 1996, that rate declined to 2.6% (Johnston 1996).

Physiological Effects Although PCP may have hallucinogenic effects, it can also cause a host of other physiological actions, including stimulation, depression, anesthesia, and analgesia. The effects of PCP on the central nervous system vary greatly. At low doses, the most prominent effect is similar to that of alcohol intoxication, with generalized numbness. As the dose of PCP is increased, the person becomes even more insensitive and may become fully anesthetized. Large doses can cause coma, convulsions, and death (American Psychiatric Association 1994).

The majority of peripheral effects are apparently related to activation of the sympathetic nervous system (see Chapter 6). Flushing, excess sweating, and a blank stare are common, although the size of the pupils is unaffected. The cardiovascular system reacts by increasing blood pressure and heart rate. Other effects include side-to-side eye movements (called *nystagmus*), muscular incoordination, double vision, dizziness, nausea, and vomiting (Gorelick and Balster 1995). These symptoms occur in many people taking medium to high doses.

Psychological Effects PCP has unpleasant effects most of the time it is used. Why, then, do people use it repeatedly as their drug of choice?

PCP has the ability to alter markedly the person's subjective feelings; this effect may be reinforcing, even though the alteration is not always positive. There is an element of risk, not knowing how the "trip" will turn out. PCP may give the user feelings of strength, power, and invulnerability. One user describes the effects of PCP as follows: "I felt like I didn't have a care in the world. It made me feel like God, like I was powerful. I felt superhuman" (Sanchez 1988). Other positive effects include heightened sensitivity to outside stimuli, a sense of stimulation and mood elevation, and dissociation from surroundings. Also, PCP is a social drug; virtually all users report taking it in groups rather than during a solitary experience. PCP also causes serious perceptual distortions. Users cannot accurately interpret the environment and as a result may walk in front of moving cars or jump off buildings, feeling indestructible or weightless (Goldstein 1995). High oral doses have been used to commit suicide; respiratory depression is the specific cause of death.

Chronic users may take PCP in "runs" extending over two to three days, during which time they do not sleep or eat. In later stages of chronic administration, users may develop outright paranoia and unpredictable violent behavior, as well as auditory hallucinations (American Psychiatric Association 1994). Law enforcement officers claim to be more fearful of suspects on PCP than of suspects on other drugs of abuse. Often such people appear to have superhuman strength and are totally irrational and very difficult, even dangerous, to manage (Sanchez 1988).

"PCP" has no equal in its ability to produce brief psychoses similar to schizophrenia. The psychoses—induced with moderate doses given to normal, healthy volunteers—last about two hours and are characterized by changes in body image, thought disorders, estrangement, autism, and occasionally rigid inability to move (**catatonia,** or catalepsy). Subjects report feeling numb, have great difficulty differentiating between themselves and their surroundings, and complain afterward of feeling extremely isolated and apathetic. They are often violently paranoid during the psychosis (American

catatonia

a condition of physical rigidity, excitement, and stupor

Psychiatric Association 1994; *Medical Letter* 1996b). When PCP was given experimentally to hospitalized chronic schizophrenics, it made them much worse not for several hours but for six weeks. "PCP is not just another hallucinogen, to be warned about in the same breath as LSD. . . . PCP is far more dangerous to some individuals than the other abused drugs" (Luisada 1978; Goldstein 1995).

Medical Management The diagnosis of a PCP overdose is frequently missed because the symptoms often closely resemble those of an acute schizophrenic episode.

Simple, uncomplicated PCP intoxication can be managed with the same techniques used in other psychedelic drug cases. It is important to have a quiet environment, limited contact with an empathic person capable of determining any deterioration in the patient's physical state, protection from self-harm, and the availability of hospital facilities. "Talking down" is not helpful; the patient is better off isolated from external stimuli as much as possible.

Valium is often used for its sedating effect to prevent injury to self and to staff and also to reduce the chance for severe convulsions. An antipsychotic agent (for example, Haldol) is frequently administered to make the patient manageable (Jaffe 1990).

The medical management of a comatose or convulsing patient is more difficult. The patient may need external respiratory assistance and external cooling to reduce fever. Blood pressure may have to be reduced to safe levels and convulsions controlled. Restraints and four to five strong hospital aides are often needed to prevent the patient from injuring himself or herself or the medical staff. After the coma lightens, the patient typically becomes delirious, paranoid, and violently assaultive.

Effects of Chronic Use Chronic PCP users may develop a tolerance to the drug; thus, a decrease in behavioral effects and toxicity can occur with frequent administration. Different forms of dependence may occur when tolerance develops. Users may complain of vague cravings after cessation of the drug. In addition, long-term difficulties in memory, speech, and thinking persist for 6 to 12 months in the chronic user (Jaffe 1990). These functional changes are accompanied by personality deficits such as social isolation, states of anxiety, nervousness, and extreme agitation (American Psychiatric Association 1994).

Marijuana In high doses, marijuana use can result in image distortions and hallucinations (Abood and Martin 1992). Some users claim that marijuana can enhance hearing, vision, and skin sensitivity, although these claims have not been confirmed in controlled laboratory studies. As one 19-year old man described:

> When you are stoned your body has control, but your mind and thinking [are] altered. I slowly felt my legs rising towards the ceiling. I wasn't nervous anymore, I was very relaxed. I gazed up at the ceiling and watched the glowing stars move. I began to get very tired and closed my eyes.

> *From Venturelli's files, 1995–1996*

Although typical marijuana use does not appear to cause severe emotional disorders like the other hallucinogens, some experts suggest it can aggravate underlying mental illness such as depression. Each month, an estimated 5000 people seek professional treatment due to marijuana-related problems (Brown 1991). In contrast to other hallucinogens that have a combination of stimulant and psychedelic effects, high doses of marijuana cause a combination of depression and hallucinations and enhance the appetite (Goldstein 1995). Marijuana is discussed thoroughly in Chapter 14.

Inhalants Abuse of inhalants is highest by eighth-graders and includes 20% of all adolescents in the United States (*Prevention Pipeline* 1995). Because of the potential for serious health consequences, this high rate of abuse by young people is very alarming. In fact, a recent report claims that inhalants killed more than 1000 adolescents in 1994 (Vaughn 1995).

These substances are popular for several reasons:

▲ They are readily available in most households.

▲ They are inexpensive.

▲ They are easy to conceal.

▲ They are not illegal.

▲ Most users are uninformed about the potential dangers (*Prevention Pipeline* 1995).

Inhalants are gases that can be introduced into the body through the pulmonary (lungs) route. This category of drugs includes an array of different compounds and can be classified into three major groups: **volatile** solvents, anesthetics, and nitrites (Swan 1993; *Medical Letter* 1996a). Most of the inhalants can cause hallucinations as well as create intoxicating and euphorigenic effects.

volatile
readily evaporated at low temperatures

Sniffing Out the Inhalants: Signs of Abuse

The following are common signs found in children who are frequent users of inhalants:

▲ Collect an unusual assortment of chemicals (such as glues, paints, thinners and solvents, nail polish, liquid eraser, and cleaning fluids) in bedroom or with belongings.

▲ Breath occasionally smells of solvents.

▲ Often has sniffles similar to a cold, but without other symptoms of the ailment.

▲ Appears drunk for short periods of time (15–60 minutes), but recovers quickly.

▲ Doesn't do well in school and usually is unkempt.

▲ Smell of inhalants or solvents in unusual containers around the house, such as soda cans and plastic bags or on rags and bandannas.

▲ If sniffing continues for extended time, there may be physical signs such as a rash around the mouth and nose, frequent headaches, nausea, slurred speech, nose bleeds, and loss of weight (Vaughn 1995). ■

Volatile Solvents Many of these substances were never intended to be used by humans as drugs; consequently, they are often not thought of as having abuse potential. For example, inhalants include some solvents, glue, paint thinner, aerosols from paints, hairsprays, cookware coating agents, liquid paper correction fluid, nail polish remover, felt-tip marking pens, lighter and cleaning fluids, and gasoline (U.S. Department of Justice 1991b). These chemicals are not regulated like other drugs of abuse, so they are readily available to young people. Consequently, children and teenagers (7 to 17 years) are most likely to abuse the volatile solvents (Swan 1993). Parents should be particularly cautious about making sure their children are not inadvertently exposed to these chemicals (see the Here and Now box).

The effects of the volatile chemicals that are commonly abused include initial nausea with some irritation of airways causing coughing and sneezing. Low doses often bring a brief feeling of light-headedness, mild stimulation followed by a loss of control, lack of coordination, and disorientation accompanied by dizziness and possible hallucinations (Goldstein 1995). Higher doses can produce relaxation and depression leading to sleep or coma. The depression effects resemble those caused by alcohol but of a shorter duration: 15–60 minutes (U.S. Department of Justice 1991b; American Psychiatric Association 1994).

Several potential toxicities may result from inhaling large quantities of these substances. Some of these chemicals can cause heart arrhythmia, the principal cause of death from acute inhalant exposure (Jaffe 1990). In some cases, the abuser inhales the vapors from containers such as plastic bags or soda cans (called "sniffing," "snorting," or "huffing") to maximize the dose as well as from old rags or bandannas soaked in a solvent fluid (U.S. Department of Justice 1991b). If inhalation is continued, dangerous **hypoxia** may occur and cause brain damage or death (Swan 1993). For example, on December 21, 1993, in Chester, New Jersey, 16-year-old Justin and his friends were inhaling laughing gas (nitrous oxide) when Justin collapsed and instantly died. The cause of his death was either cardiac arrest or suffocation from the highly concentrated amount of nitrous oxide (adapted from *Current Health* 1995). Other potential toxic consequences of inhaling such substances include hypertension and damage to the cardiac muscle, peripheral nerves, brain, and kidneys (American Psychiatric Association 1994).

hypoxia
a state of oxygen deficiency

The potential harm from chronic use of the volatile inhalants has not been well studied. However, it appears that repeated exposure to these chemicals can cause the following problems:

1. Permanent brain damage, which interferes with reasoning, memory, and problem-solving ability.

2. Impairment of motor behavior, which results in frequent falls and accidents and an inability to do simple motor tasks.

3. Severe psychological problems, which cause a withdrawn personality frequently accompanied with severe depression.

4. Other serious health consequences such as damage to airways, lungs, kidneys, and liver.

In addition, chronic users of inhalants frequently lose their appetite, are continually tired, and experience nose bleeds. If use of inhalants persists, some of the damage becomes irreversible (U.S. Department of Justice 1991b; American Psychiatric Association 1994).

Why do children and teenagers sniff the fumes of these dangerous chemicals? Most often a friend or sibling encourages the initial exposure. Chronic inhalant users frequently have a profile like that associated with other substance abusers. That is, often they live in unhappy surroundings with severe family or school problems, they have poor self-images, and sniffing gives them a readily available escape (U.S. Department of Justice 1991b).

As with most substances of abuse, the fewer times volatile inhalants are used, the easier it is to stop and the less likely it is that severe physiological damage has been done. Although the inhalants do not tend to cause dangerous physical dependence, their chronic use can lead to an addiction, which requires professional counseling or even hospitalization (American Psychiatric Association 1994). Frequently, the young inhalant users resist treatment for their addiction, because of peer pressure (U.S. Department of Justice 1991b).

Anesthetics When used properly, other forms of inhalants with abuse potential are important therapeutic agents. Included in this category are the general anesthetics. Although all the anesthetic gases work much like the CNS depressants, only nitrous oxide (laughing gas) is available enough to be a significant abuse concern (Swan 1993). Nitrous oxide is frequently used for minor outpatient procedures in offices of both physicians and dentists. Consequently, the most likely abusers of this substance are health professionals themselves or their staff. For the most part, nitrous oxide does not pose a significant abuse problem for the general public. However, occasionally college students also abuse nitrous oxide via small cylindrical cartridges used as charges for whipped cream dispensers and referred to as "whippets" (Goldstein 1995). One student who had access to this inhalant recounts:

> A couple of times after using whippets, my nose would begin to bleed profusely. That really scared the s— out of me. After that happened a couple of times, I stopped doing the laughing gas all together.
>
> *From the files of Peter Venturelli, interview with a 20-year-old male, 1995*

Although significant abuse problems are infrequent, there are occasional reports of severe hypoxia or death due to acute overdoses with nitrous oxide or psychosis and neuronal disorders developing after chronic abuse (Dohrn 1993).

Nitrites Nitrites are chemicals that cause vasodilation and historically, have been abused by only a few, selective groups, such as gay men, to enhance "sexual stamina and pleasure." The nitrite products are referred to as "poppers" or "rush" and contain butyl and propyl nitrites. Their use has dramatically declined since these chemicals were banned in 1991 (Swan 1993).

Patterns of Inhalant Abuse Inhalant abuse is typically a problem of younger adolescents. Older teenagers often view use of inhalants with disdain and consider it unsophisticated and a "kid's" habit.

There has been a recent disturbing trend of increasing inhalant abuse by younger kids (for example, approximately 35% more eighth-graders abused inhalants in 1995 than in 1992; see Table 13.1). Much of this increase in abuse is thought to be due to more young girls starting to sniff the volatile solvents. At present, it appears that in most parts of the country, males use solvents at only a slightly higher rate than females (Swan 1993).

Survey results suggest that patterns of inhalant abuse are more dependent on socioeconomic than ethnic factors. For example, use by Hispanic adolescents is high in some low-income neighborhoods; however, their patterns of abuse are similar to other ethnic groups in intermediate- and high-income neighborhoods. Consequently, it is not surprising that Native Americans, who on average live in the worst socioeconomic conditions, also have the highest solvent abuse rates (Swan 1993).

The extent of solvent abuse in the United States is very difficult to determine accurately. Typically, inhalant abuse has an episodic pattern, with short-term outbreaks occurring at single schools or in a limited region. These isolated incidents reflect the faddish nature of inhalant use and result in a continually fluctuating level of abuse. Consequently, results from regional surveys for solvent abuse frequently are distorted and do not accurately represent the national abuse patterns for these substances. However, despite the problems of accurately determining the extent of inhalant use, it is apparent that these products are being frequently abused by many adolescents, and the result can be deadly (Swan 1993).

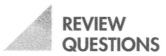

REVIEW QUESTIONS

1. Why were substances with hallucinogenic properties so popular with ancient religions and cults?

2. Why would a drug with both stimulant and hallucinogenic effects be a popular drug of abuse?

3. Why do some users find a psychedelic experience terrifying?

4. Do you think the federal government is justified in lying to the public about the dangers of hallucinogens to get people to stop using these drugs? Defend your answer.

5. How do the side effects of LSD compare to those of the CNS depressants?

6. Why is PCP more dangerous than LSD?

7. How do the effects of MDMA differ from those of LSD?

8. Why is the use of inhalants by kids especially disturbing?

9. What is the best way to convince people that hallucinogenic drugs of abuse should not be used?

10. What is a "bad trip" and how long could it last?

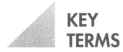

KEY TERMS

hallucinogens
psychotomimetic
psychedelic
psychotogenic
synesthesia
"flashbacks"
ergotism
mydriasis
jimsonweed
analogs
catatonia
volatile
hypoxia

WWW EXERCISES FOR THE WEB

Exercise 1: MAPS

The Multidisciplinary Association for Psychedelic Studies, MAPS, is a corporation chartered in 1986 as a membership-based research and educational organization. Currently numbering 1400 members, MAPS focuses on the development of beneficial, socially-sanctioned uses of psychedelic drugs and marijuana. Such uses may include psychotherapeutic research and treatment, treatment of addiction, pain relief, spiritual exploration, shamanic healing, psychic research, brain physiology research and related scientific inquiries. MAPS pursues its mission by helping scientific researchers design, obtain governmental approval for, fund, conduct and report on psychedelic research in human volunteers. MAPS also publish a quarterly newsletter that is sent to its members as well as a large number of government policy makers and academic experts.

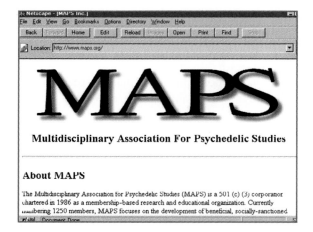

SUMMARY

1 Many drugs can exert hallucinogenic effects. The principal hallucinogens include LSD types, phenylethylamines, and anticholinergic agents. The four major effects that occur from administering LSD include (a) heightened senses, (b) a loss of sensory control, (c) self-reflection or introspection, and (d) a loss of identity or sense of cosmic merging.

2 The recent resurgence in LSD abuse likely reflects its perceived safety and a lack of education about its dangers.

3 Hallucinogens exaggerate sensory input and cause vivid and unusual visual and auditory effects.

4 The classical hallucinogens, such as LSD, cause predominantly psychedelic effects. Phenylethylamines are related to amphetamines and cause varying combinations of psychedelic and stimulant effects. Anticholinergic drugs are also psychedelic in high doses.

5 One of the prominent effects of hallucinogens is to cause self-reflection. The user becomes aware of thoughts and feelings that had been forgotten or repressed. Some experiences help to clarify motives and relationships and cause periods of greater openness. These effects have been claimed by some psychiatrists to provide valid insights useful in psychotherapy.

6 The classical hallucinogens do not cause physical dependence. Although some tolerance can occur to the hallucinogenic effects of drugs like LSD, withdrawal effects are usually minor.

7 The environment plays a major role in determining the sensory response to hallucinogens. Environments that are warm, comfortable, and hospitable tend to create a pleasant sensory response to the psychedelic effects of these drugs. In contrast, threatening, hostile environments are likely to lead to intimidating, frightening "bad trips."

8 In some users, high doses of LSD can cause a terrifying destruction of identity, resulting in panic and severe anxiety that resembles schizophrenia. Another psychological feature commonly associated with LSD is the "flashback" phenomenon. LSD use can cause recurring, unexpected visual and time distortions that last a few minutes to several hours. Flashbacks can occur months to years after use of the drug.

9 Hallucinogens purchased on the "street" are often poorly prepared and contaminated with adulterant substances. This practice of cutting with other substances also makes use of street hallucinogens very dangerous.

10 PCP differs from the other traditional hallucinogens in several ways: (a) It is a general anesthetic in high doses. (b) It causes schizophrenia-like psychosis. PCP can cause incredible strength and extreme violent behavior, making users very difficult to manage. (c) Management of the severe psychological reactions to PCP requires drug therapy, whereas treatment of other hallucinogens often only requires reassurance, "talking down," and supportive therapy. (d) Reactions to overdoses include fever, convulsions, and coma.

11 The commonly abused inhalants are volatile substances that can cause hallucinations, intoxication, and euphoria. These substances include volatile solvents, anesthetics, and nitrites. These chemicals are typically abused by children and teenagers due to their ready availability. The effects of inhalant drugs are mild stimulation, lack of motor control, dizziness, and hallucinations. High doses can cause violent behavior, heart arrhythmia, unconsciousness, and even death.

REFERENCES

Abood, M., and B. Martin, "Neurobiology of Marijuana Abuse." *Trends in Pharmacological Sciences* 13 (May 1992): 201–6.

Abraham, H., A. Aldridge, and P. Gogia. "The Psychopharmacology of Hallucinogens." *Neuropharmacology* 14 (1996): 285–98.

Adler, J. "Getting High on Ecstasy." *Newsweek* (15 April 1985): 15.

American Medical News (14 June 1985).

American Psychiatric Association. "Substance-Related Disorders." *Diagnostic Statistical Manual of Mental Disorders,* 4th ed. *[DSM-IV]*, A. Frances, Chairperson, 175–272. Washington, DC: American Psychiatric Association, 1994.

Associated Press. "Timothy Leary, 1960s LSD Guru, Succumbs to Cancer." *Salt Lake Tribune* 252 (June 1, 1996): A-6.

Becenti, D. "American Indians Get OK to Use Peyote." *Salt Lake Tribune* 249 (October 30, 1994): A10.

Brown, M. *Guide to Fight Substance Abuse.* Nashville, TN: International Broadcast Services, 1991.

Burger, A., ed. "Quotes from Albert Hofmann." *Drugs Affecting the Central Nervous System.* Psychotomimetic Agents, vol. 2. New York: Dekker, 1968.

Carlini, E. "Preliminary Note: Dangerous Use of Anticholinergic Drugs in Brazil." *Drugs and Alcohol Dependence* 32 (1993): 1–7.

"Celebration #1." *New Yorker* 42 (1966): 43.

Claus, E. P., V. E. Tyler, and L. R. Brady. *Pharmacognosy,* 6th ed. Philadelphia: Lea & Febiger, 1970.

Creighton, F., D. Black, and C. Hyde. "'Ecstasy' Psychosis and Flashbacks." *British Journal of Psychiatry* 159 (1991): 713–5.

Current Health, 1995.

De Ropp, R. S. *Drugs and the Mind.* New York: Grove, 1975.

Dishotsky, N. I., W. D. Loughman, R. E. Mogar, and W. R. Lipscomb. "LSD and Genetic Damage." *Science* 172 (1971): 431–40.

Dohrn, C., J. Lichtor, D. Coalson, A. Uitvlugt, H. deWit, and J. Zachny. "Reinforcing Effects of Extended Inhalation of Nitrous Oxide in Humans." *Drugs and Alcohol Dependence* 31 (1993): 265–80.

Goldstein, A. *Addiction from Biology to Drug Policy.* New York: Freeman, 1994.

Goldstein, F. "Pharmacological Aspects of Substance Abuse." In *Remington's Pharmaceutical Sciences,* 19th ed., edited by A. R. Genaro. Easton, PA: Mack, 1995: 780–794.

Gorelick, D., and Balster, R. "Phencyclidine (PCP)." In *Psychopharmacology: The 4th Generation of Progress,* edited by F. Bloom and D. Kupfer, 1767–76. New York: Raven Press, 1995.

Greenhouse, C. "NIDA Lays Plans for Quicker Response to Drug Crises." *NIDA Notes* 7 (January–February 1992): 20–2.

Greer, G., and R. Tolbert. "The Therapeutic Use of MDMA." In *Ecstasy: The Clinical, Pharmacological and Neurotoxicological Effects of the Drug MDMA,* edited by S. J. Peroutka. Boston: Kluwer, 1990.

Grob, C., G. Bravo, R. Walsh, and M. Liester. "The MDMA-Neurotoxicity Controversy: Implications for Clinical Research with Novel Psychoactive Drugs." *Journal of Nervous and Mental Disease* 180 (1992): 355–6.

Hofmann, A. "Psychotomimetic Agents." In *Drugs Affecting the Central Nervous System,* vol. 2, edited by A. Burger, 169–235. New York: Dekker, 1968.

Huxley, A. *The Doors of Perception.* New York: Harper, 1954.

Iwersen, S., and H. Schmoldt. "Two Very Different Fatal Cases Associated with the Use of Methylenedioxyethylene." *Clinical Toxicology* 34 (1996): 241–4.

Jaffe, J. "Drug Addiction and Drug Abuse." In *The Pharmacological Basis of Therapeutics,* 8th ed., edited by A. Gilman, T. Rall, A. Nies, and P. Taylor. New York: Pergamon, 1990: 522–573.

Johnston, L. University of Michigan New Release, December 19, 1996.

Johnston, L., P. O'Malley, and J. Bachman. *National Survey Results on Drug Use from Monitoring the Future Study,* 1975–1994, vol. 2. University of Michigan, NIDA, NIH Publication no. 96-4027. Washington, DC: National Institute on Drug Abuse, 1996.

Jones, W. H. S. *Natural History.* Cambridge, MA: Harvard University Press, 1956.

Leary, T., R. Metzner, and R. Alpert. *The Psychedelic Experience.* New Hyde Park, NY: University Books, 1964.

Letters (to the editor). "Many Were Lost Because of Leary." *USA Today* 14 (June 3, 1996): 12A.

Luisada, P. V. "The Phencyclidine Psychosis: Phenomenology and Treatment." In *Phencyclidine (PCP) Abuse: An Appraisal,* edited by R. C. Petersen and R. C. Stillman. NIDA Research Monograph no. 21. Washington, DC: National Institute on Drug Abuse, U.S. Department of Health, Education, and Welfare, 1978.

Marken, P., S. Stoner, and M. Bunker. "Anticholinergic Drug Abuse and Misuse." *CNS Drugs* 5 (1996): 190–9.

Marquardt, G. M., V. DiStefano, and L. L. Ling. "Pharmacological Effects of (S)-, and (R)-MDA." In *The Psychopharmacology of Hallucinogens,* edited by R. C. Stillman and R. E. Willette. New York: Pergamon, 1978.

Mathias, R. "NIDA Research Takes a New Look at LSD and Other Hallucinogens." *NIDA Notes* 8 (March–April 1993): 6.

McGlothin, W., S. Cohen, and M. S. McGlothin. "Long-Lasting Effects of LSD on Normals." *Archives of General Psychiatry* 17 (1967): 521–32.

Medical Letter. "Volatile Inhalants." 38 (May 10, 1996a): 45.

Medical Letter. "Phencyclidine (PCP)." 38 (May 10, 1996b): 45.

Nadis, S. "After Lights." *Omni* (February 1990): 24.

Naranjo, C., A. T. Shulgin, and T. Sargent. "Evaluation of 3,4-Methylenedioxyamphetamine (MDA) as an Adjunct to Psychotherapy." *Medicina et Pharmacologia Experimentalis* 17 (1967): 359–64.

O'Brien, C. "Drug Addiction and Drug Abuse." In *The Pharmacological Basis of Therapeutics,* 9th ed., edited by J. Hardman and L. Limbird, 557–77. New York: McGraw-Hill, 1996.

Pahnke, W. N., A. A. Kurland, S. Unger, C. Savage, and S. Grof. "The Experimental Use of Psychedelic (LSD) Psychotherapy." In *Hallucinogenic Drug Research: Impact on Science and Society,* edited by J. R. Gamage and E. L. Zerkin. Beloit, WI: Stash, 1970.

Pahnke, W. N., and W. A. Richards. "Implications of LSD and Experimental Mysticism." *Journal of Religion and Health* 5 (1966): 175–208.

Prevention Pipeline. "Target: Inhalants." 8 (July/August 1995): 24.

Randall, T. "Ecstasy-Fueled 'Rave' Parties Become Dances of Death for English Youth." *Journal of the American Medical Association* 268 (1992a): 1505.

Randall, T. "'Rave' Scene, Ecstasy Use, Leap Atlantic." *Journal of the American Medical Association* 268 (1992b): 1505.

Sanchez, E. "PCP Users Are Courting Fire." *Washington Post* (7 March 1988): A-1.

Schultes, R. E. "The Plant Kingdom and Hallucinogens (Part III)." *Bulletin on Narcotics* 22, No. 1 (1970): 25–53.

Schultes, R. E. "Ethnopharmacological Significance of Psychotropic Drugs of Vegetal Origin." In *Principles of Psychopharmacology,* 2d ed., edited by W. G. Clark and J. del Giudice. New York: Academic Press, 1978.

Schultes, R. E., and A. Hofmann. *The Botany and Chemistry of Hallucinogens.* Springfield, IL: Thomas, 1973.

Schultes, R. E., and A. Hofmann. *The Botany and Chemistry of Hallucinogens,* 2d ed. Springfield, IL: Thomas, 1980.

Shulgin, A. "History of MDMA." In *Ecstasy: The Clinical, Pharmacological, and Neurotoxicological Effects of the Drug MDMA,* ed. by S. J. Peroutka. Boston: Kluwer, 1990.

Snyder, S. H. *Madness and the Brain.* New York: McGraw-Hill, 1974.

Stone, J. "Turn On, Tune In, Boot Up." *Discover* 12 (June 1991): 32–33.

Swan, N. "Inhalant Abuse and Its Dangers Are Nothing to Sniff at." *NIDA Notes* 8 (July–August 1993): 15.

Taylor, J. "All-New MDMA FAQ." *Internet* (computer networking service), usenet News, sci.med.pharmacy (27 May 1994).

Toufexis, A. "A Crackdown on Ecstasy." *Time* (10 June 1985): 64.

Tucker, R. "Acid Test." *Omni* (November 1987): 16.

U.S. Department of Justice. "It Never Did Go Away—LSD, A Sixties Drug, Attracts Users in the Nineties." Pamphlet from DEA. Washington, DC, 1991a.

U.S. Department of Justice. "Let's All Work to Fight Drug Abuse." Pamphlet from DEA published by L.A.W. Publications and distributed with permission by International Drug Education Association, 1991b.

Vaughn, K. (Knight-Ridder News Service). "Inhalants Killing Teens by Hundreds." Salt Lake Tribune, 249 (April 13, 1995) A7.

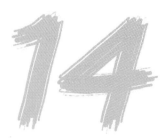

Marijuana

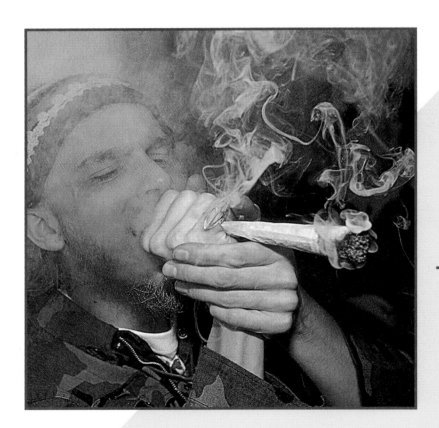

On completing this chapter
you will be able to:

- Today, marijuana is about 20 times more potent than the marijuana on the street in the 1960s and 1970s.
- Chronic marijuana users are more likely to have impaired lung capacity.
- More than 20 million Americans are current marijuana users, making this drug the most frequently used illicit substance of abuse.
- In some states, marijuana is one of the largest cash-producing crops.
- Marijuana still grows wild in many American states today.
- Research shows that many users have difficulty learning and remembering what they have learned when they are "high."
- The first known record of marijuana use is in the *Book of Drugs,* written in 2737 B.C. in China.
- An early use of marijuana plants was to make rope and cloth.
- THC, the main psychoactive chemical in marijuana, is what produces the "high;" it is available by prescription in a drug called Marinol.
- THC remains stored for a long period in body fat; complete elimination can take up to 30 days.
- THC reaches the brain within 14 seconds after inhalation.
- A typical "high" from one marijuana cigarette lasts two to three hours.
- Surveys indicate that 60% to 80% of marijuana users sometimes drive when "high."
- Cannabis has been used to treat extreme nausea, glaucoma, pain, and convulsions.
- George Washington grew marijuana plants at Mount Vernon for medicine and rope-making.

Learning Objectives

- Explain what marijuana is.
- Define the "amotivational syndrome" for marijuana.
- Explain the patterns of marijuana use in the United States.
- Discuss the link between marijuana use and progression to other, more serious drugs.
- Define *hashish* (or *hasheesh*), *ganja, sinsemilla,* and *bhang.*
- Describe the effects that high and low doses of marijuana have on the body.
- Summarize how THC affects the body overall and the respiratory system, blood pressure, sexual behavior, and growth and development in particular.
- Describe how tolerance and dependence affect the response to marijuana and its use.
- Describe how marijuana has been prescribed for therapeutic purposes.
- Summarize the effects of marijuana on motor functions.

I've used marijuana so long that, while I know it's illegal to use it, I really don't care what the laws are—I just simply enjoy it and always will. I work at home and usually finish a day's work usually around 1:00 A.M. or 2:30 A.M. I enjoy a few good hits of grass with a couple of beers or some fine rosé wine. After having been able to finally unwind, I then go to bed relaxed. Now tell me, why should this be illegal?

> *From Venturelli's research files, interview with a 40-year-old male working as a freelance writer, residing in major midwestern city, September 9, 1996*

We used to have one great big bong and fill it with dope [referring to marijuana], and all of us in someone's fraternity room would each take hits from the bong. Today, it's a different life all together. I am working three different jobs, one teaching at a junior high school, [one] working at a film production studio, and my third claim to fame is my job as part-time waiter. . . . I feel that I wasted many nights by just "smokin," "dopin," and "drinkin" back during those college days. I sometimes think that I could have accomplished a lot more if I would not have inhaled so much dope. If I had to do it over again I would not have wasted so much time.

> *From Venturelli's research files, interview with a 28-year-old male, August 9, 1996*

The interview excerpts above illustrate two contrasting views regarding marijuana usage as a subcultural phenomenon. The first interview presents a "die-hard" user who refuses to relinquish his use of this drug. This individual has been using marijuana for many years and considers it an essential recreational drug. Conversely, the second interviewee expresses some regret over the time "wasted" while becoming intoxicated with marijuana when he could have been pursuing other, more career-oriented activities.

Introduction

Although marijuana is one of the least seriously addicting drugs of abuse used in the United States, perhaps no other substance has been the object of so much research and controversy. It is difficult to wade through the emotion, politics, and rigidity found in writings on marijuana to tease out the objective, clinical reality. Extreme views go back to the 1930s, when the film "Reefer Madness" portrayed an after-school marijuana "club" for high-school students in suits and ties who became hallucinatory, homicidal, and suicidal. In the same decade, the Rastafarian religion spread among Jamaican agricultural workers, who named marijuana as a "holy plant."

Marijuana is simply the hemp plant, *Cannabis sativa*, which has been cultivated for thousands of years. When smoked, the dried and crushed leaves, stems, and seeds of cannabis produce sedative and mind-altering effects, which vary according to the potency of the variety of plant used. Usage in the United States began in the 1920s, rose in the 1960s and 1970s, and fell in every year from 1978 until 1991. From 1991 on, however, usage began to climb.

In this chapter, we will review the history and trends of marijuana use, attitudes and controversies surrounding this drug (including the amotivational syndrome and the recent debate inspired by proposals for medical legalization), and its physiological and behavioral effects.

History and Trends in Marijuana Use

In many societies, marijuana has historically been a valued crop. It is called *hemp* because the woody fibers of the stem yield a fiber that can be made into cloth and rope. The term *cannabis* comes from the Greek word for *hemp*.

Cannabis was apparently brought to the Western hemisphere by the Spaniards as a source of fiber and seeds. For thousands of years, the seeds have been pressed to extract a red oil used for medicinal and euphorigenic purposes (Iversen 1993; Abood and Martin 1992). The plant (both male and female) also produces a resin with active ingredients that affect the central nervous system (CNS). Marijuana contains hundreds of chemical compounds, but only a few found in the resin are responsible for producing the euphoric "high."

The first known record of marijuana use is the *Book of Drugs* written about 2737 B.C. by the Chinese Emperor Shen Nung; he prescribed marijuana for treating gout, malaria, gas pains, and absentmindedness. The Chinese apparently had much respect for the plant. They obtained fiber for clothes and medicine from it for thousands of years. The Chinese named the plant *ma* (*maw*), which means "valuable" or "endearing." The term "ma" was still used as late as 1930.

Around the year 500 B.C., another Chinese book of treatments referred to the medical use of marijuana. Nonetheless, the plant got a bad name from the moralists of the day, who claimed that youngsters became wild and disrespectful from the recreational use of *ma*. They called it the "liberator of sin" because, under its influence, the youngsters refused to listen to their elders and did other scandalous things. Marijuana was banned in China but because of rampant use was later legalized.

India also has a long and varied history of marijuana use. It was an essential part of Indian religious ceremonies for thousands of years. The well-known Rig Veda and other chants describe the use of *soma*, which some believe was marijuana. Early writings describe a ritual in which resin was collected from the plants. After fasting and purification, certain men ran naked through the cannabis fields. The clinging resin was scraped off their bodies, and cakes were made from it and used in feasts. For centuries, missionaries in India tried to ban the use of marijuana, but they were never successful; its use was too heavily ingrained in the culture.

Records for Assyria in 650 B.C. refer to a drug called *azulla* that was used for making rope and cloth and was consumed to experience euphoria. The ancient Greeks also knew about marijuana. Galen described the general use of hemp in cakes, which when eaten in excess were narcotic. Herodotus described the Scythian custom of burning marijuana seeds and leaves to produce a narcotic smoke in steambaths. It was believed that breathing the smoke from the burning plants would cause frenzied activity. Groups of people stood in the smoke and laughed and danced as it took effect.

One legend about cannabis is based on the travels of Marco Polo in the twelfth century.

Marco Polo told of the legendary Hasan Ibn-Sabbah, who terrorized a part of Arabia in the early 1100s. His men were some of the earliest political murderers and were supposed to kill under the influence of hashish, a strong, unadulterated cannabis derivative. The cult was called the *hashishiyya,* from which came the word *hashish.* (The word *assassin* may be derived from the name of *Sheik Hasan,* who was a political leader in the tenth century.)

It is unlikely, however, that using hashish can turn people into killers. Experience suggests that people tend to become sleepy and indolent rather than violent after eating hashish or another of the strong cannabis preparations available in Arabia (Abel 1989).

Napoleon's troops brought hashish to France after their campaign in Egypt at the beginning of the nineteenth century, despite Napoleon's strict orders to the contrary. By the 1840s, the use of hashish, as well as opium, was widespread in France, and efforts to curb its spread were unsuccessful.

In North America, hemp was planted near Jamestown in 1611 for use in making rope. By 1630, half the winter clothing at this settlement was made from hemp fibers. There is no evidence that hemp was used medicinally at this time. Hemp was also valuable as a source of fiber for clothing and rope for the Pilgrims at Plymouth. To meet the demand for fiber, a law was passed in Massachusetts in 1639, requiring every household to plant hemp seed. However, it took much manual labor to get the hemp fiber into usable form, resulting in a chronic shortage of fiber for fish nets and the like (Abel 1989).

George Washington cultivated a field of hemp at Mount Vernon, and there is some indication that it was used for medicine as well as for making rope. In his writings, Washington once mentioned that he forgot to separate the male and female plants, a process usually done because the female plant gave more resin if unpollinated.

In the early 1800s, U.S. physicians used marijuana extracts to produce a tonic intended for both medicinal and recreational purposes. This practice changed in 1937 with passage of the Marijuana Tax Act, which prohibited its use as an intoxicant and regulated its use as a medicine.

Most of the abuse of marijuana in the United States during the early part of the twentieth century occurred near the Mexican border and in the ghetto areas of major cities. Cannabis was mistakenly considered a narcotic, like opium, and legal authorities treated it as such (Abood and Martin 1992). In 1931, Harry Anslinger, who was the first appointed head of the Bureau of Narcotics and later would become responsible for the enforcement of marijuana laws, thought that the problem was slight. By 1936, however, he claimed that the increase in the use of marijuana was of great national concern (Anslinger and Cooper 1937). Anslinger set up an informational program that finally led to the federal law that banned marijuana. The following sensationalized statement was part of Anslinger's campaign to outlaw the drug:

> What about the alleged connection between drugs and sexual pleasure? . . . What is the real relationship between drugs and sex? There isn't any question about marijuana being a sexual stimulant. It has been used throughout the ages for that: in Egypt, for instance. From what we have seen, it is an aphrodisiac, and I believe that the use in colleges today has sexual connotations. (Anslinger and Cooper 1937)

Also during this time, some usually accurate magazines reported that marijuana was partly responsible for crimes of violence. In 1936, *Scientific American* reported that "marijuana produces a wide variety of symptoms in the user, including hilarity, swooning, and sexual excitement. Combined with intoxicants, it often makes the smoker vicious, with a desire to fight and kill" ("Marijuana Menaces Youth" 1936). A famous poster of the day, called "The Assassination of Youth," was effective in molding attitudes against drug use.

Largely because of the media's effect on public opinion, Congress passed the Marijuana Tax Act in 1937. However, the drug was declared unconstitutional in 1969. Marijuana has not been classified as a narcotic since 1971.

Prior to the 1960s, marijuana use was largely confined to small segments of African-American urban youth, jazz musicians, and "bohemians," particularly artists and writers who belonged to the 1950s' "beat generation." Use rose tremendously in the 1960s, when it was closely associated with the "hippie" counterculture, in which marijuana was categorized as a psychedelic (consciousness-expanding) sacrament. It spread into other youth categories during the 1970s, until approximately 1978. In each year from 1978 until 1991, marijuana use proceeded to fall. After 1991, researchers and prevention specialists were astounded to see a rise in usage among youth. The National Institute on Drug Abuse's (NIDA's) 1995 *Monitoring the Future Study* found that from 1991 to 1995, marijuana use rose from 29.9% to 34% among the nation's twelfth-graders, from 16.5% to 28.7% among tenth-graders, and perhaps most alarmingly, from 6.2% to 15.8% among eighth-graders. Although marijuana use is not typically implicated in medical or psychiatric emergencies, figures for marijuana and hashish-related emergency room visits, as seen in Figure 14.1, reflect a rise in overall marijuana use, although a rise in potency may also be a factor.

Teenagers' perception of drug use as being "dangerous" has declined since 1993. When asked, in 1993, "Does taking drugs scare you?", 47% of teenagers said "yes." Since 1993, however, only 36% of respondents have answered "yes." Similarly, 33% of teenagers said that "being high feels good" in 1993. Since then, 45% of teenagers responded affirmatively to the same question (Wren 1996, 1).

Marijuana still grows wild in many American states today. Curiously, one reason for the survival

---

Figure 14.1

This antimarijuana poster was distributed by the Federal Bureau of Narcotics in the late 1930s.

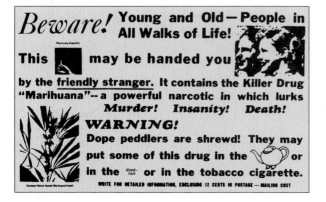

Figure 14.2

Number of
Marijuana/Hashish-
Related Episodes by
Age, 1988–1994

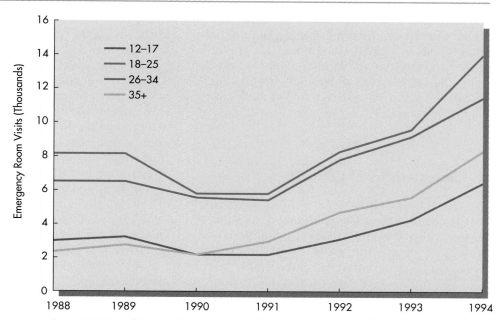

Source: L. McCaig and Substance Abuse and Mental Health Services Administration, Office of Applied Statistics (SAMHSA/OAS). *Preliminary Estimates from the Drug Abuse Warning Network.* Advance Report no. 11. Rockville, MD: SAMHSA, Office of Applied Statistics, November 1995.

Between 1993 and 1994, marijuana/hashish-related emergency department episodes rose from 28,900 to 40,100, an increase of 39%. Since 1990, marijuana/hashish-related episodes have increased 155% (from 15,700 to 40,100). Use of marijuana/hashish by itself accounted for 24% of the increase. Between 1993 and 1994, increases in marijuana/hashish-related episodes were observed in all age groups, with episodes among persons aged 12 to 17 years increasing by 50% (from 4200 to 6400).

of this supply is that, during World War II, the fiber used to make rope (sisal) was hard to import, so the government subsidized farmers to grow hemp. Much of today's crop comes from these same plants. Another reason for the spread of the plants is that, until recently, the seeds were used in birdseed. Leftover seed was discarded in the garbage and thus spread to landfill dumps, where it sprouted. Birdseed containing marijuana seeds is still available, but the seeds are sterilized so they cannot germinate.

The Indian Hemp Drug Commission Report in the 1890s and the 1930 Panama Canal Zone Report on marijuana stressed that available evidence did not prove marijuana to be as dangerous as it was popularly thought; these reports were given little publicity, however, and for the most part disregarded. In 1944, a report was issued by the LaGuardia Committee on Marijuana, which consisted of 31 qualified physicians, psychiatrists,

psychologists, pharmacologists, chemists, and sociologists appointed by the New York Academy of Medicine. They stated in one key summary that marijuana was not the killer many thought it to be:

> It was found that marijuana in an effective dose impairs intellectual functioning in general. . . . Marijuana does not change the basic personality structure of the individual. It lessens inhibition and this brings out what is latent in his thoughts and emotions but it does not evoke responses that would otherwise be totally alien to him.
>
> . . . Those who have been smoking marijuana for years showed no mental or physical deterioration that may be attributed to the drug. (Solomon 1966)

Much of the early research conducted did not consider the potency of marijuana. As a result, findings from various studies are often conflicting and difficult to compare (Chait and Pierri 1992).

Because the quality of marijuana varies so greatly, it is impossible to know the amount of drug taken without analyzing the original material and the leftover stub, or "roach." Conditions such as type of seed, soil moisture and fertility, amount of sunlight, and temperature all have an effect on the amounts of active ingredients found in the resulting marijuana plant.

◢ Characteristics of Cannabis

In 1753, Carolus Linnaeus, a Swedish botanist, classified marijuana as **Cannabis sativa.** *Cannabis sativa* is a plant that grows readily in many parts of the world. Most botanists agree that there is only one species (*sativa*) and that all the variants (*indica, americana,* and *africana*) belong to that species; others believe that the variants are three distinct species (Schultes 1978). *Indica* is considered to have the most potent resin, but climate, soil, and selective plant breeding all influence potency.

cannabis sativa

the biological species name for the variety of hemp plant known as marijuana

Cannabis is *dioecious,* meaning that there are male and female plants (see Figure 14.3). After the male plant releases its pollen, it usually dies. Cultivators of marijuana often eliminate or remove the male plants once the female plant has been pollinated. The world's record marijuana plant was 39 feet tall, and its woody stem was nearly 3 inches in diameter.

There are more than 400 different chemicals in the cannabis plant, many of which have not yet been identified. Delta-9-tetrahydrocannabinol, or THC, is the primary mind-altering (psychoactive) agent in marijuana (Abood and Martin 1992; Swan 1996, 15) and appears to be important for the reinforcing properties of this substance (Kelly et al. 1994). THC is most highly concentrated in the flowering tops and upper leaves of the female plant. When crushed or eaten, these flowering tops produce a resin in which the psychoactive ingredient THC is found.

In cultivated marijuana crops, male plants are eradicated from the growing fields so that they cannot pollinate the female plants. The lack of pollination makes the potency of female plants increase dramatically. In the United States, this method produces a type of marijuana known as **sinsemilla** (meaning "without seeds" in Spanish). This type of marijuana is made from the buds of flowering tops of female plants. The average concentration of THC is 7.5%, but can reach as high as 24%. Sinsemilla is one of the most potent varieties of marijuana available.

sinsemilla

one of the most potent types of marijuana available; means "without seeds"

Native U.S. cannabis is sometimes considered inferior because of a low concentration of THC, usually less than 0.5%. THC levels in Jamaican, Colombian, and Mexican varieties range between 0.5% and 7%.

In the United States, the amount of THC found in "street"-sold marijuana ranges broadly from 0.5% to 11%. Most ordinary marijuana averages 3% THC. Reports that the amount of THC in marijuana has risen dramatically since the 1960s appear to be true (Kaplan and Whitmire 1995, A4). "More efficient agriculture—new methods of harvesting and processing marijuana plants—has made pot about 20 times more potent than the marijuana on the street in the 1960s and 1970s, drug treatment experts and law officials say" (Henneberger 1994, F18). Further, the quantities of other more potent types of marijuana like sinsemilla are more readily available in illegal drug markets. The actual potencies of the more generic types of marijuana have remained the same in the last 30 years.

As mentioned earlier, *hashish* (or *hasheesh*) is another cannabis derivative that contains the purest form of resin. The sticky resin from the female plant flowers averages 2% to 8% THC and can contain as much as 20% THC (Swan 1996, 15). Historically, hashish users have represented a somewhat small percentage of the cannabis user population in the United States, while in Europe it is much more readily available. Hashish is produced in Lebanon, Afghanistan, and Pakistan.

Figure 14.3

Male and female marijuana plants

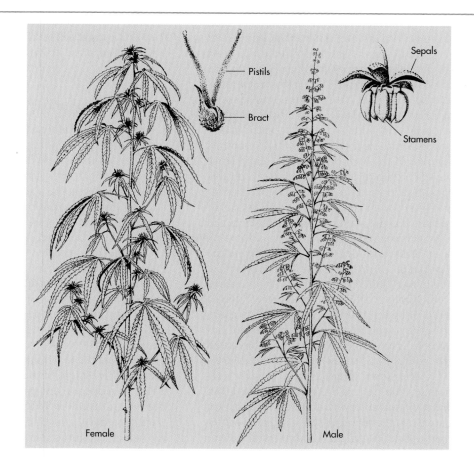

A third derivative of the cannabis plant is *ganja* in India. This preparation consists of the dried tops of female plants.

Finally, the weakest form of marijuana is known as *bhang*, popularly called *"ditch weed"*; it is made from parts of the cannabis plant that contain the least amount of THC. Some members of drug-using subcultures grind this type of marijuana as well as more potent types of marijuana into a powder and mix it into drinks, teas, and cookie and brownie batter. Bhang is rarely found in the United States, largely because it is very weak and considered low-grade, usually containing less than 1% or 2% THC.

The Behavioral Effects of Marijuana Use

The "High"

In the 1930s, it was believed that the acute effects of marijuana were very devastating and that marijuana use could suddenly lead to violent and even promiscuous behavior. Publications forecasted that marijuana use would lead to madness (Rowell and Powell 1939) and that it was the "assassin of youth" (Anslinger and Cooper 1937).

These concerns are no longer considered valid for casual or occasional use. In most individuals, low to moderate doses of cannabis produce euphoria and a pleasant state of relaxation (Goldstein 1994). What are the common effects experienced from marijuana use? After a few minutes of forcibly withholding the smoke in the lungs, most users suddenly experience the "high." During this state, the user experiences a dry mouth, elevated heartbeat, some loss of coordination and sense of balance, coupled with slower reaction times and a feeling of euphoria (mild to elevated intoxication). Blood vessels in the eyes expand, which accounts for reddening of the eyes. Some people experience slightly elevated blood pressure, which can double the normal heart rate. These effects can become intensified when other drugs, such as LSD and/or psychedelic ("magic") mushrooms, are combined with the marijuana (Swan 1996, 15).

The state of euphoria that results from the "high" is usually mild and short-lived; a typical "high" from one "joint" may last from two to three hours. Subjectively, the user experiences altered perception of space and time, impaired memory of recent events, and impaired physical coordination (more of these subjective effects are discussed at length in the next section) (Abood and Martin 1992). An occasional "high" is not usually hazardous unless the person attempts to drive a car, operate heavy machinery, fly a plane, or function in similar ways requiring coordination, good reflexes, or quick judgment (Nahas and Latour 1992). Even low doses of marijuana adversely affect perception, such as being able to judge the speed of an approaching vehicle or how much to slow down on an exit ramp.

An acute dose of cannabis can produce adverse reactions, ranging from mild anxiety to panic and paranoia in some users. A few rare cases exhibit psychoses characterized by detachment from reality, delusional and bizarre behavior, and hallucinations (Abood and Martin 1992). These reactions occur most frequently in individuals who are under stress, or who are anxious, depressed, or borderline schizophrenic (Nahas and Latour 1992); such effects may also be seen in normal users who accidentally take much more than their usual dose.

Extreme reactions also can occur as a result of ingesting marijuana treated (or "laced") with such things as opium, PCP, or other additives. Based on limited evidence from survey studies, mild, often adverse reactions are experienced on one or more occasions by more than one-half of regular users; they are mainly self-treated and usually go unreported. (See "Case in Point," page 373.)

Subjective Euphoric Effects

A **subjective euphoric effect** associated with marijuana use is the ongoing social and psychological experiences incurred while intoxicated with marijuana. It includes both the user's altered state of consciousness and his or her perceptions while intoxicated.

> **subjective euphoric effect**
>
> ongoing social and psychological experiences incurred while intoxicated with marijuana

Subjective effects include a general sense of relaxation and tranquility, coupled with heightened sensitivity to sound, taste, and emotionality. Some users report occasional similarities to the typical hallucinogenic "high." How closely the marijuana "high" resembles a hallucinogenic "high" depends on the amount of THC absorbed from marijuana. For example, higher amounts of THC found in more potent plants of marijuana, like sensimilla and *kine bud,* more clearly mimic a hallucinogenic "high." This relationship is especially evident when considering the extent to which the senses of hearing, vision, sound, and taste are distorted by use of highly potent forms of marijuana.

Among marijuana users, those who are very attached to these euphoric effects are referred to as "connoisseurs." Such users often pride themselves on their extensive knowledge of this drug. Devotees keep up with developments in the marijuana field by avidly reading monthly issues of *High Times* and *Hemp News* and frequently scanning the World Wide Web for information on the best varieties of marijuana, growing techniques, announcements of hemp festivals, and advice and information regarding current laws, fines, and other information.

Why is marijuana so attractive to so many individuals? One quote from an interview illustrates the extensive psychological and social reinforcement experienced by marijuana users:

Specific Signs of Marijuana Use

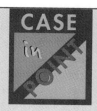

▲ A sweet odor similar to burnt rope in room, on clothes, etc.

▲ Roach: The small butt end of a marijuana cigarette.

▲ Joint: Looks like a hand-rolled cigarette, usually the ends are twisted or crimped.

▲ Roach clips: Holders for the roach could be any number of common items such as paper clips, bobby pins, or hemostats. They could also be of a store-bought variety in a number of shapes and disguises.

▲ Seeds or leaves in pockets or possession.

▲ Rolling papers or pipes, usually hidden somewhere.

▲ Eye drops: for covering up red eyes.

▲ Excessive use of incense, room deodorizers, or breath fresheners.

▲ Devices for keeping the substance such as boxes, cans, or a concealed container like a soft drink can with a screw-off lid.

▲ Eating binges: an after-effect for some marijuana users.

▲ Appearance of intoxication, yet no smell of alcohol.

▲ Excessive laughter.

▲ Yellowish stains on finger tips from holding the cigarette.

Source: L.A.W. Publications, "Let's All Work to Fight Drug Abuse," rev. ed. Addison, TX: C&L Printing, 1985, p. 39. Used with permission of the publisher.

It's the high that I particularly like. Everything becomes more mellow. Everyday tensions are released or submerged by more inner-like experiences. I can review the day and how happy or miserable I feel. Actually, when I am thinking and I am high on grass, I always feel that my thoughts are profound. You think from another perspective, one that numbs the more reality-based everyday strains. On the other hand, there are moments when this drug affects your mood and channels it [in] different ways. You have moments when you either feel sad, happy, angry (in a more contemplative way), or worried. These moods are both good and bad. If for the moment you feel good, then your mood is positive. If you feel down, your mood is negative in a particular way. If I am with friends and we are all sharing the bong or joint or pipe, we laugh a lot together. It's a type of drug that makes you more jovial, more introspective, and friendly, gregarious. . . .

From Venturelli's research files, 40-year-old male personnel manager, August 20, 1996

Despite a large difference in age, a 24-year-old male graduate student at a university in a major metropolitan city in the Midwest revealed strikingly similar views about this drug:

I use grass or marijuana because usually everything is cool. It changes my mood when I am partying and even working around the house. I get bored easily and grass has a way of removing most of the boredom. I use it often because I like it. I also think a lot about things and try to solve personal problems that occur from time to time. Like right now, I am broke with no extra spending money for about six months, and smoking grass is certainly less expensive than going out to bars at night. I just drink and smoke at home, many times by myself.

From Venturelli's research files, August 20, 1996

Intense attachment to passionate feelings surrounding the use of marijuana is quite common. As explained in Chapter 2, largely through the reinforcement of pleasurable feelings, the drug user becomes addicted—that is, attached or bound to the drug. If these subjective euphoric experiences were to become largely negative, attachment to and repeated use of this drug would cease. Thus, the theory of **differential reinforcement** applies to the two interviewees. Developed by Edwin Sutherland in 1939 and revised in 1947, this theory attempts to understand delinquent behavior. Differential reinforcement is the process by which individuals are socialized into the perceptions and values of a cultural group. In the case of marijuana, the group reinforces the perception that marijuana is "cool" and provides euphoria. The individual learns drug-using behavior from the group, and is reinforced in continuing its use.

> **differential reinforcement**
>
> taking on ways of thinking and acting held by a subcultural group within society

Driving Performance

Evidence shows that the ability to perform complex tasks, such as driving, is strongly impaired while under the influence of marijuana (Goldstein 1994; Mathias 1996a, 6). This effect has been demonstrated in laboratory assessments of driving-related skills such as eye–hand coordination and reaction time, in driver simulator studies, in test course performance, and in actual street-driving situations (Chait and Pierri 1992; Mathias 1996a, 6).

In limited surveys, from 60% to 80% of marijuana users indicate that they sometimes drive while high. A study of drivers involved in fatal accidents in the greater Boston area showed that marijuana smokers were overrepresented in fatal highway accidents as compared with a control group of nonusers of similar age and gender. A 1989 study found that, of nearly 1800 blood samples taken from drivers arrested for driving while intoxicated, 19% tested positive for marijuana.

Further, "figures from previous studies of automobile accident victims show that from 6% to 12% of nonfatally injured drivers and 4% to 16% of fatally injured drivers had THC . . . in their bloodstream," (Mathias 1996a, 6). Another study showed that 32% of drivers in shock trauma had marijuana in their bloodstream. One problem with this study, however, is that individuals testing positive for THC also had alcohol in their bloodstream, making it impossible to determine whether THC or alcohol directly caused the car accident.

Another study tested the effects of known amounts of marijuana, alcohol, or both on driving. The subjects drove a course rigged with various traffic problems. There was a definite deterioration in driving skills among those who had used either drug, but the greatest deterioration was in subjects who had taken both. In another test, 59 subjects smoked marijuana until they were high and then were given sobriety tests on the roadside by highway patrol officers. Overall, 94% of the subjects didn't pass the test 90 minutes after smoking, and 60% failed at 150 minutes, even though the blood THC was much lower at this time (Hollister 1986). Other studies on driving show this same inability to drive for as long as 12 to 24 hours after marijuana use.

Because some perceptual or other performance deficits resulting from marijuana use may persist for some time after the high, users who attempt to drive, fly, operate heavy machinery, and so on may not recognize their impairment because they do not feel intoxicated. States such as California have established testing procedures to detect the presence of THC in urine or blood samples from apparently intoxicated drivers.

If the use of marijuana becomes more socially acceptable (or perhaps even legal) and penalties for simple possession become more lenient, it is likely that individuals will feel less inclined to hide their drug use. Unfortunately, it follows that these individuals may also be more inclined to drive while high, endangering themselves and others.

Critical Thinking Skills

Marijuana has been found to have a negative impact on critical thinking skills. Recent research by the NIDA shows that heavy marijuana use impairs critical skills related to attention, memory, and learning. Impairment continues even after discontinuing this drug's use for at least 24 hours (Brown and Massaro 1996).

In the same study, researchers compared 65 "heavy users" (using approximately every other day) with "light users" (using once or twice per week). "Heavy users" made more mistakes and had a greater difficulty in sustaining attention, shifting attention to meet demands of challenges in the environment, and with registering, processing, and using information (Brown and Massaro 1996) compared with the group dubbed "light users." In addition, "heavy users" had greater difficulty in completing the tests, which specifically measured aspects of attention, memory, and learning, such as intellectual functioning, abstraction ability, attention span, verbal fluency, and learning and recalling abilities (Brown and Massaro 1996). One researcher stated, "If you could get heavy users to learn an item, then they could remember it; the problem was getting them to learn it in the first place" (Brown and Massaro 1996). The researchers surmised that marijuana alters brain activity because residues of the drug persist in the brain or because a withdrawal syndrome follows after the euphoric effects of the marijuana wear off. In another study, researchers tested the cognitive functioning of 65 marijuana-using college students. Residual impairments were seen on the day (24 hours) after use in terms of sustaining attention, shifting attention, and hence in registering, organizing, and using information (Pope and Yurgulen-Todd 1996). This study, which was undertaken during the 1990s, is significant because it was carefully controlled. The unresolved question is whether these memory impairments are short-term or long-term. These noteworthy findings complement many other similar findings that identified protracted cognitive impairment among heavy marijuana users.

The Amotivational Syndrome

The so-called **amotivational syndrome** (sometimes referred to as "antimotivational syndrome") is a flashpoint of controversy about marijuana, although not as newsworthy as that regarding medical legalization. Amotivational syndrome characterizes regular users of marijuana who experience a lack of motivation and reduced productivity. Specifically, users show apathy, poor short-term memory, difficulty in concentration, and a lingering disinterest in pursuing goals (Abood and Martin 1992).

> **amotivational syndrome**
>
> a lack of motivation and reduced productivity caused by regular marijuana use

This syndrome has received considerable attention. People who are high, or "stoned," lack the desire to perform hard work and are not interested in doing difficult tasks (Brown and Massaro 1996). There is some evidence of this behavior in regular marijuana users (Nahas and Latour 1992). Overall, though not solely *caused* by cannabis use, chronic users have lower grades in school, are more likely to be absent from classes, and are likely not to complete assignments and to drop out of school (Liska 1990; Henneberger 1994). In terms of age, the earlier someone begins smoking marijuana, the more likely the amotivational characteristics will prevail and the more difficult it will be to cease using this drug.

While the effects of marijuana per se are somewhat responsible for creating this syndrome, other factors contribute as well. For instance, marijuana users are more likely to associate with peers who are also users. Surveys show that members of these peer groups tend to be alienated from society and are likely to be classified as nonconformers and/or rebellious youths. Imagine how an entire group of marijuana users can exert a profound effect on one another. They perpetuate a subculture emphasizing pleasure and nonconformity rather than goal-directed behavior.

Advocates of marijuana legalization stress data that might tend to debunk research on amotivational syndrome. One institute that supports legalization, the Lindesmith Center, published a study asserting that college students who are users have *higher* grades than nonusers (Morgan and Zimmer 1995, 12). How can we account for the discrepancies between this study and others, not to mention the clinical experience of student assistance professionals, who often report academic repercussions of heavy use? One factor in the explanation is sociocultural:

> In the New York–New Jersey metro region, there are "druggy" schools and "drinking" schools. The "druggy" schools are more upper-middle-class, liberal arts schools, artsy types, latter-day hippies, etc. The boozer campuses are filled with blue-collar and lower-middle-class kids—sometimes big fraternity schools. Frontloading at basketball games, comas after pledge parties. . . Not as good educational backgrounds as the artsy potheads, who went to better schools, private schools, read a lot, or heard a lot at dinner before college, so they get by with their profs. But the potheads ratchet down into easier majors, and they get crummier grades as they get into regular use.

> *Interview with Pearl Mott, prevention specialist, Drug Prevention Programs in Higher Education, Washington, D.C., October 1994, for a prevention newsletter*

At a symposium among college prevention and student assistance personnel of the Higher Education Consortium for Drug Abuse Prevention in Northern New Jersey, a majority of the staff agreed with the statement quoted above.

A second methodological factor complicating drug research among such students is simply that academic failures stay in "F" categories for only one or two semesters. Many then disappear from statistics entirely, via academic attrition.

A more serious challenge to the notion of amotivational syndrome comes from ethnographic research. The most well known of these investigations was carried out by Vera Rubin and Labros Comitas, as reported in their book *Ganja in Jamaica* (1975). Follow-up studies were done in Jamaica (Dreher 1982) and Costa Rica (Carter 1980). None of these works found that chronic use impaired occupational or other functioning; in fact, the main point of the Jamaican studies was that users defined this drug as helpful and motivating for work—a *motivational* syndrome." This work is often cited to counter antimotivational syndrome claims. By this logic, dropping out of the "rat race" is a cultural posture, with marijuana being secondary to, or, at most, reinforcing the

drift away from a mainstream lifestyle. The Jamaican and Costa Rican subjects, however, were not observed engaging in an academic, cognitively complex, or rapid reflex activity, nor were they found in occupations that are competitive and striving for mobility. Rather, these subjects were involved in repetitive, physical labor such as sugarcane cutting. In such a context, marijuana drug use functions to provide a pleasant sedation that counters the monotony and physical discomfort of such labor.

In the 1990s, we have the opportunity to see the perception of the drug by adolescents, unvarnished by psychedelic mythologizing (users in the 1960s would be horrified at the pot and beer parties of later decades):

> **Burnt** v. **1.** past tense and past participle of burn **2.** (colloq.) var. of burned out or burnt-out **3.** (colloq.) adolescent slang denoting behavioral qualities of chronic marijuana users; an apathetic, dulled, unintelligent quality

> Excerpt from "A Street-Wise Student Dictionary," *Truth About Substance Abuse* student newsletter, Essex County College, Newark, NJ, 1995

As one student explains:

> It was fun hanging out and smoking weed. But it made me stupid and depressed after a while. And I needed to finish school and get a job. It was getting ridiculous. And the posse got sort of boring. They didn't care about anything except getting zonked. I stopped hanging with them.

> *From Peter Myers' files, interview with a 20-year-old female, 1992*

Young people who have never heard of amotivational syndrome may have experienced burnout, which is very much like amotivational syndrome. In the above quote from a 20-year-old woman, who is quite representative of a subgroup of former marijuana users, we can infer several reasons why a young person might "mature out" of chronic use on his or her own. First, the novelty of early use becomes routine and humdrum, sure to disenchant adolescents, unless other risk factors for abuse are present. Second, many of these users report a depressive "hangover." Third, the overall effects on concentration, memory, and "get up and go" do not fit needs of occupational attainment or upward mobility. At 19, you may not want to be identified as a "loser."

The Physiological Effects of Marijuana Use

When marijuana smoke is inhaled into the lungs, THC, the psychoactive ingredient, leaves the blood rapidly through metabolism and through efficient uptake into the tissues. THC and its metabolites tend to bind to proteins in the blood and remain stored for long periods in body fat. Five days after a single injection of THC, 20% remains stored, whereas 20% of its metabolites remain in the blood (Indiana Prevention Resource Center 1996). Complete elimination of a single dose can take up to 30 days. Measurable levels of THC in blood from chronic users can often be detected for several days or even weeks after their last marijuana cigarette.

In smokers, lung absorption and transport of THC to the brain are rapid; THC reaches the brain within as little as 14 seconds after inhalation. Marijuana is metabolized more efficiently through smoking than intravenous injection or oral ingestion. It is also three to five times more potent (Jones 1980; Kaplan 1995).

Some effects of cannabis described in the following sections are unquestionably toxic in that they can either directly or indirectly produce adverse health effects. Other effects may be beneficial in treating some medical conditions. The uses of marijuana, THC, and synthetic cannabinoids, either alone or in combination with other drugs, are currently being investigated for use in treating pain, inflammation, glaucoma, nausea, and muscle spasms (Iversen 1993).

Effects on the Central Nervous System

The primary effects of marijuana—specifically, THC—are on CNS functions. The precise CNS effects of consuming marijuana or administering THC can vary according to the expectations of the user, the social setting, the route of administration, and previous experiences (Jaffe 1990; Abood and Martin 1992). Smoking a marijuana cigarette can alter mood, coordination, memory, and self-perception. Usually, such exposure causes some euphoria, a sense of well-being, and relaxation. Marijuana smokers often claim heightened sensory awareness and **altered perceptions** (particularly a slowing of time), associated with hunger (the "**munchies**") and a dry mouth (Abood and Martin 1992; Swan 1994).

altered perceptions
changes in the interpretation of stimuli, resulting from marijuana

"munchies"
hunger experienced while under the effects of marijuana

High doses of THC or greater exposure to marijuana can cause hallucinations, delusions, and paranoia (American Psychiatric Association 1994; Goldstein 1995). Some users describe anxiety after high-dose exposure. Due to the availability and widespread use of marijuana, psychiatric emergencies from marijuana overdose are becoming somewhat common. Long-term, chronic users often show decreased interest in personal appearance or goals (part of the "amotivational syndrome" discussed earlier in this chapter) as well as an inability to concentrate, make appropriate decisions, and remember (Abood and Martin 1992; Block 1996, 560).

The precise classification of THC is uncertain because the responses to marijuana are highly variable and appear to have elements of all three major groups of drugs of abuse. Consequently, marijuana use can cause euphoria and paranoia (like stimulants), drowsiness and sedation (like depressants), and hallucinations (like psychedelics). It is possible that THC alters several receptor or transmitter systems in the brain; this action would account for its diverse and somewhat unpredictable effects. However, the recent dramatic discovery of a specific receptor site in the brain for THC, called the "cannabinoid" receptor, suggests that a selective endogenous marijuana system exists in the brain and is activated by THC when marijuana is consumed (Hudson 1990). Some researchers speculate that an endogenous fatty-acid–like substance called **anandamide** naturally works at these marijuana sites; efforts are being made to characterize this substance, which perhaps is a neurotransmitter (Iversen 1993). It is possible that, from this discovery, a group of new therapeutic agents will be developed that can selectively interact with the marijuana receptors, resulting in medical benefits without the side effects that generally accompany marijuana use (Iversen 1993; Swan 1993).

> **anandamide**
>
> a possible neurotransmitter acting at the marijuana (cannabinoid) receptor

Effects on the Respiratory System

Marijuana is often smoked like tobacco, and like tobacco can cause serious damage to the lungs (Consroe and Sandyk 1992). In smoking tobacco, for example, nearly 70% of the total suspended particles in the smoke are retained in the lungs. Because marijuana smoke is inhaled more deeply than tobacco smoke, even more tar residues may be retained with its use.

Smoke is a mixture of tiny particles suspended in gas, mostly carbon monoxide. These solid particles combine to form a residue called *tar*. Cannabis produces more tar (up to 50% more) than an equivalent weight of tobacco and is smoked in a way that increases the accumulation of tar (Jones 1980).

Over 150 chemicals have been identified in marijuana smoke and tar. A few are proven carcinogens; many others have not yet been tested for carcinogenicity. The carcinogen benzopyrene, for example, is 70% more abundant in marijuana smoke than in tobacco smoke. When cannabis tar is applied to the skin of experimental animals, it causes precancerous lesions similar to those caused by tobacco tar. Similarly, whenever isolated lung tissue is exposed to these same tars, precancerous changes result (Jones 1980; Turner 1980; Hollister 1986).

Special white blood cells in living lung tissue—*alveolar macrophages*—play a role in removing debris from the lungs. When exposed to smoke from cannabis, these cells are less able to remove bacteria and other foreign debris.

Smoking only a few marijuana cigarettes a day for six to eight weeks can significantly impair pulmonary function. Laboratory and clinical evidence often indicates that heavy use of marijuana causes cellular changes and that users have a higher incidence of such respiratory problems as laryngitis, pharyngitis, bronchitis, asthmalike conditions, cough, hoarseness, and dry throat (Hollister 1986; Goldstein 1995). Recent reports emphasize the potential damage to pulmonary function that can occur from chronic marijuana use (NIDA 1991). Evidence suggests that many 20-year-old smokers of both hashish and tobacco have lung damage comparable to that found in heavy tobacco smokers over 40 years of age. It is believed that the tar from tobacco and marijuana have damaging effects, but it is not known whether smokers who use both products suffer synergistic or additive effects (Jones 1980; Hollister 1986).

Effects on the Cardiovascular System

In humans, cannabis causes both vasodilation (enlarged blood vessels) and an increase in heart rate related to the amount of THC consumed (Abood and Martin 1992). The vasodilation is responsible for a reddening of the eyes often seen in the marijuana smoker. In physically healthy users, these effects, as well as slight changes in heart rhythm, are transitory and do not appear to be significant. In patients with heart disease, however, the increased oxygen requirement due to the accelerated heart rate may have serious consequences. The effect of cannabis on people with heart rhythm irregularities is not known.

Because of vasodilation caused by marijuana use, abnormally low blood pressure can occur when standing. In addition, if a user stands up quickly after smoking, a feeling of lightheadedness or fainting may result. Chronic administration of large doses of THC to healthy volunteers shows that tolerance develops to the increase in heart rate and vasodilation.

People with cardiovascular problems seem to be at an increased risk when smoking marijuana (Hollister 1986). Marijuana products also bind hemoglobin, limiting the amount of oxygen that can be carried to the heart tissue. This deficiency could trigger heart attacks in susceptible people (Palfai and Jankiewicz 1991). The National Academy of Science's Institute of Medicine recommends that people with cardiovascular disease avoid marijuana use because there are still many unanswered questions about its effects on the cardiovascular system.

Effects on Sexual Performance and Reproduction

Drugs may interfere with sexual performance and reproduction in several ways. They may alter sexual behavior, affect fertility, damage the chromosomes of germ cells in the male or female, or adversely affect fetal growth and development.

The Indian Hemp Commission, which wrote the first scientific report on cannabis, commented that it had a sexually stimulating effect, like alcohol. However, the report also said that cannabis was used by Asian Indian ascetics to destroy the sexual appetite. This apparent discrepancy may be a dose-related effect. Used occasionally over the short term, marijuana may act as an **aphrodisiac** by releasing CNS inhibitions. In addition, the altered perception of time under the influence of the drug could make the pleasurable sensations appear to last longer than they actually do.

> **aphrodisiac**
>
> a substance that stimulates or intensifies sexual desire

Marijuana affects the sympathetic nervous system, increasing vasodilation in the genitals and delaying ejaculation. High doses over a period of time lead to depression of libido and impotence—possibly due to the decreased amount of testosterone, the male sex hormone.

Cannabis has several effects on semen. The total number of sperm cells and the concentration of sperm per unit volume is decreased during ejaculation. Moreover, there is an increase in the proportion of sperm with abnormal appearance and reduced motility. These qualities are usually associated with lower fertility and a higher probability of producing an abnormal embryo should fertilization take place.

Despite these effects, there are no documented reports of children with birth defects in which the abnormality was linked to the father's smoking marijuana. It is possible that damaged sperm cells are incapable of fertilization (so that only normal sperm cells reach the egg) or that the abnormal sperm appearance is meaningless in terms of predicting birth defects. When marijuana use stops, the quality of semen gradually returns to normal over several months (Harclerode 1980; Institute of Medicine 1982).

Less reliable data are available on the effects of cannabis on female libido, sexual response (ability to respond to sexual stimulation with vaginal lubrication and orgasm), and fertile reproductive (menstrual) cycles ("Marijuana" 1987; Consroe and Sandyk 1992). Preliminary data from the Reproductive Biology Research Foundation show that chronic smoking of cannabis (at least three times per week for the preceding six months) adversely affects the female reproductive cycle. Results with women were correlated with work in rhesus monkeys; it was found that THC blocks ovulation (due to effects on female sex hormones).

Data on effects of marijuana use during pregnancy and lactation are inconclusive. Some evidence suggests that the use of this drug by pregnant women can result in intrauterine growth retardation, which is characterized by prolonged labor, low birthweight, and behavioral abnormalities in newborns and increased fetal mortality (Roffman and George 1988, Nahas and Latour 1992; Fernandez-Ruiz et al. 1992).

Pregnant rhesus monkeys treated with THC levels equivalent to those associated with moderately heavy marijuana use (according to U.S. standards) had an abortion and fetal death rate about four times higher than the drug-free control monkeys. THC and other cannabinoids pass through the blood–placenta barrier and concentrate in the fetus's fatty tissue, including its brain. Ethical considerations prevent duplication of the experiment in humans.

Women who smoke marijuana during pregnancy also often use other drugs—such as alcohol, tobacco, and cocaine—that are known to have adverse effects on the developing fetus. Because multiple drugs are used, it is difficult to isolate the

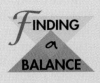

Can There Be "Moderate Drug Abuse"?

Britt's first awareness of drugs began at about age six, when she realized that her mother was a cocaine addict. Living in south Miami, she explained, is just like the situation depicted in television shows and the national news. Drugs are everywhere! Her family life was similar to that portrayed on television, too. In fact, her first stepfather is now serving time in jail in Colombia for drug-running. In an effort to reclaim her life, Britt's mother moved to Chicago, but her cocaine use only continued there. Consequently, Britt became a "parent" to her mother, cleaning the house, washing the dishes, doing the laundry, and making her school lunch. "I was 14 and even then my mother thought I didn't know about her use. My childhood was spent as an adult, even my friends were my mother's age."

Britt's teenaged years weren't particularly difficult, but for anyone in high school they can prove challenging. Because of what she observed with her mother, cocaine use was totally out of the question for Britt. Instead, she became attracted to marijuana. She smoked her first joint during her senior year in high school, but developed a real habit when she started college at the University of Colorado in Boulder. "People smoke a lot of pot in this town. And out here, there [are] really good-quality strains."

Recreational use became a daily affair after her freshman year when she moved out of the dorms and into an apartment with several friends who shared a similar devotion to pot. It didn't take long for Britt to become a connoisseur as well. "I don't smoke shwag pot [low-quality stuff] because it would get me really stoned where I would lose all motivation and focus. My pot of choice was kine bud. It's really good. It's beautiful. The THC crystals inside the bud resonate. It is so relaxing. It really opens up your mind. That's what I like about it. My problem was I didn't use it in moderation. After my freshman year I was a 24–7 [24 hours per day, 7 days per week]. For me MJ wasn't a party drug. it was a lifestyle drug. I had a pot jonesing [craving] for sure."

Eventually the drug use affected Britt's academics, which became a wake-up call of sorts. "I didn't realize it was a problem until my grades dropped. I realized that pot and school don't go well together." Confronted by friends and even her parents, Britt

---

specific effects of marijuana during pregnancy. Like many other substances, THC is taken up by the mammary glands in lactating females and is excreted in the milk. Effects on human infants due to the presence of marijuana in the maternal milk have not been determined (Christina 1994; Murphy and Bartke 1992).

In studies on mice and rats (but not humans), the addition of THC to pregnant animals lowered litter size, increased fetal reabsorption, and increased the number of reproductive abnormalities in the surviving offspring (Dewey 1986). The offspring of the drug-treated animal mothers had reduced fertility and more testicular abnormalities. The dose of cannabinoids used in these studies was proportionally higher than that used by humans. Clearly, pregnant women should be advised against using marijuana, even though there are few direct data on its prenatal effects in humans (Dewey 1986; Murphy and Bartke 1992).

Tolerance and Dependence

It has been known for many years that tolerance to some effects of cannabis builds rapidly in animals—namely, the drug effect becomes less intense with repeated administration. Frequent use of high doses of marijuana or THC in humans produces similar tolerance. For example, increasingly higher doses must be given to obtain the same intensity of subjective effects and increased

saw she was headed in the wrong direction. "You can lie to other people, but you cannot lie to yourself. Eventually you have to face the truth. My parents thought I was on coke, but I told them it was only pot. They didn't become harsh, but they did encourage me to stop doing so much."

Britt also took a good look at the friends she associated with and didn't like what she saw. "Pot-heads think they are so in touch, but they are in denial. Real pot-heads have no goals or ambitions in life. I want certain things in life, I want to do well in school, and I want to have a career. There is another aspect of pot that I didn't like. A quarter ounce is $100, so you have to buy it in quantity. In effect, you have to start selling. I was headed there. It becomes a lifestyle, one that I didn't want and I said to myself, Britt, you are doing this too much."

Britt got another wake-up call when her apartment was robbed—not once, but twice. For Britt, the winds of change were in the air.

The stress management term *social engineering* is an expression used to describe making specific changes in one's behavior, not so much to avoid problems, but to steer clear of them. In essence, it involves navigating the shoals of life without running aground. It is what people like Britt find themselves doing to put their lives back on track. Social engineering is a common coping technique in drug intervention and addiction treatment. And it is exactly what Britt did.

I had to change my environment. I had to move out and find a new place to live. I realized, I don't want to be around those people.

Britt will tell you that smoking pot is not physically addictive, but it is psychologically addictive. She acknowledges that she was addicted. "This is not to say that pot is bad. I am a firm advocate of hemp," she says. "But it must be used in moderation. That was my downfall. I'll tell you what really saddens me. I see kids at the local high school [ages] 13 and 14, and these kids are pot-heads. They are at an age when their brains aren't fully developed, and look what they're doing to themselves. They don't even know who they are. That much pot smoking at a young age hinders your thinking process. At least my brain was completely formed. I learned a lot about myself."

Recently Britt went home to Chicago for a funeral. She has seen a lot of drug-related death through her mother's friends. Today her mother is clean, and Britt explains with a smile, "This time when I was home, she did the laundry and the cooking. It was a really nice change." ■

heart rate that occur initially with small doses (Abood and Martin 1992).

Frequent high doses of THC also can produce mild physical dependence. Healthy subjects who smoke several "joints" a day or who are given comparable amounts of THC orally experience irritability, sleep disturbances, weight loss, loss of appetite, sweating, and gastrointestinal upsets when drug use is stopped abruptly. This mild form of withdrawal is not experienced by all subjects, however. It is much easier to show psychological dependence in heavy users of marijuana (Hollister 1986; Abood and Martin 1992).

Psychological dependence involves an attachment to the euphoric effects of the THC content in marijuana and may include "craving." The subjective effects of marijuana intoxication include a heightened sensitivity to and distortion of sight, smell, taste, and sound; mood alteration; and diminished reaction time.

So how to get over, how to get by? /I wish I had a joint to get me high.

These lyrics from the song "I Need a Joint," by the rap group Basehead, reflect the psychological dependence many users have developed on *marijuana.*

Diagnosis: Cannabis Dependence In general, outright cannabis addiction, with obsessive drug-seeking and compulsive drug-taking behavior, is relatively rare with low-THC cannabis, but much more common with THC special-variety marijuana and high-dose hashish (Gardner 1992). Because the less potent forms of marijuana are most readily available in the United States, most chronic users in this country would have little problem controlling or eliminating their cannabis habit if they so desired (Abood and Martin 1992; Christina 1994).

The *Diagnostic and Statistical Manual of Mental Disorders,* fourth edition *(DSM-IV),* recognizes a diagnosis of cannabis dependence. It is characterized by "compulsive use" and spending hours per day acquiring and using the substance. These users persist in their use despite knowledge of physical problems (for example, chronic cough related to smoking) or psychological problems (for example, excessive sedation resulting from repeated use of high doses) (American Psychiatric Association 1994, 216). In *DSM-IV,* Cannabis dependence is distinguished from cannabis abuse and cannabis intoxication.

Chronic Use

Research on chronic use of marijuana (repeated daily use of this drug) in the 1970s and 1980s indicated the possibility of three types of damage: (1) chromosomal damage (Stenchever et al. 1974); (2) cerebral atrophy (shrinking of the brain) (Campbell et al. 1971); and (3) lowered capacity of white blood cells to fight disease (Nahas et al. 1974). These findings have all been contradicted or otherwise refuted by subsequent research. The only finding that appears very creditable is that chronic use of this drug impairs lung capacity (Oliwenstein 1988; Bloodworth 1987; Swan 1994; Kaplan 1995; Henneberger 1994).

Other evidence indicates that chronic, heavy use of cannabis can lead to persistent and troublesome behavioral changes in some users (see the Case in Point box). We have pointed out that marijuana produces a variety of psychoactive effects. One of those effects is sedation of unwanted emotional states such as anxiety, which are inevitable given the conflicts and turmoil of adolescent development. As with the chronic use of any psychoactive drug that produces sedating effects,

normal psychosocial development can be arrested by heavy marijuana consumption. As the proverb states, "a flower doesn't grow in a closed box." A youth who is usually "high" at a party will avoid the anxieties and embarrassments of interpersonal interactions, developing romantic and sexual involvements, and so on. Former users also report a chronic depressant effect from such drug use.

In a similar vein, marijuana appears to compromise cognitive functions such as memory, concentration, problem solving, and thought. Educational attainment and overall intellectual development may be held back in the chronic user.

The amotivational syndrome can, in fact, be "deconstructed" into the sedation, depression, and cognitive impairment discussed throughout this chapter. The user who is experiencing a subjective euphoric effect, enjoying the presence and social reinforcement of peers, "feeling no pain," and remaining cognitively unfocused finds it difficult to intellectually grasp these abstract concepts of developmental delays and amotivational syndrome. While many do "mature out" of use, this step may occur only after years of development have slipped away. Sometimes treatment interventions are necessary to get the subject into a drug-free state, with nonusing peer influences brought to bear, to bring this awareness.

Therapeutic Uses

Cannabis was used to treat a variety of human ills in folk and formal medicine for thousands of years in South Africa, Turkey, South America, and Egypt as well as such Asian countries as India, the Malays, Burma, and Siam. As recently as 1937, tinctures of cannabis were still cited in the *U.S. Pharmacopeia and National Formulary,* which listed current therapeutic drugs.

After marijuana was legally classified as a narcotic and the Marijuana Tax Act of 1937 required that its use be reported, medical use of this substance effectively ceased. Only in the past decade has there been organized renewed interest in possible medical uses for cannabis. A few therapeutic applications have been demonstrated, and others are being investigated to a limited extent. Because

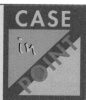

Chronic Marijuana Use

CASE IN POINT

The following comments show how marijuana use can become a disturbing habit:

I guess you could say it was peer pressure. Back in 1969, I was a sophomore in college, and everyone was smoking "dope." The Vietnam War was in progress, and most students on college campuses were heavily involved in the drug scene. I first started smoking marijuana when my closest friends did. I was taught by other students who already knew how to enjoy the effects of "pot."

I recall that one of my fellow students used to supply me with "nickel bags," and many users nicknamed him "God." How did he get such a name? Because he sold some very potent marijuana that at times caused us to hallucinate.

I used pot nearly every day for about a year and a half, and hardly an evening would pass without smoking dope and listening to music. Smoking marijuana became as common as drinking alcohol. I used it in the same manner a person has a cocktail after a long day. At first, I liked the effects of being "high," but later, I became so accustomed to the stuff that life appeared boring without it.

After graduating, my college friends went their separate ways, and I stopped using marijuana for a few years. A year later, in graduate school, a neighborhood friend reintroduced me to the pleasure of smoking pot. I began using it again but not as often. Whenever I experienced some pressure, I would use a little to relax.

After finishing my degree, I found myself employed at an institution that at times was boring. Again, I started using pot at night to relax, and somehow it got out of control. I used to smoke a little before work and sometimes during lunch. I thought all was going well until one day I got fired because someone accused me of being high on the job.

Soon afterward, I came to the realization that the use of marijuana can be very insidious. It has a way of becoming psychologically addictive, and you don't even realize it. When I was high, I thought that no one knew and that I was even more effective with others. Little did I know, I was dead wrong and fooling no one. ∎

Source: Peter Venturelli, interview with a 39-year-old male, May 1990.

---

of potential clinical uses for marijuana, enforcement of laws prohibiting the use of this substance can be awkward and very controversial (see "Fighting the Drug War," page 384). One of the problems with trying to determine the clinical usefulness of cannabis is that the effectiveness of this substance decreases with repeated use (tolerance develops). In addition, effective doses vary according to routes of administration (smoking versus oral ingestion), and responses are highly variable among users (Goldstein 1995).

The use of marijuana, TCH, or related drugs for treatment of the extreme nausea and vomiting that often accompany cancer chemotherapy is an example of a beneficial application of this drug. Consequently, the FDA has approved the use of purified THC as the drug called **Marinol** (dronabinol) for antiemetic treatment in cancer patients (Sewester 1993). Although the use is not FDA-approved, some have argued that administration of THC by smoking a marijuana product is a particularly useful form of administering this drug in nauseated and vomiting patients receiving chemotherapy (Gavzer 1994). Another FDA-approved application for THC is to stimulate appetite in patients with advanced AIDS who are suffering from severe anorexia (Sewester 1993).

Marijuana has been shown to be effective in the treatment of several other medical conditions; because other medicines are available that are at least as effective and without abuse potential, none

Marinol
FDA-approved THC in capsule form (dronabinol)

FIGHTING THE DRUG WAR

In San Francisco, a small underground shop called the Cannabis Buyers' Club flourishes. Writer Richard C. Paddock describes a typical scene: "Dozens of people sit on rummage-sale couches and folding chairs, smoking high-grade marijuana. A dozen more line up at the counter, fingering the day's sample buds and buying their ration of weed." Although this setting may sound enticing to the average pot smoker, chances are he or she would be leery of partaking in this scene; as Paddock tells us, " . . . doing your shopping here means you are sick or dying."

The Cannabis Buyers' Club is just one flourishing underground trend directed toward granting sick or dying people the right to use marijuana. Thousands of people stricken with such ailments as AIDS, cancer, glaucoma, epilepsy, and multiple sclerosis use marijuana every day to treat their sicknesses or allay their pains. Regarding the San Francisco scene, 1995 Mayor Frank Jordan (formerly a police chief) said, "I have not problem whatsoever with the use of marijuana for medical purposes . . . we should bend the law."

Marijuana has been used for medical purposes for at least 5000 years, across cultures and generations; such a strong grounding in history would seem to grant a certain credibility to this drug as being medically beneficial. Unfortunately for proponents of medical cannabis use, the United States has been reluctant to permit studies on possible ways to allow open use of marijuana for medical reasons. For over three years, Donald Abrams of the University of California, San Francisco, a respected AIDS researcher, has been seeking government permission to conduct a " . . . clinical trial to determine whether smoking marijuana can help patients overcome the deadly AIDS wasting syndrome." To date, Abrams has been unsuccessful in his attempts. Abrams predicts that he will be able to do his research if science can survive the politics.

Bob Randall, one of the eight people in the United States who can legally smoke marijuana, is quoted by Paddock as saying, "In a sane society, the prospect of an easy-to-grow plant that could ease suffering and prolong life would be a cause for celebration."

Source: R. C. Paddock. "'Drag Stores' Fill Prescriptions with Pot, Not Pills." *Salt Lake Tribune* 249, (March 1, 1995): A-1

---

of these applications are currently FDA sanctioned. According to researchers (Iversen 1993; Abood and Martin 1992; Consroe and Sandyk 1992), the unauthorized therapeutic benefits for marijuana include the following:

Reduction in intraocular (eye) pressure. Marijuana lowers **glaucoma**-associated intraocular pressure, even though it does not cure the condition or reverse blindness (Goldstein 1995). Use of marijuana to treat this eye disease is not widespread.

glaucoma

an eye disease manifested by increased intraocular pressure

Antiasthmatic effect. Some research indicates that short-term smoking of marijuana has improved breathing for asthma patients. Marijuana smoke dilates the lung's air passages (bronchodilation). Findings also show, however, that the lung-irritating properties of marijuana smoke seem to offset its benefits. Regardless, marijuana may still prove useful when other drugs are not effective because of a different mode of action in causing bronchodilation.

Muscle-relaxant effect. Some studies indicate that muscle spasms are relieved when patients with muscle disorders, such as multiple sclerosis, use marijuana.

Antiseizure effect. Marijuana has both convulsant and anticonvulsant properties and has been considered for use in preventing seizures associated with epilepsy. In animal experimentation, the cannabinoids reduced or increased seizure activities, depending on how the experiments were conducted. One or more of the marijuana components may be useful in combination with other standard antiseizure medication, although at present their value seems limited.

Antidepressant effect. Cannabis and the synthetic cannabinoid synhexyl have been used successfully in Great Britain as specific euphorants for the treatment of depression.

Analgesic effect. Published testimonials have reported that marijuana can relieve the intense pain associated with migraine and chronic headaches or inflammation. In South Africa, native women smoke cannabis to dull the pain of childbirth (Solomon 1966). The pain-relieving potency of marijuana has not been carefully studied and compared with other analgesics such as the narcotics or aspirin-type drugs.

Whether THC or a similar drug is accepted as a legitimate medicine depends on several considerations. For example, it must be determined whether the pharmaceutically desirable effects are useful for treating chronic conditions because tolerance develops rapidly to many of the actions of THC. Like any other medication, marijuana and related products must be carefully tested for toxicity and therapeutic effectiveness. This process is time-consuming, expensive, and is not worthwhile if other drugs are already available that offer therapeutic efficacy comparable to, or better than, the marijuana substances. In addition, concerns about abuse potential and the social stigmas associated with marijuana need to be considered.

In 1996, voters in Arizona and California approved propositions permitting physicians to prescribe marijuana for medical problems, with the idea that terminally ill patients could be given the option of smokable marijuana as opposed to the already-approved Marinol (dronabinol). This event triggered a major response by the federal government. President Clinton, the Secretary of Health and Human Services, and the U.S. Attorney General all made pronouncements reiterating the negative effects of marijuana, its abuse potential, and the danger of sending a "pro-use message" or one that suggested use was not outside the pale of accepted behavior. The government warned that physicians who availed themselves of the permission given in these new state regulations would be prosecuted, lose their privilege of writing prescriptions, and be excluded from Medicare and Medicaid reimbursement. The entire legislative initiative was cast as being a smokescreen for legalization, with the federal government purporting that those who supported it were "closet" marijuana advocates or, at best, legalization advocates.

Physicians responded indignantly to what they considered a heavy-handed attempt to overrule their medical judgments, and to smear them unfairly, especially when most of them were neither pro-use or even pro-legalization, except in this one medical exception. An editorial in the prestigious *New England Journal of Medicine,* titled "Federal Foolishness and Marijuana" (Kassirer 1997), claimed that it was hypocritical to allow physicians to prescribe the highly addicting opiates morphine or meperidine, which cause death at doses not much greater than those that relieve pain, but not marijuana, which is far less addictive and does not cause death. The purpose of the legislative initiative, the editorial pointed out, was to alleviate the suffering of terminally ill patients, for whom long-term abuse potential is irrelevant. Many of these patients perceive the smokable form of THC as being more effective than Marinol, a factor that is difficult to measure in experimental procedures. This debate was, a few joked, a rerun of "Reefer Madness."

◢ Marijuana and Youth

Marijuana: Assassin of Youth?

In the late 1930s, the poster "Marijuana: Assassin of Youth" made a clever play on words, bringing up reminders of the Middle Eastern "hashashin" cult, whose terrible exploits were attributed to their use of hashish (marijuana resin).

At the time, marijuana was even incorrectly classified as a narcotic like opium and morphine.

Amotivational syndrome, lassitude, poor driving the day after smoking, educational failure, and dependence may not quite add up to "assassination," as wildly exaggerated in "Reefer Madness," but the poster was right in associating use of this drug with young people.

As the data in Table 14.1 show, the frequency of marijuana use is strongly correlated to age. Lifetime rates found in 1994 for 12- to 17-year-olds (11.7%) were the lowest of all age groups reported; they were sharply higher in successive age groups. The age group reporting the highest lifetime use was 26–34-year-olds (59.2%). For past-year and past-month usage, the 18–25-year-olds reported the highest use. Marijuana use dropped sharply in the 35 and older age group across all usage time periods (lifetime 26.6%, past year 4.0%, and past month 2.3%). Overall, the heaviest users are between 18 and 34 years old.

Crunching numbers to show the statistical association of marijuana with youth must be followed up with an examination of social groups in which marijuana is customary, both in local peer groups and broad youth cultures of which they are a part.

Peer Influences

As discussed in the early chapters of this text, the mass media and parental role models have a significant impact on the attitudes that youth develop regarding drug use. However, peers may exert the most influence of all (Heitzeg 1996; Tudor et al. 1987; Norem-Hebeisen and Hedlin 1983).

Research shows that it is very unlikely that an individual will use drugs when his or her peers do not use drugs. Marijuana use, in particular, is a group occurrence and thus is strongly affected by peer pressure and influence. Learning theory (see Chapter 2) shows how peers can influence one another; drug-using peer members serve as role models, legitimizing this form of deviant behavior. Peers in such groups are in effect saying, "It's OK to use drugs," and they make drugs available. Heavy drug users are likely to belong to drug-using groups; in contrast, people who do not use drugs belong to groups where drug use is perceived as a very deviant form of social recreation.

Including and in addition to peer influences, Radosevich et al. (1980) have highlighted three different factors that determine marijuana use patterns: (1) structural factors, such as age, gender, social class, and ethnicity or race; (2) social and interactional factors, such as type of interpersonal relationships, friendship cliques, and drug use within the peer group setting; and (3) attitudinal factors, such as personal attitudes toward the use of drugs. Keep in mind that these factors can easily overlap; they are not separate and distinct.

Sociologists have long studied "youth cultures" (Coleman 1961). In the 1970s, sociologists began to examine different subcultures of youth in terms of the behaviors that symbolically represent the group, where participation in drug use is a ritual that marks off entrance into the group and out of childhood—a "rite of passage." Typically, American high school culture includes a "leading" clique, often associated with team sports, whose

---

| Table 14.1 | Marijuana Use Reported in 1994 by Americans during Lifetime, Past Year, and Past Month, According to Age |

Age	Lifetime	Past Year	Past Month
12–17 years	11.7%	10.1%	6.0%
18–25	47.4	22.9	12.1
26–34	59.2	13.8	6.9
35+	26.6	4.0	2.3

Source: Substance Abuse and Mental Health Services Administration, Office of Applied Studies. *National Household Survey on Drug Abuse. Preliminary Estimates from the 1994 National Household Survey on Drug Abuse,* Advance Report Number 10. Rockville, MD: U.S. Department of Health and Human Services, September 1995.

members might be called "jocks," "collegiates," or "rah-rahs," and a marginal, deviant, rebellious group (Eckert 1989, 2–10). In some cases, the latter group is associated with marijuana use. In the mid-1960s "hippies" were perceived as committed counterculturalists who espoused pacifism and communalism in addition to psychedelic drugs; by 1970, this name denoted broader segments of youth who adhered merely to "hippie" styles of clothing and drug use (Buff 1970). By the 1980s, marijuana use was identified with subgroups of youth often called "burnouts." In some communities, such as two in New Jersey and Michigan that were studied by sociologists, "burnouts" came from socioeconomically lower strata of their community, and were marginal and/or rebellious within the educational system, if not dropouts (Eckert 1989, Gaines 1992). Membership in such marijuana-using subcultures can be a pathway into other drugs.

The Role of Marijuana as a Gateway Drug

Gateway drugs are drugs that serve as the "gate" or path that almost always precedes the use of illicit drugs such as marijuana, heroin, and LSD (Indiana Prevention Resource Center 1995). Gateway drugs, or drugs-of-entry, serve to initiate a novice user into the drug-using world. While the linkage is not biochemical, common gateway drugs include tobacco, inhalants, alcohol, and anabolic steroids. The claim that marijuana use leads to the use of other more serious drugs, such as heroin, is controversial (Gardner 1992). Although it is true that many heroin addicts began drug use with marijuana, it is also true that many, if not most, also used coffee and cigarettes. Millions of marijuana users never go beyond this drug. As one study reports, "There are only a few thousand opiate addicts in Great Britain, yet there are millions who have tried cannabis" (Gossop 1987).

> **gateway drugs**
>
> drugs that often lead to the use of more serious drugs. Alcohol, tobacco, and marijuana are the most commonly used gateway drugs.

Nevertheless, some explanation is needed for the small percentage of marijuana users who do progress to such hard drugs as heroin. It is not likely that the use of marijuana is the principal cause of moving to harder drugs, but much more important factors are the personality of the users as well as their social environment. As described in Chapter 17, youth who turn to drugs are usually slightly to seriously alienated individuals. Thus, progression from marijuana to other drugs is more likely to depend on peer group composition, family relationships, social class, and the age at which drug use begins (Indiana Prevention Resource Center 1995).

It is important to note, however, that people can leave both drug-using groups and drug-using behavior, a process sometimes called "maturing out." The 20-year-old female interviewed earlier in the section on amotivational syndrome was one such individual. Penelope Eckert documents some young "burnouts" quitting marijuana smoking without sacrificing group membership (Eckert 1989, 154–5).

Inaccuracy in Estimates of Marijuana Use

In a world where marijuana can be considered either an "assassin" or a "sacrament," and where it is associated with membership in prized or despised peer groups, it is not surprising that estimates of its use will vary widely and inaccurately. Parents, for example, tend to underestimate their children's use of drugs. In one study, "Only 14% of the parents interviewed thought their children had experimented with marijuana while 38% of the teenagers said they had tried it" (Wren 1996, 1). In the same survey, 52% of teenagers reported having been offered drugs, while 34% of the parents thought their children may have been offered drugs.

On the other hand, college students tend to have exaggerated misperceptions of use, believing that their peers use marijuana much more than is true (Berkowitz 1991). For example, at one campus in northern New Jersey, two-thirds of students reported never using marijuana, yet most students polled believed that the average student uses marijuana once per week.

EXERCISES FOR THE WEB

Exercise 1: NORML

Since its founding in 1970, the National Organization for the Reform of Marijuana Laws (NORML) has been the principal national advocate for legalizing marijuana. During the 1970s, NORML led the efforts to decriminalize successfully minor marijuana offenses in 11 states and significantly lower penalties in all others. Though the decriminalization movement eventually fell victim to the "War on Drugs," NORML has remained the nation's principal organization dedicated to ending marijuana prohibition.

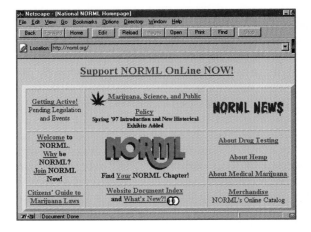

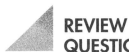 **REVIEW QUESTIONS**

1. Why do you think that marijuana has become the most frequently used illicit substance in the United States?

2. Do you believe that prosecution for marijuana possession should be more or less rigid than it currently is? Why?

3. How do one's surroundings and personality affect the response to cannabis?

4. Sometimes use of marijuana can cause relaxation and sedation. How does marijuana differ from typical CNS depressants in terms of tolerance, dependence, and withdrawal?

5. Explain why a user of cannabis might develop psychological dependence.

6. Do you believe that use of marijuana is more or less harmful than use of tobacco products? Should they be regulated differently? Explain your response.

7. Why do you think that there is so much controversy concerning the effects of marijuana on fetal development and sexual behavior?

8. What effects does marijuana have on the cardiovascular and respiratory systems?

9. What is the drug Marinol, and what are its FDA-approved uses?

10. Why does the FDA refuse to approve marijuana for clinical uses?

11. What are the potential effects of chronic, high-dose cannabis use?

12. What is the *amotivational syndrome,* and how does it occur?

13. What are the most important factors in determining the pattern of marijuana use?

14. How are the patterns of marijuana use affected by factors such as gender, geographic location, and college education?

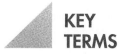

KEY TERMS

Cannibis sativa
sinsemilla
subjective euphoric effect
amotivational syndrome
altered perceptions
"munchies"
anandamide
aphrodisiac
Marinol
glaucoma
gateway drugs

SUMMARY

1 Marijuana consists of the dried and crushed leaves, flowers, stems, and seeds of the *Cannabis sativa* plant. THC (delta-9-tetrahydrocannabinol) is the primary mind-altering (psychoactive) ingredient in marijuana.

2 Chronic, heavy use of marijuana can cause an "amotivational syndrome" in some users. This syndrome consists of a lack of desire to pursue goals, apathy, a noncaring attitude about others and an inability to concentrate at work, in school, or during other activities that require attention.

3 *Hashish, ganja, sinsemilla,* and *bhang* are all derivatives of the cannabis plant; of these hashish (or *hasheesh*) is the strongest derivative and *bhang* is the weakest.

4 Effects of marijuana can vary according to expectations and surroundings. At low doses, such as when smoked or eaten, marijuana often has a sedative effect. At higher doses, it can produce hallucinations and delusions.

5 As with tobacco, smoking marijuana can impair pulmonary function, cause chronic respiratory diseases (such as bronchitis and asthma), and promote lung cancer. Marijuana causes vasodilation and a compensatory increase in heart rate. The effects of marijuana on sexual performance and reproduction are controversial. Some studies have suggested this substance enhances sexual arousal but may retard fetal growth if smoked during pregnancy.

6 Tolerance to the CNS and cardiovascular effects of marijuana develops rapidly with repeated use. Although physical dependence and associated withdrawal are minor, psychological dependence can be significant in chronic, heavy users.

7 The active ingredient in marijuana, THC, has been used as treatment for a variety of seemingly unrelated medical conditions. Because of its clinical potential, THC is available as the FDA-approved product Marinol. This drug is indicated for treatment of nausea and vomiting in cancer patients receiving chemotherapy and to treat anorexia (lack of appetite) in AIDS patients. Other potential therapeutic uses for THC include relief of intraocular pressure associated with glaucoma, as an antiasthmatic drug, for muscle relaxation, as prevention for some types of seizures, as an antidepressant, and as an analgesic to relieve migraines and other types of pain.

8 *Highs* from using marijuana can impair motor coordination and cause perceptual and performance deficits, especially when the user engages in complex activities, such as driving a motor vehicle.

REFERENCES

Abel, E. L. *Marijuana: The First Twelve Thousand Years.* New York: Plenum, 1989.

Abood, M., and B. Martin. "Neurobiology of Marijuana Abuse." *Trends in Pharmacological Sciences* 13 (May 1992): 201–6.

American Psychiatric Association. *Diagnostic and Statistical Manual of Mental Disorders,* 4th ed., *[DSM-IV],* chairman Allen Frances. Washington, DC: APA, 1994.

Anslinger, H. J., and C. R. Cooper. "Marijuana: Assassin of Youth." *American Magazine* 124 (July 1937): 18–19, 150–3.

Berkowitz, A. "Following Imaginary Peers: How Norm Misperceptions Influence Student Substance Abuse." Module no. 2 in *Project Direction,* edited by G. Lindsay and G. Rulf. Muncie, IN: Bali State University, 1991: 12–15.

Block, R. I. "Does Heavy Marijuana Use Impair Human Cognition and Brain Function?" *Journal of the American Medical Association* 275, no. 7 (21 February 1996).

Bloodworth, R. C. "Major Problems Associated with Marijuana Use." *Psychiatric Medicine* 3, no. 3 (1987): 173–84.

Brown, M. W., and S. Massaro. *Attention and Memory Impaired in Heavy Users of Marijuana.* Rockville, MD: NIDA, 20 February 1996. Available http://www/health.org/pressrl/heavymar.html.

Buff, J. "Greasers, Dopers, and Hippies: Three Responses to the Adult World." In *The White Majority,* edited by L. Howe, 60–70. New York: Random House, 1970.

Campbell, A. G., M. Evans, J. L. Thomson, and M. J. Williams. "Cerebral Atrophy in Young Cannabis Smokers." *Lancet* (1971): 1219–25.

Carter, E. *Cannabis in Costa Rica.* Philadelphia: Institute for the Study of Human Issues, 1980.

Chait, L., and J. Pierri. "Effect of Smoked Marijuana on Human Performance: A Critical Review." In *Marijuana/Cannabinoids, Neurobiology and Neurophysiology,* edited by L. Murphy and A. Bartke, 387–424. Boca Raton, FL: CRC Press, 1992.

Christina, D. *Marijuana: Personality and Behavior.* Tempe, AZ: Do It Now, 1994.

Coleman, J. S. *The Adolescent Society.* New York: Free Press of Glencoe, 1961.

Consroe, P., and R. Sandyk. "Potential Role of Cannabinoids for Therapy of Neurological Disorders." In *Marijuana/Cannabinoids, Neurobiology and Neurophysiology,* edited by L. Murphy and A. Bartke, 459–524. Boca Raton, FL: CRC Press, 1992.

Dewey, W. L. "Cannabinoid Pharmacology." *Pharmacological Reviews* 38, no. 2 (1986): 48–50.

Dreher, M. Philadelphia: Institute for the Study of Human Issues, Philadelphia, 1982.

Eckert, P. *Jocks and Burnouts: Social Categories and Identity in the High School.* New York: Teachers College, Columbia University, 1989.

Epidemiology Report. "Marijuana Use Is Up Again." *NIDA Notes* 9 (February–March 1994): 12, 13.

Farley, C. "Hello Again, Mary Jane." *Time* (April 1993).

Fernandez-Ruiz, J., F. Rodriguez de Fonseca, M. Navarro, and J. Ramos. "Maternal Cannabinoid Exposure and Brain Development: Changes in the Ontogeny of Dopaminergic Neurons." In *Marijuana/Cannabinoids, Neurobiology and Neurophysiology,* edited by L. Murphy and A. Bartke, 118–64. Boca Raton, FL: CRC Press, 1992.

Gaines, G. *Teenage Wasteland: Suburbias Dead-End Kids.* New York, Harper Perennial, 1992.

Gardner, E. "Cannabinoid Interaction with Brian Reward Systems: The Neurobiological Basis of Cannabinoid Abuse." In *Marijuana/Cannabinoids, Neurobiology and Neurophysiology,* edited by L. Murphy and A. Bartke, 275–335. Boca Raton, FL: CRC Press, 1992.

Garzer, B. "Should Marijuana Be Legal?" *Parade Magazine* (12 June 1994): 4–7.

Goldstein, A. *Addiction from Biology to Drug Policy.* New York: Freeman, 1994: 169–177.

Goldstein, F. "Pharmacological Aspects of Substance Abuse." In *Remington's Pharmaceutical Sciences,* 19th ed. Easton, PA: Mack, 1995.

Gossop, M. *Living with Drugs,* 2nd ed. Aldershot, England: Wildwood House, 1987.

Harclerode, J. "The Effect of Marijuana on Reproduction and Development." In *Marijuana Research Findings: 1980,* edited by R. C. Petersen. NIDA Research Monograph no. 31. Washington, DC: National Institute on Drug Abuse, 1980.

Health and Human Services (HHS). Substance Abuse—A National Challenge. 6 May 1996. Available www.os.dhhs.gov/news/press/1996pres/960506b.html.

Heitzeg, N. *Deviance: Rulemakers and Rulebreakers.* St. Paul, MN: West Publishing, 1996.

Henneberger, M. "Pot Surges Back, It's Like a Whole New World." *New York Times* (6 February 1994).

Hollister, L. E. "Health Aspects of Cannabis." *Pharmacological Reviews* 38 (1986): 39–42.

Hudson, R. "Researchers Identify Gene That Triggers Marijuana's 'High.'" *Wall Street Journal* (9 August 1990): B-2.

Indiana Prevention Resource Center. *Factline on: Gateway Drugs.* Bloomington, IN: Indiana Prevention Resource Center, June 1995.

Indiana Prevention Resource Center. *Factline on: Marijuana.* Bloomington, IN: Indiana Prevention Resource Center, 1996.

Institute of Medicine, National Academy of Sciences. *Marijuana and Health.* Washington, DC: National Academy Press, 1982.

Iversen, L. "Medicinal Use of Marijuana." *Nature* 365 (1993): 12–13.

Jaffe, J. H. "Drug Addiction and Drug Abuse." In *The Pharmacolocial Basis of Therapeutics,* 8th ed., edited by A. Gilman, T. Rall, A. Nies, and P. Taylor. New York: Pergamon, 1990.

Johnston, L., P. O'Malley, and J. Bachman. *National Survey Results from The Monitoring the Future Study,* 1975–1992. Rockville, MD: National Institute on Drug Abuse, 1992, 1993, and 1994.

Jones, R. T. "Human Effects: An Overview." In *Marijuana Research Findings: 1980,* NIDA Research Monograph no. 31. Washington, DC: National Institute on Drug Abuse, 1980.

Kaplan, L. F., and R. Whitmire. "Pot—It's Potent, Prevalent and Preventable." *Salt Lake Tribune* 250 (21 May 1995).

Kassirer, J. "Federal Foolishness and Marijuana" (editorial). *New England Journal of Medicine* 336, No. 5 (January 30, 1997).

Kearns, R. "Legalize Drugs? Elders Sparks Firestorm." *Salt Lake Tribune* 247 (9 December 1993): A-18.

Kelly, T., R. Foltin, C. Enurian, and M. Fischman. "Effects of THC on Marijuana Smoking, Drug Choice and

Verbal Report of Drug Liking." *Journal of Experimental Analysis of Behavior* 61 (1994): 203–11.

Knight-Ridder News Service. "Time to Make Drugs Legal? Many Say Yes." *Salt Lake Tribune* 244 (21 September 1992).

L.A.W. Publications. *Let's All Work to Fight Drug Abuse,* 3rd ed. Addison, TX: C&L Printing, 1985.

Liska, K. *Drugs and the Human Body,* 3rd ed. New York: Macmillan, 1990.

"Marijuana." *Harvard Medical School Mental Health Letter* 4, no. 5 (November 1987): 1–4.

"Marijuana Menaces Youth." *Scientific American* 154 (1936): 151.

Mathias, R. "NIDA Survey Provides First National Data on Drug Use During Pregnancy." *NIDA Notes* 10, no. 1 (January/February 1995).

Mathias, R. "Marijuana Impairs Driving-Related Skills and Workplace Performance." *NIDA Notes* 11, no. 1 (January/February 1996a): 6.

Mathias, R. "Studies Show Cognitive Impairments Linger in Heavy Marijuana Users." *NIDA Notes* 11, no. 3 (May/June 1996b).

McCaig L., and Substance Abuse and Mental Health services Administration, Office of Applied Statistics (SAMHSA/OAS). Preliminary Estimates from the Drug Abuse Warning Network. Advance Report no. 11. Rockville, MD: SAMHSA/OAS, November 1995.

Murphy, L., and A. Bartke. "Effects of THC on Pregnancy, Puberty, and the Neuroendocrine System." In *Marijuana/Cannabinoids, Neurobiology and Neurophysiology,* edited by L. Murphy and A. Bartke, 539. Boca Raton, FL: CRC Press, 1992.

Nahas, G., and C. Latour. "The Human Toxicity of Marijuana." *Medical Journal of Australia* 156 (April 1992): 495–7.

Nahas, G. G., et al. "Inhibition of Cellular Immunity in Marijuana Smokers." *Science* 183 (1 February 1974): 149–20.

National Institute on Drug Abuse (NIDA). *Drug Abuse and Drug Abuse Research,* DHHS Publication no 91-1704. Washington, DC: U.S. Department of Health and Human Services, 1991.

Norem-Hebeisen, A., and D. P. Hedlin. "Influences on Adolescent Problem Behavior: Causes, Connections, and Contexts." In *Adolescent Substance Abuse: A Guide to Prevention and Treatment,* edited by R. Isralowitz and M. Singer. New York: Haworth, 1983.

Oliwenstein, L. "The Perils of Pot." *Discover* 9, no. 6 (1988): 18.

Palfai, T., and H. Jankiewicz. *Drugs and Human Behavior.* Dubuque, IA: Brown, 1991.

Pope, H. G., Jr., and D. Yurgulen-Todd. "The Residual Cognitive Effects of Heavy Marijuana Use in College Students." *Journal of the American Medical Association* 275 (1996): 521–7.

Radosevich, M., L. Lanza-Kaduce, R. L. Akers, and M. D. Krohn. "The Sociology of Adolescent Drug and Drinking Behavior: Part II." *Deviant Behavior* 1 (January–March 1980): 145–69.

Roffman, R. A., and W. H. George. "Cannabis Abuse." In *Assessment of Addictive Behaviors,* edited by D. M. Donovan and G. A. Marlatt. New York: Guilford, 1988.

Rowell, E., and R. Powell. *On the Trail of Marijuana: The Weed of Madness.* Mountain View, CA: Pacific, 1939.

Rubin, V. and L. Comitas. *Ganja in Jamaica.* The Hague: Mouton, 1975.

Schultes, R. E. "Ethnopharmacological Significance of Psychotropic Drugs of Vegetal Origin." In *Principles of Psychopharmacology,* 2nd ed., edited by W. G. Clark and J. del Giudice. New York: Academic Press, 1978.

Sewester, S. *Drug Facts and Comparisons.* St. Louis: Kluwer, 1993: 259h–59k.

Solomon, D., ed. *The Marihuana Papers.* New York: New American Library, 1966.

Stenchever, M. A., T. J. Kunysz, and M. A. Allen. "Chromosome Breakage in Users of Marijuana." *American Journal of Obstetrics and Gynecology* 118 (January 1974): 106–13.

Substance Abuse and Mental Health Services Administration (SAMHSA), Office of Applied Studies (OAS). *Preliminary Estimates from the 1993 National Household Survey on Drug Abuse.* Advance Report no. 7. Rockville, MD: U.S. Department of Health and Human Services, July 1994.

Substance Abuse and Mental Health Services Administration (SAMHSA), Office of Applied Studies (OAS). *Preliminary Estimates from the 1994 National Household Survey on Drug Abuse.* Advance Report no. 10. Rockville, MD: U.S. Department of Health and Human Services, September 1995.

Swan, N. "A Look at Marijuana's Harmful Effects." *NIDA Notes* 9 (February/March 1994).

Swan, N. "Facts About Marijuana and Marijuana Abuse. *NIDA Notes* 11 (March/April 1996): 15.

Swan, N. "Researchers Make Pivotal Marijuana and Heroin Discoveries." *NIDA Notes* 8 (10 September 1993): 1.

Tudor, C. G., D. M. Petersen, and K. W. Elifson. "An Examination of the Relationships Between Peer and Parental Influences and Adolescent Drug Use." In *Chemical Dependencies: Patterns, Costs, and Consequences,* edited by C. D. Chambers, J. A. Inciardi, D. M. Petersen, H. A. Siegal, and O. Z. White. Athens, OH: Ohio University Press, 1987.

Turner, C. E. "Chemistry and Metabolism." In *Marijuana Research Findings: 1980.* NIDA Research Monograph no. 31. Washington, DC: National Institute on Drug Abuse, 1980.

Wren, C. S. "Youth Marijuana Use Rises." *Themes of the Times, New York Times.* 20 February 1996: 1.

15

Over-the-Counter (OTC)
and Prescription Drugs

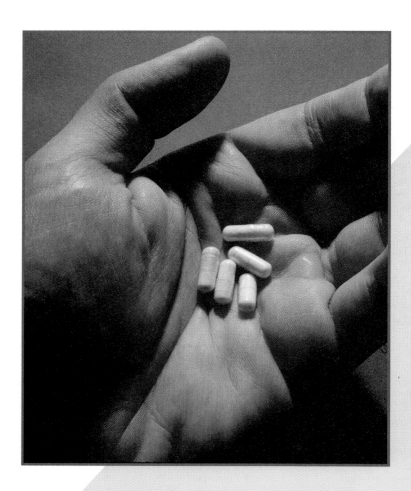

**On completing this chapter
you will be able to:** ▶

- The public can be much more confident of the effectiveness and safety of OTC drugs today than prior to 1972.
- Pharmacists can provide useful counseling in selecting appropriate OTC products.
- Excessive use of some OTC medications can cause physical dependence, tolerance, and withdrawal symptoms.
- OTC drugs can interact with prescription drugs in a dangerous and sometimes even lethal manner.
- Even though there are hundreds of different brands of OTC analgesics, there are really only three different types of active analgesic ingredients in these medications.
- OTC cold medications do not alter the course of the common cold but might relieve symptoms such as nasal congestion, muscle aches, and coughing.
- Frequent use of OTC antacids can be habit-forming.
- Herbal remedies are often drug products available without a prescription that are not regulated by the FDA.
- Melatonin is a hormone sold OTC to treat jet-lag, but its safety for this application has not been tested.
- More people die in the United States from adverse reactions to legal medications than succumb to all illegal drug use.
- Most generic drugs are as effective as, but substantially less expensive than, their proprietary counterparts.
- Pharmacists are required by law to counsel patients concerning the use and safety of prescriptions that they fill.

Learning Objectives

- Outline the general differences between prescription and nonprescription drugs.
- Explain the rationale for the switching policy of the Food and Drug Administration (FDA).
- Identify some of the drugs that the FDA recently made available over the counter (OTC).
- Discuss the potential problems of making more effective OTC drugs available to the public for self-care.
- Describe the type of information that is included on the labels of nonprescription medicines.
- State the rules for safe use of nonprescription drugs.
- Classify the principal drug groups that are available OTC.
- Discuss the type of information that should be communicated between doctor and patient to improve the quality of drug treatment.
- Explain why people are asking for FDA regulation of herbal medicines.
- Explain the differences between, as well as the advantages and disadvantages of, generic and proprietary drugs.
- Classify the most frequently prescribed drug groups.

Prescription and nonprescription (over-the-counter, or OTC) drugs have been viewed differently by the public since these classifications were established by the Durham-Humphrey Amendment of 1951. In general, we view OTC medications as minimally effective, relatively free from side effects, and rarely abused; in contrast, we often think of prescription drugs as much more potent and frequently dangerous. However, distinctions between prescription and nonprescription drugs, which at one time appeared to be clear-cut, have become blurred by changes in public demand and federal policies. Because of escalating health costs and a growing interest in self-care, people today want access to effective medications, and governmental agencies such as the FDA are responding to their demands. Consequently, the FDA is actively involved in switching effective and relatively safe prescription medications to OTC status. It is clear that in the future, many more drugs will be removed from behind the pharmacist's counter and made available for public access as nonprescription medication. These changes emphasize the arbitrary nature of classifying drugs as prescription and OTC, and remind us that similar care should be taken with all medications to achieve maximal benefit and minimal risk.

In this chapter, we begin by discussing OTC or nonprescription drugs. The first topic discusses policies regarding OTC drug regulation followed by a discussion of safe self-care with nonprescription drug products. A short explanation of some of the most common medications in this category, including herbal remedies, concludes the section on OTC drugs. The second part of this chapter gives a general overview of prescription drugs. The consequences of misusing prescription drugs, as well as ways for you to avoid such problems, are discussed. A brief presentation of some of the most commonly prescribed drugs ends the chapter.

◢ OTC Drugs

Each year the United States spends over $14 billion on drug products that are purchased over the counter (OTC), and this market is projected to reach $28 billion by the year 2010 (Covington 1993; Greenberg 1996). Today, more than 300,000 different OTC products are available to treat everything from age spots to halitosis; they comprise 60% of the annual drug purchases in this country (Greenberg 1996). An estimated three out of four people routinely self-medicate with these drug products (Greenberg 1996). The major drug classes currently approved for OTC status are shown in Table 15.1.

OTC remedies are nonprescription drugs that may be obtained and used without the supervision of a physician or other health professional. Nevertheless, some OTCs may be dangerous when used alone or in combination with other drugs. Although some OTC drugs are very beneficial in the self-treatment of minor to moderate uncomplicated health problems, others are of questionable therapeutic value, and their usefulness is often misrepresented by manufacturers.

Abuse of OTC Drugs

During 1996 spring break, Peter Schlendorf, a 20-year-old student, was found dead in his motel room in Panama City, Florida, only hours after consuming eight pills of Ultimate Xphoria. This herbal stimulant is manufactured by Alternate Research (Tempe, Arizona) and contains the amphetamine-related drug, ephedrine. Although a medical examiner's report on the Schlendorf case was not made public, friends and family claimed that Peter was in good health and had not used other drugs or alcohol prior to consuming the stimulant. Because herbal medicines are generally exempt from FDA regulation and available as OTC products by mail order, counterculture shops, or "health nutrition stores," the possible abuse of these potentially dangerous drugs is of concern to federal and state authorities ("New York County" 1996; Lane 1996).

This account gives only one example of problems associated with misuse or abuse of OTC products. Because these drugs are usually available on demand, perceived as being exceptionally safe, and poorly understood by the general public, their abuse patterns differ somewhat from those seen with the so-called "hard core" drugs of abuse; nev-

| Table 15.1 | Major Drug Classes Approved by the FDA for OTC Status |

Drug Class	Effects
Analgesics and anti-inflammatories	Relieve pain, fever, and inflammation
Cold remedies	Relieve cold symptoms
Antihistamines and allergy products	Relieve allergy symptoms
Stimulants	Diminish fatigue and drowsiness
Sedatives and sleep aids	Promote sleep
Antacids	Relieve indigestion from rebound acidity
Laxatives	Relieve self-limiting constipation
Antidiarrheals	Relieve minor, self-limiting diarrhea
Emetics and antiemetics	Induce or block vomiting (respectively)
Antimicrobials	Treatment of skin infections
Bronchodilators and antiasthmatics	Assist breathing
Dentrifices and dental products	Promote oral hygiene
Acne medications	Treat and prevent acne
Sunburn treatments and sunscreens	Treat and prevent skin damage from ultraviolet rays
Dandruff and athlete's foot medications	Treat and prevent specific skin conditions
Contraceptives and vaginal products	Prevent pregnancy and treat vaginal infections
Ophthalmics	Promote eye hygiene and treat eye infections
Vitamins and minerals	Provide diet supplements
Antiperspirants	Promote body hygiene

Source: W. Gilbertson. "The FDA's OTC Drug Review." In *Handbook of Nonprescription Drugs,* 10th ed. Washington, DC: American Pharmaceutical Association, 1993.

ertheless, they can be equally harmful. Even though the OTC products generally have a greater margin of safety than their prescription counterparts, issues of abuse need to be considered. For example, many OTC drugs can cause physical and psychological dependence. Nonprescription products that can be severely habit-forming include nasal and ophthalmic (eye) decongestants, laxatives, antihistamines, sleep aids, and antacids. Of particular abuse concern are the OTC stimulants, such as ephedrine, which can either be severely toxic by themselves (see the account above) or can be used as precursors to the synthesis of the extremely addicting and dangerous amphetamines.

Because use of OTC products is unrestricted, the patterns of abuse are impossible to determine accurately. However, these products are more likely to be abused by members of the unsuspect-ing general public who inadvertently become dependent due to excessive self-medication than by hard-core drug addicts who secure the most potent drugs of abuse by illicit means.

Federal Regulation of OTC Drugs

In the United States, the Food and Drug Administration (FDA) is responsible for regulating OTC drugs. However, many critics claim that this federal agency has not satisfactorily fulfilled its regulatory responsibility in regard to these products (Schwartz and Rifkin 1991).

The active ingredients in OTC drugs have been, and continue to be, evaluated and classified according to their effectiveness and safety (Gilbertson 1993; Holt 1996). At this time, most principal ingredients included in nonprescription drug products are category I (that is, they are considered safe and effective). As recently as August 1992, however, the FDA banned over 400 ingredients from seven categories of OTC products (Lamy 1993). In addition, the FDA is attempting to make even more drugs available to the general public by switching some frequently used and safe prescription medications to OTC status. This policy is in response to public demand to have access to effective drugs for self-medication and has resulted in over 63 switched ingredients (Schwartz 1996). This policy helps to cut medical costs by eliminating the need for costly visits to health providers for treatment of minor, self-limiting ailments (Hsu 1994). A few of the more notable drugs that have been switched to nonprescription status since 1985 (Gilbertson 1993; Slezak 1996) are naprosyn (analgesic, anti-inflammatory: Aleve); ketoprofen (analgesic: Orudis); diphenhydramine (antihistamine: Benadryl); hydrocortisone (anti-inflammatory steroid: Cortaid); loperamide (antidiarrheal: Imodium); clotrimazole (vaginal antifungal: Gyne-Lotrimin); adrenaline (bronchodilator: Bronkaid Mist); miconazole (antifungal: Monistat 7); cimetidine (heartburn medication: Tagamet); minoxidil (hair growth stimulant: Rogaine); and nicotine patch (smoking cessation aid: Nicotrol).

A major concern of health professionals is that reclassification of safe prescription drugs to OTC status will result in overuse or misuse of these agents. The switched drugs may tempt individuals to self-medicate rather than seek medical care for potentially serious health problems or encourage the use of multiple drugs at the same time, increasing the likelihood of dangerous interactions (Stewart 1995). However, the FDA has proceeded cautiously and the majority of consumers support the switching policy (Slezak 1996). As of yet, few major problems have been identified, and the switched products have been well received by the public.

It is likely that effective and safe prescription drugs will continue to be made available OTC, and it is hoped the public will be prepared to use them properly. In fact, the FDA is considering another group of drugs currently available by prescription for OTC status in the next several years. Drugs being evaluated for reclassification include those that lower cholesterol, inhaled nasal steroids for allergies, and new topical antibiotics (Slezak 1996).

OTC Drugs and Self-Care

More than one-third of the time people treat their routine health problems with OTC medications to receive symptomatic relief from their ailments (McCormick 1992). This fact demonstrates the popularity of the OTC drugs and reflects the public enthusiasm for medical self-care. Self-care with nonprescription medications occurs because we decide that we have a health problem that can be adequately self-medicated without involving a health professional. Proper self-care assumes that the individual has made a correct diagnosis of the health problem and is informed enough to select the appropriate OTC product. If done correctly, self-care with OTC medications can provide significant relief from minor, self-limiting health problems at minimal cost. However, a lack of understanding about the nature of the OTC products—what they can and cannot do—and their potential side effects can result in harmful misuse. For this reason, it is important that those who consume OTC medications be fully aware of their proper use. This goal usually can be achieved by reading product labels carefully and asking questions of health professionals such as pharmacists and physicians (Klein-Schwartz and Hoopes 1993).

OTC Labels Information about proper use of OTC medications is required to be cited on the drug label and is regulated by the FDA (see Figure 15.1 for an example). Required label information includes (1) approved uses of the product, (2) detailed instructions on safe and effective use, and (3) cautions or warnings to those at greatest risk when taking the medication (Greenberg 1996).

Many consumers experience adverse side effects because they either choose to ignore the warnings on OTC labels or simply do not bother to read them. For example, excessive or inappropriate use of some nonprescription drugs can cause drug dependence; consequently, people who

Figure 15.1

Label information controlled by the FDA

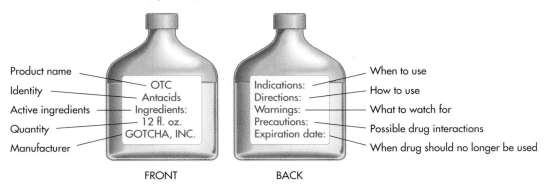

Product name
Identity
Active ingredients
Quantity
Manufacturer

OTC
Antacids
Ingredients:
12 fl. oz.
GOTCHA, INC.

FRONT

Indications:
Directions:
Warnings:
Precautions:
Expiration date:

When to use
How to use
What to watch for
Possible drug interactions
When drug should no longer be used

BACK

are always dropping medication in the eyes "to get the red out" or popping antacids like dessert after every meal are likely addicted. They continue to use OTC products to avoid unpleasant eye redness or stomach acidity, which are actually withdrawal consequences of excessive use of these medications.

Rules for Proper OTC Drug Use The OTC marketplace for drugs operates differently than does its prescription counterpart. The use of OTC drugs is not restricted, and consumers are responsible for making correct decisions about these products. Thus, the consumer sets policy and determines use patterns.

Because there are no formal controls over the use of OTC drugs, abuse often occurs. In extreme situations, the abuse of OTC medication can be very troublesome, even causing structural damage to the body. Proper education about the pharmacological features of these agents is necessary if consumers are to make intelligent and informed decisions about OTC drug use. To reduce the incidence of problems, the following rules should be observed when using nonprescription products:

1. *Always know what you are taking.* Identify the active ingredients in the product.

2. *Know the effects.* Be sure you know both the desired and potential undesired effects of each active ingredient.

3. *Read and heed the warnings and cautions.* The warnings are not intended to scare but to protect.

4. *Don't use anything for more than one to two weeks.* If the problem being treated persists beyond this time, consult a health professional.

5. *Be particularly cautious if also taking prescription drugs.* Serious interactions between OTC and prescription medications frequently occur. If you have a question, be sure to find the answer.

6. *If you have questions, ask a pharmacist.* Pharmacists are excellent sources of information about OTC drugs. They possess up-to-date knowledge of OTC products and can assist consumers in selecting correct medications for their health needs. Ask them to help you.

7. Most importantly: *If you don't need it, don't use it!*

Types of OTC Drugs

It is impossible to provide a detailed description of the hundreds of active ingredients approved by the FDA for OTC distribution; however, the following includes a brief discussion of the most common OTC drugs available in this country.

Internal Analgesics

We spend more than $2 billion on internal (taken by mouth) **analgesics,** the largest sales category of OTC drugs in the United States. Most of the money is for **salicylates** (aspirin products—Anacin, Bayer), acetaminophen (Tylenol, Datril, Pamprin, Panadol), ibupro-
fen (Advil, Nuprin), and ibuprofen-like drugs such as naproxen (Alleve) and ketoprofen (Orudis). The compositions of common OTC internal analgesics are given in Table 15.2.

> **analgesics**
> drugs that relieve pain while allowing consciousness
>
> **salicylates**
> asprin-like drugs

Therapeutic Considerations   The internal analgesic products are effective in treating several common ailments.

▲ *Analgesic Action.* The OTC analgesics effectively relieve mild to moderate somatic pain associated with musculoskeletal structures such as bones, skin, teeth, joints, and liga-
ments. Pains that are relieved by the use of these drugs include headaches, toothaches, earaches, and muscle strains. In contrast, these drugs are not effective in the treatment of severe pain or pain associated with internal organs, such as the heart, stomach, and intestines ("Acetaminophen" 1996).

▲ *Anti-inflammatory Effects.* Use of high doses (two to three times the analgesic dose) of the salicylates and ibuprofen relieves the symptoms of inflammation such as those associated with arthritis (Tyle 1993). In contrast, even high doses of acetaminophen have little **anti-inflammatory** action (Engle 1992). Because of this anti-inflammatory effect, these drugs are frequently compared to a group of natural, very potent anti-inflamma-

> **anti-inflammatory**
> relieves symptoms of inflammation
>
> **steroids**
> potent hormones released from the adrenal glands

Table 15.2   **Compositions of OTC Internal Analgesics** (dose per unit)

Product	Salicylate	Acetaminophen	Ibuprofen	Other
Anacin	400 mg	—	—	Caffeine
Anacin (Maximum Strength)	500	—	—	Caffeine
Bayer	325	—	—	—
Empirin	325	—	—	—
Alka-Seltzer (Extra Strength)	500	—	—	Antacid
Ecotrin	325	—	—	Coated tablet
Excedrin (Extra Strength)	250	250 mg	—	Caffeine
Tylenol, Regular Strength	—	325	—	—
Tylenol, Children's	—	80	—	—
Advil	—	—	200 mg	—
CoAdvil	—	—	200	Decongestant
Motrin IB	—	—	200	—
Motrin, Children's	—	—	100	—
Nuprin	—	—	200	—
Alleve	—	—	—	Naproxen (200 mg)
Orudis	—	—	—	Ketoprofen (12.5 mg)

Source: S. Greenberg. *Physician's Desk Reference for Nonprescription Drugs,* 17th ed. Oradell, NJ: Medical Economics Data, 1996.

tory compounds, the **steroids.** To distinguish drugs such as the salicylates and ibuprofen from steroids, these drugs are often called the **nonsteroidal anti-inflammatory drugs (NSAIDs).**

> **nonsteroidal anti-inflammatory drugs (NSAIDs)**
> anti-inflammatory drugs that do not have steroid properties

▲ *Antipyretic Effects.* The OTC analgesics, such as aspirin and acetaminophen, reduce fever but do not alter normal body temperature (Tyle 1993). Such drugs are called **antipyretics.** The frequent use of these drugs to eliminate fevers is very controversial. Some clinicians believe that fever may be a defense mechanism that helps destroy infecting microorganisms such as bacteria and viruses; thus, interfering with fevers may hamper the body's ability to rid itself of infection-causing microorganisms.

> **antipyretics**
> drugs that reduce fevers

Because no serious problems are associated with fevers of 102°F or less, they are probably better left alone (Lackner 1990).

▲ *Side Effects* When selecting an OTC analgesic drug for relief of pain, inflammation, or fever, possible side effects should be considered. Al-

though salicylates such as aspirin are frequently used, they can cause problems for both children and adults (see Table 15.3). Because of their side effects, salicylates are not recommended for (1) children, because of the potential for **Reye's syndrome;** (2) people suffering gastrointestinal problems, such as ulcers; or (3) people with bleeding problems, who are taking anticlot medication, who are scheduled for surgery, or who are near term in pregnancy, because salicylates interfere with clotting in the blood and prolong bleeding. Consider the following incident:

> **Reye's syndrome**
> a potentially fatal complication of colds, flu, or chicken-pox in children

A 34-year-old woman suffered blood clots during the delivery of her last child. She was put on the anticlotting drug warfarin to prevent additional clots. The following week, the patient experienced a headache and treated it with aspirin. She was not aware that aspirin also interferes with the formation of blood clots. The next morning, the patient slipped and fell but did not appear to be significantly injured. Later that day, she noticed large amounts of blood in her urine. Her husband rushed her to the hospital, where she was diagnosed with serious internal bleeding due to the interaction of warfarin and aspirin (Popovich 1991).

Table 15.3 **Common Side Effects of OTC NSAID Agents**

Drugs	System Affected	Side Effects
Salicylates (aspirin-like)	Gastrointestinal	Irritation, bleeding, aggravation of ulcers
	Blood	Interference with clotting; prolongs bleeding
	Ears	Chronic high doses cause ringing (tinnitis) and hearing loss
	Pediatric	Reye's syndrome
Acetaminophen	Liver	High acute doses or chronic exposure can cause severe damage
Ibuprofen (includes other, newer NSAIDs)	Gastrointestinal	Similar to salicylates but less severe
	Blood	Similar to salicylates but less severe
	Kidneys	Damage in elderly or those with existing kidney disease

For minor aches and pains, acetaminophen substitutes adequately for salicylates, has no effect on blood clotting, and does not cause stomach irritation. In addition, acetaminophen does not influence the occurrence of Reye's syndrome, a potentially deadly complication of colds, flu, and chickenpox in children (up to the age of 16 to 18 years) who are using salicylates (*Drug Facts and Comparisons* 1996).

Caffeine and Other Additives

A number of OTC analgesic products contain caffeine. Increasing evidence indicates that caffeine relieves some types of pain (Sawynok and Yaksh 1993). In addition, caffeine may relieve the aversion of pain due to its stimulant effect, which may be perceived as pleasant and energizing. The combination of caffeine with OTC analgesics may enhance pain relief (Abramowicz 1993) and be especially useful in treating vascular headaches because of the vaso-constrictive properties on cerebral blood vessels caused by this stimulant. In most OTC analgesic products, the amount of caffeine is less than that found in one-fourth to one-half cup of coffee (about 30 milligrams/tablet; for example, Anacin, Excedrin). Other ingredients—such as antacids, antihistamines, and decongestants—sometimes included in OTC pain-relieving products have little or no analgesic action and usually add little to the therapeutic value of the medication.

Cold, Allergy, and Cough Remedies

The common cold accounts for 20% of all acute illness in the United States. It is also the single most expensive ailment in the country (Sause and Mangione 1991; Bryant and Lombardi 1993). More time is lost from work and school due to the common cold than from all other diseases combined. About one-half of all absences and approximately one-fourth of total work time lost each year in industry is due to cold symptoms (Sause and Mangione 1991). Americans spend nearly $4 billion annually for cough, cold, allergy, hay fever, and sinus products (Vaczek 1996).

The incidence of the common cold varies with age. Children between 1 and 5 years are most susceptible; each child averages 6 to 12 respiratory illnesses per year, most of which are common colds. Individuals 25 to 30 years old average about 6 respiratory illnesses a year, and older adults average 2 or 3. The declining incidence of colds with age is due to the immunity that occurs after each infection with a cold virus; thus, if reinfected with the same virus, the microorganism is rapidly destroyed by the body's defense and the full-blown symptoms of a cold do not occur (Sause and Mangione 1991).

Most colds have similar general symptoms: the first stage, in which the throat and nose are dry and scratchy, and the second stage, in which secretions accumulate in the air passages, nose, throat, and bronchial tubes. The second stage is marked by continuous sneezing, nasal obstruction, sore throat, coughing, and nasal discharge. There may be watering and redness of the eyes and pain in the face (particularly near the sinuses) and ears. One

The common cold accounts for 20% of all acute illnesses in the United States.

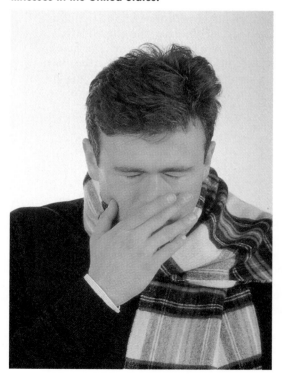

of the most bothersome symptoms of the common cold is the congestion of the mucous membranes of the nasal passages, due in part to capillary dilation, which causes them to enlarge and become more permeable. Such vascular changes allow fluids to escape, resulting in drainage and also inflammation due to fluid-swollen tissues (Bryant and Lombardi 1993).

Decongestants The cold and allergy products we use are formulated with such drugs as decongestants (sympathomimetics), antihistamines (chlorpheniramine or pheniramine), analgesics (aspirin or acetaminophen), and an assortment of other substances (vitamin C, alcohol, caffeine, and so on). Table 15.4 lists the ingredients found in many common OTC cold and allergy products.

Antihistamines reduce congestion caused by allergies, but their effectiveness in the treatment of virus-induced colds is controversial (Consumer Report Books 1989). In high doses, the anticholinergic action of antihistamines (see Chapter 5) also decreases mucus secretion, relieving the runny nose; however, this action is probably insignificant at the lower recommended doses of OTC preparations (Sause and Mangione 1991). An anticholinergic drying action may actually be harmful because it can lead to a serious coughing response. Due to anticholinergic effects, antihistamines also may cause dizziness, drowsiness, impaired judgment, constipation, and dry mouth; they sometimes are abused because of psychedelic effects resulting from high-dose consumption. Because of the limited usefulness and the side effects of antihistamine for treating colds, decongestant products without such agents are usually preferred for these viral infections. In contrast, antihistamines are very useful in relieving allergy-related congestion and symptoms.

The sympathomimetic drugs used as decongestants cause nasal membranes to shrink because of their vasoconstrictive effect, which reduces the congestion caused by both colds and allergies. Such drugs can be used in the form of sprays or

---

Table 15.4 **Compositions of Common OTC Cold and Allergy Products** (dose per tablet)

Product	Sympathomimetic	Antihistamine	Analgesic
Actifed	Pseudoephedrine (30 mg)	Triprolidine (2.5 mg)	—
Allerest Maximum Strength	Pseudoephedrine (30 mg)	Chlorpheniramine (2 mg)	—
Chlor-trimeton	—	Chlorpheniramine (4 mg)	—
Contac Maximum Strength	Phenylpropanolamine (75 mg)	Chlorpheniramine (12 mg)	—
Contac Day & Night	Pseudoephedrine (60 mg)	—	Acetaminophen (650 mg)
Dimetapp Extentabs	Phenylpropanolamine (75 mg)	Brompheniramine (12 mg)	—
Dristan Cold	Phenylephrine (5 mg)	Chlorpheniramine (2 mg)	Acetaminophen (325 mg)
Sudafed 12 Hour	Pseudoephedrine (120 mg)	—	—

Source: S. Greenberg. *Physician's Desk Reference for Nonprescription Drugs,* 17th ed. Oradell, NJ: Medical Economics Data, 1996.

drops (topical decongestants) or systemically (oral decongestants) (see Table 15.5). FDA-approved sympathomimetics include pseudoephedrine, phenylpropanolamine, phenylephrine (probably the most effective topical), naphazoline, oxymetazoline, and xylometazoline (Bryant and Lombardi 1993).

If you use decongestant nasal sprays frequently, you can experience **congestion rebound** due to tissue dependence. After using a nasal spray regularly for longer than the recommended period of time, the nasal membranes adjust to the effect of the vasoconstrictor and become very congested when the drug is not present. You may become "hooked" and use the spray more and more with less and less relief, until your tissues no longer respond and the sinus passages become almost completely obstructed. Allergists frequently see new patients who are addicted to nasal decongestant sprays and are desperate for relief from congestion (Bryant and Lombardi 1993). This problem can be prevented by using nasal sprays sparingly and for no longer than the recommended time.

> **congestion rebound**
>
> withdrawal from excessive use of a decongestant, resulting in congestion

Orally ingested sympathomimetic drugs give less relief from congestion than the topical medications but do not cause rebound effects. In contrast, systemic administration of these drugs is more likely to cause cardiovascular problems (that is, to stimulate the heart, cause arrhythmia, increase blood pressure, and cause stroke).

Antitussives   Other drugs used to relieve the common cold are intended to treat coughing. The cough reflex helps clear the lower respiratory tract of foreign matter, particularly in the later stages of a cold. There are two types of cough: productive and nonproductive. A *productive* cough removes mucus secretions and foreign matter so that breathing becomes easier and the infection clears up. A *nonproductive,* or dry, cough causes throat irritation; this type of cough is of little cleansing value. Some types of cough suppressant **(antitussive)** medication are useful for treating a nonproductive cough but should not be used to suppress a productive cough ("A Hacker's Guide" 1995).

> **antitussive**
>
> a drug that blocks the coughing reflex

Two kinds of OTC preparations are available to treat coughing:

▲ *Antitussives*—such as codeine, dextromethorphan, and diphenhydramine (an antihistamine)—that act on the central nervous system (CNS) to raise the threshold of the cough-coordinating center, thereby reducing the frequency and intensity of a cough

▲ **Expectorants,** such as guaifenesin and terpin hydrate, which theoretically (but not very effectively) increase and thin the fluids of the respiratory tract in order to soothe the irritated respiratory

> **expectorants**
>
> substances that stimulate mucus secretion and diminish mucus viscosity

---

Table 15.5   **Compositions of OTC Topical Decongestants** (Drug Concentrations)

Product	Sympathomimetic
Afrin Nasal Spray	Oxymetazoline (0.05%)
Neo-Synephrine, Maximum Strength	Oxymetazoline (0.05%)
Vicks Sinex, 12-Hour	Oxymetazoline (0.05%)

Source: S. Greenberg. *Physician's Desk Reference for Nonprescription Drugs,* 17th ed. Oradell, NJ: Medical Economics Data, 1996.

tract membranes and decrease the thickness of the accumulated secretions so that coughing becomes more productive.

Table 15.6 lists commonly used OTC antitussives and their compositions.

Often the tickling sensation in the throat that triggers a cough can be eased by sucking on a cough drop or hard candy, which stimulates saliva flow to soothe the irritated membranes. Unless the cough is severe, sour hard candy often works just as well as more expensive cough lozenges.

Cough remedies, like other medications, have a psychological value. Many patients with respiratory tract infections claim they cough less after using cough remedies, even when it is objectively demonstrated that the remedies reduce neither the frequency nor the intensity of the cough. Cough remedies work in part by reducing patients' anxiety about the cough and causing them to believe that their cough is lessening. If you believe in the remedy, you often can get as much relief from a simple, inexpensive product as from the most sophisticated and costly one. If a cough does not ease in a few days, you should consult a doctor ("A Hacker's Guide" 1995).

Although not widely known, abuse of antitussive products by teenagers is a significant problem in some regions of this country. This abuse likely relates to the fact that the antitussive ingredient, dextromethorphan, in high doses can have a phencyclidine (PCP)-like effect (White 1995).

Vitamin C   Vitamin C is found in some OTC cold remedies, although there is little evidence that it has a beneficial or preventive effect. Even so, the late Linus Pauling, a Nobel laureate, advocated using large doses of vitamin C (Bryant and Lombardi 1993). It should be noted that doses of 4 to 12 grams daily of this acidic vitamin (technically known as *ascorbic acid*) can cause kidney stones and that high levels can cause unreliable glucose tests in diabetics. Those who believe in taking vitamin C should use supplements instead of buying it mixed with a cold remedy. Better still, drinking lots of orange juice may help. Even if vitamin C does not relieve the cold, the increase in liquid intake might.

What Really Works?   With all the advances in medicine today, there is still no cure for the common cold. In most cases, the best treatment is plenty of rest, increased fluid intake to prevent dehydration and to facilitate productive coughing, humidification of the air if it is dry, gargling with diluted salt water (2 teaspoons per quart), an analgesic to relieve the accompanying headache or muscle ache, and perhaps an occasional decongestant if nasal stuffiness is unbearable. Allergy symptoms, in contrast, are best relieved by antihistamines.

Table 15.6   **Compositions of Common OTC Antitussives** (dose per unit)

Product	Dextromethorphan	Expectorant	Other
Cheracol plus	20 mg	—	Sympathomimetic; antihistamine; alcohol
Cheracol D	10	Guaifenesin	Alcohol
Novahistine DMX	10	Guaifenesin	Sympathomimetic; alcohol
Robitussin CF	10	Guaifenesin	Sympathomimetic
Vicks NyQuil	30	—	Sympathomimetic; antihistamine

Source: S. Greenberg. *Physician's Desk Reference for Nonprescription Drugs,* 17th ed. Oradell, NJ: Medical Economics Data, 1996.

Sleep Aids

In 1995, an estimated 49% of the U.S. population experienced insomnia (the inability to get to sleep or stay asleep) at least five nights each month (Shuster 1996). About 1% of the adult population routinely self-medicate their insomnia with OTC sleep aids (such as Nytol, Sleep-eze, Sominex) that are advertised as inducing a "safe and restful sleep" (Eggert and Crismon 1992). Described as non-barbiturate and non–habit-forming, these low-potency products are frequently misused (Shuster 1996). For example, the parents of a young child were going out for the evening. Their child often fussed when they were gone, so they decided to do something to keep the child from hassling the baby-sitter. They knew that cough syrup including an antihistamine caused drowsiness, so they gave the child Benylin Cough Syrup (containing the antihistamine diphenhydramine) prior to the arrival of the baby-sitter in order to make the child fall asleep (Popovich 1991). Use of these products in young children is inappropriate and can be dangerous.

The drugs commonly used in OTC sleep aids are antihistamines, particularly diphenhydramine (Shuster 1996). Although antihistamines have been classified as category I sleep aid ingredients (see Chapter 3), their usefulness in treating significant sleep disorders is highly questionable. At best, some people who suffer mild, temporary sleep disturbances caused by problems such as physical discomfort, short-term disruption in daily routines (such as jet lag), and extreme emotional upset might experience temporary relief. However, even for those few who initially benefit from these agents, tolerance develops within two to four days. For long-term sleep problems, OTC sleep aids are of no therapeutic value and are rarely recommended by health professionals. Actually, their placebo benefit is likely more significant than their actual pharmacological benefit. Usually counseling and psychotherapy are more effective approaches for resolving chronic insomnia than OTC or even prescription sleep aid drugs (Eggert and Crismon 1992).

Because antihistamines are CNS depressants, in low doses, they can cause sedation and antianxiety action (see Chapter 6). Although in the past, some OTC products containing antihistamines were promoted for their relaxing effects (for example, Quietworld, Compoz), currently, no sedatives are approved for OTC marketing. The FDA decided that the earlier products relieved anxiety by causing drowsiness, so, in fact, they were not legitimate sedatives. Because of this ruling, medications that are promoted as antianxiety products are no longer available without a prescription. However, antihistamines have been added to an array of other OTC drug products marketed for the purpose of causing relaxation or promoting sleep; such products include analgesics (Excedrin P.M.) and cold medicines (Tylenol Sinus Nighttime). The rationale of such combinations is questionable and their therapeutic value unsubstantiated.

Melatonin   The hormone melatonin is currently being used by millions to induce sleep or to help the body's natural clock readjust after the effects of jet lag. Melatonin has been referred to as the "all-natural nightcap of the 1990s." Sales of melatonin reached an estimated $140 million in 1995. Although most users of this hormone want assistance in falling asleep, melatonin is also claimed to slow the aging process, stimulate the immune system, and enhance the sex drive. Besides being a naturally occurring hormone, melatonin is found in some foods. Under the 1994 Dietary Supplement and Education Act, it is considered a dietary supplement and is not regulated by the FDA. Despite the popularity of melatonin products, little is known about the benefits or the potential adverse effects of this hormone; consequently, these products should be used cautiously, if at all (Klepacki 1996).

Stimulants

Some OTC drugs are promoted as stay-awake (No Doz) or energy-promoting (Vivarin) products. In general, these medications contain high doses of caffeine (100 to 200 milligrams per tablet). (Caffeine and its pharmacological and abuse properties were discussed at length in Chapter 11.) Although it is true that CNS stimulation by ingesting significant doses of caffeine can increase the state of alertness during periods of drowsiness, the usefulness of such an approach is highly suspect (Crismon and Jermain 1993).

For example, many college students rely on such products to enhance mental endurance during cramming sessions for exams. In fact, at one western U.S. university, the back page of a quarterly class schedule, printed and distributed by the university, included a full-page advertisement for the OTC stimulant Vivarin with the caption, "Exam Survival Kit." The implications of such promotion are obvious and disturbing. Due to the objections of the faculty, the ad was not run again at this university.

Routine use of stay-awake or energy-promoting products to enhance performance at work or in school can lead to dependence, resulting in withdrawal when the person stops using the drug. Most health professionals agree that there are more effective and safer ways to deal with fatigue and drowsiness—for example, get plenty of rest.

"Look-Alike" and "Act-Alike" Drugs Mild OTC stimulants have been marketed as safe substitutes for more potent and illicit stimulants of abuse. Known as "look-alike" stimulants, these products have been made to appear as real amphetamines and are intended to give a mild lift or sense of euphoria. The principal drugs found in the look-alikes are phenylpropanolamine, ephedrine, and caffeine. The same drugs are routinely found in OTC decongestants and diet aids (Gauvin 1993).

As mentioned in Chapter 11, some states have outlawed look-alike medications, but products, called *act-alikes*, have taken their place. Act-alikes do not resemble the restricted amphetamine drugs. Even so, these minor stimulants are sold on the streets as "speed" and "uppers," especially to young users, and are promoted by drug dealers as being legal and harmless.

Although much less potent than amphetamines, when used in high doses look-alikes and act-alikes can cause anxiety, restlessness, throbbing headaches, breathing problems, and tachycardia (rapid heartbeat). There have even been reports of death due to heart arrhythmia and cerebral hemorrhaging. The availability of these drugs encourages their routine use and the development of dependence. Thus, they can serve as "gateway" drugs, leading to abuse of more potent compounds.

The manufacturers of the look-alike and act-alike drugs unscrupulously advertise in college newspapers, handbills posted at truckstops, and unsolicited literature from mail order companies.

Gastrointestinal Medications

The gastrointestinal (GI) system consists principally of the esophagus, stomach, and intestines and is responsible for the absorption of nutrients and water into the body, as well as the elimination of body wastes. The function of the GI system can be altered by changes in eating habits, stress, infection, and diseases, such as ulcers and cancers. Such problems may affect appetite, cause discomfort or pain, result in nausea and vomiting, and alter the formation and passage of stools from the intestines.

A variety of OTC medications are available to treat GI disorders such as indigestion (antacids), constipation (laxatives), and diarrhea (antidiarrheals). However, before individuals self-medicate with nonprescription drugs, they should be certain that the cause of their GI problem is minor, self-limiting, and does not require professional care. Because antacids are the most frequently used of the GI nonprescription drugs, they are discussed.

Antacids and Anti-Heartburn Medication

Over $1 billion is spent annually on antacid preparations that claim to give relief from heartburn and indigestion caused by excessive eating or drinking, and for long-term treatment of chronic peptic ulcer disease (Cramer 1992). It is estimated that as much as 50% of the population has had one or more attacks of **gastritis,** often referred to as *acid indigestion, heartburn, upset stomach,* and *sour or acid stomach.* These are often due to acid rebound, occurring one to two hours after eating; by this time, the stomach contents have

> **gastritis**
> inflammation or irritation of the gut

passed into the small intestines, leaving the gastric acids to irritate or damage the lining of the empty stomach. Heartburn, or gastroesophageal reflux, occurs after exposure of the lower esophagus to these very irritating gastric chemicals.

Some cases of severe, chronic acid indigestion may progress to peptic ulcer disease. Peptic ulcers (open sores) most frequently affect the duodenum (first part of the intestine) and the stomach. Although this condition is serious, it can be treated effectively with antacids often combined with drugs available OTC or by prescription, such as cimetidine (Tagamet), ranitidine (Zantac), and famotidine (Pepcid). A person with acute, severe stomach pain; chronic gastritis; blood in the stools (common ulcer symptoms); diarrhea; or vomiting should see a physician promptly and should not attempt to self-medicate with OTC antacids.

Most bouts of acid rebound, however, are associated with overeating or consuming irritating foods or drinks; these self-limiting cases can usually be managed safely with OTC antacids (such as sodium bicarbonate, calcium carbonate, aluminum salts, and magnesium salts). Because of their alkaline (opposite of acidic) nature, the nonprescription products neutralize gastric acids and give relief.

Generally speaking, OTC antacid preparations are safe for occasional use at low recommended doses, but excessive use can cause serious problems. In addition, all antacids can interact with other drugs; they may alter the gastrointestinal ab-

sorption or renal elimination of other medications. For example, some antacids inhibit the absorption of tetracycline antibiotics; thus, these products should not be taken at the same time. Consequently, patients using prescription drugs should consult with their physicians before taking OTC antacids (Pinson and Weart 1993).

Heartburn can be effectively treated by low doses of Tagamet, Zantac, or Pepcid. These drugs were recently switched to OTC status and help reduce gastric secretions.

Diet Aids

In U.S. society, being slim and trim are prerequisites to being attractive. It is estimated that approximately 25%–30% of the people in the United States are obese (with body fat in excess of 20% of normal) and 50% are overweight. Being obese has been linked to cardiovascular disease, some cancers, diabetes, chronic fatigue, and an array of aches and pains, not to mention psychological disorders such as depression. Popular remedies for losing weight often come as fad diets advertised in supermarket journals, expensive weight loss programs, or the use of both prescription and OTC diet aids.

Using drugs as diet aids is highly controversial (Doheny 1993). Most experts view them as useless or even dangerous. These drugs are supposed to depress the appetite, which helps users maintain low-calorie diets. The most effective of these agents are called **anorexiants.** Potent anorexiants, such as amphetamine-like drugs (including the popular diet aid, Phen-fen), can cause dangerous side effects (see Chapter 11) and are available only by prescription.

anorexiants
drugs that suppress the activity of the brain's appetite center, causing reduced food intake

The appetite suppression effects of prescription anorexiants are usually temporary, after which time tolerance often occurs. Thus, even prescription diet aid drugs are usually effective for only a short period. There are no wonder drugs to help the obese lose weight permanently (Doheny 1993).

Approximately 25% to 30% of the people in the United States are obese and 50% are overweight.

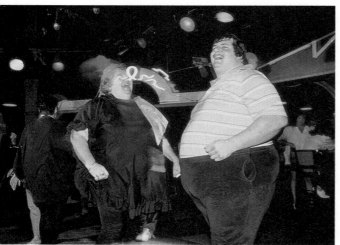

The most potent and most frequently used OTC diet aid ingredient is the sympathomimetic phenylpropanolamine (Acutrim, Dexatrim). Estimates show that, when taken as recommended, even the best of the OTC products significantly reduce appetite in less than 30% of the users, and tolerance occurs in one to three days of use (Consumer Report Books 1989). Clearly, such products are of no value in the treatment of significant obesity. Despite their questionable value, frequent use of high doses of the OTC diet aid products is a common practice by weight-conscious female high school and college students. As one college sophomore who routinely carried a package of Dexatrim in her purse said, "Popping two or three of these before an important date helps me to eat like a bird and appear more petite" (interview with Dr. Glen Hanson, 1996). Interestingly, this same woman also occasionally induced vomiting after eating because of her fear that she was gaining weight. Such weight-management practices are extremely worrisome.

Skin Products

Because the skin is so accessible and readily visible, most people are sensitive about its appearance. These cosmetic concerns are motivated by attempts to look good and preserve youth. Literally thousands of OTC skin products with cosmetic and health objectives are available to consumers. Only a few of the most commonly used products will be mentioned here: acne medications, sun products, and basic first-aid products.

Acne Medications Acne is a universal skin problem that occurs most frequently during puberty in response to the secretion of the male hormone androgen (both males and females have this hormone) (Zander and Weisman 1992). Acne is usually chronic inflammation caused by bacteria trapped in plugged sebaceous (oil) glands and hair follicles. This condition consists of whiteheads, pimples, nodules, and in more severe cases, pustules, cysts, and abscesses. Moderate to severe acne can cause unsightly scarring on the face, back, chest, and arms and should be treated aggressively by a dermatologist with drugs such as antibiotics

(tetracycline) and potent **keratolytics,** such as Retin A (retinoic acid or vitamin A) or Accutane (isotretinoin). Usually, minor to moderate acne does not cause scarring or permanent skin damage and often can be safely self-medicated with over-the-counter acne medications (Billow 1990).

> **keratolytics**
> caustic agents that cause the keratin skin layer to peel

Several nonprescription approaches to treating mild acne are available:

1. *Sebum removal.* Oil and fatty chemicals (sebum) can accumulate on the skin and plug the sebaceous glands and hair follicles. Use of OTC products such as alcohol wipes can help remove such accumulations (for example, Stri Dex).

2. *Peeling agents.* The FDA found several keratolytic agents safe and effective for treatment of minor acne: benzoyl peroxide (Oxy 5 and Oxy 10), salicylic acid (Oxy Medicated Pads), resorcinol, and sulfur (Acnemol), alone or in combination. These drugs help to prevent acne eruption by causing the **keratin layer** of the skin to peel or by killing the bacteria that cause inflammation associated with acne. If multiple concentrations of a keratolytic are available (such as Oxy 5 and Oxy 10), it is better to start with a lower concentration and move up to the higher one, allowing the skin to become accustomed to the caustic action of these products. The initial exposure may worsen the appearance of acne temporarily; however, with continual use, the acne usually improves.

> **keratin layer**
> the outermost protective layer of the skin

Sun Products The damaging effects of sun exposure on the skin have been well publicized in recent years. It is now clear that the ultraviolet (UV) rays associated with sunlight have several adverse effects on the skin. It has been demonstrated that almost one million cases of skin cancer each year in the United States are a direct consequence of exposure to UV rays (Debrovner 1994b). Almost one of six people will experience

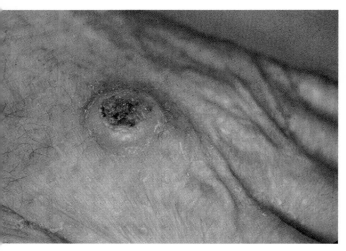

This sore is skin cancer caused by excessive exposure to ultraviolet light.

some form of skin cancer during his or her lifetime (Simonsen 1993).

The majority of these will be cancers of skin cells called *basal cell* or *squamous cell carcinomas* (Rigel 1991). These cancers usually are easily removed by minor surgery and have a good prognosis for recovery. About 0.5% of the population will suffer a much more deadly form of skin cancer called *melanoma.* It is estimated that, because people today tend to spend so much time outdoors, by the year 2000, the risk of this cancer will reach 1 in 75 Americans (Ritter 1991). Melanomas are cancers of the pigment-forming cells of the skin, called *melanocytes,* and spread rapidly from the skin throughout the body, causing death in 20%–25% of the cases (DeSimone 1993).

Another long-term concern (to some people, considered worse than cancer) related to UV exposure is premature aging. Skin frequently exposed to UV rays, such as during routine tanning, experiences deterioration associated with the aging process. Elastin and collagen fibers are damaged, causing a loss of pliability and elasticity in the skin and resulting in a leathery, wrinkled appearance (Simonsen 1993).

Because of these damaging effects of sun exposure, an array of protective sunscreen products are available OTC. Most sunscreens are formulated to

screen out the shorter UV-B rays. These products have deliberately been designed to allow passage, in varying degrees, of the UV-A rays because researchers once thought that these longer rays would help skin to tan without causing damage. Now it appears scientists were mistaken and due to deep penetration in the skin, UV-A rays likely contribute to melanoma as well as chronic skin damage, causing wrinkling, sagging skin, and loss of skin tone (Simonsen 1993; Debrovner 1994b).

The protection afforded by sunscreens is designated by an **SPF (sun protection factor) number.** This designation tells users the relative length of time they can stay in the sun before burning and varies from 2 to 46. For example, proper application of a product with an SPF of 10 allows users to remain in the sun without burning 10 times longer than if it wasn't applied. It is important to remember that the SPF designation does not indicate protection against UV-A rays. Although there currently is no convenient rating system to assess UV-A screening, products with SPF ratings of 15 or greater usually offer some protection against the longer UV radiation. In addition, a compound called *avobenzone* appears to offer the fullest protection against UV-A rays. Two FDA-approved products that contain avobenzone are Photoplex and Shade UVAGUARD. Both are classified as broad-spectrum screens as they also protect against UV-B and have an SPF designation of 15 ("Full Sun Protection" 1993).

Because the natural pigment in the skin affords some UV protection, people with fair skin complexion (less skin pigmentation) require products with higher SPF numbers than do dark-skinned people.

People who want complete protection from UV-B exposure can use OTC sunblockers, which prevent any tanning. Sunscreen ingredients in high concentrations essentially become sunblockers (for example, Presun 46). In addition, an opaque zinc oxide ointment is a highly effective and inexpensive sun-blocking product and is available OTC.

> **SPF (sun protection factor) number**
> a designation to indicate a product's ability to screen UV rays

Skin First-Aid Products

A variety of unrelated OTC drugs are available as first-aid products for the self-treatment of minor skin problems. Included in this category of agents are the following products:

1. *Local anesthetics,* such as benzocaine (such as Americaine First Aid Spray or Dermoplast) to relieve the discomfort and pain of burns or trauma

2. *Antibiotics and antiseptics,* such as bacitracin (Polysporin), neomycin (Neosporin), betadine, and tincture of iodine to treat or prevent skin infections

3. *Antihistamines* (Benadryl) or corticosteroids (hydrocortisone—Cortaid and Caldecort) to relieve itching or inflammation associated with skin rashes, allergies, or insect bites

These first-aid skin products can be effective when used properly. In general, side effects to such topical products are few and minor when they occur.

OTC Herbal Products

Herbal products are a unique category of OTC remedies that account for almost $1.5 billion a year in U.S. sales (Foreman 1997). They are unique because, despite the presence of active ingredients, there is little or no federal regulation due to a 1994 law, supported by the dietary-supplement industry, called the Dietary Supplement Health and Education Act (Cowley 1996). This law requires the government to demonstrate that substances in the herbal products are harmful before such products can be removed from the market ("New York County" 1996). This lack of government involvement has led to unproven claims for these remedies, such as a "legal high," a "natural boost" in energy, weight reduction, or sexual euphoria (Lane 1996). These products, which are typically merchandised through the mail or at health food, counterculture, or alternative-health stores, are sold with brand names such as Cloud 9, Herbal Ecstasy, Up Your Gas, Ripped Fuel, and Ultimate Xphoria (Lane 1996).

The responses to these herbal products can vary considerably, as illustrated by the following two Internet accounts of young adult users (Internet address http://www.hyperreal.com/drugs/mdma/cloud 9). Jonathan writes, "A friend of mine purchased and tried Cloud 9. I read the brochure its distributors mail out on request, and it is very vague . . . and tries to make this herbal placebo sound like a good replacement for MDMA (Ecstasy). Not a chance . . . [My friend] bought the caplets from a health food store, for around $10 apiece. He said it produced a definite warmth sensation, but it was very minimal, and that a cup of coffee was way more psychoactive. He said it was a total waste of money . . . It's a placebo sugar pill." In contrast, Chico responds, "[Cloud 9] is fairly new, so there is no law against it yet. I took one dose . . . it's very similar to Ecstasy . . . It [causes] a very mild dreamy feeling, kind of like coke, but without guilt, and without angst. Just try some . . . "

While use of most herbal products is relatively safe (Crowley 1996), the lack of understanding by users that some of these products contain very active drugs has led to fatal consequences. For example, the stimulants ephedrine, ephedra, or ma huang (a Chinese herb) are included in dozens of popular herbal remedies. They and other chemically related stimulants have been linked to at least 15 deaths, 400 serious adverse events, and likely many more unreported negative incidents (Lane 1996). These drugs, like other stimulants, can provoke insomnia, heart attacks, strokes, tremors, and seizures ("New York County" 1996). Consequently, even though the federal government is limited in its ability to restrict these products, states such as Ohio and Texas have banned the ephedrine-containing stimulants ("New York County" 1996).

◢ Prescription Drugs

The Durham-Humphrey Amendment of 1951 established the criteria that are still used today to determine if a drug should be used only under the direction of a licensed health professional, such as a physician. According to this piece of legislation, drugs are controlled with prescriptions if they are (1) habit-forming, (2) not safe for self-medication, (3) intended to treat ailments that require the supervision of a health professional, and/or (4) new and without an established safe track record. There currently are more than 10,000 prescription products sold in the United States, representing approximately 1500 different drugs, with 20 to 50 new medications approved each year by the FDA (*Physician's Desk Reference* 1997).

Because of their specialized training, physicians, dentists, and, under certain conditions, podiatrists, physician assistants, nurse practitioners, pharmacists, and optometrists are granted drug-prescribing privileges. The health professionals who write prescriptions are expected to accurately diagnose medical conditions requiring therapy, consider the benefits and risks of drug treatment to the patient, and identify the best drug and safest manner of administering it. The responsibility of the health professional does not conclude with the writing of a prescription; in many ways it only just begins. Professional monitoring to ensure proper drug use and to evaluate the patient's response is crucial for successful therapy.

Prescription Drug Abuse

Dealing with suspected abuse of prescription medication can pose a difficult management problem for physicians and pharmacists (see "Fighting the Drug War," page 411). It has become such a major issue that some third-party payers (that is, health insurance companies) have implemented tight monitoring procedures. Abusing patients often employ manipulative tactics to gain access to drugs for which they have developed severe dependence. For example, a woman who became loud and abusive when a pharmacist questioned the validity of her prescription for a narcotic claimed a taxicab was waiting in the front to take her to a family emergency; her prescription was subsequently found to be fraudulent (Wick 1995). Illicit use of prescription drug products may be prompted by any of several reasons (Wick 1995): (1) to relieve withdrawal caused by drug habits (for example, benzodiazepines are used to relieve alcohol withdrawal); (2) to treat infections

caused by drug abuse (for example, antibiotics are used to treat injection infections); (3) to provide a source of fresh, clean needles for injecting drugs of abuse (for example, via insulin syringes); and (4) to prolong the high caused by drugs of abuse (for example, appetite suppressants are taken to enhance effects of stimulants of abuse).

Abusers of prescription drugs often have multiple addictions, including dependence on caffeine, nicotine, or both. In addition, once a pharmacy is recognized as an easy target, word spreads and other abusers often begin to frequent the same store (Wick 1995). Signs of patients with drug-seeking behavior include the following:

▲ Use of altered or forged prescriptions

▲ Claims that a prescription has been lost and a physician is unavailable for confirmation

▲ Frequent visits to emergency rooms or clinics for poorly defined health problems

▲ Visits made to a pharmacy late in the day, on weekends, or just prior to closing

▲ Alteration of doses on a legitimate prescription

▲ Loud, abusive, and insulting behavior

▲ Use of several names

▲ Being particularly knowledgeable about drugs

Proper Doctor–Patient Communication

Many unnecessary side effects and delays in proper care are caused by poor communication between the health professional and the patient when a drug is prescribed. The smaller a drug's margin of safety (the difference between therapeutic and toxic doses), the greater the need for direction from a health professional concerning its proper use. The following is a brief overview of principles to help ensure that satisfactory communication takes place between the health professional and the patient.

Doctor–patient communication must be reciprocal. We tend to think that patients listen while doctors talk when it comes to deciding on the best medication for treatment. To ensure a proper diagnosis, precise and complete information from the patient is also essential. In fact, if a doctor is to

FIGHTING THE DRUG WAR

Anyone taking a drug prescribed by his or her physician—and the numbers of such users are growing—would probably not think that ordinary prescriptions could grow into an illegal market for abused drugs. Yet the marketing and consumption of illegally obtained prescription drugs by criminal abusers is becoming increasingly common, and equally difficult to control.

According to a *Los Angeles Times* article published in 1996, prescription painkillers, stimulants, and tranquilizers are believed to be among the most extensively abused substances in the United States—even rivaling the estimated volume for cocaine and crack. Nevertheless, only a few agents investigate the illegal trafficking of prescription drugs. Special Agent Walter Allen III of the California Bureau of Narcotic Enforcement, quoted in the *Times* article, said, "There is just no glory in it—no guns, no piles of coke, and no bundles of cash to stack up for the TV cameras."

In the late 1990s, an estimated 2.6 million people in the United States used prescription medications for "nonmedical" purposes. Users ranged from teenagers to street addicts to senior citizens. Some combined prescription drugs with illicit narcotics to enhance the latter's effects. Others used tranquilizers to soften the crash from cocaine and heroin. And for some, pharmaceuticals were just their drugs of choice—often because of their purity, their predictable effect, and their low cost relative to illicit drugs.

A number of factors have combined in recent years to create this problem. First is the sheer volume of prescription drugs, which some have projected to double within one year. A second issue is the demands imposed on primary care doctors by insurance companies to increase the number and reduce the length of patient visits, which can cause doctors to prescribe medication too quickly.

These conditions make life easy for con artists garnering illegal drug prescriptions through practice of "doctor shopping"—tricking doctors and pharmacists, using a variety of different ailments and self-inflicted injuries, to collect marketable prescriptions. Other drug peddlers find it easier to bypass doctors completely and merely fill forged prescriptions. In addition, some unscrupulous doctors, dentists, and pharmacists prescribe drugs dishonestly, are grossly negligent in prescribing them, or knowingly fill fraudulent prescriptions—at tremendous profit. Depending on the drug, a prescription could sell for $200 to $250.

Because these drugs are legal, and because prosecuting medical professionals is problematic, the illegal prescription drug market is growing at a healthy pace. Some states have tried to attack the problem of fraudulent prescriptions by a system of registering and tracking. This paper-copy system requires that for Schedule II drugs—a federal ranking for medications with a high potential for abuse—doctors and dentists should issue the order on "triplicate" forms; one copy would stay with the doctor, one would go the pharmacy, and a third would be sent to the state agency that monitors controlled substances. While proponents of the practice claim that triplicates facilitate identification of drug-dealing professionals and people using fraudulent prescriptions, many physicians see the system as a government intrusion into their practice and their patients' privacy. For their part, pharmaceutical companies see this system as a threat to patients and to their own profitability. Secure and private electronic tracking systems might possibly overcome some of these objections, but such enforcement is never trouble-free.

Even with the use of triplicates, some continue to feel that the federal government could do more to control prescription drug abuse. Of the $13 billion to $14 billion allocated annually to the war on drugs, a mere $70 million is spent on investigating prescription drug offenses. Law and health officials are hoping that stronger efforts to monitor the practices of nontraditional drug traffickers, such as medical professionals, will provide the means to end this type of drug abuse. ∎

Sources: Marsa, L. "Hey, Who Needs a Prescription?" *Los Angeles Times Magazine* (September 29, 1996).
Weikel, D. "Prescription for Abuse." *Maine Sunday Telegram* (August 25, 1996).
Weikel, D. "Doctor Accused of Aiding Large Narcotics Ring." *Los Angeles Times* (January 7, 1997): B-1.

select the best and safest drug for a patient, he or she needs to know everything possible about the medical problems to be treated. In addition, the patient should provide the doctor with a complete medical and drug history, particularly if there has been a problem with the patient's cardiovascular system, kidneys, liver, or mental functions. Other information that should be shared with the doctor includes previous drug reactions as well as a complete list of drugs routinely being used, both prescription and nonprescription.

The patient needs to be educated about proper drug use. If the doctor does not volunteer this information, the patient should insist on answers to the following questions:

▲ *What is being treated?* This question doesn't require a long, unintelligible scientific answer. It should include an easy-to-understand explanation of the medical problem.

▲ *What is the desired outcome?* The patient should know why the drug is prescribed and what the drug treatment is intended to accomplish. It is difficult for the patient to become involved in therapy if he or she is not aware of its objectives.

▲ *What are the possible side effects of the drug?* This answer does not necessitate an exhaustive list of every adverse reaction ever recorded in the medical literature; however, it is important to realize that adverse drug reactions to prescription drugs are very common. In the United States more people die from adverse reactions to legal medications than succumb to all illegal drug use (Fried 1994). In general, if the incidence is more than 1% of the users, it should be mentioned to the patient. In addition, the patient should be made aware of ways to minimize the occurrence of side effects (for example, an irritating drug should not be taken on an empty stomach to minimize nausea) as well as what to do if a side effect occurs (for example, if a rash occurs, call the doctor immediately).

▲ *How should the drug be taken to minimize problems and maximize benefit?* This answer should include details on how much, how often, and how long the drug should be taken.

Although it is a health professional's legal and professional obligation to communicate this information, patients frequently leave the doctor's office with a prescription that gives them legal permission to use a drug, but without the knowledge of how to use it properly. Because of this all-too-common problem, pharmacists have been mandated by legislation referred to as the Omnibus Budget Reconciliation Act of 1990 (OBRA 90) to provide the necessary information to patients on proper drug use (Zak 1993) (see "Here and Now," page 413). Patients should be encouraged to ask questions of those who write and fill prescriptions.

Drug Selection: Generic Versus Proprietary

Although it is the primary responsibility of the doctor or health care provider to decide which drug is most suitable for a treatment, often an inexpensive choice can be as effective and safe as a more costly option. This statement frequently is true when choosing between generic and proprietary drugs. The term **generic** is used by the public to refer to the common name of a drug that is not subject to trademark rights; in contrast, **proprietary** denotes medications marketed under specific brand names. For example, diazepam is the generic designation for the proprietary name Valium. Often the most common proprietary name associated with a drug is the name given when it is newly released for marketing. Because such drugs are almost always covered by patent restrictions for several years when first sold to the public, they become identified with their first proprietary names. After the patent lapses, the same drug often is also marketed by its less-known generic designation.

Because the pharmaceutical companies that market the generic products have not invested in the discovery or development of the drug, they

generic
the official, nonpatented, nonproprietary name of a drug

proprietary
a brand or trademark name that is registered with the U.S. Patent Office

OBRA 90–The Evolving Role of Pharmacists in Drug Management

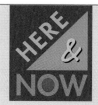

In 1990, the U.S. Congress passed section 4401 of the Omnibus Budget Reconciliation Act (commonly referred to as OBRA 90), which substantially altered the role of pharmacists in drug management. This act designated the pharmacist as the key player in improving the quality of drug care for patients in this country. Because OBRA 90 is federal legislation, it can require drug-related services for Medicare patients only; however, most states have recognized that similar services should be made available to all patients and have enacted legislation to that end. OBRA 90 requires pharmacists to conduct a **drug use review (DUR)** for each prescription to improve the outcome of drug therapy and reduce adverse side effects. The DUR program describes four basic professional services that a pharmacist must render whenever a drug prescription is filled:

1. Prescriptions and patients' records must be screened to avoid problems caused by drug duplications, adverse drug–drug interactions, medical complications, incorrect drug doses, and incorrect duration of drug treatment.

2. Patients should be counseled regarding

   ▲ How to safely and effectively administer the drug

   ▲ Common adverse effects and interactions with other drugs, food, and so forth

   ▲ How to avoid problems with the drug

   ▲ How to monitor the progress of drug therapy

   ▲ How to store the drug properly

   ▲ Whether a refill is intended

   ▲ What to do if a dose is missed

3. Patient profiles, including information on disease, a list of medications, and the pharmacist's comments relevant to drug therapy, must be maintained. This information should be stored in computer files for future reference.

4. Documentation must record if the patient refuses consultation from the pharmacist, or if a potential drug therapy problem is identified and the patient is warned. ■

Source: R. Abood. *"OBRA 90: Implementation and Enforcement."* NABP U.S. Pharmacists, State Boards—a Continuing Education Series. Park Ridge, IL: National Association of Boards of Pharmacy, 1992.

---

drug use review (DUR)

a process conducted by pharmacists to improve the outcome of prescription drug therapy

often charge much less for their version of the medication. This situation contrasts with that of the original drug manufacturer, which may have invested up to $500 million for research and development (see Chapter 3). Even though the generic product frequently is less expensive, the quality usually is not inferior to the related proprietary drug; thus, substitution of generic for proprietary products rarely compromises therapy. It should be noted that occasionally an inferior generic drug product

is marketed in order to increase profit margins for the manufacturer and is not therapeutically equivalent to the proprietary drug product; however, physicians and pharmacists should be aware of these differences and prescribe accordingly. If a patient alerts the physician to concerns about drug costs, less expensive generic brands often can be substituted.

Because of reduced cost, generic products have become very popular. Currently, generic drugs account for over 30% of all prescription drug sales amounting to approximately $10 billion (Simonsen 1993a). Because of the great demand, all states have laws that govern the use and substitution of generic drugs; unfortunately, the laws are not all the same. Some states have positive laws that require pharmacists to substitute a generic product unless the physician gives specific instructions not to do so. Other states have negative laws that forbid substitution without the physician's permission. Some physicians use convenient prescription forms with "May" or "May Not" substitution boxes that can be checked when the prescription is filled out.

Common Categories of Prescription Drugs

Of the approximately 10,000 different prescription drugs available in the United States, the top 50 drugs in sales account for almost 30% of all new and refilled prescriptions ("Top 200 Drugs" 1996). As an example, a list of the 30 top-selling prescription drugs in 1995 is shown in Table 15.7. The following includes a brief discussion of drug groups represented in the 30 most frequently prescribed medications. This list is not intended to be all inclusive, but gives only a sampling of common prescription products.

Analgesics The prescription analgesics consist mainly of narcotic and NSAID (nonsteroidal anti-inflammatory drug) types. The narcotic analgesics most often dispensed to patients by prescription are (1) the low-potency agents propoxyphene (Darvon) and codeine, (2) the moderate-potency agents pentazocine (Talwin) and oxycodone (Percodan), and (3) the high-potency drug meperidine (Demerol). All narcotic analgesics are scheduled drugs because of their abuse potential and are effective against most types of pain. The narcotic analgesic products are often combined with aspirin or acetaminophen (for example, Percocet is a combination of oxycodone and acetaminophen) to enhance their pain-relieving actions. For additional information on the narcotics, see Chapter 10.

The NSAIDs constitute the other major group of analgesics available by prescription. The pharmacology of these drugs is very similar to that of the OTC compound ibuprofen, discussed earlier in this chapter. These medications are used to relieve inflammatory conditions (such as arthritis) and are effective in relieving minor to moderate musculoskeletal pain (pain associated with body structures such as muscles, ligaments, bones,

teeth, and skin). These drugs have no abuse potential and are not scheduled; several are also available OTC (see the discussion of OTC analgesics). The principal adverse side effects include stomach irritation, kidney damage, tinnitus (ringing in the ears), dizziness, and swelling from fluid retention. Most prescription NSAIDs have similar pharmacological and side effects. Included in the group of prescription NSAIDs are ibuprofen (Motrin), naproxen (Anaproxyn), indomethacin (Indocin), sulindac (Clinoril), mefenamic acid (Ponstel), tolmetin (Tolectin), piroxicam (Feldene), and ketoprofen (Orudis) (*Drug Facts and Comparisons* 1996).

Antibiotics Drugs referred to by the layperson as **antibiotics** are more accurately described by the term **antibacterials,** although the more common term will be used here. For the most part, antibiotics are effective in treating infections caused by microorganisms classified as bacteria. Bacterial infections can occur anywhere in the body, resulting in tissue damage, loss of function, and, if untreated, ultimately death. Even though bacterial infections continue to be the most common serious diseases throughout the world and in the United States today, the vast majority of these can be cured with antibiotic treatment. There are currently close to 100 different antibiotic drugs, which differ from one another in (1) whether they kill bacteria (**bactericidal**) or stop their growth (**bacteriostatic**), and (2) the species of bacteria that are sensitive to their antibacterial action (Mills et al. 1992). Antibiotics that are effective against many species of bacteria are classified as **broad-spectrum** types,

> **antibiotics**
> common drugs used to control infections
>
> **antibacterials**
> drugs used to control bacterial infections

> **bactericidal**
> kills bacteria
>
> **bacteriostatic**
> stops replication and growth of bacteria

> **broad-spectrum**
> effective against many species of bacteria
>
> **narrow-spectrum**
> effective against only a few species of bacteria

Table 15.7 **The 30 Top-Selling Prescription Drugs of 1995** (based on new and refill prescriptions)

Ranking	Proprietary Name	Generic Name	Principal Clinical Use
1	Premarin	Estrogen	Relieve symptoms of menopause
2	Trimox	Amoxicillin	Antibiotic
3	Synthroid	Levothyroxin	Replace thyroid hormone
4	Zantac	Ranitidine	Relieve ulcers
5	Amoxil	Ampicillin	Antibiotic
6	Lanoxin	Digoxin	Relieve heart failure
7	Vasotec	Enalapril	Reduce hypertension
8	Procardia	Nifedipine	Relieve angina pectoris
9	Prozac	Fluoxetine	Antidepressant
10	Proventil	Albuterol	Open air passages
11	Cardizem	Diltiazem	Reduce hypertension
12	Coumadin	Warfarin	Prevent blood clots
13	Zoloft	Sertraline	Antidepressant
14	Biaxen	Clarithromycin	Antibiotic
15	Hydrocodone	Same	Narcotic analgesic
16	Augmentin	Amoxicillin	Antibiotic
17	Zestril	Lisinopril	Reduce hypertension
18	Triamterene	Same	Diuretic for hypertension
19	Cipro	Ciprofloxacin	Antibiotic
20	Amoxicillin	Same	Antibiotic
21	Prilosec	Omeprazole	Relieve ulcers
22	Ventolin	Albuterol	Open air passages
23	Norvasc	Amlodipine	Reduce hypertension
24	Acetaminophen/codeine	Same	Analgesic
25	Veetids	Penicillin	Antibiotic
26	Furosemide	Same	Diuretic
27	Claritin	Loratidine/pseudoephedrine	Decongestant
28	Mevacor	Lovastatin	Lower cholesterol
29	Propoxyphene	Same	Narcotic analgesic
30	Dilantin	Phenytoin	Reduce seizures

Source: "Top 200 of 1995." *Pharmacy Times* (April 1996): 29.

whereas those antibiotics that are relatively selective and effective against only a few species of bacteria are considered **narrow-spectrum** drugs. Although most antibiotics are well tolerated by patients, they can cause very serious side effects, especially if not used properly. For example, the penicillins have a very wide margin of safety for most patients, but 5% to 10% of the population is allergic to these drugs and life-threatening reactions can occur in sensitized patients if penicillins are used. The most common groups of antibiotics include penicillins (for example, ampicillin—Amoxil, Augmentin, and Trimox), cephalosporins (such as cefaclor—Ceclor), fluoroquinolones (such as ciprofloxacin—Cipro), tetracyclines (such as minocyclin—Minocin), aminoglycosides (such as streptomycin), sulfonamides (such as sulfamethoxazole—Bactrim and Septra), and macrolides (such as erythromycin—E-mycin).

Antidepressants Severe depression is characterized by diminished interest or pleasure in normal activities accompanied by feelings of fatigue, pessimism, and guilt as well as sleep and appetite disturbances and suicidal desires (American Psychiatric Association 1994). Severe depression afflicts approximately 5% to 6% of the population at any one time, and it is estimated that about 10% of the population will become severely depressed during their life (Debrovner 1994a). This high prevalence makes depression the most common psychiatric disorder (Hollister 1992). According to the classification of the *Diagnostic and Statistical Manual of Mental Disorders (DSM-IV)* of the American Psychiatric Association, several types of depression exist, based on their origin: (1) endogenous major depression, a genetic disorder that can occur spontaneously and is due to transmitter imbalances in the brain; (2) depression associated with bipolar mood disorder (that is, manic-depressive disorder); (3) reactive depression, the most common form of depression, which is a response to situations of grief, personal loss, illness, or other very stressful situations. Antidepressant medication is typically used to treat endogenous major depression, although on occasion these drugs also are used to treat other forms of depression if they are resistant to conventional therapy (Hollister 1992).

Several groups of prescription antidepressant medication are approved for use in the United States (Grinspoon 1995). The most commonly used category is the **tricyclic antidepressants.** Included in this group are drugs such as amitryptyline (Elavil), imipramine (Tofranil), and nortryptyline (Pamelor). Although usually well tolerated, the tricyclic antidepressants can cause annoying side effects due to their anticholinergic activity. These adverse reactions include drowsiness, dry mouth, blurred vision, and constipation. Tolerance to these side effects usually develops with continued use. The second group of drugs used to treat depression is referred to as the **monoamine oxidase (MAO) inhibitors.** Historically, these agents have been

> **tricyclic antidepressants**
>
> most commonly used group of drugs to treat severe depression

> **monoamine oxidase (MAO) inhibitors**
>
> groups of drugs used to treat severe depression

backup drugs for the tricyclic antidepressants. Because of their annoying and sometimes dangerous side effects as well as problems with interacting with other drugs or even food, the MAO inhibitors have become less popular with clinicians. Drugs belonging to this group include phenelzine (Nardil) and tranylcypromine (Parnate). Agents from a third, somewhat disparate, group of antidepressants have been recently approved by the FDA. Supposedly safer and with fewer side effects than the tricyclic or MAO inhibitor antidepressants, drugs in this third generation of antidepressants are rapidly gaining in popularity. They include fluoxetine (Prozac), sertraline (Zoloft), paroxetine (Paxil), fluvoxamine (Luvox), bupropion (Wellbutrin), and trazodone (Desyrel). Although side effects and the margin of safety of these groups of antidepressants may differ, in general they all appear to have similar therapeutic benefits.

Of this third group of antidepressants, Prozac is the best known. Ironically, Prozac is the most frequently prescribed antidepressant (in 1995 it was the eighth most frequently prescribed drug in the United States—see Table 15.7), as well as the most controversial (Stanford 1996). Reports began to surface in 1990 that use of Prozac caused some patients to commit suicide or murder. One report described six patients who experienced intense preoccupation with suicide only after beginning treatment with Prozac (Masand et al. 1991). It was discovered that much of the early anti-Prozac propaganda was orchestrated by the "Citizens Commission on Human Rights," a nonmedical organization described by the television program "60 Minutes" as a front group for the Church of Scientology, a religious group that opposes the use of medications to treat many illnesses (Debrovner 1994a). Since these early findings and anti-Prozac campaigns, close scrutiny of Prozac has not revealed this drug to be any more likely than other antidepressants to cause dangerous emotional problems in severely depressed patients (American Hospital Formulary Service [AHFS] 1996). Although most commonly used to treat depression, Prozac has also been prescribed by physicians to treat over 30 other conditions ranging from drug addiction (such as cocaine dependence) to kleptomania. The vast majority of these uses are not proven to be effective nor are they approved by the FDA (Sewester 1995).

Antidiabetic Drugs **Diabetes mellitus** afflicts millions of people in the United States and is the result of insufficient activity of insulin, a hormone secreted from the pancreas (Davis and Granner 1995). Due to the lack of insulin, untreated diabetics have severe problems with metabolism and elevated blood sugar (called **hyperglycemia**). The two major types of diabetes are type I (or juvenile type) and type II (or adult-onset type). **Type I diabetes** is caused by total destruction of the insulin-producing cells in the pancreas and usually begins in juveniles, but occasionally begins during adulthood. In contrast, **type II diabetes** occurs most often after 40 years of age and is frequently associated with obesity: in these patients the pancreas is able to produce insulin, but insulin receptors no longer respond normally to this hormone (Davis and Granner 1995). In both types of diabetes mellitus, drugs are administered to restore proper insulin function.

> **diabetes mellitus**
> disease caused by elevated blood sugar due to insufficient insulin
>
> **hyperglycemia**
> elevated blood sugar

> **diabetes, type I**
> associated with complete loss of insulin-producing cells in the pancreas
>
> **diabetes, type II**
> usually associated with obesity; does not involve a loss of insulin-producing cells

Because of the inability to produce or release insulin in the type I diabetic, these patients are universally treated with subcutaneous injections of insulin 1–3 times a day, depending on their needs. Usually the levels of sugar (glucose) in the blood are evaluated to determine the effectiveness of treatment. Insulin products are characterized by their onset of action and duration of effects. Three types of insulin are used: short-acting (regular), medium-acting (NPH and lente) and long-acting (ultralente) types.

The strategy for treating type II diabetics is somewhat different. For many of these patients, the

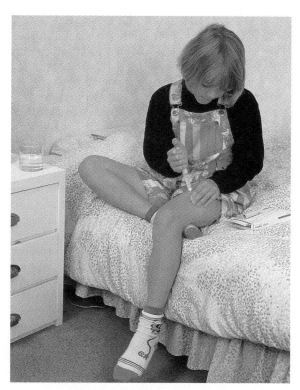

Insulin is self-administered by diabetic patients in subcutaneous injections.

symptoms of diabetes subside with proper diet, weight, and exercise management. If an appropriate change in lifestyle is insufficient to correct the diabetes-associated problems, drugs called **oral hypoglycemics** (meaning they are taken by mouth and lower blood sugar) are often prescribed. These drugs, which stimulate the release of additional insulin from the pancreas, include glyburide (Micronase) and tolbutamine (Orinase). If the diabetic symptoms are not adequately controlled with the oral hypoglycemic drugs, type II diabetics are treated with insulin injections, as are type I patients.

> **oral hypoglycemics**
> drugs taken by mouth to treat type II diabetes

Antiepileptic Drugs Approximately 1% of the population in the United States has some form of **epilepsy.** Although appropriate medication can

epilepsy

disease consisting of spontaneous, repetitive seizures

control the disease in 80% of these patients, many people in this country with epilepsy are inadequately treated. Epilepsy is a neurological condition characterized by recurring seizures (that is, uncontrolled hyperactivity of the brain). Seizures are classified according to the region of the brain involved and how far the hyperactivity spreads. Thus, seizures are considered to be either partial (brain involvement stays local) or generalized (brain involvement is widespread) and can involve severe motor activity (for example, grand mal seizures) or few motor symptoms (such as petit mal seizures). Because of the diverse nature of different types of epilepsy, several drugs are used as antiepileptics. Thus, phenytoin (Dilantin), carbamazepine (Tegretal), and phenobarbital are prescribed to control partial and grand mal seizures while ethosuximide (Zarontin) and valproic acid (Depakene) are used to treat generalized and petit mal seizures.

Antiulcer Drugs **Peptic ulcers** are sores that recur in the lining of the lower stomach (gastric ulcer) or most often in the upper portion of the small intestines (duodenal ulcer). It is apparent that secretions of gastric acids and digestive enzymes are necessary for ulcer development. Because gastric secretions are involved in developing peptic ulcers, several drug types are useful in ulcer treatment.

peptic ulcers

open sores that occur in the stomach or upper segment of the small intestine

Antacids help to relieve acute discomfort due to ulcers by neutralizing gastric acidity. These drugs are discussed in greater detail in the OTC section of this chapter. Prescription drugs that block gastric secretion have been the mainstay of ulcer treatment. Because the endogenous chemical histamine is important in regulating gastric secretions, drugs that selectively block the activity of gastric histamine (called H_2 blockers) substantially reduce secretion of gastric acids and digestive enzymes. The very popular prescription drugs cimetidine (Tagamet), ranitidine (Zantac) and Pepcid function in this manner (Babe and Serafin

1995). Because Tagamet, Zantac, and Pepcid are used so frequently, they have been switched to OTC status by the FDA—not to treat ulcers, though, but for relieving heartburn (esophageal reflux).

Although the exact causes of peptic ulcers are not completely understood, a role for the bacteria *Helicobacter pylori* is now widely accepted. Because of the involvement of these microorganisms, most clinicians treat patients with recurring ulcers with multiple antibiotics to eliminate these bacteria (Altman 1995).

Bronchodilators Of the top 30 prescription drugs in 1995, two (Proventil and Ventolin) are drugs that widen air passages (that is, bronchi) to facilitate breathing in patients with air passage constriction or obstruction ("Top 200 Drugs" 1996). These drugs are called **bronchodilators** and are particularly useful in relieving respiratory difficulty associated with asthma. Asthmatic patients frequently experience bouts of intense coughing, shortness of breath, tightness in the chest, and wheezing.

bronchodilators

drugs that widen air passages

Many of the symptoms of asthma are due to an increased sensitivity of the airways to irritating substances (Boushey 1992) and can result in serious asthma attacks that are life-threatening if not treated promptly. Two major categories of bronchodilators include sympathomimetics known as β-**adrenergic stimulants**—for example, isoproterenol (Isuprel) and albuterol (Proventil and Ventolin)—and xanthines (caffeine-like drugs) such as theophylline and its derivatives. These drugs relax the muscles of the air passages, cause bronchodilation, and facilitate breathing. In the early 1990s, some bronchial dilator medications were switched to OTC status, such as Bronkaid Mist and Primatene Mist.

β-**adrenergic stimulants**

drugs that stimulate a subtype of adrenaline and noradrenaline receptors

Cardiovascular Drugs Cardiovascular disease has been the number one cause of death in the United States for the past several decades. Consequently, of the 30 top-selling drugs in this country, nine are medications for diseases related to the cardiovascular system. The following are brief discussions of the major categories of cardiovascular drugs.

Antihypertensive Agents It is estimated that 15% of American adults require treatment for **hypertension** (persistent elevated high blood pressure; Benowitz 1992). Because hypertension can result in serious damage to heart, kidneys, and brain, this condition needs to be treated aggressively. Treatment should consist of changes in lifestyle, including exercise and diet, but usually also requires drug therapy. Two of the principal antihypertensive agents are diuretics and direct vasodilators (Oates 1995):

> **hypertension**
> elevated blood pressure

1. *Diuretics* are drugs that lower blood pressure by eliminating sodium and excess water from the body. Included in this category is hydrochlorothiazide (Dyazide).

2. *Direct vasodilators* reduce blood pressure by relaxing the muscles in the walls of blood vessels that cause vasoconstriction, thereby dilating the blood vessels and decreasing their resistance to the flow of blood. Drugs included in this category are calcium-channel blockers (diltiazem or Cardizem; verapamil or Calan; nifedipine or Procardia); inhibitors of the enzyme that synthesizes the vasoconstricting hormone, angiotensin II (enalapril or Vasotec); and drugs that block the vasoconstricting action of the sympathetic nervous system (clonidine or Catapres; prazosin or Minipress).

Antianginal Agents When the heart is deprived of sufficient blood (a condition called **ischemia**), the oxygen requirements of the cardiac muscle are not met and the breakdown of chemicals caused by the continual activity of the heart results in pain; this viselike chest pain is called

> **ischemia**
> tissue deprived of sufficient blood and oxygen

angina pectoris. The most frequent cause of angina is obstruction of the large coronary vessels (Katzung and Chatterjee 1995). Angina pectoris frequently occurs in patients with hypertension; left untreated, the underlying blockage of coronary vessels can result in heart attacks. All the drugs used to relieve, or prevent, angina decrease the oxygen deficit of the heart by either decreasing the amount of work required of the heart during normal functioning or by increasing the blood supply to the heart (Katzung and Chatterjee 1995). The three types of drugs prescribed for treating angina pectoris are (1) calcium-channel blockers (for example, verapimil or Calan, and diltiazem or Cardizem), (2) nitrates and nitrites (for example, amylnitrite or Vaporate, and nitroglycerin or Transderm-nitro), and (3) blockers of the sympathetic nervous system, specifically classified as β-adrenergic blockers (for example, atenolol or Tenormin, and propranolol or Inderal).

> **angina pectoris**
> severe chest pain usually caused by a deficiency of blood to the heart muscle

Drugs to Treat Congestive Heart Failure When the cardiac muscle is unable to pump sufficient blood to satisfy the oxygen needs of the body, **congestive heart failure** occurs. This condition causes an enlarged heart, decreased ability to exercise, shortness of breath, and accumulation of fluid (**edema**) in the lungs and limbs (Katzung and Parmley 1995). The principal treatment for congestive heart failure consists of drugs that improve the heart's efficiency, such as digoxin (Lanoxin).

> **congestive heart failure**
> heart is unable to pump sufficient blood for the body's needs
>
> **edema**
> swollen tissue

Drugs that cause vasodilation are also sometimes used successfully to reduce the work required of the heart as it pumps blood through the body. Among the drugs causing vasodilation are those already discussed in conjunction with other heart conditions such as hypertension and angina pectoris (for example, enalapril or Vasotec, and captopril or Capoten).

Cholesterol and Lipid-Lowering Drugs Cholesterol and some types of fatty (lipid) molecules can accumulate in the walls of arteries and narrow the openings of these blood vessels. Such arterial changes cause hypertension, heart attacks, strokes, and heart failure and are the leading cause of death in the United States and other Western countries (Witztum 1995). These health problems can often be avoided by adopting a lifestyle that includes a low-fat and low-cholesterol diet combined with regular, appropriate exercising. However, sometimes lifestyle changes are insufficient; in such cases, cholesterol-lowering drugs can be used to prevent the damaging changes in blood vessel walls. The drugs most often used include lovastatin (Mevacor), cholestyramine (Questran), and niacin (vitamin B₃).

Hormone-Related Drugs As explained in Chapter 6, hormones are released from endocrine (ductless) glands and are important in regulating metabolism, growth, tissue repair, reproduction, and other vital functions. When there is a deficiency or excess of specific hormones, body functions can be impaired, causing abnormal growth, imbalance in metabolism, disease, and often death. Hormones, or hormone-like substances, are sometimes administered as drugs to compensate for an endocrine deficiency and to restore normal function. This is the case for (1) insulin used to treat diabetes (see the earlier discussion for more details), (2) levothyroxin (Synthroid, an artificial thyroid hormone) to treat **hypothyroidism** (insufficient activity of the thyroid gland), and (3) conjugated estrogens (Premarin) to relieve the symptoms caused by estrogen deficiency during menopause.

hypothyroidism
thyroid gland does not produce sufficient hormone

Hormones can also be administered as drugs to alter normal body processes. Thus, drugs containing the female hormones, estrogen and progesterone (norethindrone mestranol, ethynyl estradiol or Ortho Novum), can be used as contraceptives to alter the female reproductive cycles and prevent pregnancy. Another example involves drugs related to corticosteroids (hormones from the cortex of the adrenal glands), which are often prescribed because of their immune-suppressing effects. In high doses, the corticosteroid drugs (for example, triamcinolone or Kenalog) reduce symptoms of inflammation and are used to treat severe forms of inflammatory diseases, such as arthritis (Goldfien 1992).

Sedative-Hypnotic Agents The sedative-hypnotics are discussed in considerable detail in Chapter 7. Because of the high incidence of anxiety and sleep disorders in the United States (Shuster 1996), drugs that encourage relaxation and drowsiness are frequently prescribed and are usually included in the list of top-selling prescription drugs ("Top 200 Drugs" 1996). For 1995, the benzodiazepine drug alprazolam (Xanax) was listed as the thirty-sixth most prescribed drug in the United States. Other benzodiazepines commonly prescribed are clonazepam (Klonapin), and lorazepam (Ativan) ("Top 200 Drugs" 1996).

Drugs to Treat HIV Although not included in the top 30 list of prescription drugs (see Table 15.7), medications to treat human immunodeficiency virus (HIV) infection are of special relevance to drug abuse because of the high prevalence of infection by this deadly virus in intravenous drug addicts. The issue of acquired immunodeficiency syndrome (AIDS) and drug abuse is discussed at length in Chapter 16; of relevance to our discussion on prescription drugs are recent advances in pharmacological management of this disease. Although no cure for HIV or immunization against this virus is available yet, some drug therapies can delay the onset, or slow the progression, of this infection. The first drugs to be used effectively in AIDS therapy are the "transcriptase inhibitors" such as AZT (zidovudine) and Stavudine, which block a unique enzyme essential for HIV replication (Hayden 1996). A recently developed group of anti-AIDS drugs called the "protease inhibitors" prevent HIV maturation; they include the recently approved drug, Saquinar. The protease inhibitors are particularly effective when

FINDING a BALANCE

The Process of Acceptance: A Way to Counter Life-Stress and Drug Dependency

As a child, Sean used to sit in a classroom and look out the window, daydreaming for what seemed like hours. Living in a coastal town in New England, he often found that his mind would set sail for lands far away, enchanted by the lure of the sea. Once in high school, Sean's mind didn't drift away so much in the form of daydreaming. He simply had problems concentrating, and at times his behavior could best be described as "antsy." Studying was always difficult for him, and as he explains quite candidly, "My grades were nothing to brag about."

At the time that Sean was in grade school, it was rather uncommon to diagnose children with low cognitive skills. Typically kids at this young age are labeled as hyperactive. It wasn't until Sean turned 18 that he learned his concentration problem had a name: attention deficit disorder, more commonly known as ADD. "I was a textbook case of ADD," Sean explained. "I hated school. I had marginal grades, I had no interest, and I was completely distracted."

To an extent, being diagnosed as ADD had its benefits. Sean was soon prescribed Ritalin and almost immediately noticed a difference. Studying for college courses in his major of biology became much easier. "Taking Ritalin really helped me concentrate. I could do in a half-hour what it would take me hours to accomplish in terms of school work. It's unfortunate that it was so late in life that I was diagnosed."

Like most drugs, Ritalin is associated with side effects. While Sean's concentration skills improved exponentially, the drug has affected him negatively as well. The result is best described as a "mixed blessing."

"Ritalin puts a lot on one's body. Not only does it kill my appetite," he explains, "but it keeps me up so I cannot sleep. My mouth gets dry, my eyes get weird—and they're bad to begin with. Ritalin is really a form of speed. It's an upper. It brings the synaptic firing up to a certain level so I can study better, but at the same time . . . " Sean pauses, and then explains that, on average, he loses five pounds when taking the drug regularly; he admits, "I cannot afford to lose one pound." Hearing him describe its use, you can tell immediately that he does not truly enjoy taking this medication.

"Both my parents are schoolteachers. My mom teaches elementary school. She sees kids on Ritalin all the time. She says she can see dramatic changes in their behavior. For this reason, and my own experience, I am skeptical about its use. I don't really think we know the long-term effects because it hasn't been on the market that long. I have heard of people 35–40 who are taking it. I don't plan to take it my entire life. I don't even take it in the summers."

Slowly Facing the Inevitable. Whether facing a diagnosis of ADD or something else that appears to be a pothole in the road of life, Sean has decided that there are some things we cannot change. We just have to accept them as they are. Acceptance is a coping strategy that does not come easily, however, nor does it deliver results with immediate gratification. Rather, acceptance is a process that must be practiced regularly, especially when encountering things in life that simply cannot be changed. Sean has not only accepted his condition, but has also learned to make the most of it. His grades are good, his disposition is fair, and his outlook on life is promising.

Once he is finished with school, Sean has no plans to continue taking Ritalin. He will graduate with a degree in biology, and he doesn't plan to sit behind a desk for ten hours a day, reading reports and writing proposals. He hopes to pursue a career in marine biology. The sea still holds a sense of enchantment for him and most likely it will be enough to claim his attention for a long time to come. ■

used in combination with the transcriptase inhibitor drugs (Hayden 1996).

Common Principles of Drug Use

Probably the most effective way to teach people not to use drugs improperly is to help them understand how to use drugs correctly. This goal can be achieved by educating the drug-using public about both prescription and OTC drug products. If people can appreciate the difference between the benefits of therapeutic drug use and the negative consequences of drug misuse or abuse, they are more likely to use medications in a cautious and thoughtful manner (see "Finding a Balance," page 421). To reach this level of understanding, patients must be able to communicate freely with health professionals. Before prescription or OTC drugs are purchased and used, patients should have all questions answered about the therapeutic objective, the most effective mode of administration, and side effects. Education about proper drug use greatly diminishes drug-related problems and unnecessary health costs.

To minimize problems, before using any drug product, the patient should be able to answer the questions:

1. Why am I using this drug?

2. How should I be taking this drug?

3. What are the active ingredients in this drug product?

4. What are the most likely side effects of the drug?

5. How long should the drug be used?

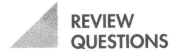

REVIEW QUESTIONS

1. What types of prescription drugs would be appropriate for switching to OTC status? Why?

2. What should the FDA use as a standard of *effectiveness* when evaluating OTC and prescription drugs?

3. What role should the pharmacist play in providing information about OTC and prescription drugs to patients?

4. What type of formal training should be required before a health professional is allowed to prescribe drugs?

5. Should health professionals other than physicians be allowed to prescribe drugs?

6. What can a health professional do to ensure that a patient has sufficient understanding concerning a drug to use it properly and safely?

7. Why are there so many different brands of OTC analgesics when there are only three basic types of drugs used in these products? Describe some of the differences among these types of drugs.

8. Should the FDA require that generic and proprietary versions of the same drug be exactly the same?

9. Even though some antibiotics have a wide margin of safety, currently there is no systemic antibiotic available OTC. Why is the FDA not willing to make some of these drugs nonprescription?

10. Should herbal remedies be required to be safe and effective by the FDA like other OTC drug products?

EXERCISES FOR THE WEB

Exercise 1: Health Touch

"Health Touch On-line" provides information about over-the-counter and prescription drugs. You can type in an over-the-counter drug and pull up information related specifically to that drug.

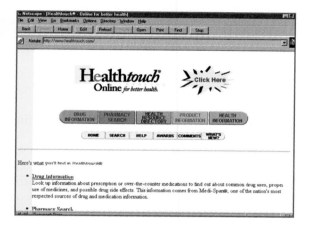

Exercise 2: FDA

The Food and Drug Administration's job is to ensure that the food we eat is safe and wholesome; that the cosmetics we use will not hurt us; that the medicines and medical devices we use are safe and effective; that radiation-emitting products, such as microwave ovens, are not harmful. Food and drugs for pets and farm animals also fall under FDA scrutiny. FDA also ensures that all of these products are labeled truthfully, providing the information that people need to use these products properly.

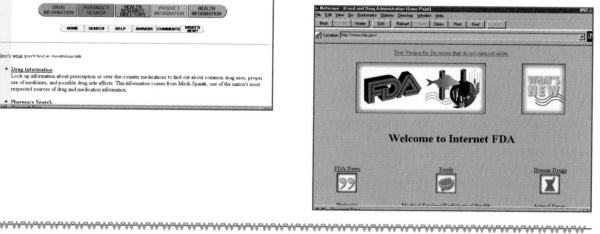

 KEY TERMS

analgesics
salicylates
anti-inflammatory
steroids
nonsteroid anti-inflammatory drugs (NSAIDs)
antipyretics
Reye's syndrome
congestion rebound
antitussive

expectorants
gastritis
anorexiants
keratolytics
keratin layer
SPF (sun protection factor) number
generic
proprietary
drug use review (DUR)
antibiotics
antibacterials
bactericidal
bacteriostatic
broad-spectrum

narrow-spectrum
tricyclic antidepressants
monoamine oxidase (MAO) inhibitors
diabetes mellitus
hyperglycemia
diabetes, type I
diabetes, type II
oral hypoglycemics
epilepsy
peptic ulcers
bronchodilators
β-adrenergic stimulants
hypertension
ischemia
angina pectoris
congestive heart failure
edema
hypothyroidism

SUMMARY

1 Prescription drugs are available only by recommendation of an authorized health professional, such as a physician. Nonprescription (over-the-counter, or OTC) drugs are available on request and do not require approval by a health professional. In general, OTC medications are safer than their prescription counterparts but often less effective.

2 The switching policy of the FDA is an attempt to make available more effective medications to the general public on a nonprescription basis. This policy has been implemented in response to the interest in self-treatment by the public and in an attempt to reduce health care costs.

3 Drugs recently switched by the FDA to OTC status include ulcer medications, such as Tagamet and Zantac, and the hair-growing medication, Rogaine.

4 Potential problems with making more effective drugs available OTC include overuse and inappropriate use, leading to dependence and other undesirable side effects. These more effective drugs could encourage self-treatment of medical problems that require professional care.

5 Information on OTC product labels is crucial for proper use of these drugs and thus is regulated by the FDA. Product labels must list the active ingredients and their quantities in the product. Labels must also provide instructions for safe and effective treatment with the drug as well as cautions and warnings.

6 Although OTC drug products can be useful for treatment of many minor to moderate, self-limiting medical problems, when used without proper precaution they can cause problems.

7 The principal drug groups available OTC are used in the treatment of common, minor medical problems and include analgesics, cold remedies, allergy products, mild stimulants, sleep aids, antacids, laxatives, antidiarrheals, antiasthmatics, acne medications, sunscreens, contraceptives, and nutrients.

8 Even though herbal remedies often contain active drugs, they are usually exempt from FDA regulation and are available to the general public without restrictions. This lack of governmental control has led to hundreds of experiences with serious side effects and several documented deaths.

9 In order for drugs to be prescribed properly, patients need to provide complete and accurate information about their medical condition and medical history to their physicians. In turn, the provider needs to communicate to the patient what is being treated, why the drug is being used, how it should be used for maximum benefit, and what potential side effects can occur.

10 Proprietary drug names can only be used legally by the drug company that has trademark rights. Often the original proprietary name becomes the popular name associated with the drug. Because the pharmaceutical manufacturer that develops a drug is trying to recover the investment, a newly marketed proprietary drug is expensive. Once the patent rights expire, other drug companies can also market the drug, but under a different name; often the common, generic name is used because it cannot be trademarked. The generic brands are less expensive because the manufacturers do not need to recover any significant investment. Generally, the less expensive generic drug is as effective and safe as the proprietary counterpart.

11 Of the approximately 1500 different prescription drugs currently available in the United States, the most commonly prescribed groups are analgesics, antibiotics, antidepressants, drugs used for diabetes, antiulcer drugs, antiepileptic drugs, bronchodilators, drugs used to treat cardiovascular diseases, hormone-related drugs, and sedative-hypnotics.

12 Abuse of prescription drugs is a serious problem in the United States. Some patients try to persuade clinicians or pharmacists to make prescription medication available by using deceit or intimidation. Legal drugs obtained in this manner are often used to relieve drug dependence or to reduce withdrawal symptoms from illicit substances.

REFERENCES

Abramowicz, M. "Drugs for Pain." *Medical Letter* 3 (8 January 1993): 6.

"Acetaminophen, NSAIDs and Alcohol." *Medical Letter* (June 21, 1996): 55, 56.

"A Hacker's Guide to Cough Remedies." *Wellness Letter* (UC Berkley). (October 1995): 3.

Altman, D. "Drugs Used in Gastrointestinal Diseases." In Basic & Clinical Pharmacology, 6th ed., edited by B. Katzung, 949–961. Norwalk, CT: Appleton & Lange, 1995.

American Hospital Formulary Service (AHFS), edited by G. McEvoy, 1401. Bethesda, MD: American Society of Hospital Pharmacists, 1996.

American Psychiatric Association. *Diagnostic and Statistical Manual of Mental Disorders,* 4th ed. *[DSM-JV].* American Psychiatric Association, Washington, D.C. (1994) pp. 317–391.

Associated Press. "Warning: Abusing OTC Drugs Can Be Hazardous to Health." *Salt Lake Tribune* 244 (29 April 1992): 1A.

Babe, K., and W. Serafin. "Histamine, Bradykinin, and Their Antagonists." In *The Pharmacological Basis of Therapeutics,* 9th ed., edited by J. Hardman and L. Limbird, 581–600. New York: McGraw-Hill, 1995.

Benowitz, N. "Antihypertensive Agents." In *Basic and Clinical Pharmacology,* 5th ed., edited by B. Katzung, 139–61. Norwalk, CT: Appleton & Lange, 1992.

Berkowitz, B., and B. Katzung. "Basic and Clinical Evaluations of New Drugs." In *Basic and Clinical Pharmacology,* 5th ed., edited by B. Katzung, 60–8. Norwalk, CT: Appleton & Lange, 1992.

Billow, J. "Acne Products." In *Handbook of Nonprescription Drugs,* 10th ed., edited by T. Covington, 511–20. Washington, DC: American Pharmaceutical Association, 1993.

Boushey, H. "Bronchodilators and Other Agents Used in Asthma." In *Basic and Clinical Pharmacology,* 5th ed., edited by B. Katzung, 278–93. Norwalk, CT: Appleton & Lange, 1992.

Bryant, B., and J. Lombardi. "Cold, Cough and Allergy Products." In *Handbook of Nonprescription Drugs,* 10th ed., edited by T. Covington, 89–115. Washington, DC: American Pharmaceutical Association, 1993.

Consumer Report Books. *The New Medicine Show.* New York: Consumer Report Books (51 East 42nd St., New York, NY), 1989.

Covington, T. "Trends in Self-Care: The Rx to OTC Switch Movement." *Drug Newsletter* 12 (February 1993): 15–6.

Covington, T. "Introduction." In *Handbook of Nonprescription Drugs,* 10th ed., edited by T. Covington, Washington, DC: American Pharmaceutical Association, 1993.

Cowley, G. "Herbal Warning." *Newsweek* (May 6, 1996): 61–8.

Davis, S., and D. Granner. "Insulin, Oral Hypoglycemic Agents, and the Pharmacology of the Endocrine Pancreas." In *The Pharmacological Basis of Therapeutics,* 9th ed., edited by J. Hardman and L. Limbird, 1487–1517. New York, McGraw-Hill, 1995.

Debrovner, D. "Here Comes the Sun." American Druggist (May 1994b): 30–34.

Debrovner, D. "Mind Menders." American Druggist (April 1994a): 20–26.

DiSomone, E. "Sunscreen and Suntan Products." In Handbook of Nonprescription Drugs, 10th ed., edited by T. Covington, Washington, DC: American Pharmaceutical Association, 1993: 575–588.

Doheny, K. "The Skinny on Diet Pills." *American Druggist* (February 1993): 32–36

Drug Facts and Comparisons. St Louis: Lippincott, 1996.

Eggert, A., and L. Crismon. "Dealing with Insomnia." *American Druggist* (May 1992): 83–96.

Engle, J. "Internal Analgesics II." *American Druggist* (July 1992): 81–2.

Foreman, J. "Ginseng: $350 Million for Not Much." *Boston Globe* (February 3, 1997): C4.

Fried, S. "Prescription for Disaster." *Washington Post Magazine* (3 April 1994): 13–6.

"Full Sun Protection." *Wellness Letter* (June 1993): 4–5.

Garnett, W. "Antacid Products." In *Handbook of Nonprescription Drugs,* 9th ed., edited by T. Covington. Washington, DC: American Pharmaceutical Association, 1990: 243–281.

Gauvin, D., K. Moore, B. Youngblood, and F. Holloway. "The Discriminative Stimulus Properties of Legal OTC Stimulants Administered Singly and in Binary and Ternary Combinations." *Psychopharmacology* 110 (1993): 309–19.

Gilbertson, W. "The FDA's OTC Drug Review." In *Handbook of Nonprescription Drugs,* 10th ed., edited by T. Covington, 21–37. Washington, DC: American Pharmaceutical Association, 1993.

Goldfien, A. "Adrenocorticosteroids and Adrenocortical Antagonist." In *Basic and Clinical Pharmacology,* 5th ed., edited by B. Katzung, 543–57. Norwalk, CT: Appleton & Lange, 1992.

Greenberg, S. *Physician's Desk Reference for Nonprescription Drugs,* 17th ed. Oradell, NJ: Medical Economics Data, 1996.

Grinspoon, L. "Update on Mood Disorders—Part II." *Harvard Medical Letter* 11 (January 1995): 1–4.

Hayden, F. "Antimicrobial Agents." In *The Pharmacological Basis of Therapeutics,* 9th ed., edited by J. Hardman and L. Limbird, 1191–1223. New York: McGraw-Hill, 1996.

Hollister, L. "Antidepressant Agents." In *Basic and Clinical Pharmacology,* 5th ed., edited by B. Katzung, 410. Norwalk, CT: Appleton & Lange, 1992.

Holt, C. "The Evolution of the OTC Drug History." *American Druggist* 213 (1996): 51–60.

Hsu, I. "Prescription to Over-the-Counter Switches." *American Druggist* (July 1994): 57–64.

Katzung, B., and K. Chatterjee. "Vasodilators and the Treatment of Angina Pectoris." In *Basic and Clinical Pharmacology,* 4th ed., edited by B. Katzung, 171–87. Norwalk, CT: Appleton & Lange, 1995.

Katzung, B., and W. Parmley. "Cardiac Glycosides and Other Drugs Used in Congestive Heart Failure." In *Basic and Clinical Pharmacology,* 6th ed., edited by B. Katzung, 188–204. Norwalk, CT: Appleton & Lange, 1995.

Klepacki, L. "Melatonin: Nightcap of the '90s." *American Druggist* (September 1996): 43–6.

Klein-Schwartz, W., and J. Hoopes. "Patient Assessment and Consultation." In *Handbook of Nonprescription Drugs,* 10th ed., edited by T. Covington, 11–20. Washington, DC: American Pharmaceutical Association, 1993.

Lackner, T. "Antipyretic Drug Products." In *Handbook of Nonprescription Drugs,* edited by E. Feldman 91–118. Washington, DC: American Pharmaceutical Association, 1990.

Lamy, P. " . . . And on Nonprescription Products." *Elder Care News* 9 (Summer 1993): 17.

Lane, E. "On 'Cloud 9'? Loose Regulation of Ephedrine." *Ogden Standard-Examiner* (April 21, 1996): 5E.

Laskoski, G. "Rx to OTC." *American Druggist* (December 1992): 47–50.

Masand, P., S. Gupta, and M. Dewan. "Suicidal Ideation Related to Fluoxetine Treatment." *New England Journal of Medicine* 324 (1992): 420.

McCormick, E. "Rx to OTC: A Growth Industry?" *Pharmacy Times* (December 1992): 69–74.

Mills, J., S. Barriere, and E. Jawetz. "Clinical Use of Antimicrobials." In *Basic and Clinical Pharmacology,* 5th ed., edited by B. Katzung, 695–711. Norwalk, CT: Appleton & Lange, 1992.

"New York County Bans Herbal Stimulant." *Pharmacy Times* 62 (May 1996): 8.

Oates, J. "Antihypertensive Agents and the Drug Therapy of Hypertension." In *The Pharmacological Basis of Therapeutics,* 9th ed., edited by J. Hardman and L. Limbird, 780–808. New York: McGraw-Hill, 1995.

Physician's Desk Reference, 51st ed. Oradell, NJ: Medical Economics Data, 1997.

Physician's Desk Reference for Nonprescription Drugs, 15th ed. Oradell, NJ: Medical Economics Data, 1994.

Pinson, J., and C. Weart. "Antacid Products." In *Handbook of Nonprescription Drugs,* 10th ed., edited by T. Covington, 147–79. Washington, DC: American Pharmaceutical Association, 1993.

Popovich, N. "Not All Over-the-Counter Drugs Are Safe." *American Journal of Pharmaceutical Education* 55 (1991): 166–72.

Rigel, D. "Malignant Melanoma in the 1990s." *Pharmacy Times* (May 1991): 33–9.

Ritter, M. "Risk of Sometimes-Fatal Skin Cancer Rising." *Salt Lake Tribune* (13 June 1991): D10.

Sause, R., and R. Mangione. "Cough and Cold Treatment with OTC Medicine." *Pharmacy Times* (February 1991): 108–17.

Sawynok, J., and T. Yaksh. "Caffeine as an Analgesic Adjuvant: A Review of Pharmacology and Mechanisms of Action." *Pharmacology Review* 45 (1993): 43–85.

Schwartz, R., and S. Rifkin. "No More Paper Tiger." *American Druggist* (June 1991): 26–34.

Schwartz, R. "NMDA Exec Reflects on 18 Years of Changes." *American Druggist* (August 1996): 12.

Sewester, S. "Fluoxetine: Unlabeled Uses and Dosage Range." *Drug Newsletter* 14 (March 1995): 24.

Shuster, J. "Insomnia: Understanding Its Pharmacological Treatment Options." *Pharmacy Times* 62 (August 1996): 67–76.

Simonsen, L. "Generic Prescribing and RPh Substitution Continue to Climb." *Pharmacy Times* (October 1993a): 29.

Simonsen, L. "Sun Exposure: The Stakes Are Rising." *Pharmacy Times* (May 1993b): 25–31.

Slezak, M. "Steering Patients to Switches." *American Druggist* (July 1996): 32–5.

Stanford, S. "Prozac: Panacea or Puzzle." *Trends in Pharmacological Sciences.* 17 (April 1996): 150–4.

Stewart, R. "Adverse Drug Reactions." In *Remington's Pharmaceutical Sciences,* 19th ed. Mack, edited by A. Gennaro, 1995.

"Top 200 Drugs of 1995." *Pharmacy Times* 62 (April 1996): 29.

Tyle, W. "Internal Analgesic Products." In *Handbook of Nonprescription Drugs,* 10th ed., edited by T. Covington, 49–64. Washington, DC: American Pharmaceutical Association, 1993.

Vaczek, D. "Assisting the Cough/Cold Patient." *Pharmacy Times* 9 (September 1996): 34–48.

White, W. "The Dextromethorphan FAQ." Internet: Usenet alt.drugs, 1995.

Wick, J. "Outsmarting Prescription Fraud." *Pharmacy Times* 61 (April 1995): 33–6.

Witztum, J. "Drugs Used in the Treatment of Hyperlipoproteinemias." In *The Pharmacological Basis of Therapeutics,* 9th ed., edited by J. Hardman and L. Limbird, 875–97. New York: McGraw-Hill, 1995.

Zak, J. "OBRA '90 and DUR." *American Druggist* (October 1993): 57.

Zander, E., and S. Weisman. "Self-Medication of Acne with Topical Salicylic Acid." *Pharmacy Times* (May 1992): 114–8.

16

Drug Use
Within Subcultures

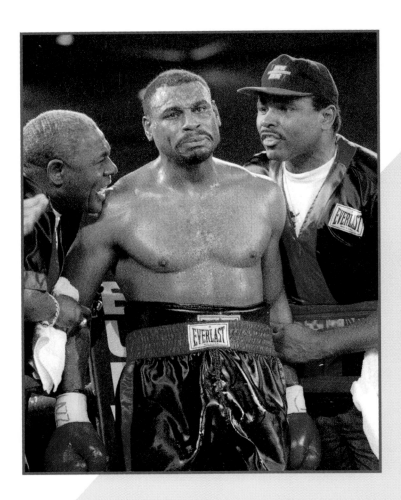

On completing this chapter
you will be able to:

- Athletes are no more likely than nonathletes to abuse alcohol, marijuana, or cocaine.
- If used during puberty, anabolic steroids will stunt growth.
- Women are more likely than men to be adversely affected by alcohol consumption.
- Male college students are more likely to smoke cigarettes on a daily basis than female college students.
- Women are less likely than men to seek therapy for their drug abuse problems.
- More males than females report using an illicit drug during the prior year.

- Research continues to show that the most important factor in adolescent drug use remains the peer group.
- Adolescents continue to learn their most influential attitudes toward drug use from family relationships (bonds).
- Recent surveys found that by eighth grade approximately 55% of children had used alcohol, 46% had used cigarettes, 22% had used inhalants, and 20% had used marijuana.
- Teenage gangs have emerged as major players in the drug trade.

- Drug abuse is more likely to be associated with criminal behavior in adolescents than in adults.
- People who were victims of incest as children are more likely to abuse drugs than the general population.
- Use of protease inhibitor medications has, in many cases, resulted in miraculous remissions of AIDS patients.
- In a recent study undertaken by Columbia's Center on Addiction and Substance Abuse, 76% of 12–17-year-olds indicated that the entertainment industry encourages illegal drug use.

Learning Objectives

- Know which drugs are most likely to be abused by athletes and why.
- Describe the use of drug testing in athletic competitions.
- Explain why adolescents use substances of abuse.
- Describe the type of parents most likely to have drug-abusing children.
- Identify drugs that are most likely to be abused by adolescents.
- Explain the relationship between adolescents' involvement with drug abuse and gangs.

- Explain the best predictor for recreational drug use in college.
- Explain how "smart drugs," also known as nootropic drugs, and the sedative Rohypnol are used by college students.
- Compare patterns of drug use in females and males.
- Explain why the unique socioeconomic roles of women make them vulnerable to drug abuse problems.
- Describe how drug treatment programs can meet the needs of female patients.

- Explain how drug abuse contributes to the spread of AIDS.
- List major strategies to prevent contracting AIDS.
- Describe the importance of protease inhibitors.
- Briefly describe the major findings about drug use in entertainment subcultures.
- Explain the latest subculture that has developed and how it contributes to drug use knowledge.

Although similarities appear in the patterns of addiction among drug users, the development of initial use and eventual abuse varies immensely from individual to individual. When attempting to understand common causes and patterns of drug use, examining subcultures often provides a semblance of commonality. A **subculture** is defined as a subgroup within the population whose members share similar values and patterns of related behaviors that differ from the larger population. When defining a subculture, some sociologists refer to it as a "world within a world." Subcultures create and provide their members with lifestyle patterns that are observable, fairly consistent, and interwoven. Overall, viewing a group as a subculture offers a way to look at distinctive patterns of drug use.

> **subculture**
>
> subgroup within the population whose members share similar values and patterns of related behaviors that differ from the larger population

Let's first examine why individuals within various subcultures would initially turn to drugs. The two types of forces that affect members of a subculture are internal and external subcultural forces, both of which affect these individuals' drug use behavior. *Internal subcultural forces* include: (1) shared attitudes toward drug users and nonusers; (2) compatibility with other members of the peer group (often peer members share complementary personality traits); (3) shared attitudes favorable to drug use despite conventional society's view that such behavior constitutes deviant behavior; (4) addiction to drugs or, at minimum, habitual drug usage; and (5) a common secrecy about drug use. *External subcultural forces* include: (1) preoccupation with law enforcement while procuring the drugs and while under the effects of illicit drugs; (2) a desire to identify sellers of illicit drugs and verify the dependability of the drug dealer; and (3) preoccupation with getting caught using or acting high in public, at work, at school, or at a social function where drug use would be perceived as deviant social behavior.

To further understand how drug use and/or abuse is affected by membership in a subculture, this chapter examines drug use and potential abuse in the following five subcultures: sport/athletic, women, adolescent, college student, HIV-positive, and entertainment subcultures. It also considers a new media subculture that has arisen in recent years.

Athletes and Drug Abuse

The Canadian sprinter, Ben Johnson, once known as the fastest human in history, was banned for life from competitive running in March 1993 (Hoberman and Yesalis 1995, 81). Five years earlier, Johnson was stripped of a world's record for the 100-meter dash at the 1988 Seoul Olympics and forfeited the gold medal when he tested positive for steroids in his urine. Because of the first incident, Johnson was suspended from competition for two years. However, in 1992 the 31-year-old sprinter was attempting a comeback, with speeds that approached his world record times. In January 1993, a routine urine test determined Johnson was again using steroids to enhance his athletic performance (Ferrente 1993).

Widely publicized incidents such as this one concerning illicit use of so-called **ergogenic** (performance-enhancing) drugs by professional and amateur athletes have created intense interest in the problems of drug abuse in sports (Merchant 1992). To understand why athletes are willing to risk using these drugs, it is necessary to understand the sports mind-set. Young athletes receive exaggerated attention and prestige in almost every university or college, high school, and junior high school in the United States. Pressure to excel or "be the best" is placed on athletes by parents, peers, teachers, coaches, school administrators, the media, and surrounding community. The importance of sports is frequently distorted and even used by some to evaluate the quality of educational institutions (Lawn 1984) or the quality of living conditions in a city. Athletic success can determine the level of financial support for these institutions by local and state governments, alumni, and other private donors; thus, winning in athletics often translates into fiscal stability and institutional prosperity.

> **ergogenic**
>
> drugs that enhance athletic performance

For the athlete, success in sports means psychological rewards such as the admiration of peers, school officials, family, and community. In addition, athletic success can mean financial rewards such as scholarships, paid living expenses in college, advertising endorsement opportunities, and, for a few, incredible salaries as professional athletes. With the rewards of winning, athletes have to deal with the added pressures of not winning, such as "What will people think of me if I lose?"; "When I lose, I let everybody down"; or "Losing shows that I am not as good as everyone thinks." These pressures on young, immature athletes can result in poor coping responses. Being better than competitors, no matter the cost, becomes the driving motivation, and *doing one's best* is no longer sufficient. Such attitudes may lead to serious risk-taking behavior in order to develop an advantage over the competition; this situation can include using drugs to improve performance. (See "Finding a Balance," page 432.)

Drugs Used by Athletes

Yes, the steroids I used certainly made me get bigger. I was going out for football and I had just made the team, so I kept using them and the results were phenomenal. Now two years later, I won't be graduating. Several months ago, they removed a tumor on my liver, but they didn't get all the cancer. I am going home at the end of this semester. My parents want me to stay with them for the time I have left. When I go, I only have one wish—I want to die big and always be known as big Jim.

From Venturelli's research files, interview with a 20-year-old male, December 13, 1996

Studies have shown that athletes are not more likely than nonathletes to use some drugs of abuse such as marijuana, alcohol, barbiturates, cocaine, and hallucinogens (Samples 1989; Hoberman and Yesalis 1995). However, athletes are much more likely than other populations to take drugs that enhance (physically or psychologically), or are thought to enhance, competitive performance; these drugs include stimulants such as the amphetamines and an array of drugs with presumed ergogenic effects, such as anabolic steroids (Bell 1987). Some of the drugs that are abused by athletes are listed in Table 16.1, along with their desired effects. The following sections discuss the drugs that are most frequently self-administered by athletes in an effort to improve their competitive performance.

Table 16.1 **Partial List of Ergogenic Substances and Expected Effects**

Drugs	Expected Results
Amino acids	Stimulate natural production of growth hormone
Amphetamines and cocaine	Increase strength, alertness, and endurance
Anabolic steroids	Increase muscle mass and strength
B-complex vitamins	Enhance body metabolism and increase energy
Caffeine	Reduce fatigue
Chromium	Enhance carbohydrate metabolism
Ephedrine	Improve breathing
Asthma medication	Improve breathing
OTC decongestants	Increase endurance
Thyroid hormone	Enhance metabolism and energy
β-blockers	Reduce hand tremor and stimulate growth hormone
Methylphenidate	Enhance alertness and endurance
Furosemide	Mask steroid use and enable rapid weight loss

Source: R. Harlan and M. Garcia. "Neurobiology of Androgen Abuse." In *Drugs of Abuse*, edited by R. Watson, 185–201. Boca Raton, FL: CRC Press, 1992.

The lure of a high-profile life can mean pressures and risks for a young guy on the go like Jason. It seems that becoming a model takes more than good looks, a pearl-white smile, and ambition. Today, it can also take steroids and amphetamines. Suddenly Jason's budding career had sucked him into the vortex of abuse—big time.

Jason's modeling career began in New York. He was dating a model and one day accompanied her on a shoot. As luck would have it, the photographer needed a filler, and Jason was asked to step in. He agreed, and his lucrative career as a model had begun. The pay was good and, of course, so was the prestige. Within a few months, Jason had relocated to Denver to continue his new profession. But it didn't take long to notice a change—not only in the altitude, but also in the modeling climate.

> In New York it was very different. Here in Denver, I got into the scene with a guy who was my new agent and one of the first things he said was, "You got to get in better shape. Modeling is a very funny business. You could be modeling jackets one day and underwear the next, so you've got to look good in next to nothing. The look is lean and muscular. This is what sells." There is incredible pressure to be in good shape,

so my agent said I should start taking injections. It's called "low-balling." Low-balling is not a typical steroid; it doesn't build up muscle. It makes you look lean, well-cut, and low on fat—dangerously low.

Having spent time working out with weights, Jason was no stranger to the drug scene. "Speed is very prevalent. There is a lot of denial, no one wants to admit it, but when you see a guy put on 30 pounds of muscle in three months, you know he's doing something." Jason acknowledged the psychological addiction to speed and steroids among his peers. "You start doing 'roids because you want to look good, and you want to lift more. But you become dependent on them more and more. Whatever you do is never enough. D-balling [anabolic steroid use] is tough. Nowadays, people are taking growth hormone, but it's not pure, it's mixed with other stuff, things you don't want in your body."

Jason was doing normal weight workouts and supplementing his diet with amino acids. Nevertheless, according to his agent, it wasn't enough to get "the look." So at the age of 28, Jason found himself low-balling, doing injections—one injection per week for a three-week period, followed by one injection every day for a nine-week cycle. "You do these injections in the butt before a workout. It feels like injecting hot syrup. One of the immediate side

Anabolic Steroids Anabolic steroids consist of a group of natural and synthetic drugs that are chemically similar to cholesterol and related to the male hormone testosterone (Lukas 1993). Naturally occurring male hormones, or **androgens,** are produced by the testes in males. These hormones are essential for normal growth and development of male sex organs as well as secondary sex characteristics such as muscular development, male hair patterns, voice changes, and fat distribution. The androgens are also necessary for appropriate growth spurts during adolescence (*Drug Facts and Comparisons* 1994). The

androgens
naturally occurring male hormones, such as testosterone

principal accepted therapeutic use for the androgens is for hormone replacement in males with abnormally functioning testes. In such cases, the androgens are administered prior to puberty and for prolonged periods during puberty to stimulate proper male development (*Drug Facts and Comparisons* 1994).

Abuse of Anabolic Steroids by Athletes Under some conditions, androgen-like drugs can increase muscle mass and strength; for this reason, they are referred to as **anabolic** (able to stimulate the conversion of nutrients into tissue)

anabolic steroids
androgen-like drugs that can increase muscle mass and strength

effects is scar tissue buildup, which causes you to massage your butt constantly."

One day his agent brought in a shipment of drugs from Mexico. "It was a type of asthma medication to increase heart rate and burn fat. I took that for two months. I'd take [the drugs] before I went to sleep and they would kick in by the time I was pumping weights the next day. You drive on the shakes. If you weren't vibrating, then you were upset. When you start taking this stuff, your body goes out of balance, and it quits making hormones. I got the desired effect, lean muscle mass, but I lost the edge. My weight would fluctuate 5 pounds a day. I always felt like people were looking at me. And I was always going to the bathroom to urinate. I'd eat a huge meal, and an hour later still be hungry."

Seeking self-esteem. The more Jason worked on his body image, the worse he felt about himself. If there is a bottom line to dealing with stressors in life, most likely it's related to self-esteem. Self-esteem consists of how you value yourself as a result of how you are valued by others. It isn't just based on good looks or the approval of others about one's physical appearance. Instead, experts say that self-esteem is nurtured through four aspects: uniqueness (characteristics that make you feel special), connectedness (people who make up your support group), power (those things you feel empowered about), and role

models (aspects of people whom you wish to emulate to reach your potential). When these four components are addressed positively, self-esteem is high. When they are neglected, self-esteem bottoms out, and stress ensues. Self-esteem can be augmented with positive self-talk, where you listen to the voice of conscience and begin to believe in yourself rather than the voice of the negative critic, which says that you're just not good enough.

One day Jason took a good look at the guys in his modeling agency and didn't like what he saw. "They were freaking out, acting super-macho, and they never sat still, just [remained] hyper. The drugs don't so much bring out feelings of anger as they block the ability to rationalize. They keep the body in a constant state of stress." Weeks behind the other models in the cycle, Jason was able to see where he was headed if he continued in their footsteps. It wasn't a direction he wanted to take. So at the age of 30, Jason quit his modeling career and decided to return to college. His desire to know more about human performance had steered him toward the field of kinesiology. He still lifts weights, but without the help of drugs.

"I'm glad I am not doing it anymore," he says with a smile. "I better appreciate my body and, although it takes longer to make the gains, it's more solid and the recovery time is quicker." ◼

steroids (because chemically, they are similar to the steroids produced in the adrenal glands) and are used by many athletes to improve performance (Burke and Davis 1992). It is estimated that as many as 1 million Americans have used or are currently using these drugs to achieve a "competitive edge" or for other purposes (Welder and Melchert 1993), see Figure 16.1. Studies suggest that approximately 2% of college-age men and 6.7% of male high school students use anabolic steroids (Harlan and Garcia 1992). Although the vast majority of anabolic steroid users are male, women involved in body building or strength and endurance sports also abuse these drugs. Thus, as many as 1% of the female high school students have used these drugs sometime during their life (Lukas 1993).

The first report of use of anabolic steroids to improve athletic performance was in 1954 by the Russian weight-lifting team. These drugs' performance-enhancing advantages were quickly recognized by other athletes, and it has been estimated that as many as 90% of the competitors in the 1960 Olympic games used some form of steroid (Toronto 1992). Because of the widespread misuse and associated problems with the use of these drugs, anabolic steroids were classified as Schedule III controlled drugs on 27 February 1991 (Merchant 1992).

Due to federal regulations, individuals convicted of a first offense of trafficking with anabolic steroids can be sentenced to a maximum prison term of 5 years and a $250,000 fine. For a second

Figure 16.1

Reasons for nonmedicinal steroid use by college students

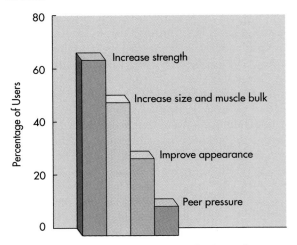

Source: R. Harlan and M. Garcia. "Neurobiology of Androgen Abuse." In *Drugs of Abuse,* edited by R. Watson, 186. Boca Raton, FL: CRC Press, 1992.

offense, the prison term can increase to 10 years with a $500,000 fine. Even possession of illicitly obtained anabolic steroids can result in a 1-year term with at least a $1000 fine (U.S. Department of Justice 1991–1992).

Patterns of Abuse Geographical factors appear to have little to do with the use of anabolic steroids among athletes in both inner-city and suburban schools; all are equally attracted to these drugs. However, some athletes are more inclined to abuse anabolic steroids than others; for example, football players have the highest rate of abuse, while track and field athletes have the least. In addition, the likelihood of abusing these drugs increases as the level of competition increases. Usage rates were approximately 14% in the National Collegiate Athletic Association (NCAA) Division I athletes and 30% to 75% in professional athletes (Lukas 1993).

Usage patterns for the anabolic steroids can vary considerably according to the objectives of the athlete. The pattern usually consists of self-administering doses that are 10 to 200 times greater than dosages used for legitimate medical conditions (Welder and Melchert 1993), see Table 16.2. **Stacking** is the use of several types of steroids together with the intent of maximizing their muscle-building effects and minimizing their adverse side effects; the use of different steroids taken singly but in sequence is called **cycling**. It is believed that tolerance to the effects of anabolic steroids or **plateauing** can be avoided by staggering the different steroids with an overlapping dosing pattern during the cycle. In general, *power* athletes prefer the stacking approach, while body builders prefer cycling (Lukas 1993).

Now that steroid use has been prohibited by almost all legitimate sporting organizations, urine testing just prior to the athletic event has become commonplace (Lukas 1993). Steroid-using athletes attempt to avoid detection by trying to fool the tests. These highly questionable strategies include the following (Lukas 1993; Merchant 1992):

> **stacking**
> use of several types of steroids together

> **cycling**
> use of different types of steroids singly, but in sequence

> **plateauing**
> developing tolerance to the effects of anabolic steroids

▲ Using the steroid only during training for the athletic events, but discontinuing its use several weeks before the competition to allow the drug to disappear from the body. Because oral steroids are cleared from the body faster than the injectable types, they are usually discontinued two to four weeks while the injection steroids are stopped three to six weeks before competition.

▲ Taking drugs, such as probenecid, that block the excretion of steroids in the urine.

▲ Using diuretics and drinking large quantities of water to increase the urine output and dilute the steroid so it cannot be detected by the test.

▲ Adding adulterant chemicals to the urine, such as Drano, Chlorox, ammonia, or Murine Eye Drops to invalidate the tests.

Table 16.2	Typical Patterns of Anabolic Steroid Use

Use	Steroid	Dosing	Duration
Light	Methandrostenolone (Dianabol)	15 mg, oral	6 weeks
Moderate	Methandrostenolone	20 mg, oral	10
	Nandrolone decanoate (Deca-durabolin)	200 mg, intramuscular	10
	Testosterone cypionate (Depo-Testosterone)	200 mg, intramuscular	10
Intense	Methandrostenolone	40 mg, oral	16
	Oxandrolone (Anavar)	40 mg, oral	16
	Nandrolone decanoate	600 mg, intramuscular	16
	Boldenone undecylenate (Vebonol)	8 ml/week, intramuscular	16
	Methenolone enanthate	4 ml/week, intramuscular	16

Note: Moderate to intense doses are 10 to 100 times typical medical doses.
Source: R. Harlan and M. Garcia. "Neurobiology of Androgen Abuse." In *Drugs of Abuse,* edited by R. Watson, 187. Boca Raton, FL: CRC Press, 1992.

Although these techniques may make the analysis of steroids in the urine more difficult, they usually are not sufficient to prevent detection by carefully conducted urine drug testing.

Effects of Anabolic Steroids Low to moderate doses of the anabolic steroids have little effect on the strength or athletic skills of the average adult. However, these drugs cause significant gains in lean body mass (that is, muscle) and strength, while decreasing fat when high doses are used by athletes during intense training programs (Lukas 1993). Because most of these effects are transient and will disappear when steroid use is stopped, athletes feel compelled to continue their use, and become psychologically *hooked* (Toronto 1992). The effect of anabolic steroids on athletic performance and skills is not clear and is difficult to measure (Lukas 1993). The drugs are most likely beneficial in contact and strength sports where increased muscle mass provides an advantage, such as weight lifting and football; they are less likely to benefit the athlete involved in sports requiring dexterity and agility, such as baseball or tennis.

The risks caused by the anabolic steroids are not completely understood. Most certainly, the higher the doses and the longer the use, the greater the potential damage these drugs can do to the body. Some of the adverse effects thought to occur with heavy steroid use (10 to 30 times the doses used therapeutically) include the following:

▲ Increases in the blood cholesterol, which could eventually clog arteries and cause heart attacks and strokes (Burke and Davis 1992).

▲ Increased risk of liver disorders, such as jaundice and tumors (Lukas 1993).

▲ Psychological side effects, including irritability, outbursts of anger ("roid rage"), mania, psychosis, and major depression (Lukas 1993; Burke and Davis 1992).

▲ Possible psychological and physical dependence with continual high-doses use, resulting in withdrawal symptoms such as steroid craving (52%), fatigue (43%), depression (41%), restlessness (29%), loss of appetite (24%), insomnia (20%), diminished sex drive (20%), and headaches (20%) (Lukas 1993).

▲ Alterations in reproductive systems and sex hormones, causing changes in sex-related characteristics (Burke and Davis 1992) such as breast enlargement in males and breast reduction in females, infertility in both sexes, and changes in genitalia in both sexes.

▲ Changes in skin and hair in both sexes, such as increased incidence and severity of acne, male pattern baldness, and increased body hair (Burke and Davis 1992).

▲ Other changes, including stunted growth in adolescents, deepening of voice in females, and water retention, causing bloating (Burke and Davis 1992).

Sources of Steroids Where do the anabolic steroids come from? About 50% of the anabolic steroids used in this country are prescribed by doctors; the other 50% are obtained from the black market. Black market sources of steroids include drugs diverted from legitimate channels, smuggled from foreign countries—for example, Brazil, Italy, Mexico, Great Britain, Portugal, France, and Peru (NIDA 1996), designated for veterinarian use or inactive counterfeits (U.S. Department of Justice 1991–1992). Several different types of commonly used anabolic steroids are listed in Table 16.2. Some health food stores and mail-order firms also offer products with names like the prescription anabolic steroids, such as Dynabdin, Metrobolin, and Diostero. These "sham steroids" contain only vitamins, amino acids, or micronutrients (Merchant 1992).

Stimulant Use Among Athletes

A month rarely passes in which the media do not report a football, basketball, or baseball player who has tested positive in a drug-screening evaluation or who has been suspended from competition due to stimulant abuse. For example, as noted earlier, Ben Johnson was stripped of his gold medal in the Seoul Olympics after he tested positive for anabolic steroids (Hoberman and Yesalis 1995). Sometimes the stories are more tragic. In 1986, reports of cocaine-related deaths of sports figures included basketball star Len Bias and professional football player Don Rogers. Perhaps such sports tragedies helped convince some U.S. youth of the dangers of stimulant abuse and contributed to the decline in drug abuse in the late 1980s (Johnston et al. 1993). Clearly, no one—not even an athlete—is immune from the risks of these drugs.

Amphetamines and cocaine are abused to improve athletic skills (McDonald 1995, C1). However, it is not clear if stimulants actually enhance athletic performance or merely the athlete's *perception* of performance. Many athletes believe these drugs promote quickness, enhance endurance, delay fatigue, increase self-confidence and aggression, and mask pain (Hoberman and Yesalis 1995). In fact, some studies have shown that stimulants can improve some aspects of athletic performance, especially in the presence of fatigue (NIDA 1996). However, the risk of using stimulants in sports is substantial because these drugs mask extreme fatigue, increase the risk of heat exhaustion, and can have severe cardiovascular consequences, such as heart attacks, strokes, and failure of the cardiovascular system (Bell 1987). (See "Case in Point," page 437.)

Although some athletes would never consider using the *hard* stimulants, such as cocaine and the amphetamines, milder stimulants that are legal and available OTC's may be thought acceptable. Such stimulants include caffeine and OTC decongestants (for example, phenylpropanolamine and phenylephrine). Use of these drugs can be a double-edged sword for the athlete; their use can reduce fatigue, give a sense of energy, and even mask pain. But in high doses, especially when combined, they can cause nervousness, tremors, and restlessness, impair concentration, accelerate dehydration, and interfere with sleep ("OTC Drugs and Athletes" 1992). Some athletic competitions limit permissible blood levels of caffeine (Bell 1987) and do not allow the use of OTC stimulants such as decongestant drugs (Merchant 1992).

Miscellaneous Ergogenic Drugs

Most athletic organizations have banned the use of anabolic steroids and stimulants and are using more effective screening procedures to detect offenders. A result of this clamp-down has been the search for alternative performance-enhancing drugs by athletes who feel a need for such pharmacological assistance. The following are brief discussions of a few of these substitute ergogenic substances (for a more complete list, see Table 16.1).

Clenbuterol At the 1992 Olympic Games in Barcelona, Spain, at least four athletes, including German world sprint champion Katrina Krabbe, were disqualified from competition for using the drug clenbuterol to enhance their

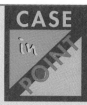

When Drugs Enter the Boxing Ring

When Oliver McCall entered the boxing ring to fight for the heavyweight championship on February 7, 1997, he was not alone. With him came the spectre of years of drug abuse.

Just seven weeks before, McCall had been arrested for swinging a Christmas tree around a hotel lobby while in a drug-induced haze. A few years earlier, he was found in a crack house after having been mugged by a fellow addict, to whom he lost the $1.5 million check he had carried with him in a sock to buy drugs. These events were just two of many drug-related occurrences on his record. His most recent arrest, however, had been followed by a drug treatment program, which he attended daily.

But something went wrong the night of February 7. After having announced to a friend, "I want my title. I'm fighting for my life," McCall seemed to want to get knocked out. In the third round, in the middle of the ring, in front of a packed audience, he listlessly walked around as his opponent, Lennox

Lewis, threw punches at him. McCall dodged and bobbed his head, yet refused to fight back. After the fourth round, McCall stood alone, away from his corner, sobbing uncontrollably, seemingly having a nervous breakdown in front of a worldwide cable television audience. Fifty-five seconds into the fifth round, referee Mills Lane stopped the fight. Lewis was the winner. McCall, in more ways than one, was not.

While drugs have been an unwelcome part of sports in recent sports, there are few cases where the consequences became more publicly evident. Here was a great contradiction for the world to see: Oliver McCall, the athlete who had never been knocked down, and Oliver McCall, the man floored by the pain and drugs in his life. McCall's trainer, George Benton, said, "It was hard to watch, but it could be the best thing that ever happened to the human race. Now a father can tell his kids, 'You see what you saw on T.V.? You see what happens on drugs?' It was a hell of a lesson."

Sources: Boston Globe (February 8, 1997). *New York Times* (February 9, 1997).

---

athletic performance (Merchant 1992). Not available in the United States, this drug is known as Doper's Delight and is supposed to improve breathing and increase strength. Currently it is tested for in most athletic urine examinations.

Erythropoietin Clinically, erythropoietin is a drug used to treat patients with anemia. Because it stimulates the production of red blood cells (the oxygen-carrying cells in the blood), it is thought that this drug enhances oxygen use and produces additional energy. Erythropoietin is being used as a substitute for *blood doping*—athletes' attempts to increase the number of red blood cells by reinfusing some of their own blood (which has been stored) prior to an athletic event. Erythropoietin is impossible to detect and has been reported to be used by athletes engaged in endurance activities such as long-distance cycling. The use of

erythropoietin by athletes is extremely dangerous and is thought to be responsible for several deaths. It is also very expensive, which likely has helped to limit its abuse (Merchant 1992).

Human Growth Factor and Human Growth Hormone Relatively recently, athletes have begun to abuse two types of steroids known as **human growth factor (HGF)** and its "designer drug" synthetic version, **human growth hormone (HGH).** HGF, also known as *somatotropin,* is a hormone naturally secreted by the pituitary gland at the base of the brain that helps to achieve normal growth potential of muscles, bones,

> **human growth factor (HGF)**
> a hormone that stimulates normal growth
>
> **human growth hormone (HGH)**
> a "designer drug" synthetic version of HGF

and internal organs. Some athletes claim that release of natural HGF can be simulated by using drugs such as levadopa (which is used to treat Parkinson's disease), clonidine (used to treat hypertension), and amino acids. Athletes use commercially prepared HGF because it cannot be distinguished from naturally occurring HGF. Use of this hormone by athletes is limited, however, by its high cost. The benefits of HGF to athletic performance are very controversial, although the potential side effects are substantial, including abnormal growth patterns (called *acromegaly*), diabetes, thyroid gland problems, heart disease, and loss of sex drive (Merchant 1992).

In recent years, the synthetic HGH has become available in the form of a newly structured steroid-type analog sold in vials; this product is used to build muscle tissue, with corresponding decreases in body fat, without exercise (McDonald 1995, C1). HGH is probably the most potent anabolic agent ever discovered. It is reportedly very expensive, affordable only to a select group such as Olympic athletes. In fact, HGH is so expensive that until recently, " . . . its use in the United States has been confined to pediatric endocrinologists who treat undersized children" (McDonald 1995, C1). To date, no tests have proved capable of detecting HGH in the blood or urine. Also, the side effects of this drug remain largely unknown. As a result, this drug is highly vulnerable to abuse.

Beta-Adrenergic Blockers The beta-adrenergic blockers are drugs that affect the cardiovascular system and are frequently used to treat hypertension. They have been used in sports because they reduce the heart rate and signs of nervousness, which in turn quiets hand tremors. Consequently, these drugs are most likely to be used by individuals participating in sports that require steady hands, such as competitive shooting. The use of these drugs is prohibited by most athletic organizations (Merchant 1992).

Gamma-Hydroxybutyrate The substance gamma-hydroxybutyrate (GHB) is found naturally in the brain and has been used in England to treat insomnia. Athletes and body builders have used GHB to increase muscle mass and strength. Although the actual effects of the compound are not known, it has been reported to cause euphoria and increase the release of growth hormone. Acute poisoning with GHB has occurred, causing hospitalization; other adverse effects can include headaches, nausea, vomiting, muscle jerking, and even short-term coma, though full recovery has been universal ("Bodybuilding Drug" 1992; "Multistate Outbreak" 1994). Prolonged use may cause withdrawal (insomnia, anxiety, and tremor). GHB is especially dangerous when combined with CNS stimulants such as amphetamines and cocaine.

Prevention and Treatment

If the problem of drug abuse among athletes is to be dealt with effectively, sports programs must be designed to discourage inappropriate drug use and assist athletes who have developed drug abuse problems. Coaches and administrators should make clear to sports participants that substance abuse will never give an athlete a competitive advantage in their program and will not be tolerated. The following are specific suggestions for sports leaders to discourage drug abuse in their programs (Lawn 1984):

1. Make it known publicly that you recruit non–drug-using athletes to your programs, to exert pressure on team members who use these substances.

2. Rigidly enforce training rules and don't make exceptions, even for the "stars."

3. Select team captains and leaders who are opposed to drug use and require from them a commitment to help enforce training rules with teammates.

4. Be open about drug abuse incidents: don't avoid the subject but communicate to the athletes your concern for users. However, be sensitive to the need for confidentiality and the emotional and social needs of offenders.

5. Be educated about which drugs athletes typically abuse, how they are abused, and what

their effects are. With such knowledge, coaches and trainers are better prepared to recognize drug abuse symptoms, such as mood swings, changes in personality, impaired coordination, and sudden increases in muscle size and strength.

6. Have a definite plan in mind when an athlete gets caught abusing drugs. Ignoring the incident does not help the athlete to deal with his or her problems. The athlete should be confronted directly, and the family should be encouraged to get involved in the solution.

7. Establish and enforce a consequence or punishment for violating training rules by using drugs. However, after the rule has been enforced, the athlete should not be rejected, but encouraged.

It is essential that coaches and trainers be selected for their ability to be good role models for the athletes. They should encourage athletes to keep sports in perspective and should help the student athlete understand that many things in life are more important than success on the playing field (Lawn 1984).

◢ Drug Use Among Women

Little is known about how and why drugs are abused specifically by women. In general, most clinical drug abuse research is either conducted in male populations and the results are extrapolated to women, or the research is done in general populations with little regard to gender influences (Brady et al. 1993; Alexander 1994; Dicker and Leighton 1994; Lin 1994, 27). Even basic research into drug abuse mechanisms generally prefers male animal models in order to avoid the hormonal complexities that are inherent with female laboratory animals. However, a growing concern for the importance of unique emotional, social, biochemical, and hormonal features in females has caused researchers to acknowledge the importance of gender differences; consequently, scientists now are encouraged to determine the influences of gender differences in drug abusing subcultures.

Patterns of Drug Use: Comparing Females with Males

Recent surveys comparing male and female drug use patterns confirm that differences exist among the licit and illicit drug-using populations. Table 16.3 compares annual female and male drug use. In addition, results from a national survey (Johnston, O'Malley, and Bachman 1996, 64–5) and other research findings indicate the following gender-related differences in drug use:

1. Overall, females consistently use fewer licit and illicit drugs (23% of females versus 31% of males).

2. More males (4.5%) than females (1.4%) use marijuana daily. Also, on a daily basis, males consume alcohol more often (2.1% of females and 6.7% of males) and binge drink (five or more drinks in a row) more frequently (23% of females and 43% of males). Lifetime rates of cocaine and marijuana use show higher prevalence among white females compared with either black or Hispanic females (Alexander 1994b).

3. Use of stimulants is nearly equal among males and females in high school and about equal in post–high-school period (annual prevalence of 4.6% of men versus 3.5% of women).

4. Crystal methamphetamine (known as ice) is used by small percentages of both males (1.0% annual prevalence) and females (0.6%).

5. In the 1990s, small differences have emerged regarding cigarette use by high school seniors; past-month prevalence is 33% for males compared with 29% for females.

6. Steroid use among young adults is much more prevalent among males than females. Among high school seniors, 2.1% of the males reported steroid use in the past year versus 0.5% of females.

7. MDMA (Ecstasy) use is higher among males than females in the young adult sample (annual prevalence is 0.9% for males versus 0.3% for females).

Although some similarities appear in gender drug usage rates for specific types of drugs, the

Table 16.3   **Annual Use of Various Types of Drugs, by Sex, 1994** (percent of population)

	Females	Males	Total
Any illicit drug	**23.4**	**31.2**	**26.9**
Any illicit drug other than marijuana	**10.3**	**15.4**	**12.6**
Marijuana	20.0	28.6	23.8
Inhalants	1.0	2.5	1.7
Hallucinogens	2.2	6.1	3.9
LSD	1.9	4.9	3.2
PCP	0.2	0.3	0.3
Cocaine	3.0	6.7	4.6
Crack	0.7	1.8	1.2
Other cocaine	2.4	5.8	3.9
MDMA (Ecstasy)	0.3	0.9	0.6
Heroin	0.1	0.2	0.2
Other opiates	1.9	2.8	2.3
Stimulants	3.5	4.6	4.0
Crystal methamphetamine (ice)	0.6	1.0	0.8
Barbiturates	1.3	2.2	1.7
Tranquilizers	2.7	3.4	3.0
Steroids	0.1	0.6	0.3
Alcohol	81.9	85.6	83.6
5+ drinks in a row in the last 2 weeks	22.6	43.4	31.8
Cigarettes	34.9	37.6	36.1
Half-pack or more per day	15.0	16.8	15.8

Source: Modified from L. D. Johnston, P. O. O'Malley, and J. G. Bachman. *National Survey Results from The Monitoring the Future Study, 1975–1994.* Rockville, MD: National Institute on Drug Abuse, 1996: 64–5.

general differences in the prevalence rates for females and males compel researchers to look for explanations so that we can better understand and deal with gender-related drug abuse problems.

Female Roles and Drug Addiction

Women are expected to take on more responsibilities than in my mother's days. Not only are we expected to work like men, but also take care of the house, worry about the children, and get dinner on the table. If the house needs cleaning, everyone looks at the woman of the house. Men still have these expectations. I know things are changing with more equality between the sexes, but real equality of responsibilities has yet to occur. After everyone gets to bed on weekdays, I have a few drinks in order to calm me down before I go to bed.

From Venturelli's research files, interview with a 43-year-old female, employed full-time, June 30, 1996

To appreciate the impact of drug abuse on women, it is necessary to understand the uniqueness of female roles in our society. Relative to drug abuse problems, women are often judged by a double standard, and thus women suffering from drug addictions are often perceived less tolerantly than comparably addicted men (Erickson and Murray 1989). Because of these social biases, women are afraid of being condemned and are less likely to seek professional help for their drug abuse problems. In addition, family, friends, and associates are less inclined to provide drug-dependent women with important emotional support (Alexander 1994).

Due to their unique socioeconomic and family roles, women are especially vulnerable to emotional disruptions resulting from divorce, loneliness, and professional failures. Studies suggest that such stresses aggravate tendencies for women to abuse alcohol and other substances (Korolenko and Donskih 1990). In addition, drug addiction can occur in some women due to domestic adversities. Consequently, there is a high prevalence of drug dependence in women who are victims of sexual and/or physical abuse (Ladwig and Anderson 1989). These emotional traumas are the result of, or precursors to, factors leading to drug abuse, such as low self-esteem, self-condemnation, anxiety, and personal conflicts (Alexander 1994). In addition, because of their crucial nurturing roles, drug abuse problems in women can be particularly damaging to family stability.

Another unique role for women in drug abuse situations is that of a spouse, "significant other," or mother to a drug addict. Often, in both traditional and nontraditional family relationships, women are expected to be nurturing, understanding, and willing to sacrifice in order to preserve the "family integrity." If a family member becomes afflicted by drug dependence, the wife or mother is viewed as a failure. In other words, if the woman had maintained a good home and conducted her domestic chores properly, the family member would not have been driven to drugs (Alexander 1994).

Despite the disruption and considerable stress caused by drug addiction in the home, women continue to bear the burden of raising children, performing domestic chores, and keeping the family together (Alexander 1994). In addition, women in such circumstances frequently are put at great physical risk from an addicted spouse who becomes abusive to his partner or from exposure to sexually transmitted diseases, such as HIV infection or hepatitis, transmitted by a careless infected partner. The anxiety and frustrations resulting from these stressful circumstances can encourage women themselves to become dependent as they seek emotional relief by using drugs.

Women's Unique Response to Drugs

Relatively little drug research specifically evaluates women's response to substances of abuse. Often in drug abuse studies, female populations are deliberately avoided and the effects of the drugs in men are extrapolated to females. Even when drug abuse research is conducted on women, frequently the woman's response is not of primary concern but the objective is to determine the effects on a fetus during pregnancy or an infant during nursing (Alexander 1994). Although it generally can be assumed that the physiological and drug responses of men and women are similar, some distinctions should be recognized. For example, a recent study compared the risk for lung cancer in men and women after a lifetime of cigarette smoking. It was found that female smokers were twice as likely to get lung cancer as comparable males who had smoked an identical number of cigarettes in their lifetime ("Women Smokers Run Higher Risk for Lung Cancer" 1994). These differences suggest cigarette smoking may be more dangerous for women than men.

Drug Abuse and Reproduction A very important physiological distinction that sets women apart from men in regard to taking drugs is their reproductive capabilities. Because of this unique function, women have different endocrine (hormone) systems, organs, and structures and varied drug responses according to their reproductive state. These unique features can have a substantial impact on the response to drug abuse in the presence and absence of pregnancy.

Drug abuse patterns can influence the outcome of pregnancy even if they occur prior to the pregnant state. For example, women who are addicted to heroin are more likely to have poor health, including chronic infections, poor nutrition, and sexually transmitted diseases, such as human immunodeficiency virus (HIV) infection, that can damage the offspring if pregnancy occurs (American College of Obstetricians 1986; Black et al. 1994, 44c). If substances are abused during pregnancy, they may directly affect the fetus and adversely alter its growth and development. The incidence of substance abuse during pregnancy is not known precisely, but undoubtedly hundreds of thousands of children have been exposed to these drugs in utero—while in the uterus during pregnancy (Alexander 1994). The effects of individual drugs of abuse taken during pregnancy are discussed in detail in the corresponding chapters, but several specific observations merit reiteration.

1. Cocaine is a substantial threat for both the pregnant woman and the fetus. Although a number of specific claims for the fetal effects of cocaine are controversial (see Chapter 11), several observations appear legitimate. Cocaine increases the likelihood of miscarriage when used during pregnancy. Use of cocaine in the late stages of pregnancy can cause cardiovascular or CNS complications in the offspring at birth and immediately thereafter. Due to its vasoconstrictor effects, cocaine may deprive the fetal brain of oxygen, resulting in strokes and permanent physical and mental damage to the child (Alexander 1994).

2. The impact of alcohol consumption during pregnancy has been well documented and publicized (Mathias 1995, 6). Alcohol crosses the placenta when consumed by the mother, but the effect of this drug on the fetus is highly variable and depends on the quantity of drug consumed, timing of exposure, maternal drug metabolism, maternal state of health, and the presence of other drugs (Alexander 1994). A particularly alarming consequence of high alcohol intake during pregnancy is an aggregate of physical and mental defects known as the fetal alcohol syndrome (FAS). Characteristics included in this syndrome are low birth weight, abnormal facial features, mental retardation, and retarded sensorimotor development (Alexander 1994). For additional details, see Chapters 8 and 9.

In addition to direct effects on the fetus, alcohol has played a major role in many unwanted pregnancies or has resulted in women's exposure to sexually transmitted diseases such as AIDS. As a CNS depressant, alcohol impairs judgment and

reason, in turn encouraging sexual risk taking that normally would not be considered. The results are all too frequently tragic for women (Alexander 1994).

3. Tobacco use during pregnancy is particularly rampant in the United States. Specifically, 20% of the smoking female adult population are pregnant. Some experts suggest smoking cigarettes during pregnancy may be a greater risk to the fetus than taking cocaine. Tobacco use by pregnant women may interfere with blood flow to the fetus and deprive it of oxygen and nutrition and disrupt development of fetal organs, particularly the brain ("Cigarettes May Pose a Greater Risk" 1994). Also of significant concern is the possibility that exposure of nonsmoking pregnant women to second-hand tobacco smoke may be damaging to the fetus.

4. Other drugs of abuse that have been associated with abnormal fetal development when used during pregnancy include the barbiturates, benzodiazepines, amphetamines, marijuana, LSD, and even caffeine when consumed in high doses.

Clearly, women should be strongly urged to avoid all substances of abuse, especially during pregnancy.

Women and Alcohol Alcohol is the drug most widely used and abused by women in the United States. As reported in Table 16.3, in 1994, approximately 82% of women drank alcohol and approximately 23% binged on alcohol. According to the National Institute on Alcohol Abuse and Alcoholism, 5% of U.S. women have a serious drinking problem (Alexander 1994). Alcohol abuse is also a major problem for women on college campuses, although male college students are more likely than their female counterparts to use alcohol on a daily basis.

Usually, women are less likely than men to develop severe alcohol dependence; thus, only 25% of the alcoholics in America are female. Women are also likely to initiate their drinking patterns later in life than men (Alexander 1994). Interesting ethnic patterns of alcohol consumption have been reported in females, with black and white women manifesting similar drinking patterns. While the proportions of black and white females drinking alcohol are similar, however, black women are more likely to completely abstain from alcohol than white women.

Women who are dependent on alcohol are usually judged more harshly than men with similar difficulties (Alexander 1994). Alcoholic males are more likely to be excused because their drinking problems are often perceived as being caused by frustrating work conditions, family demands, economic pressures, or so-called nagging wives and children. In contrast, women with drinking problems are often perceived as spoiled or pampered, weak, deviant, or immoral. Such stigmas, referred to as labels in Chapter 2 (see labeling theory), cause women to experience more guilt and anxiety about their alcohol dependence and discourage them from admitting their drug problems and seeking professional help (Alexander 1994).

The principal reasons for excessive alcohol consumption in women range from loneliness, boredom, and domestic stress in the "housewife drinker" to financial problems, sexual harassment, lack of challenge, and discrimination and powerlessness for career women. Depression often is associated with alcohol problems in women, although it is not clear whether this condition is a cause or an effect of the excessive drug use.

Women's Unique Physiological Responses to Alcohol

Health consequences for excessive alcohol consumption appear to be more severe for women than for men. For example, alcoholic women are more likely to suffer premature death than alcoholic men. In addition, liver disease is more common and occurs at a younger age in female drinkers than in male alcoholics (Alexander 1994). In general, higher morbidity rates are experienced by alcoholic women than their male counterparts.

Several explanations have been suggested for the greater adverse effects seen in female alcoholics. Their higher blood alcohol concentrations may be due to a smaller blood volume and more rapid absorption into the bloodstream after drinking. Alternatively, slower alcohol metabolism in the stomach and liver might cause more alcohol to reach the brain and other organs as well as prolong exposure to the drug following consumption (Goldstein 1995). Studies have shown that for a woman of average size, one alcoholic drink has effects equivalent to two drinks in an average-size man (see Chapter 8).

Dealing with Women's Alcohol Problems

Alcoholic consumption varies considerably in women, ranging from total abstinence or an occasional drink to daily intake of large amounts of alcohol. Clearly, much is yet to be learned about the cause of some women's excessive drinking of, and dependence on alcohol. The role of genetic factors in predisposing women to alcohol-related problems is still unclear. Female alcoholics are less likely than male alcoholics to have had alcoholic parents or siblings (Alexander 1994a), suggesting that heredity may be less important in female drinkers than in male alcoholics. Environment certainly is a major factor contributing to excessive alcohol consumption in women. It is well established that depression, stress, and trauma encourage alcohol consumption, because of the antianxiety and amnesic properties of this drug. Because of unreasonable societal expectations and numerous socioeconomic disadvantages, women are especially vulnerable to the emotional upheavals that encourage excessive alcohol consumption.

As with all drug dependence problems, prevention is the preferred solution to alcohol abuse by women. Alcohol usually becomes problematic when it is no longer used occasionally to enhance social events, but its consumption becomes a daily exercise to deal with personal problems. Such alcohol dependence can best be avoided by using constructive techniques to manage stress and frustrations. Because of unique female roles, women especially need to learn to be assertive with family members, associates in the workplace (including bosses), and other contacts in their daily routines (also see Chapter 4). By expecting and demanding equitable treatment and consideration in personal and professional activities, stress and anxiety can often be reduced. Education, career training, and development of communication abilities can be particularly important in establishing a sense of self-worth (see Chapter 17). With these skills and confidence, women are better able to manage problems associated with their lives and less likely to resort to drugs for solutions.

Women and Prescription Drugs Women are more likely than men to suffer mental disorders such as depression, anxiety, and panic attacks (Brady 1993). Consequently, they are also more likely to take and become addicted to the prescription drugs used in treating these disorders. Because these drugs are used as part of the psychiatric therapy and under the supervision of a physician, drug dependence frequently is not recognized and may be ignored for months or even years. This type of "legitimate" drug abuse occurs most often in elderly women and includes the use of sedatives, hypnotics, and antianxiety medications; elderly women are prescribed these types of medications 2.5 times more often than are elderly men (Alexander 1994b). Excessive use of these drugs by older women results in side effects such as insomnia, mood fluctuations, and disruption of cognitive and motor functions that can substantially compromise the quality of life.

Treatment of Drug Dependency in Women

As previously discussed, women are less likely than men to seek treatment for, and rehabilitation from, drug dependence (Alexander 1994b). Possible reasons for their reluctance are as follows:

1. In more traditional families, women have unique roles with high expectations. They have demanding and ongoing responsibilities, such as motherhood, child rearing, and family maintenance, that cannot be postponed and often cannot be delegated, even temporarily, to others. Consequently, many women feel that they are too essential for the well-being of other family members to leave the home and seek time-consuming treatment for drug abuse problems.

2. Drug treatment centers often are not designed to handle the extensive and unique health requirements of females. Women have been shown to have greater health needs than men due to more frequent respira-

genitourinary

having to do with the reproductive and urinary systems

tory, **genitourinary** (associated with the sex and urinary organs), and circulatory problems. If drug treatment centers are not capable of providing the necessary physical care, women are less likely to participate in associated drug abuse programs.

3. Drug-dependent women are more inclined to be unemployed than male counterparts and more likely to be receiving public support (Alexander 1994b). The implications of this difference are twofold. First, because concerns about one's job often motivate drug-dependent workers to seek treatment, this issue is less likely to be a factor in unemployed women. Second, without the financial security of a job, unemployed women may feel that good treatment for their drug problems is unaffordable. (For more on treatment, see Chapter 4.)

The unique female requirements must be recognized and considered if women are to receive adequate treatment for drug dependence. Some considerations to achieve this objective include the following:

1. The role of motherhood needs to be used in a positive manner in drug treatment strategies. For most women, motherhood is viewed with high regard and linked to their self-esteem. Approximately 90% of female drug abusers are in their childbearing years, and many have family responsibilities. Consequently, treatment approaches need to be tailored to allow women to fulfill their domestic responsibilities and satisfy their maternal obligations.

2. Employment and independence may be especially crucial for drug-dependent females. Helping women to gain control of their own lives by developing skills or careers and becoming financially independent can be important steps in helping them gain a sense of worth and inner strength. With self-confidence comes the belief that success and satisfaction are possible without drugs.

3. Women dependent on drugs often lack important coping skills. Because many women lead restricted, almost isolated lives that focus entirely on domestic responsibilities, they

have limited alternatives for dealing with stressful situations. Under these restrictive circumstances, the use of drugs to cope with anxieties and frustrations is very appealing. In order to enhance their ability to cope, drug-dependent women need to develop communication skills and assertiveness; they need to be encouraged to control situations rather than allowing themselves to be controlled by the situation. Specific techniques useful in coping management are exercise (particularly relaxation types), relaxing visual imagery, personal hobbies, and outside interests that require active participation. Many drug-dependent women require experiences that divert their attention from the source of their frustrations while affording them an opportunity to succeed and develop a sense of self-worth.

Prevention of Drug Dependence in Women

The best treatment for drug addiction is prevention. To help prevent drug problems in women, socioeconomic disadvantages need to be recognized as factors that make women more vulnerable to drug dependence, especially from prescription medication, than men. Women need to learn that nondrug approaches are often more desirable for dealing with situational problems than prescribed medications. For example, for older women suffering loneliness, isolation, or depression, it is better to encourage participation in outside interests, such as hobbies and service activities. In addition, social support and concern should be encouraged from family, friends, and neighbors. Such nonmedicinal approaches are preferred over prescribing sedatives and hypnotics to cope with emotional distresses. Similarly, medical conditions such as obesity, constipation, or insomnia should be treated by changing lifestyle, eating, and exercise habits rather than using drug "bandage therapy."

When women are prescribed drugs, they should ask about the associated risks, especially as they relate to drug abuse potential. Frequently, drug dependency develops insidiously and is not recognized by either the patient or attending physician until it is already firmly established. If a woman taking medication is aware of the potential for becoming dependent and is instructed on how to avoid its occurrence, the problems of dependence and abuse can frequently be averted. See Chapter 17 for more on prevention and education.

◢ Drug Use in Adolescent Subcultures

Hell yeah! Any chance I get away from my mom, especially when she has to be at work, I always go out lookin' to get high. When I get with my friends we usually run around, party at someone's house, or end up having sex with someone.

From Venturelli's research files, interview with a 15-year-old male high school sophomore residing in a smaller Midwestern city, December 16, 1996

From ages 13 through 18, many adolescents experience heightened psychological, social, and biological changes. Oftentimes, such internal and external changes are manifested by emotional outbursts. Why do such changes and urges arise? The adolescent's body is stretching, growing, and sometimes screaming out of control due to the hormonal changes of puberty. Adolescents are uncertain and confused about not knowing who or what they are becoming. They are often confused as to their worth to family, peers, society, and even to themselves.

Adding to the frustration of growing up, the cultural status of adolescents is poorly defined. They find themselves trapped in a "no-man's land" between the acceptance, simplicity, and security of childhood, and the stress, complexities, expectations, independence, and responsibilities of adulthood. Not only do adolescents have difficulty deciding who and what they are, but adults are also equally unsure as to how to deal with these transitional human beings. While the grownup world tries to push adolescents out of the secure nest of childhood, it isn't willing to bestow the full membership and rights of adulthood (Archambault 1992; Johnson et al. 1996).

Because of their uniquely rapid development, several developmental issues are particularly important to evolving adolescents (Elmen and Offer 1993; Johnson et al. 1996):

▲ Discovering and understanding their distinctive identities

▲ Forming more intimate and caring relationships with others

▲ Establishing a sense of autonomy

▲ Coming to terms with the hormone-related feelings of puberty and expressing their sexuality

▲ Learning to become productive contributors to society

Due to all this developmental confusion, normal behavior for the adolescent is difficult to define precisely. Experts generally agree that persistent low self-esteem, depression, and other severe emotional disturbances can be troublesome for teenagers. Most adolescents are relatively well adjusted and are able to cope with sociobiological changes. Emotionally stable adolescents relate well to family and peers, and function productively within their schools, neighborhoods, and communities. The majority of adolescents experience transient problems, which they are able to resolve, while others become deeply disturbed and are unable to grow out of their problems without help (Elmen and Offer 1993). Those adolescents who are unable or unwilling to ask for assistance often turn to destructive devices, such as drugs, for relief from their emotional dilemmas.

Why Adolescents Use Drugs

Although there is no such thing as a "typical" substance-abusing adolescent, there are physiological, psychological, and sociological factors that are often associated with drug problems in this subculture (Lawson and Lawson 1992; Johnson et al. 1996). However, it is important to remember that not all drug use by adolescents means therapy is necessary or even desirable. Most excessive drug use and abuse by adolescents results from the desire to experience new behaviors and sensations, a passing fancy of maturation, an attempt to relieve peer pressure, or an inclination to enhance a social setting with chemistry. Most of these adolescent users will not go on to develop problematic dependence on drugs and, for the most part,

should be watched but not aggressively confronted or treated. The adolescents who usually have significant difficulty with drug use are those who turn to drugs for extended support as coping devices and become drug-reliant because they are unable to find alternative, less destructive solutions to their problems. Several major factors can contribute to serious drug dependence in adolescents (Archambault 1992; Walsh and Scheinkman 1992; Johnson et al. 1996).

Most recent research indicates that the most important factor influencing drug use among adolescents is peer drug use (Swadi 1992, 253; Bahr et al. 1995; Kandel 1980). Consequently, eventual transition to heavier substance use is also a result of this factor (Steinberg et al. 1994, 1063). Conversely, individuals whose peer groups do not use or abuse drugs are less likely to use drugs themselves. Research has identified a correlation between strong family bonds and non–drug-using peer groups. "Adolescents with higher family bonds are less likely than adolescents with lower bonds to have close friends who use drugs" (Bahr et al. 1995, 466). In addition, family bonding is highly correlated with educational commitment. In essence, family bonding influences choice of friends and educational goals and aspirations (Bahr et al. 1995, 466).

Three noteworthy differences exist between male and female adolescents: (1) males demonstrate a stronger association between educational achievement and family bonds; (2) among females, peer drug use is negatively associated with family bonds, so peer drug use and family bonds are not likely to influence the use of licit and illicit drugs by females; and (3) the impact of age on peer drug use (the younger the age, the more vulnerable to peer pressure) and on the amount of alcohol consumed can be predicted with slightly greater accuracy for males than females.

Many adolescents use drugs to help cope with unpleasant feelings, emotions, and stress or to relieve depression and reduce tension. Psychological differences among adolescents who are frequent drug users, experimenters, and abstainers often can be traced to early childhood, the quality of parenting in their homes, and their home environment. It has been suggested that certain types of parents are more likely to raise children at high risk for substance abuse (Archambault 1992). For example, an alcoholic adolescent usually has at least one parent of the following types:

Alcoholic. This parent serves as a negative role model for the adolescent. The child sees the parent dealing with problems by consuming drugs. Even though drinking alcohol is not illegal for adults, it sends the message that drugs can solve problems. The guilt-ridden alcoholic parent is unable to provide the child with a loving supportive relationship. In addition, the presence of the alcoholic parent is often disruptive or abusive to the family and creates fear or embarrassment in the child.

Nonconsuming and condemning. This type of parent not only chooses to abstain from drinking, but is also very judgmental about drinkers and condemns them for their behavior. Such persons, who are often referred to as *teetotalers,* have a rigid, moralistic approach to life. Their black-and-white attitudes frequently prove inadequate and unforgiving in an imperfect, gray world. Children in these families can feel inferior and guilty when they are unable to live up to parental expectations, and they may resort to drugs to cope with their frustrations.

Overly demanding. This type of parent forces unrealistic expectations on his or her children. These parents often live vicariously through their children and require sons and daughters to pursue endeavors where the parents were unable to succeed. Particular emphasis may be placed on achievements in athletics, academics, or career selections. Even though the parents' efforts may be well intended, the children get the message that their parents are more concerned about "what they are" than "who they are." These parents frequently encourage sibling rivalries to enhance performance, but such competitions always yield a loser.

Overly protective. These types of parents do not give their children a chance to develop a sense of self-worth and independence. Because the parents deprive their children of the opportunities to learn how to master their abilities within their surroundings, the children are not able to develop confidence and a positive self-image. Such children are frequently unsure about who they are and what they are capable of achieving. Parents who use children to satisfy their own ego needs or are trying to convince themselves that they really do like their children tend to be overly protective.

The principal influence for learned behavior is usually the home; therefore, several other family-related variables can significantly affect adolescents' decision to start, maintain, or cease a drug habit (Lawson and Lawson 1992). For example, adolescents usually learn their attitudes about drug use from family models. In other words, what are the drug-consuming patterns of parents and siblings? Adolescents are more likely to develop drug problems if other members of the family (1) are excessive in their drug (legal or illegal) consumption, (2) approve of the use of illicit drugs, or (3) use drugs as a problem-solving strategy.

Sociological factors that damage self-image can also encourage adolescent drug use. Feelings of rejection cause poor relationships with family members, peers, school personnel, or co-workers. In a racist society, ethnic differences sometimes contribute to a poor self-image because people of minority races or cultures are frequently socially excluded and are viewed as being inferior and undesirable by the majority population. This type of negative message is very difficult for adolescents to deal with. Sometimes to ensure acceptance, adolescents adopt the attitudes and behavior of their affiliated groups. If a peer group, or a *gang,* views drug use as *cool,* desirable, or even necessary behavior, members (or those desiring membership) feel compelled to conform and become involved in drugs.

Patterns of Drug Use in Adolescents

For many adolescents in the United States, the first drug exposure occurs at a very early age. Recent surveys regarding drug user patterns found that by eighth grade, approximately 55% of children had used alcohol, 46% had used cigarettes, 22% had used inhalants, and 20% had used marijuana (see

Table 16.4). The 1995 Monitoring the Future study conducted by the National Institute on Drug Abuse (NIDA) reported the following findings (Mathias 1996, 8–9):

1. Marijuana use had the sharpest increase, and more of the nation's eighth-, tenth-, and twelfth-grade students also reported using other illicit drugs in 1995.

2. From 1991 to 1995, the percentage of eighth-graders who used an illicit drug almost doubled, rising from 11.3% to 21.4%.

3. Since 1992, annual use of any illicit drug has risen from 21.4% to 33.3% of tenth-graders and from 29.4% to 39% of high school seniors.

4. Cigarette smoking rose significantly among tenth- and twelfth-graders. The proportion of tenth-graders who reported smoking cigarettes in the 30 days prior to the survey (referred to as current use) rose from 25.4% in 1994 to 29.9% in 1995. Current use of cigarettes among twelfth-graders climbed from 31.2% to 33.5%.

5. Rates of alcohol use held steady among students in all three grades in 1995.

6. The *perceived* risks of using marijuana have sharply declined at all three grade levels. (Interestingly, the decrease in the perceived risks of using marijuana has been countered by a dramatic increase in self-reported marijuana usage.)

Adolescent Versus Adult Drug Abuse   Adolescent patterns of drug abuse are very different from drug use patterns in adults (Moss et al. 1994). The uniqueness of adolescent drug abuse means that drug-dependent teenagers usually are not successfully treated with adult-directed therapy. For example, compared with adults who abuse drugs, drug-using adolescents are (1) more likely to be involved in criminal activity; (2) more likely to get involved in criminal activity at a very early age; (3) more likely to have other members of the family who abuse drugs; (4) more likely to be associated with a dysfunctional family that engages in emotional and/or physical abuse of its members; and (5) more likely to begin their drug use because of curiosity or peer pressure (Segal et al. 1982; Daily

1992b; Hoshino 1992; Steinberg et al. 1994; Bahr et al. 1995). Differences such as these need to be considered when developing adolescent-targeted treatment programs.

Consequences and Coincidental Problems

Researchers have concluded that the problem of adolescent drug use is a symptom and not a cause of personal social maladjustment. Even so, because of the pharmacological actions of drugs, routine use can contribute to school and social failures, unintended injuries (usually automobile-related), criminal and violent behavior, sexual risk taking, depression, and suicide (Hernandez 1992; Curry and Spergel 1997).

It is important to realize that, because serious drug abuse is usually the result of emotional instability, consequences of the underlying disorders may be coexpressed with chemical dependence, making diagnosis and treatment more difficult. The undesirable coincidental problems may include self-destruction, risk taking, abuse, or negative group behaviors. Some of these adolescent problems and their relationship to drug abuse are discussed in the following sections.

Adolescent Suicide   Adolescents are particularly vulnerable to suicide actions; in fact, white males between 14 and 20 years are the most likely to commit suicide in the United States (Daily 1992b). Further, the teenage suicide rate has doubled since 1980 (Siegel and Senna 1997). The result is that suicide is now the second leading cause of death among persons 15 to 24 years of age. Twenty to thirty-six percent of suicide victims have a history of alcohol abuse or were drinking shortly before their suicide. Some experts have described severe chemical dependence as a form of slow drug-related suicide. Clearly, many teenagers who abuse alcohol and other drugs possess a self-destructive attitude. These adolescents often (1) feel insecure and inferior, (2) demonstrate risk-taking behaviors, and (3) have little concern for their own health or physical well-being.

Beside posing a direct health threat because of their physiological effects, drugs of abuse can precipitate suicide attempts due to their pharmacological impact. A number of studies have found a

Table 16.4

Drug Use among Eighth-, Tenth-, and Twelfth-graders Data shows the percentages of 8th-, 10th-, and 12th-graders who used drugs, including alcohol and tobacco, in the past three years. The University of Michigan's Institute for Social Research has conducted the survey each year since 1975 among a representative sample of 12th-graders; 8th- and 10th-graders were surveyed for the first time in 1991.

	8th Graders			10th Graders			12th Graders		
	1993	1994	1995	1993	1994	1995	1993	1994	1995
Alcohol[†]									
Lifetime	55.7	55.8	54.5	71.6	71.1	70.5	80.0	80.4	80.7
Annual	45.4	46.8	45.3	63.4	63.9	63.5	72.7	73.0	73.7
30-Day	24.3	25.5	24.6	38.2	39.2	38.8	48.6	50.1	51.3
Daily	1.0	1.0	0.7	1.8	1.7	1.7	3.4	2.9	3.5
Cigarettes (any use)									
Lifetime	45.3	46.1	46.4	56.3	56.9	57.6	61.9	62.0	64.2
30-Day	16.7	18.6	19.1	24.7	25.4	27.9	29.9	31.2	33.5
Daily	8.3	8.8	9.3	14.2	14.6	16.3	19.0	19.4	21.6
1/2 Pack+ per day	3.5	3.6	3.4	7.0	7.6	8.3	10.9	11.2	12.4
Marijuana/hashish									
Lifetime	12.6%	16.7%	19.9%	24.4%	30.4%	34.1%	35.3%	38.2%	41.7%
Annual	9.2	13.0	15.8	19.2	25.2	28.7	26.0	30.7	34.7
30-Day	5.1	7.8	9.1	10.9	15.8	17.2	15.5	19.0	21.2
Daily	0.4	0.7	0.8	1.0	2.2	2.8	2.4	3.6	4.6
Inhalants									
Lifetime	19.4	19.9	21.6	17.5	18.0	19.0	17.4	17.7	17.4
Annual	11.0	11.7	12.8	8.4	9.1	9.6	7.0	7.7	8.0
30-Day	5.4	5.6	6.1	3.3	3.6	3.5	2.5	2.7	3.2
Daily	0.3	0.2	0.2	0.2	0.1	0.1	0.1	0.1	0.1
Stimulants									
Lifetime	11.8	12.3	13.1	14.9	15.1	17.4	15.1	15.7	15.3
Annual	7.2	7.9	8.7	9.6	10.2	11.9	8.4	9.4	9.3
30-Day	3.6	3.6	4.2	4.3	4.5	5.3	3.7	4.0	4.0
Daily	0.1	0.1	0.2	0.3	0.1	0.2	0.2	0.2	0.3
Hallucinogens									
Lifetime	3.9	4.3	5.2	6.8	8.1	9.3	10.9	11.4	12.7
Annual	2.6	2.7	3.6	4.7	5.8	7.2	7.4	7.6	9.3
30-Day	1.2	1.3	1.7	1.9	2.4	3.3	2.7	3.1	4.4
Daily	0.1	0.1	0.1	0.1	0.1	*	0.1	0.1	0.1
Cocaine									
Lifetime	2.9	3.6	4.2	3.6	4.3	5.0	6.1	5.9	6.0
Annual	1.7	2.1	2.6	2.1	2.8	3.5	3.3	3.6	4.0
30-Day	0.7	1.0	1.2	0.9	1.2	1.7	1.3	1.5	1.8
Daily	0.1	0.1	0.1	0.1	0.1	0.1	0.1	0.1	0.2
Crack cocaine									
Lifetime	1.7	2.4	2.7	1.8	2.1	2.8	2.6	3.0	3.0
Annual	1.0	1.3	1.6	1.1	1.4	1.8	1.5	1.9	2.1
30-Day	0.4	0.7	0.7	0.5	0.6	0.9	0.7	0.8	1.0
Daily	0.1	*	*	*	*	*	0.1	0.1	0.1
Steroids									
Lifetime	1.6	2.0	2.0	1.7	1.8	2.0	2.0	2.4	2.3
Annual	0.9	1.2	1.0	1.0	1.1	1.2	1.2	1.3	1.5
30-Day	0.5	0.5	0.6	0.5	0.6	0.6	0.7	0.9	0.7
Daily	0.1	*	*	*	0.1	0.1	0.1	0.4	0.2
Heroin									
Lifetime	1.4	2.0	2.3	1.3	1.5	1.7	1.1	1.2	1.6
Annual	0.7	1.2	1.4	0.7	0.9	1.1	0.5	0.6	1.1
30-Day	0.4	0.6	0.6	0.3	0.4	0.6	0.2	0.3	0.6
Daily	*	0.1	*	*	*	*	*	*	0.1

(*) Indicates less than 0.05%. (†) Starting in 1993, the question was changed slightly to indicate that a "drink" meant "more than a few sips."
Source: "Drug Use Among 8th, 10th, and 12th Graders." *NIDA Notes* 11 (January/February 1996): 15.

very high correlation between acute suicidal behavior and drug use (Buckstein et al. 1993). One report noted that adolescent alcoholics have a suicide rate 58 times greater than the national average. In another study, 30% of adolescent alcoholics had made suicide attempts, while 92% admitted to a history of having suicidal thoughts (Daily 1992b).

It has been speculated that the incidence of suicide in drug-consuming adolescents is high because both types of behavior are the consequence of their inability to develop fundamental adult attributes of confidence, self-esteem, and independence. When drug use does not satisfy the need for these characteristics, the resulting frustrations are intensified and ultimately played out in the suicide act.

Most adolescents experiment with drugs for reasons not related to antisocial or deviant behavior but rather due to curiosity, desire for recreation, boredom, desire to gain new insights and experiences, or the urge to heighten social interactions. These adolescents are not likely to engage in self-destructive behavior. In addition, adolescents from "healthy" family environments are not likely to attempt suicide. Specifically, families least likely to have suicidal members are those that (Daily 1992b)

▲ Express love and show mutual concern

▲ Are tolerant of differences and overlook failings

▲ Encourage the development of self-confidence and self-expression

▲ Have parents who assume strong leadership roles, but are not autocratic

▲ Have interaction characterized by humor and good-natured teasing

▲ Are able to serve as a source of joy and happiness to their members

Suicide is more likely to be attempted by those adolescents who turn to alcohol and other drugs to cope with serious emotional and personality conflicts and frustrations. These susceptible teenagers represent approximately 5% of the adolescent population (Beschner and Friedman 1985; Siegel and Senna 1997).

Wright (1985) found in his studies that four features significantly contribute to the likelihood of suicidal thought in high school students:

1. Parents with interpersonal conflicts who often use an adolescent child with drug problems as the scapegoat for family problems.

2. Fathers who have poor, and often confrontational, relationships with their children

3. Parents who are viewed by their adolescent children as being emotionally unstable, usually suffering from perpetual anger and depression

4. A sense of frustration, desperation, and inability to resolve personal and emotional difficulties through traditional means

Clearly, it is important to identify those adolescents who are at risk for suicide and to provide immediate care and appropriate emotional support.

Sexual Violence and Drugs Alcohol use has been closely associated with almost every type of sexual abuse wherein the adolescent is victimized. For example, alcohol is by far the most significant factor in date, acquaintance, and gang rapes involving teenagers (Parrot 1988; Prendergast 1994). The evidence for alcohol involvement in incest is particularly overwhelming. Approximately 4 million children in America live in incestuous homes with alcoholic parents. In addition, 42% of drug-abusing female adolescents have been victims of sexual abuse (Daily 1992a). It is estimated that almost half of the offenders consume alcohol before molesting a child and at least a third of the perpetrators are chronic alcoholics. Finally, 85% of child molesters were sexually abused themselves as children, usually at the same age as their victims, and the vast majority of these molesters abused drugs as adolescents (Daily 1992a).

These very disturbing associations illustrate the relationship between drugs and violent sexual behavior both in terms of initiating the act and as a consequence of the act. The effects of such sexual violence are devastating and far reaching. Thus, incest victims are themselves more likely than the general population to abuse drugs as adolescents and engage in antisocial delinquency, prostitution, depression, and suicide (Daily 1992a).

Gangs and Drugs The very disturbing involvement of adolescents in gang organizations and gang-related activities and violence is a social phenomenon that first became widely recognized in the 1950s and 1960s. Hollywood, for example, introduced America to the problems of adolescent gangs in the classic movies "Blackboard Jungle" and "West Side Story." Although the basis for gang involvement has not changed over the years, the level of violence and public concern have increased dramatically. Many communities consider gang-related problems to be their number one social issue. Access to sophisticated weaponry and greater mobility have drawn unsuspecting neighborhoods and innocent bystanders into the often violent clashes of **intragang** and **intergang** warfare. Individuals and communities have been reacting angrily to this growing menace. To deal effectively with the threats of gang-initiated violence and crime, however, it is important to understand why gangs form, what their objectives are, how they are structured, and how to discourage adolescent involvement.

> **intragang**
> rivalry between members of the same gang
>
> **intergang**
> rivalry between members of different gangs

Gang members are often neglected by their parents, lack positive role models, and fail to receive adequate adult supervision. Other motivations for joining a gang include peer pressures, low self-esteem, and perceived easy acquisition to money from gang-related drug dealing and other criminal activities.

In comparison to traditional, formal youth organizations, juvenile gangs may appear disorganized. Research shows, however, that verbal rules, policies, customs, and hierarchies of command are rigidly observed within the gang. Thus, common values and attitudes exist. For example,

1. Gang membership is usually defined in socioeconomic, racial, and ethnic terms, and adolescents involved have similar backgrounds.

2. Gang members are distinguished by a distinctive and well-defined dress code. Violation of this code by members, or mimicking of the dress code by nongang members can result in ostracism, ridicule, physical abuse, and violence.

3. Leadership and seniority within the gang are defined by vested time in belonging to the gang, age, loyalty, and demonstrated delinquent cleverness (often related to drug dealing and other crimes).

4. Gang members use gang slang to ensure *camaraderie* and group loyalty.

Although a stable home life does not ensure that an adolescent won't become involved with gang-related activity, a strong family environment and guidance from respected parents and guardians are clearly deterrents (Lale 1992). Many gang members are children from dysfunctional, broken, or single-parent homes. Many parents are aware of their children's gang involvement but they lack the skill, confidence, and authority to deter the gang or curtail drug involvement of their teenagers. To make matters worse, ineffective parents often discourage or even interfere with involvement by outside authorities due to misdirected loyalty to their children and/or to avoid embarrassment to their family and community.

Because troubled adolescents are often estranged from their families, they are particularly influenced by their peer groups. These teenagers are most likely to associate with groups who have similar backgrounds and problems, and who make them feel accepted. Because of this vulnerability, adolescents may become involved with local gangs.

In summary, gangs offer

▲ Fellowship and camaraderie

▲ Identity and recognition

▲ Membership and belonging

▲ Family substitution and role models

▲ Security and protection

▲ Diversion and excitement

▲ Friendships and structure

▲ Money and financial gain for relatively little effort

▲ Ability to live the crazy life (*vida loca*) (Sanders 1994, 71)

Research shows that teenage gangs are becoming major players in the drug trade (Siegel and Senna 1997, 408). Two of the largest gangs in Los

Angeles, the Bloods and Crips, are examples of this trend. Estimated membership in these two gangs exceeds 20,000. In the past, organized crime families maintained a monopoly on the Asian heroin market. Today, youth gangs have entered this trade, for two reasons: (1) recent efforts and successes in prosecuting top mob bosses by criminal justice officials have created opportunities for new players, and (2) demand has grown for cocaine and synthetic drugs that are produced locally in many U.S. cities. In Los Angeles, drug-dealing gangs maintain "rock houses" or "stash houses" (where "crack" cocaine is used and sold) that serve as selling and distribution centers for hard drugs. The "crack" cocaine found in these "rock houses" is often supplied or run by gang members (Siegel and Senna 1997, 408).

To a lesser extent, other less violent gangs with smaller memberships are also involved in drug dealing. Recent research shows that the percentage of gangs involved in drug dealing may be exaggerated by the media. Citywide drug dealing by tightly organized "super" gangs appears to be on the decline and is being superseded by the activities of loosely organized, "neighborhood-based

groups" (Siegel and Senna 1997, 409). The main reason for this shift is that federal and state law enforcement of drug laws forced drug dealers to become " . . . flexible, informal organizations [rather] than rigid vertically organized gangs with . . . [leaders] . . . who are far removed from day-to-day action [on the street]" (Siegel and Senna 1997, 409).

Drug use and gang-related activities are often linked but the relationship is highly variable (Fagan 1990; Curry and Spergel 1997). Clearly, problems with drugs exist without gangs and gang-related activities can occur despite the absence of drugs; however, because they have common etiologies, their occurrences are often intertwined. Most adolescents who are associated with gangs are knowledgeable about drugs. Many gang members have experimented with drugs, much like other adolescents their age. However, the hard-core gang members are more likely to be engaged not only in drug use, but also in drug dealing as a source of revenue to support the gang-related activities (Lale 1992; Siegel and Senna 1997). The types of drugs used and their significance and functions vary from gang to gang

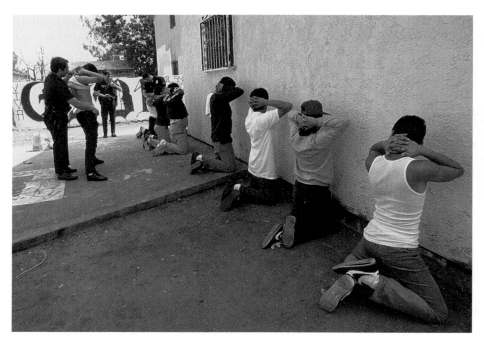

The very disturbing involvement of adolescents in gang organizations and violence is a social phenomenon that first became widely recognized in the 1950s and 1960s, but has increased dramatically in the 1990s.

(Fagan 1990; Siegel and Senna 1997). For example, many Latino gangs do not profit from drug trafficking but are primarily interested in using hardcore drugs such as heroin and PCP. In contrast, African-American gangs tend to be more interested in the illicit commercial value of drugs and often engage in dealing "crack" and other cocaine forms.

Prevention and Intervention

The most effective way to prevent adolescent gang involvement is to identify, at an early age, those children at risk and provide them with lifestyle alternatives. Important components of such strategies are as follows:

▲ Encourage parental awareness of gangs and teach parents how to address problems in their own families that encourage gang involvement.

▲ Provide teenagers with alternative participation in organizations or groups that satisfy their needs for camaraderie, participation, and emotional security in a constructive way. These groups can be organized around athletics, school activities, career development, or service rendering.

▲ Help children to develop coping skills that will enable them to deal with the frustration and stress in their personal lives.

▲ Educate children about gang-related problems and help them understand that, like drugs, gangs are the result of problems and are not the solutions.

Prevention and Treatment of Adolescent Drug Problems

As with most health problems, the sooner drug abuse is identified in the adolescent, the greater the likelihood that the problem can be resolved. It can be difficult to recognize signs of drug abuse in teenagers because their behavior can be so erratic and unpredictable even under the best of circumstances. In fact, many of the behavioral patterns that occur coincidentally with drug problems are also present when drugs are not a problem. How-

ever, frequent occurrence or clustering of these behaviors may indicate the presence of substance abuse. The behaviors that can be warning signs include the following (Archambault 1992):

▲ Abruptly changing the circle of friends

▲ Experiencing major mood swings

▲ Continually challenging rules and regulations

▲ Overreacting to frustrations

▲ Being particularly submissive to peer pressures

▲ Sleeping excessively

▲ Keeping very late hours

▲ Withdrawing from family involvement

▲ Letting personal hygiene deteriorate

▲ Becoming isolated

▲ Engaging in unusual selling of possessions

▲ Manipulating family members

▲ Becoming easily frustrated and angered

▲ Developing abusive behavior to other members of the family

▲ Frequently coming home at night "high"

Prevention of Adolescent Drug Abuse Logically, the best treatment for drug abuse is to prevent the problem from starting. This approach, referred to as **primary prevention,** has been typically viewed as total abstinence from drug use (see Chapter 17). Informational scare tactics are frequently used as a component of primary prevention strategies. These messages often consist of focusing on a dangerous (although in some cases, rare) potential side effect and presenting the warning against drug use in a graphic and frightening fashion. Although this approach may scare naive adolescents away from drugs, many adolescents today, especially if they are experienced, question the validity of the scare tactics and ignore the message.

Another form of primary prevention is to encourage adolescents to become involved in formal

> **primary prevention**
> prevention of any drug use

groups, such as structured clubs (such as athletic or fine arts teams at school) or organizations (such as outdoor or scouting groups), in order to reduce the likelihood of substance abuse (Howard 1992). Group memberships can help develop a sense of belonging and contributing to a productive, desirable objective. This involvement can also provide strength in resisting undesirable peer pressures. In contrast, belonging to informal groups such as gangs—groups with loose structures and ill-defined, often antisocial, objectives—can lead to participation in poorly controlled parties, excessive sexual involvement, and nonproductive activities. Adolescent members of such poorly defined organizations tend to drink alcohol at an earlier age and are more likely to use other substances of abuse (Howard 1992).

Some experts claim that primary prevention against drug use is unrealistic for many adolescents. They believe that no strategy is likely to stop adolescents from experimenting with alcohol or other drugs of abuse, especially if these substances are part of their home environment (for example, if alcohol or tobacco is routinely used) and are viewed as normal, acceptable, even expected, behavior (Howard 1992). For these adolescents, it is important to recognize when drug use moves from experimentation or a social exercise to early stages of a problem, and to prevent serious dependence from developing. This approach, referred to as **secondary prevention,** consists of (1) teaching adolescents about the early signs of abuse, (2) teaching adolescents how to assist peers and family members with drug problems, and (3) teaching them how and where help is available for people with drug problems (Archambault 1992). Regardless of the prevention approach used, adolescents need to understand that drugs are never the solution for emotional difficulties nor are they useful long-term coping techniques.

> **secondary prevention**
>
> prevention of casual drug use from progressing to dependence

Treatment of Adolescent Drug Abuse To provide appropriate treatment for adolescent drug abuse, the severity of the problem must be ascertained. The criteria for such assessments include

▲ Differentiating between abuse and normal adolescent experimentation with drugs

▲ Distinguishing between minor abuse and severe dependency on drugs

▲ Distinguishing between behavioral problems resulting from (1) general behavioral disorders, such as juvenile delinquency; (2) mental retardation; and (3) drugs of abuse

There is no single best approach for treating adolescent substance abuse. Occasionally the troubled adolescent is admitted to a clinic and treated on an inpatient basis. The inpatient approach is very expensive and creates a temporary "artificial" environment that may be of limited value in preparing adolescents for the problems to be faced in their real homes and neighborhoods. However, the advantage of an inpatient approach is that adolescents can be managed better and the behavior can be more tightly monitored and controlled (Hoshino 1992).

A more practical and routine treatment approach is to allow adolescents to remain in their natural environment and to provide the necessary life skills to be successful at home, in school, and in the community. For example, adolescents being treated for drug dependence should be helped with

▲ Schoolwork, so appropriate progress toward high school graduation occurs

▲ Career skills, so adolescents can become self-reliant and learn to care for themselves and others

▲ Family problems and learning to communicate and resolve conflicts.

If therapy is to be successful, it is important to improve the environment of the drug-abusing adolescent. This aspect of treatment includes dissociation of the adolescent from groups (such as gangs) or surroundings that encourage drug use and encourages association with healthy and supportive groups (such as a nurturing family) and experiences (such as athletics and school activities). Although desirable, such separation is not always possible, especially if the family and home environment are factors that encourage abuse; the likelihood of therapeutic success is substantially diminished under these circumstances.

Often therapeutic objectives are facilitated by positive reinforcement that encourages life changes that eliminate access to and use of drugs. This goal can frequently be achieved by association with peers who have similar drug and social problems, but are motivated to make positive changes in their life. Group sessions with such peers are held under the supervision of a trained therapist and consist of members sharing problems and solutions (Hoshino 1992).

Some other recent options include holistic therapies such as acupuncture, homeotherapy, massage therapy, aromatherapy, yoga, nutrition therapy, and many more options that were once marginalized by the medical profession (Apostolides 1996, 35).

Another useful approach is to discourage use of drugs by reducing their reinforcing effects. This result can sometimes be achieved by substituting a stronger positive or a negative reinforcer. For example, if adolescents use drugs because they believe these substances cause good feelings and help cope with emotional problems, it may be necessary to replace the drug behavior with other activities that make the adolescent feel good without the drug (such as participation in sports or recreational activities). Negative reinforcers, such as parental discovery and punishment or police apprehension, may discourage drug use by teenagers who are willing to conform and respect authorities. However, negative approaches are ineffective deterrents for nonconforming, rebellious adolescents. Negative reinforcers also do not tend to discourage adolescent use of substances that are more socially acceptable, such as alcohol, tobacco, and even marijuana (Howard 1992).

Regardless of the treatment approach, several basic objectives must be accomplished if therapy for adolescent drug dependence is to be successful (Daily 1992b). Adolescents must

▲ Realize that "drugs do not solve problems"— they only make the problems worse.

▲ Understand why they turned to drugs in the first place.

▲ Be convinced that abandoning drugs grants them greater independence and control over their own lives.

▲ Understand that drug abuse is a symptom of underlying problems that need to be resolved.

Summary of Adolescent Drug Abuse

Drug abuse by adolescents is particularly problematic in the United States. The teenage years are filled with experimentation, searching, confusion, rebellion, poor self-image, and insecurity. These attributes, if not managed properly, can cause inappropriate coping maneuvers and lead to problems such as drug dependence, gang involvement, violence, criminal behavior, and suicide. Clearly, early detection of severe underlying emotional problems and applications of effective early preventive therapy are important for proper management. Approaches to treatment of drug abuse problems must be individualized because each adolescent is a unique product of physiological, psychological, and environmental factors.

Almost as important as early intervention for adolescent drug abuse problems is recognizing when treatment is unnecessary. We should not be too quick to label all young drug users as antisocial and emotionally unstable. In most cases, teenagers who have used drugs are merely experimenting with new emotions or exercising their new-found freedom. In such situations, nonintervention is usually better than therapeutic meddling. For the most part, if adolescents are given the opportunity, they will work through their own feelings, conflicts, and attitudes about substance abuse, and will develop a responsible philosophy concerning the use of these drugs.

◢ Drug Use in College Student Subcultures

Chapter 9 includes a lengthy discussion of alcohol use and abuse by college students. This section will focus on college undergraduate use of alcohol not discussed in that chapter, with additional emphasis on the use and abuse of illicit drugs by college students currently attending institutions of higher education. Table 16.5 compares trends in the

Table 16.5 **Annual Prevalence for Various Types of Drugs, 1994: Full-time College Students Versus Others** (Among respondents one to four years beyond high school)

	Full-Time College Students	Others
Any illicit drug*	31.4%	32.5%
Any illicit drug*other than marijuana	12.2	16.4
Marijuana	29.3	29.2
Inhalants†	3.0	3.2
Hallucinogens	6.2	7.2
LSD	5.2	6.7
Cocaine	2.0	5.1
Crack	0.5	1.9
MDMA (Ecstasy)#	0.5	1.2
Heroin	0.1	0.2
Other opiates§	2.4	3.3
Stimulants, adjusted§,°	4.2	6.6
"Ice"#	0.8	0.9
Barbiturates§	1.2	3.2
Tranquilizers§	1.8	2.9
Alcohol	82.7	79.5
Cigarettes	37.6	47.1
Approximate weighted N =	(1410)	(1450)

(*) Use of "any illicit drug" includes use of marijuana, hallucinogens, cocaine, or heroin, or any use of other opiates, stimulants, barbiturates, or tranquilizers not under a doctor's orders.
(†) This drug was included in five of the six questionnaire forms. Total N in 1994 for college students is approximately 1175.
(#) This drug was included in two of six questionnaire forms. Total N in 1994 for college students is approximately 470.
(§) Only drug use that was not under a doctor's orders is included here.
(°) Based on the data from a revised question, which attempts to exclude the inappropriate reporting of nonprescription stimulants.
Source: National Institute on Drug Abuse (NIDA). "Annual Prevalence for Various Types of Drugs, 1994: Full-Time College Students vs. Others." Capsule 49. Rockville, MD: NIDA, 1996.

annual use of various licit and illicit drugs by full-time college students with trends in other groups. Overall, full-time college students were less likely to use any illicit types of drugs in 1994 when compared to others. Alcohol was the only licit drug that was more frequently used when compared to others (by 87.2% of full-time college students versus 79.5% of other college-age individuals).

Table 16.6 shows yearly trends in drug use among U.S. college students from 1980 through 1994. This population of students consisted of 1200 full-time college students one to four years past high school. The study measured the percentage who used licit and illicit drugs in the past 12 months before the survey was administered. The main finding was that, with exceptions for some slight increases in the use of marijuana/hashish since 1991 and in the use of hallucinogens and LSD since 1993, use of all licit and illicit drugs by college students steadily declined from 1980 through 1994.

Other Noteworthy Findings Regarding Drug Use by College Students

The following sections describe recent significant studies and findings regarding the use of drugs by college students.

Patterns of Alcohol and Other Drug Use Research reviewing recent literature on undergraduates' substance use and abuse, and the prevalence patterns of alcohol and other drug use, found that the most popular substance used by undergradu-

Table 16.6 **Trends in Annual Prevalence of Various Types of Drugs Among College Students One to Four Years Beyond High School** (Percentage who used in the past 12 months)*

The following table describes partial results from the nationwide survey of drug use among high school students and young adults, conducted annually for the National Institute on Drug Abuse by the University of Michigan Institute for Social Research. Each year since 1977, some participants from all previously graduated high school classes have been followed through the use of mailed questionnaires. The followup surveys include a sample of about 1200 full-time college students one to four years past high school.

	1980	1982	1984	1986	1988	1990	1992	1994
Approximate weighted N =	(1040)	(1150)	(1110)	(1190)	(1310)	(1400)	(1490)	(1410)
Any illicit drug	56.2%	49.5%	45.1%	45.0%	37.4%	33.3%	30.6%	31.4%
Any illicit drug other than marijuana	32.3	29.9	27.2	25.0	19.2	15.2	13.1	12.2
Marijuana/hashish	51.2	44.7	40.7	40.9	34.6	29.4	27.7	29.3
Inhalants	3.0	2.5	2.4	3.9	4.1	3.9	3.1	3.0
Hallucinogens	8.5	8.7	6.2	6.0	5.3	5.4	6.8	6.2
LSD	6.0	6.3	3.7	3.9	3.6	4.3	5.7	5.2
Cocaine	16.8	17.2	16.3	17.1	10.0	5.6	3.0	2.0
Crack	NA	NA	NA	1.3	1.4	0.6	0.4	0.5
MDMA (Ecstasy)	NA	NA	NA	NA	NA	2.3	2.0	0.5
Heroin	0.4	0.1	0.1	0.1	0.2	0.1	0.1	0.1
Other opiates	5.1	3.8	3.8	4.0	3.1	2.9	2.7	2.4
Stimulants	22.4	NA	NA	NA	NA	NA	NA	NA
Stimulants	NA	21.1	15.7	10.3	6.2	4.5	3.6	4.2
Crystal methamphetamine	NA	NA	NA	NA	NA	0.1	0.2	0.8
Sedatives	8.3	8.0	3.5	2.6	1.5	NA	NA	NA
Barbiturates	2.9	3.2	1.9	2.0	1.1	1.4	1.4	1.2
Methaqualone	7.2	6.6	2.5	1.2	0.5	NA	NA	NA
Tranquilizers	6.9	4.7	3.5	4.4	3.1	3.0	2.9	1.8
Alcohol	90.5	92.2	90.0	91.5	89.6	89.0	86.9	82.7

NA indicates data not available   (*) Indicates a percentage less than 0.05%.
Source: National Institute on Drug Abuse (NIDA). *Trends in Drug Use Among College Students.* NCADI: NIDA Capsule—Monitoring the Future Study. Rockville, MD: NIDA, 1997. Available from //www.health.org/pubs/caps/NCCollegeTrends.html

ates is alcohol, which was used by about 90% of students at least once a year. Heavy alcohol use, which includes binge drinking, ranged from 20% to 40% in this group. Other results showed that alcohol use was associated with serious and acute problems (such as alcoholism, poor academic performance, drinking and driving, and criminal behavior). While overall rates of illicit drug use (other than marijuana) have been declining for undergraduates (see Table 16.6), this study found high rates of other licit and illicit drug use (Prendergast 1994).

Predicting Drug Use for First-Year College Students The best predictor of drug use for first-year college students was drug use during a typical month in the senior year of high school. Overall, college students responding to a questionnaire were found to use marijuana less frequently than they did in high school. Further, alcohol use increased early in the college years. While the frequency of alcohol use increased, however, the number of times that college students got drunk did not rise. Most of these students found new friends in college with whom they got drunk.

Alcohol and drug use depended on the choice of new college friends (Leibsohn 1994).

Dormitory for Drug-Addicted Students To date, Rutgers University is the only university with a dormitory for students who are recuperating addicts and who want to stay away from the alcohol-charged atmosphere of conventional dormitories. The dormitory at Rutgers was opened on the university campus in 1988 with strict rules and careful management (Witham 1995, A33).

Students Using Illicit Drugs In a random survey of illicit drug use conducted at a private university in 1990 whose results were compared with those from a similar survey conducted in 1986 (Cuomo et al. 1994), the following findings were made:

▲ Cocaine use declined from 39% of students in 1986 to 21% in 1990.

▲ Use of traditional amphetamines declined from 22% to 12%.

▲ No significant differences were found in the use of marijuana (68% in 1986 and 64% in 1990) or in the use of LSD (14% in 1986 and 17% in 1990).

▲ Use of mescaline/psilocybin increased from 8% of students to 24%.

▲ Use of MDMA (Ecstasy) increased from 16% to 24%.

▲ According to the 1990 study, mescaline/psilocybin and MDMA were more likely than other drugs to have been used first during the students' college years.

Increasing Popularity of Softer Drugs Marijuana and psilocybin mushrooms are two types of illicit recreational drugs whose popularity appeared to be growing in the 1990s. Referred to as "soft drugs," these substances are commonly used on most college campuses (Ravid 1995, 99).

Drug Use Abroad With regard to alcohol and drug use in the United Kingdom, recent research indicates that drug and alcohol consumption among college students in Great Britain is rising. Results from a survey of 3075 second-year university students (Webb et al. 1996) indicated that:

▲ Eleven percent of the students were nondrinkers.

▲ Cannabis and other illegal drugs were used regularly, often in combination, and mostly by white students.

▲ LSD was the most popular drug, followed by amphetamines, Ecstasy, and amyl/butyl nitrates.

▲ The primary reason for drug use was reportedly pleasure rather than social pressure or stress.

Steroid Usage Patterns With regard to undergraduate steroid users, a study of 58,625 college students from 78 colleges and universities in the United States (Meilman et al. 1995) found that:

▲ Steroid users consumed dramatically more alcohol and demonstrated higher rates of binge drinking than other students.

▲ A significantly higher percentage of steroid users than nonusers reported using tobacco, marijuana, cocaine, amphetamines, sedatives, hallucinogens, opiates, inhalants, and designer drugs.

▲ A higher percentage of steroid users than nonusers reported experiencing negative consequences as a result of substance abuse. Such negative consequences included arrest, public intoxication, driving under the influence, community service, and disciplinary actions by university officials.

▲ A greater percentage of steroid users than nonusers reported family histories of alcohol abuse and other drugs.

Rohypnol and Date Rape **Rohypnol,** also known as the date-rape drug, is currently circulating on many college campuses. The small white pills are slipped into young women's drinks at college parties, causing them to black out and forget what happens to them (including rape). A minority of undergraduates also use the drug

Rohypnol

currently known as the date rape drug, used on many college campuses to intensify the effects of marijuana and alcohol. One problem with identifying whether this drug has been given to an unwilling recipient is that Rohypnol can be detected only within 60 hours after ingestion (Lively 1996, A29).

"Smart Drugs" "Smart drugs" are a class of legally available pharmaceuticals used to treat diseases associated with mental decline or dysfunction. These agents are often referred to as **nootropic drugs.** In one study, drug use was compared to steroid users in a student population of 193 college students (Canterbury and Lloyd 1994). Results showed that 5% of the males reported casual use of nootropic drugs to increase their intelligence, enhance their memory, and make them smarter. College student usage rates were approximated at 3%.

> **nootropic drugs**
>
> also known as "smart drugs" that are legally available and used to remedy mental decline or dysfunction

Summary of Drug Use in College Student Subcultures

In summarizing these research studies regarding drug use and college students, it appears that

▲ Alcohol continues to be the most widely used and abused drug, causing a multitude of personal, social, health, academic, and legal problems (also see Chapters 8 and 9).

▲ In most cases, recreational drug use does not begin in college but has already become established in high school.

▲ Attempts to prevent alcohol abuse include designating college dormitories as "off limits" to drug use.

▲ "Softer" illicit drugs, such as marijuana and psilocybin mushrooms, remain popular on most college campuses in the 1990s despite legal warnings and penalties (also see Chapter 3).

▲ Drug use on college campuses in some foreign countries remains as problematic as the drug use on college campuses in the United States.

▲ Steroid users have a tendency to abuse other licit and illicit drugs.

▲ "Smart drugs," also known as nootropic drugs, and the sedative Rohypnol (known as the "date-rape drug") are currently being used on a number of college campuses.

▲ Drug Use in HIV-Positive Subcultures

The first described case of acquired immunodeficiency syndrome (AIDS) occurred in 1981. As of June 1994, the CDC reported a cumulative 401,749 AIDS cases, with 240,323 deaths from this cause in the United States. The Centers for Disease Control and Prevention (CDC) of the U.S. Public Health Service estimates that approximately 1 million people are infected with HIV in the United States, and most are expected to develop AIDS within 10 to 15 years.

Through June 1996, the CDC had received reports of 548,102 men, women, and children with AIDS, and 343,000 deaths among these persons. The cumulative reported AIDS cases included (CDC 1996)

▲ 540,806 adolescents and adults

▲ 452,152 men

▲ 78,654 women

▲ 7,296 children less than 13 years of age

In recent years, the incidence of AIDS has been increasing more rapidly among women than men. AIDS is now the fourth leading cause of death among women aged 25 to 44 in the United States. More than three-fourths (77%) of the female AIDS cases occurred among African-American and Hispanic women, and infection rates for black and Hispanic women were 16 times those for white women (CDC 1996). Worldwide, 73 women are infected with HIV for every 100 infected men.

In the early stages of the U.S. epidemic, most AIDS cases occurred in California and New York and were seen almost exclusively in homosexual and bisexual men. The pattern of occurrence has since changed, however. For example, AIDS now occurs everywhere. In particular, the incidence of HIV infection is greater with intravenous (IV) drug users. Approximately 30% of all AIDS patients are IV drug users (Siegal et al. 1995, 105), and these people represent the second largest group at risk for the deadly AIDS disease (Pietroski 1993; Swan 1995).

On a national scale, the spread of AIDS is more prevalent in the following metropolitan areas: San Francisco (213 cases per 100,000 population), New York City (160), and Miami (141.9). These cities have infection rates that are 8 to 15 times higher than those in cities such as Cincinnati (13.7), Detroit (15.2), and Pittsburgh (11.2) (CDC 1995).

Nature of HIV Infection and Related Symptoms

AIDS is caused by the human immunodeficiency virus (HIV). "An HIV-infected individual may not manifest symptoms of AIDS for as many as 10 to 20 years after the initial infection" (Edlin et al. 1997, 193). While the HIV-infected individual may experience no symptoms, he or she is highly contagious and able to infect others.

After an individual has become infected, he or she may have a brief flu-like illness usually 6 to 12 weeks after exposure to the virus. It is not known what determines the length of the latency period, when symptoms are not present. The asymptomatic period eventually ends, however, and signs of immune disorder appear. Initial symptoms of this disease include night-sweats, swollen lymph glands, fever, and/or headaches.

Progression of the disease brings weight loss, infections in the throat ("thrush") and skin (shingles), and other, opportunistic infections and/or cancer (for example, Kaposis Sarcoma). Basically, the immune systems of HIV-positive individuals are compromised. The damage to the immune system appears to result from the destruction of important immune cells called CD4+ helper T-lymphocytes and macrophages (see Figure 16.2). Because these immune cells are crucial in identifying and eliminating infection-causing microorganisms, such as bacteria, fungi, and viruses, their deficiency substantially increases the likelihood and severity of infectious diseases.

With the destruction of the immune cells, infections become increasingly difficult to control with antibacterial (for example, antibiotics), antifungal, and antiviral drugs; consequently, severe opportunistic infections, such as pneumonia, meningitis, hepatitis, and tuberculosis, can occur and eventually lead to death (Pietroski 1993). The likelihood of introducing these opportunistic infections in the body increases in patients who are IV drug users because they often share injection equipment, such as needles and syringes, that are contaminated with disease-causing microorganisms.

Protease Inhibitors

In 1996, the most promising drug treatment for combating the HIV virus since it was first identified in 1981 surfaced. Prior to the discovery of **protease inhibitors,** the only clinically supported drug treatment that could temporarily slow down the spread of HIV was AZT. When combined with AZT, protease inhibitors result in miraculous remissions of desperately ill AIDS patients (Crowley 1996, 68).

> **protease inhibitors**
>
> a recently discovered class of drugs used to treat HIV-infected individuals

Further, it appears that "newly infected patients are holding HIV at exceedingly low levels in their bloodstreams" (Crowley 1996).

The introduction of protease inhibitors began with saquinavir (brand name Invirase), followed by indinavir (Crixivan), and ritonavir (Norvir). "Numerous studies have now shown that when infected people combine one of the new drugs with a couple of Rt [reverse transcriptase] inhibitors [typically AZT and 3TC, another newly discovered inhibitor], the amount of virus in their blood drops precipitously—often to undetectable levels" (Crowley 1996, 69). While this drug combination does not rid the body of infected cells, current results indicate that HIV infections " . . . could become as manageable as diabetes" (Crowley 1996, 69). Largely because this new drug combination (sometimes referred to as "the cocktail") has not had the time to be thoroughly tested, some initial warnings for recipients include the possibility that this treatment program can be ineffective and toxic to some users. Side effects can include diarrhea, bone-marrow suppression, and an inability to tolerate the drugs. To date, the likelihood

Figure 16.2

Disrupting the Assembly Line
HIV survives by invading white blood cells and turning them into virus factories. The process involves several steps, and each offers a potential target for therapy. This diagram shows how HIV does its work, and how antiviral drugs do theirs.

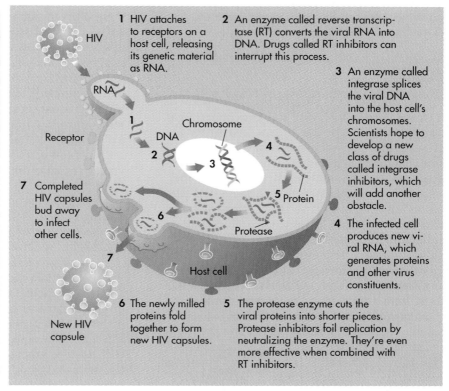

1 HIV attaches to receptors on a host cell, releasing its genetic material as RNA.

2 An enzyme called reverse transcriptase (RT) converts the viral RNA into DNA. Drugs called RT inhibitors can interrupt this process.

3 An enzyme called integrase splices the viral DNA into the host cell's chromosomes. Scientists hope to develop a new class of drugs called integrase inhibitors, which will add another obstacle.

4 The infected cell produces new viral RNA, which generates proteins and other virus constituents.

5 The protease enzyme cuts the viral proteins into shorter pieces. Protease inhibitors foil replication by neutralizing the enzyme. They're even more effective when combined with RT inhibitors.

6 The newly milled proteins fold together to form new HIV capsules.

7 Completed HIV capsules bud away to infect other cells.

Source: G. Crowley. "Targeting a Deadly Scrap of Genetic Code." Newsweek (2 December 1996): 69.

of experiencing some of these side effects has proved difficult to predict; more thorough controlled testing will clarify this issue.

Another serious problem is the prohibitive cost of these drugs. Many health insurance companies are actively issuing restrictive amendments on their policies that cap reimbursement for such expensive drug therapies. Infected individuals with extensive debt obligations and patients without health insurance are therefore unable to afford this latest drug therapy.

In the coming years, controversy is likely to continue over how to pay for the possible promise of being spared the ravages of HIV symptoms when the cure is touted as cost-prohibitive for health insurance companies. Debate is also likely regarding how to provide such drug therapy for HIV-infected individuals who are unable to pay for these drug regimens.

In summary, a current successful prognosis for HIV infection and AIDS relies on three factors: (1)

initiation of this drug regimen as soon as possible after the patient has been diagnosed as HIV-positive, which provides maximum suppression of the HIV virus; (2) strict adherence to ingesting AZT with two other protease inhibitor-type drugs on a daily basis without deviation (missing one of three required doses per day can accelerate the spread of HIV more aggressively than if the illness went untreated); and (3) maintenance of a healthy diet without drug use and abuse so as to avoid taxing the immune system when it is under attack with the virus (this step includes complete elimination of tobacco, alcohol, marijuana, and any other licit and illicit nonprescription drugs).

At the time of this writing, our ability to successfully suppress the spread of HIV over the long run remains undetermined. Short-term results since the cocktail therapy was first tried in 1996 shows that it can minimize the spread of HIV. Even in patients displaying accelerated or "full blown" symptoms of AIDS, combining protease inhibitors with AZT appears to suppress the advancement of this disease in a significant number of patients devastated by this disease.

Diagnosis

It is crucial that HIV-infected people be aware of their condition to avoid activities that might transmit the infection to others. Testing for the presence of infection has been available since 1985 and is done by determining whether the body is producing antibodies against the HIV. Further, since 1996, newspaper, magazine, radio, and television ads have been advertising a take-at-home HIV antibody test. The presence of these specific antibodies indicates HIV infection. If an individual is infected, it requires 6 to 12 weeks after the HIV exposure before the body produces enough antibodies to be detected in currently available tests. If the antibody is not present within six months after HIV exposure, infection is likely to have not occurred (Pietroski 1993).

Although the tests for HIV infection are reliable, false negatives (that is, the test says no HIV is present even though the individual is infected) and false positives (that is, the test says the individual is infected even though no HIV is present) occur in a small percentage of individuals (1 out of 30,000 tests) tested for antibodies. Because testing positive for HIV is currently perceived as eventually life-threatening and is a highly emotional diagnosis, great effort is made to ensure confidentiality of the test results. The blood specimens to be tested are coded, and the personnel conducting the tests are not allowed to divulge the results. The issue of confidentiality is very controversial, however. It is often difficult to decide who has the right to know when HIV has been detected. People who should be tested for HIV infection include individuals who participate in high-risk activities. (Specific high-risk categories are listed in the next section.)

Who Gets AIDS?

Although anyone can become infected with HIV, its routes of transmission are limited to blood, semen, vaginal fluid, and possibly some other body fluids (Grinspoon 1994). HIV is a virus that is not likely to survive outside of the body. Consequently, it is not spread by casual contact at work or school, such as by shaking hands, touching, hugging, or kissing. In addition, it is not spread through food or water, by sharing cups or glasses, by coughing and sneezing, or by using common toilets. It is not spread by mosquitoes or other insects. Thus, infection cannot occur through ordinary social contact (Goldfinger 1994). The transmission of HIV occurs most often through sexual contact; the next most likely means of transmission is by exposure to contaminated blood or blood products, usually by drug addicts sharing IV needles. HIV can also be passed from an infected mother to a child either prenatally or possibly by breastfeeding (Pietroski 1993).

Because of these limited routes of HIV transmission, the following populations are at greatest risk for contracting AIDS: (1) men with a history of homosexual or bisexual activity; (2) IV drug users and their sexual partners; (3) infants born to HIV-infected women (in approximately 25% of all HIV-positive mothers); and (4) people receiving contaminated blood products, such as for transfusions or treatment of blood disorders, although blood banks have greatly improved the screening of their blood supplies in the last five years. (See Figure 16.3 for a detailed breakdown of categories of U.S. AIDS cases by type of HIV exposure.)

Adolescents and AIDS Although people of all ages can contract AIDS, a particularly alarming trend is the high rate of HIV infection in the adolescent population. More than 75,000 adolescents in the United States have tested positive for the presence of HIV, and half of the 14 million people worldwide who are HIV-positive became infected between the ages of 15 and 24 years. Furthermore, female adolescents are now being infected at higher rates than males, and in some regions of the United States at rates higher than adults (Hein et al. 1995, 96).

As of March 1993, there had been 12,116 reported cases of AIDS among young people 13 to 24 years of age (Hein et al. 1995, 96). Research shows that three of the principal ways adolescents become infected with HIV are as follows: (1) high-risk sexual activity (unprotected sexual inter-

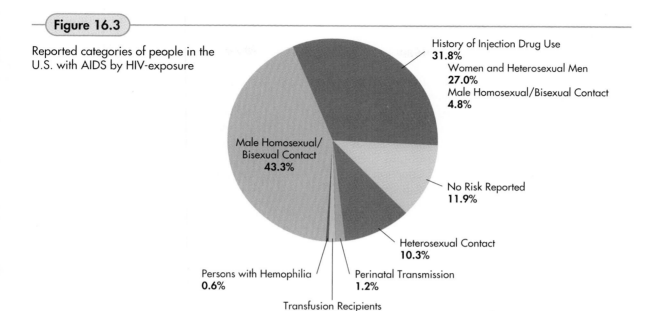

Figure 16.3

Reported categories of people in the U.S. with AIDS by HIV-exposure

History of Injection Drug Use
31.8%
Women and Heterosexual Men
27.0%
Male Homosexual/Bisexual Contact
4.8%

Male Homosexual/
Bisexual Contact
43.3%

No Risk Reported
11.9%

Heterosexual Contact
10.3%

Persons with Hemophilia
0.6%

Perinatal Transmission
1.2%

Transfusion Recipients
1.0%

Source: Centers for Disease Control and Prevention (CDC). *Morbidity and Mortality Weekly Report* 44, no. 4 (February 3, 1995). Reported U.S. AIDS Cases by HIV-Exposure Category, 1994

course is reported by over half of adolescents by the age of 19 years); (2) injection of substances of abuse; and (3) sex with multiple partners (Schafer et al. 1993). Clearly, young people must be better educated about HIV, its transmission, and potential consequences before this infection becomes disastrous to adolescents.

AIDS and Drugs of Abuse

During the past few years, the AIDS epidemic has become closely associated with drug abuse problems. Individuals addicted to illicit drugs are currently the second largest risk group for contracting AIDS (Booth et al. 1993; Grinspoon 1994; Swan 1995). AIDS in women is particularly linked to drug abuse. Nearly 70% of the female AIDS victims are infected because of IV drug use by themselves or by a sexual partner (Glave 1994). Several reasons account for the high incidence of this deadly infection in the drug-abusing population:

Intravenous Drugs Intravenous drug use has become the most important factor in the spread of AIDS in the United States. One-third of the AIDS cases reported in the United States by late 1993 were associated with injecting cocaine, heroin, or both (Landau 1994; Swan 1995). Intravenous drug use is often undertaken with little regard to hygiene, and injection paraphernalia such as needles, syringes, and cotton are frequently shared with other drug addicts (Millstein 1993). Sharing HIV-contaminated injection equipment can result in the transmission of, and infection by, this virus. The likelihood of an intravenous drug user contracting AIDS is directly correlated with (a) the frequency of drug injections, (b) the number of partners with whom injection equipment is shared, (c) the frequency of needle sharing, and (d) the frequency of injections in locations of high AIDS infection rates, such as in shooting galleries or crack houses (Booth et al. 1993).

Crack Use of drugs such as crack (Ciba Foundation 1992) and alcohol (Colthurst 1993) tends to compromise judgment and encourage high-risk activities such as IV drug use or sexual risk taking (Beard and Kunsman 1993). In particular, the use of crack has been associated with HIV infection. Crack addicts often exchange sex for drugs or money to purchase drugs (Mathias 1993). These dangerous activities frequently occur in populations with a high rate of HIV infection (Ciba Foundation 1992). Once infected, almost half of crack users continue to use sex to obtain their drugs and become a source of HIV infection for others (Diaz and Chu 1993). In general, because of the effects of cocaine on sexual activity, crack smokers also have a greater risk for HIV infection because they tend to have many sex partners during cocaine binges and frequently participate in unprotected sexual behaviors (Booth et al. 1993).

What to Do About HIV and AIDS

What can I do about being HIV-positive? I was diagnosed three years ago, and so far I am basically okay. I have started taking medication to slow down the rate of infection, but one never knows when the first symptoms suddenly pop up. My lover is clear of the infection and we are careful—usually. I am worried about my condition, but nothing can be done about it. Life is full of good luck and bad luck; so far I have been spared. Regarding tomorrow, who knows.

From Venturelli's research files, interview with a 32-year-old male hospital administrator, October 10, 1996

The discovery and use of protease inhibitors in 1996 represents the most promising treatment for combating the HIV virus since it was first identified in 1981. Although protease inhibitors do not appear to completely rid the body of HIV antibodies, this category of drugs is usually successful in holding the HIV virus at low levels in the bloodstream. The current lack of a permanent cure makes prevention the most important element in dealing with the AIDS problem. Strategies for preventing HIV can be classified into two main categories:

▲ People should be encouraged to adopt safer sexual behavior. Some of the steps to help achieve this end include (1) avoiding multiple sex partners, especially if they are strangers or only casual acquaintances; (2) avoiding risk-taking sexual behavior, which may allow HIV transmission, such as unprotected vaginal or anal intercourse; and (3) encouraging individuals who choose to continue high-risk sexual behaviors to use a condom or insist that the sexual partner use a condom (Merson 1993).

▲ Drug abusers should be educated about their risk of contracting AIDS. They should be encouraged to reduce their risk by (1) abstaining from use of drugs by injection; (2) not sharing injection paraphernalia or always using clean needles (if available through "needle exchange programs"); (3) not sharing drugs with groups with high rates of HIV infection such as shooting galleries or crack houses; and (4) disinfecting the equipment (cleaning and boiling equipment for at least 15 minutes) between uses if they continue to share injection equipment (Millstein 1993).

One of the major difficulties in controlling the AIDS epidemic is to identify where preventive efforts should be focused. Because of limited resources, it is impossible to personally educate everyone in this country about HIV and AIDS. Consequently, our most intense efforts must be targeted at populations and neighborhoods with particularly high HIV infection rates. The National Research Council has declared that, although anyone can be a victim of AIDS, a handful of neighborhoods have been devastated by this infection while most of the nation remains relatively unscathed (Kolata 1993). It has been speculated that some 25–30 large neighborhoods in the United States fuel the AIDS epidemic throughout the country; if the HIV infection could be controlled in these areas, the national epidemic would diminish significantly. Because of this hypothesis, it has been proposed that AIDS prevention efforts particularly be focused on gay men and IV drug users who have multiple sex partners in the high-density AIDS neighborhoods found in cities such as New York, New York; Memphis, Tennessee;

Miami and Ft. Lauderdale, Florida; Jersey City, New Jersey; San Francisco, California; Ann Arbor, Michigan; and Washington, D.C. (available gopher.//cdenac.org:72/11/4/Midyear 96). Even with this focused approach, no one should be fooled into thinking that the AIDS problem will be eliminated. Each person must become educated about this deadly disease and take steps to avoid HIV exposure.

◢ Promoting Drug Use in the Subculture of the Entertainment Industry and a New Media Subculture

Drug use has a tendency to be fueled by popular culture. In this section we discuss one important *genre* of popular culture—rock music. We conclude with a new media subculture that promotes drug use knowledge.

At the Lollapalooza music festival last July in Great Woods, Massachusetts, the mostly white, suburban teen crowd cheered wildly when rap group Cypress Hill pushed a six-foot-tall "bong," or water pipe, onstage. The group sold five million copies of its first two albums, one of which included songs titled "Legalize It," "Hits from the Bong," and "I Wanna Get High." (Winters 1997, 41)

In a research study for Columbia's Center on Addiction and Substance Abuse, 76% of 12–17-year-olds indicated that the entertainment industry encourages illegal drug use. One 16-year-old daily marijuana user said, "All I know is that almost every song you listen to says something about [drug use]. It puts it into your mind constantly. . . . When you see the celebrities doing it, it makes it seem okay" (Winters 1997, 41).

Recently, the rock and rap music industries have experienced a heroin epidemic. Though many other rock stars before Kurt Cobain have used and abused drugs, Cobain's struggle with heroin and his 1994 suicide appear to have glamorized the use of this drug. "The number of top alternative bands that have been linked to heroin through a member's overdose, arrest, admitted use, or recovery is staggering: Nirvana, Hole, Smashing Pumpkins, Everclear, Blind Melon,

Skinny Puppy, 7 Year Bitch, Red Hot Chili Peppers, Stone Temple Pilots, Breeders, Alice in Chains, Sublime, Sex Pistols, Porno for Pyros, and Depeche Mode. Together these bands have sold more than 60 million albums—that's a heck of a lot of white, middle-class kids in the heartland" (Schoemer 1996). Currently, factions in the music industry are attempting to curtail heroin use by rock stars. This "house cleaning" appears to have been prompted by Cobain's death.

What effect has the past glamour bestowed on serious drug use had on the young, who often memorize rock music that glorifies illicit drugs? Among eighth-graders who have used drugs in their lifetime, crack use has increased 108% from 1991 to 1995, from 1.3% of these youths in 1991 to 2.3% in 1995; marijuana use has increased from 10.2% of these children in 1991 to 19.9%, a 95% increase; and cocaine use has increased from 2.3% of this group in 1991 to 4.2% in 1995, an 83% increase. While the percentage using such drugs remains low in terms of the overall population, the fact that these percentages nearly doubled from 1991 to 1995 is alarming, as are the role models that these children chose to emulate. As indicated in a *Newsweek* article in 1996, "[A]fter a series of drug deaths, the music world wants to clear up its act. But [the larger question remains]—are teen fans still falling under the influence?" (Schoemer 1996, 50).

A New Media Subculture?

Pro-drug messages and detailed information are readily available over the recently created Internet. The Internet maintains a unique subculture of drug enthusiasts. Drug use information found in the source includes how to roll super joints, bake marijuana-laced brownies, and grow "magic" psilocybin mushrooms; where to purchase the latest equipment for indoor growing of marijuana; and where to obtain catalogs that offer drug paraphernalia for sale. Similarly, magazines such as *High Times* and *Hemp Times* claim growing numbers of subscribers. Such magazines devote most of their articles, features, advice columns, hemp festival information, and advertisements to the pleasures of drug consumption.

EXERCISES FOR THE WEB

Exercise 1: Steroids

This page focuses on information regarding anabolic steroids. Five types of steroids are described as well as what results a person should expect to see from using a particular steroid and the effects the drug has on one's body.

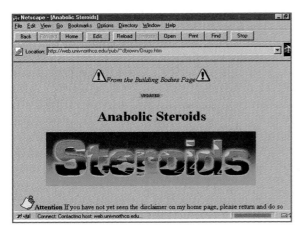

Exercise 2: Youth Drinking

A major concern among every community in the U.S. is underage drinking. A city in Wisconsin attempted a new approach to dealing with this problem and is reported by the Wisconsin Clearinghouse on Prevention Resources web page.

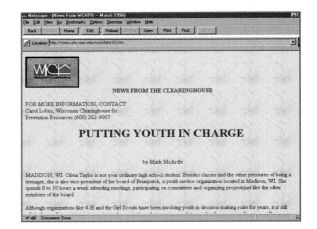

Exercise 3: AL-ANON

Alcoholism affects more than just the alcoholic. AL-ANON (and ALATEEN for younger members) is a worldwide organization that offers a self-help recovery program for families and friends of alcoholics, whether or not the alcoholic seeks help or even recognizes the existence of a drinking problem.

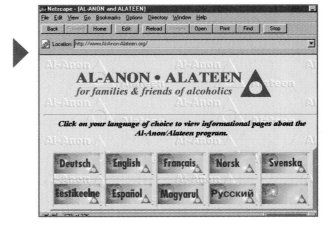

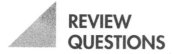

REVIEW QUESTIONS

1. What factors encourage drug use by athletes?

2. What are the principal drugs abused by athletes?

3. How are anabolic steroids used, and what are their principal effects and side effects?

4. Why are CNS stimulants used by athletes?

5. Do you think that drug testing is an effective deterrent to drug misuse in sports?

6. What type of penalties do you think should be used against athletes who abuse drugs?

7. Describe three gender differences in use patterns for drugs of abuse. Explain why these differences occur.

8. Why do you think that in the past most drug abuse research did not study female populations? Are any of these reasons justified?

9. What factors in the unique female roles encourage the use of substances of abuse?

10. What factors discourage drug-dependent women from seeking treatment?

11. Why does alcohol consumption tend to cause greater physiological damage in females than in males?

12. What are some important factors that should be considered when designing drug dependence treatment and prevention programs for women?

13. Why are adolescents especially vulnerable to drug abuse problems?

14. What types of parents are most likely to have children who develop drug abuse problems?

15. Which substances of abuse are most likely to be used by adolescents, and which are most likely to be used frequently?

16. How do adolescent drug abuse patterns differ from those in adults?

17. What coincidental problems are likely to be associated with adolescent drug abuse? Why?

18. In what way are drugs of abuse associated with juvenile gang activity?

19. Should all adolescents who use drugs of abuse be treated for drug dependence? Explain your answer.

20. Why are users of illicit drugs currently the second largest risk group for contracting AIDS?

21. What are the major preventive strategies to protect against contracting AIDS?

22. Do you think that it is realistic to expect drug abusers to change their habits in order to prevent the spread of AIDS? Why or why not?

23. How are youth affected by the current increases in heroin use in the entertainment industry? Explain your response.

24. Have the drug habits of anyone in the entertainment industry influenced your like or dislike of their celebrity status? Explain your answer.

KEY TERMS

subculture
ergogenic
androgens
stacking
cycling
plateauing
human growth factor (HGF)
human growth hormone (HGH)
genitourinary
intragang
intergang
primary prevention
secondary prevention
Rohypnol
protease inhibitors

SUMMARY

1 The most common drugs abused by athletes are the ergogenic (performance-enhancing) substances. They include the anabolic steroids, for building muscle mass and strength, and the CNS stimulants, to achieve energy, quickness, and endurance.

2 Drug testing is conducted for most athletic competitions and usually includes screens for steroids and stimulants. However, some performance-enhancing drugs, such as erythropoietin and human growth factor, are undetectable. Some athletes go to great lengths to avoid detection by these drug tests.

3 Most drugs of abuse are used more frequently by males than females. In addition, men tend to have a higher prevalence for intense drug use. An exception to this trend is the higher daily use of cigarettes by female college students than their male counterparts.

4 Because of their traditional domestic roles, women who abuse drugs are generally viewed by society less tolerantly than men. Many women also are socioeconomically disadvantaged, which creates frustrations and stress that predispose them to drug abuse. Finally, a woman's unique function in the family can create special pressures that lead to poor coping strategies such as drug dependence.

5 Drug treatment programs for women should accommodate their ongoing family responsibilities, be sensitive to their unique health needs, and provide special training for employment, coping, and the development of independence.

6 Most adolescents who use substances of abuse do so with normal psychosocial development and will not develop problematic dependence on these drugs. The adolescent users who have difficulty with drugs often lack coping skills to deal with their problems, have dysfunctional families, possess poor self-images, and/or feel socially and emotionally insecure.

7 Parents who are most likely to foster drug-abusing children are (a) drug abusers themselves, (b) excessively rigid and condemning, (c) overly demanding, (d) overly protective, (e) overwhelmed with their own personal conflicts, or

(f) unable to communicate effectively with their children.

8 The substances adolescents are most likely to abuse are alcohol, cigarettes, inhalants, marijuana, and prescription stimulants. High-frequency use is most likely to occur with cigarettes, alcohol, and marijuana.

9 Similar problems lead to both drug abuse problems and gang involvement. Gangs often use drug dealing as a means of obtaining money. Adolescent involvement in drugs and gangs can be discouraged by increasing parental awareness of the problem, providing alternative activities that help develop coping skills, and educating children about gang-related problems.

10 Two interesting findings from research regarding drug use by college student subcultures are that: (a) the best predictor of drug use for first-year college students is drug use during a typical month in the senior year of high school, and (b) recreational drug use does not begin in college but has already been established in high school. *Smart drugs,* also known as *nootropic drugs,* and the sedative *Rohypnol* (known as the "date-rape drug") are currently being used on a number of college campuses.

11 Next to homosexual men, individuals who are addicted to illicit drugs are the second largest risk group for contracting AIDS. This risk is due to sharing of blood-contaminated needles and syringes and increased involvement in sexual risk taking because of the effects of drugs or in payment for drugs.

12 Major strategies to prevent contracting HIV include (a) safer sexual behavior, (b) avoiding use of contaminated drug paraphernalia, (c) avoiding use of IV drugs, and (d) avoiding use of drugs in groups with high rates of HIV infection.

13 The music industry has been setting up drug-using celebrities as teen role models. The message conveyed by much of the music and by many bands is that drug use is acceptable. After several drug-related deaths of celebrities over the past few years, the industry is working on changing such perceptions.

14 New media influences contribute to drug use. The Internet is considered to be the latest source of information where knowledge about use of illicit drugs is burgeoning.

REFERENCES

Alexander, L. and J. LaRosa *New Dimensions in Women's Health.* Boston: Jones and Bartlett, 1994a.

"A Moving Target: CDC Still Trying to Eliminate HIV-I Prevalence." *Journal of NIH Research* 6 (June 1994): 25, 26.

Apostolides, M. "How to Quit the Holistic Way." *Psychology Today* 29 (September/October 1996): 30–43, 75–6.

Archambault, D. "Adolescence, a Physiological, Cultural and Psychological No Man's Land." In *Adolescent Substance Abuse, Etiology, Treatment and Prevention,* edited by G. Lawson and A. Lawson, 11–28. Gaithersburg, MD: Aspen, 1992.

Associated Press. "Shocking Death of Kordic Spurs NHL President to Clamp Down on Use of Anabolic Steroids." *Salt Lake Tribune* 244 (11 August 1992): C-4.

Bahr, S. J., A. C. Marcos, and S. L. Maughan. "Family, Educational and Peer Influences on Alcohol Use of Female and Male Adolescents." *Journal of Studies on Alcohol* 56 (1995): 457–69.

Beard, B., and V. Kunsman. "A Cause for Concern: Alcohol-Induced Risky Sex on College Campuses." *Prevention Pipeline* 6 (September–October 1993): 24.

Bell, J. "Athletes' Use and Abuse of Drugs." *The Physician and Sports Medicine* 15 (March 1987): 99–108.

Beschner, G., and A. Friedman. "Treatment of Adolescent Drug Abusers." *International Journal of the Addictions* 20 (1985): 977–993.

Black, M. M., P. Nair, C. Kight, R. Wachtel, P. Roby, and M. Schuler. "Parenting and Early Development Among Children of Drug-Abusing Women: Effects of Home Intervention." *Pediatrics* 94 (October 1994): 440–448.

"Bodybuilding Drug Yields 'High.'" *Pharmacy Times* (June 1992): 14.

Booth, R., J. Watters, and D. Chitwood. "HIV Risk-Related Sex Behaviors Among Injection Drug Users, Crack Smokers, and Injection Drug Users Who Smoke Crack." *American Journal of Public Health* 83 (1993): 1144–8.

Brady, K., D. Grice, L. Dustan, and C. Randall. "Gender Differences in Substances Use Disorders." *American Journal of Psychiatry* 150 (November 1993): 1707–11.

Buckstein, D., D. Brent, J. Perper, G. Moritz, M. Baugher, J. Schweers, C. Roth, and L. Balach. "Risk Factors for Completed Suicide Among Adolescents with a Lifetime History of Substance Abuse: A Case-Control Study." *Acta Psychiatry Scandinavia* 88 (1993): 403–8.

Burke, C., and S. Davis. "Anabolic Steroid Abuse." *Pharmacy Times* (June 1992): 35–40.

Caetano, R. "Drinking Patterns and Alcoholic Problems in a National Sample of U.S. Hispanics." In *The Epidemiology of Alcohol Use and Abuse Among U.S. Minorities.* NIAA Monograph no. 18 (DHHS Pub. no. ADM89-1435) 147–62. Washington, DC: U.S. Government Printing Office, 1989.

Canterbury, R. J., and E. Lloyd. "Smart Drugs: Implications of Student Use." *Journal of Primary Prevention* 14 (1994): 197–207.

Centers for Disease Control and Prevention (CDC). "HIV/AIDS." *Surveillance Reports* 8 (1996): 1–3.

Ciba Foundation. "AIDS and HIV Infection in Cocaine Users." In *Cocaine: Scientific and Social Dimensions,* 181–94. New York: Wiley, 1992.

"Cigarettes May Pose a Greater Risk in Developing Fetus Than Cocaine." *Prevention Pipeline* 7 (May–June 1994): 10, 11.

Cohen, J. "How Can HIV Replication Be Controlled?" *Science* 260 (May 1993a): 1257.

Cohen, J. "What Causes the Immune System Collapse Seen in AIDS?" *Science* 260 (May 1993b): 1256.

Colthurst, T. "HIV and Alcohol Impairment: Reducing Risks." *Prevention Pipeline* 6 (July–August 1993): 24.

Crowley, G. "Targeting a Deadly Scrap of Genetic Code." *Newsweek* (2 December 1996): 68–69.

Cuomo, M. J., P. Dyment, G. Paul, and V. M. Gammino. "Increasing Use of 'Ecstasy' (MDMA) and Other Hallucinogens on a College Campus." *Journal of American College Health* 42 (1994): 271–274.

Curry, D. G., and I. A. Spergel. "Gang Homicide, Delinquency, and Community." In *Gangs and Gang Behavior,* edited by G. Larry Mays. Chicago: Nelson-Hall, 1997: 314–336.

Daily, S. "Alcohol, Incest, and Adolescence." In *Adolescent Substance Abuse, Etiology, Treatment and Prevention,* edited by G. Lawson and A. Lawson, 251–66. Gaithersburg, MD: Aspen, 1992a.

Daily, S. "Suicide Solution: The Relationship of Alcohol and Drug Abuse to Adolescent Suicide. In *Adolescent Substance Abuse, Etiology, Treatment and Prevention,* edited by G. Lawson and A. Lawson, 233–50. Gaithersburg, MD: Aspen, 1992b.

Diaz, T., and S. Chu. "Crack Cocaine Use and Sexual Behavior Among People with AIDS." *Journal of the American Medical Association* 269 (1993): 2845–6.

Dicker, M., and E. A. Leighton. "Trends in the U.S. Prevalence of Drug-Using Parturient Women and Drug-Affected Newborns, 1979 Through 1990." *American Journal of Public Health* 84 (September 1994): 1433.

Drug Facts and Comparisons, 109–109c. St. Louis: Kluwer, 1994.

Edlin, G., E. Golanty, and K. M. Brown. *Essentials for Health and Wellness.* Sudbury, MA: Jones and Bartlett Publishers, 1997.

Elmen, J., and D. Offer. "Normality, Turmoil and Adolescence." In *Handbook of Clinical Research and Practice with Adolescents,* edited by P. Tolan and B. Cohler, 5–19. New York: Wiley, 1993.

Erickson, P. G., and G. F. Murray: "Sex Differences in Cocaine Use and Experiences: A Double Standard Revived?" *American Journal of Drug and Alcohol Abuse* 15 (1989): 135–52.

Fagan, J. "Social Processes of Delinquency and Drug Use Among Urban Gangs." In *Gangs in America*, edited by C. R. Huff, 183–213. Newbury Park, CA: Sage, 1990.

Ferrente, R. "Ben Johnson Retires from Running After Positive Test." Morning Edition on National Public Radio, 8 March 1993.

Glave, J. "Betty Ford Got Help, But Addiction Stalks Thousands of Women." *Salt Lake Tribune* 248 (3 June 1994): A-1.

Goldfinger, S. "When HIV Hits Home." *Harvard Health Letter* 19 (April 1994): 1–3.

Goldstein, F. "Pharmacological Aspects of Substance Abuse." In *Remington's Pharmaceutical Sciences,* 19th ed. Easton, PA: Mack, 1995.

Grinspoon, L. "AIDS and Mental Health—Part 1." *Harvard Mental Health Letter* 10 (January 1994): 1–4.

Harlan, R., and M. Garcia. "Neurobiology of Androgen Abuse." In *Drugs of Abuse,* edited by R. Watson, 185–201. Boca Raton, FL: CRC Press, 1992.

Harris, H. G. "Cholas, Mexican-American Girls and Gangs." In *Gangs and Gang Behavior,* edited by G. Larry Mays. Chicago: Nelson-Hall, 1997: 129–149.

Hasin, D., B. Grant, and J. Weinflash. "Male/Female Differences in Alcohol-Related Problems: Alcohol Rehabilitation Patients." *International Journal of the Addictions* 23 (1988): 437–48.

Hein, K., R. Dell, D. Futterman, M. Rotheram-Borus, and N. Shaffer. "Comparison of HIV+ and HIV– Adolescents: Risk Factors and Psychosocial Determinants." *Pediatrics* 95 (January 1995): 96–104.

Henslin, J. M. *Sociology: A Down-to-Earth Approach,* 3rd ed. Boston: Allyn and Bacon, 1997.

Hernandez, J. "Substance Abuse Among Sexually Abused Adolescents and Their Families." *Journal of Adolescent Health* 13 (1992): 658–62.

Hoberman, J. M., and C. E. Yesalis. "The History of Synthetic Testosterone." *Scientific American* (February 1995).

Hoshino, J. "Assessment of Adolescent Substance Abuse." In *Adolescent Substance Abuse, Etiology, Treatment and Prevention,* edited by G. Lawson and A. Lawson, 87–104. Gaithersburg, MD: Aspen, 1992.

Howard, M. "Adolescent Substance Abuse: A Social Learning Theory Perspective." In *Adolescent Substance Abuse, Etiology, Treatment and Prevention,* edited by G. Lawson and A. Lawson, 29–40. Gaithersburg, MD: Aspen, 1992.

Johnson, R. A., J. P. Hoffmann, and D. R. Gerstein. *The Relationship Between Family Structure and Adolescent Substance Use.* Rockville, MD: SAMHSA, Office of Applied Studies, July 1996.

Johnston, L. D., P. O'Malley, and J. G. Bachman. *National Survey Results from The Monitoring the Future Study, 1975–1992.* Rockville, MD: National Institute on Drug Abuse, 1993.

———. *National Survey Results from The Monitoring the Future Study, 1975–1994.* Rockville, MD: National Institute on Drug Abuse, 1996.

Kandel, D. B. "Drug And Drinking Behavior Among Youth." *Annual Review of Sociology* 6 (1980): 235–85.

Kolata, G. "Targeting Urged in Attack on AIDS." *New York Times* 142 (7 March 1993): 1.

Korolenko, C. P., and T. A. Donskih. "Addictive Behavior in Women: A Theoretical Perspective." *Drugs and Society* 4 (1990): 39–65.

Ladwig, G. B., and M. D. Anderson. "Substance Abuse in Women: Relationship Between Chemical Dependency of Women and Past Reports of Physical and/or Sexual Abuse." *International Journal of the Addictions* 24 (1989): 739–54.

Lale, T. "Gangs and Drugs." In *Adolescent Substance Abuse, Etiology, Treatment and Prevention,* edited by G. Lawson and A. Lawson, 267–81. Gaithersburg, MD: Aspen, 1992.

Landau, I. "Can Clean Needles Slow the AIDS Epidemic?" *Consumer Reports* (July 1994): 466–9.

Lawn, J. *Team Up for Drug Prevention with America's Young Athletes.* Drug Enforcement Administration, U.S. Department of Justice, Washington, D.C. 1984.

Lawson, G., and A. Lawson, "Etiology." In *Adolescent Substance Abuse, Etiology, Treatment and Prevention,* edited by G. Lawson and A. Lawson, 1–10. Gaithersburg, MD: Aspen, 1992.

Leibsohn, J. "The Relationship Between Drug and Alcohol Use and Peer Group Associations of College Freshmen as They Transition from High School." *Journal of Drug Education* 24 (1994): 177–192.

Lin, A. Y. F. "Should Women Be Included in Clinical Trials?" *Pharmacy Times* 10 (November 1994): 27.

Lindberg, S., and G. Agren. "Mortality Among Male and Female Hospitalized Alcoholics in Stockholm 1962–1983." *British Journal of the Addictions* 83 (1988): 1193–1200.

Lively, K. "The 'Date-Rape Drug': Colleges Worry about Reports of Growing Use of Rohypnol, a Sedative." *Chronicle of Higher Education* 42 (28 June 1996): A29.

Lukas, S. "Urine Testing for Anabolic-Androgenic Steroids." *Trends in Pharmacological Sciences* 14 (1993): 61–8.

Marsh, K. L., and D. D. Simpson. "Sex Differences in Opioid Addiction Centers." *American Journal of Drug and Alcohol Abuse* 12 (1986): 309–29.

Mathias, R. "NIDA Survey Provides First National Data on Drug Use During Pregnancy." *NIDA Notes* 10 (January/February 1995): 6–7.

———. "Students' Use of Marijuana, Other Illicit Drugs, and Cigarettes Continued to Rise in 1995." *NIDA Notes* 11 (January/February 1996): 8–9.

———. "Sex-for-Crack Phenomenon Poses Risk for Spread of AIDS in Heterosexuals." *NIDA Notes* 8 (May–June 1993): 8–11.

McDonald, M. "Fast, Strong, Dead?" *Salt Lake Tribune* 250 (22 June 1995): C1, C8.

Meilman, P. W., R. K. Grace, C. A. Presley, and R. Lyerla. "Beyond Performance Enhancement: Polypharmacy

Among Collegiate Users of Steroids." *Journal of American College Health* 44 (November 1995): 98–104.

Merchant, W. "Medications and Athletes." *American Druggist* (October 1992): 6–14.

Merson, M. "Slowing the Spread of HIV: Agenda for the 1990's." *Science* 260 (May 1993): 1266–8.

Miller, W. B. *Violence by Youth Gangs and Youth Groups as a Crime Problem in Major American Cities.* Washington, DC: U.S. Government Printing Office, 1975.

Millstein, R. *Community Alert Bulletin.* Rockville, MD: National Institute on Drug Abuse, U.S. Department of Health and Human Services, 25 March 1993.

Moss, H., L. Kirisci, H. Gordon, and R. Tarter. "A Neuropsychological Profile of Adolescent Alcoholics." *Alcoholism: Clinical and Experimental Research* 18 (1994): 159–63.

"Multistate Outbreak of Poisonings Associated with Illicit Use of GHB." *Prevention Pipeline* 7 (May–June 1994): 95, 96.

National Institute on Drug Abuse (NIDA). *Drugs and Drug Interactions in Elderly Women.* National Institute on Drug Abuse Research Monograph 65. Washington, DC: U.S. Government Printing Office, 1986.

National Institute on Drug Abuse (NIDA). *Anabolic Steroid Abuse.* Capsule 43. Rockville, MD: NIDA, 1996.

"Ongoing Program Announcement." *NIH Guide* 22 (5 November 1993): 13.

"OTC Drugs and Athletes." *Pharmacy Times* (June 1992): 16.

Parrot, A. *Date Rape and Acquaintance Rape.* New York: Rosen, 1988.

Pietroski, N. "Counseling HIV/AIDS Patients." *American Druggist* (August 1993): 50–6.

Prendergast, M. L. "Substance Use and Abuse Among College Students: A Review of Recent Literature." *Journal of American College Health* 43 (1994): 99–113.

Ravid, J. "The Hard-Core Curriculum." *Rolling Stone* 719 (19 October 1995): 99.

Sanders, W. B. *Gangbangs and Drive-bys.* New York: Aldine De Gruyter, 1994.

Sandmaier, M. *The Invisible Alcoholics.* New York: McGraw-Hill, 1980.

Samples, P. "Alcoholism in Athletes: New Directions for Treatment." *The Physician and Sports Medicine* (17 April 1989): 193–202.

Schafer, M. A., J. F. Hilton, M. Ekstrand, and J. Keogh. "Relationship Between Drug Use and Sexual Behaviors and the Occurrence of Sexually Transmitted Diseases Among High-Risk Male Youth." *Sexually Transmitted Diseases* 20 (November–December 1993): 39–47.

Schoemer, K. "Rockers, Models and the New Allure of Heroin." *Newsweek* (26 August 1996): 24–36.

Segal, B., F. Cromer, H. Stevens, and P. Wasserman. "Patterns of Reasons for Drug Use Among Detained and Adjudicated Juveniles." *International Journal of Addictions* 17 (1982): 1117–30.

Siegal, H. A., R. G. Carlson, R. S. Falck, and J. Wang. "Drug Abuse Treatment Experience and HIV Risk Behaviors Among Active Drug Injectors in Ohio." *American Journal of Public Health* 85 (1995): 105–8.

Siegel, L., and J. Senna. *Juvenile Delinquency,* 6th ed. St. Paul, MN: West, 1997.

Steinberg, L., A. Fletcher, and N. Darling. "Parental Monitoring and Peer Influences on Adolescent Substance Use." *Pediatrics* 93 (1994): 1060–4.

Swadi, H. "Relative Risk Factors in Detecting Adolescent Drug Abuse." *Drug and Alcohol Dependence* 29 (1992): 253–4.

Swan, N. "NIDA Plays Key Role in Studying Links Between AIDS and Drug Abuse." *NIDA Notes* 10 (May/June 1995): 7–10.

Toronto, R. "Young Athletes Who Use 'Enhancing' Steroids Risk Severe Physical Consequences." *Salt Lake Tribune* 244 (6 July 1992): C-5.

U.S. Centers of Disease Control and Prevention (CDC). "HIV/AIDS." *Surveillance Report* 6 (February 1995): 17–34.

U.S. Department of Health and Human Services (USDHHS). *Seventh Special Report to Congress on Alcohol and Health.* Washington, DC: National Institute on Alcohol Abuse and Alcoholism, 1990.

U.S. Department of Justice. "Anabolic Steroids and You." Washington, DC: Demand Reduction Section, Drug Enforcement Administration, 1991–1992.

Walsh, F., and M. Sheinkman. "Family Context of Adolescence." In *Adolescent Substance Abuse, Etiology, Treatment and Prevention,* edited by G. Lawson and A. Lawson, 149–71. Gaithersburg, MD: Aspen, 1992.

Webb, E., C. H. Ashton, P. Kelly, and F. Kamali. "Alcohol and Drug Use in U.K. University Students (United Kingdom)." *Lancet* 348 (5 October 1996): 922.

Weiss, R. "How Does HIV Cause AIDS?" *Science* 260 (May 1993): 1273–9.

Welder, A., and R. Melchert. "Cardiotoxic Effects of Cocaine and Anabolic-Androgenic Steroids in the Athlete." *Journal of Pharmacological and Toxicological Methods* 29 (1993): 61–8.

Wentz, A. "22.2 Million Women Just Don't Get IT." *Prevention Pipeline* 7 (May–June 1994): 127, 128.

Whitmire, R. "Don't Use Drugs While Pregnant; 25% of Moms Ignored Warning." *Salt Lake City Tribune* 248 (13 September 1994): A1–A4.

Winters, P. A. *Teen Addiction.* San Diego, CA: Greenhaven Press, 1997.

Witham, D. "Recovery in the Dorm: Rutgers University's Special Housing for Addicted Students." *Chronicle of Higher Education* 42 (10 November 1995): A33.

"Women Smokers Run High Risk for Lung Cancer." *Prevention Pipeline* 7 (May–June 1994): 7.

Wright, L. "Suicidal Thoughts and Their Relationship to Family Stress and Personal Problems Among High School Seniors and College Undergraduates." *Adolescence* 20 (1985): 575–80.

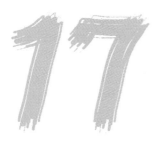

Drug Abuse

Prevention

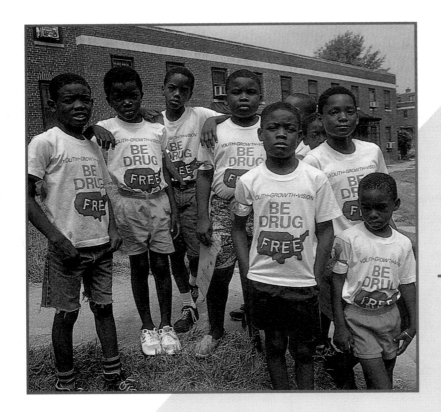

On completing this chapter
you will be able to:

Learning Objectives

- Explain and give examples of four primary prevention activities.
- Explain and give examples of two secondary prevention activities.

- Describe at least three exemplary programs in higher education drug prevention.
- Explain the difference between drug treatment and drug prevention.

- Explain why it is difficult to measure the effectiveness of drug prevention programs.
- Describe the role of peers in prevention work.
- Describe the goals and objectives of drug education.

"This is your brain ... this is your brain on drugs." Everyone has seen this television commercial—or anti-commercial—sponsored by the Partnership for a Drug-Free America, which shows an egg, first whole and then frying in a pan. It ran during the mid-1990s, and groups of marijuana-smoking teenagers laughed about it on street corners. Was it worth the millions of dollars' worth of airtime purchased? Can we even take measurements to figure out the answer to that question? In 1997, 15 states thought prevention of alcohol and other drug abuse important enough to maintain *certified prevention specialist* credentialing. A bewildering variety of programs exist from coast to coast in school districts, churches, and in communities, all with the idea of influencing people not to start drug use ("Be Smart, Don't Start"), or not to abuse drugs and subsequently get hurt ("Friends Don't Let Friends Drive Drunk").

An example of an ad developed by Partnership for a Drug-Free America

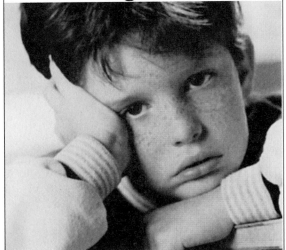

America's Drug Problem
Is Not As Big As You Think.

It can start as a dare. Or youthful curiosity. Or it may be a way to escape problems at home. Whatever the reasons, studies show that an alarming number of young children are trying drugs. Unfortunately, too many parents still do not believe that *their* kids are at risk.
The truth is, it's never too early to start teaching

your kids about the dangers of drugs. If you're not sure how to talk to them, call 1-800-624-0100 and ask for a free booklet called *Growing Up Drug-Free – A Parent's Guide To Prevention.* Call today, because if you don't take care of little problems, they can easily grow into big ones.

Partnership for a Drug-Free America®

Earlier in this text we examined risk factors for initiation of use (outlined in Chapter 2), risk factors that generate habitual use and abuse, and vicious cycles moving abusers toward addiction (outlined in Chapter 4). You've now become familiar with the dozens, if not hundreds, of reasons why people experiment with, habitually use, abuse, and become dependent on psychoactive substances. You also know that drug use involves personal, group, subcultural, societal, and institutional factors. How can we tease these influences apart enough even to think about affecting individual drug use?

Let's try to stand in the shoes of a parent and teacher committee trying to design a primary prevention program for students at Central High, in Elmtown. The group has some prevention research materials that it received from the National Clearinghouse for Alcohol and Drug Information. After some thought, most members of the committee decide not to address individual, personal risk factors (discussed in Chapters 2 and 4) that generate anxieties, conflicts, or painful or threatening feelings. Moreover, they've spoken with some concerned students, and ascertained that most of the ninth- and tenth-graders, even those who tend toward rebelliousness and avant-garde styles, don't especially *like* the idea of taking drugs. On their own, these students might not be likely to take drugs. But there are trends in the school that worry the committee members; some important eleventh- and twelfth-grade peer group leaders are pro-use, and drug sales have been seen near the school. The presence and availability of drugs, and the beginning of a "druggy" atmosphere make it more likely that some of the younger students will initiate use. In the brainstorming sessions that were conducted, different committee members suggested ways to avert initiation of drug use in this group. Depending on their thinking and theoretical bent, or their limited exposure to prevention models, members came up with the following ideas:

▲ Students need to be grounded in good, solid knowledge about the negative effects and dangers of drugs (1) As provided in a drug education course (an example is D.A.R.E., covered below) or (2) More subtly, in a curriculum infusion concerning drug effects and drug-using behaviors (also covered later, in the section on higher education).

▲ Students with low self-esteem will feel uncomfortable asserting an individual choice or point of view that deviates from those held by peers or peer leaders. Bolstering a positive self-image would allow such students to refuse the offer of drugs.

▲ Students who have low expectations regarding their ability to successfully refuse drugs will be unlikely to follow this course. We might try to increase their "self-efficacy"—that is, their belief that their behaviors are powerful and will have results.

▲ Students just don't know how to say no, and need refusal skills training.

▲ Although a clique leadership may set a pro-use tone, it is probable that the quiet antidrug students represent a silent majority. They may misperceive the real norms concerning drugs. Therefore, if their own beliefs and attitudes can be demonstrated to them, they will see that the "emperor has no clothes" (discussed in the section on higher education prevention strategies).

▲ The drugs can be removed from the environment by infiltrating the student body or using informants to gather information on who is distributing drugs. Distributors and users can then be arrested and/or expelled.

At this point, a few members of the committee become dissatisfied at what they perceive as the "soft," "wishy-washy" approach to drug abuse. Some have experienced alcoholism in their families, and see a crisis in the use patterns emerging. One asks "Why are you 'preaching to the choir'? What about the students who are experimenting? They are going to end up as drug addicts! We should put them in NA [Narcotics Anonymous]. Your programs won't be of any help to *them*."

Seeing a disaster brewing, the committee chairman makes a call to the Division of Substance Abuse Services in the state Department of Health (every state has such a division or department) and asks about drug prevention programs. The operator refers the call to the prevention specialists at the agency, who are linked nationally by

a National Prevention Network, a network of state prevention specialists within the National Association of State Alcohol and Drug Abuse Directors. The specialist schedules a meeting with the committee, where she makes the following points:

1. She proposes a prevention needs assessment, utilizing validated survey instruments, to determine the patterns of behavior and attitudes regarding drug use among the student body.

2. No discrepancy exists between the approaches of these factions. One set of strategies, reducing risk factors for use, is called **primary prevention.** It is aimed at nonusers and is intended to ensure their continued non-use. We must also address at-risk youth and those who are just beginning to abuse, an approach called **secondary prevention.** The specialist suggests a combination of sanctions and group treatment for substance abuse at an adolescent outpatient clinic, rather than a recovery fellowship for seriously addicted persons, for these students. Finally, a few truly chemically dependent students who are well on their way to addiction will be assessed and referred into inpatient treatment by the same clinic. This intervention at an advanced abuse state is called **tertiary prevention.** All three types of approaches are components of a comprehensive prevention strategy. (See Table 17.1).

primary prevention
refers to the very broad range of activities aimed at reducing the risk of drug use among non-users and assuring continued non-use

secondary prevention
targeting at-risk groups, experimenters, and early abuse populations to reverse the progression of abusive behaviors; similar to "early intervention"

tertiary prevention
intervention at an advanced state of drug abuse; basically the same as drug abuse treatment

The specialist brought along a staff member of the "local council on alcoholism and drug dependence," an affiliate of the National Council on Alcoholism and Drug Dependence (NCADD) branch serving a three-county region of the state.

Table 17.1   Levels of Drug Prevention and Suggested Activities

Primary Prevention (risk reduction before abuse)	
Intrapersonal Factors	Affective education (emotional literacy)
	Resilience training
	Values clarification
	Personal and social skills development
	Assertiveness skills training
	Refusal skills
	Drug information and education
Small Group Factors	Peer mentoring, counseling, outreach, modeling
	Conflict resolution
	Curriculum infusion
	Activities demonstrating misperception of peer norms
	Alternatives to use: recreational, cultural, athletic
	Strengthening families
Systems Level	Strengthening school–family links
	Strengthening school–community group links
	Strengthening community support systems
	Media advocacy efforts, reduce alcohol marketing
Secondary Prevention (intervening in early abuse)	Assessment strategies: identification of abuse subgroups and individual diagnoses
	Early intervention coupled with sanctions
	Teacher–counselor–parent team approach
	Developing healthy alternative youth culture
	Recovering role models
Tertiary Prevention (intervening in advanced abuse)	Assessment and diagnosis
	Referral into treatment
	Case management
	Reentry

Thousands of branches of NCADD exist in the United States, with their goal to help local groups design and implement prevention programs. Many have developed specialized programs for teens, children, women, and the elderly. The staff member conducts preliminary sessions with the prevention committee and arranges to sign an affiliation agreement with the school administration, whereby NCADD will act as consultants to the school, aiding it in designing a prevention program to fit its particular needs. It will design a project, which will be based on a needs assessment that incorporates a chemical attitudes and use survey instrument and interviews with parents,

teachers, and students. The project design will include the program objectives, a methods and management plan, a timeline, and an evaluation component. To help those members bewildered by the many possible factors identified by the committee in its brainstorming session (such as self-esteem, self-efficacy, and refusal skills), the staff member invites the committee to sample a number of available, attractive packages of "user-friendly" activities such as:

▲ "Broad-brush" packages covering a variety of personal choice and primary prevention areas (Holstein et al. 1995)

▲ More targeted strategies, which might include a component such as assertiveness training that would use a training package to be implemented by a training consultant who would need to be hired by the school district.

Assertiveness training skills, which include a variety of "personal and social skills development," enable people to communicate their needs and feelings in an open, direct, and appropriate manner, while still recognizing the needs and feelings of others. They make people feel more powerful and better about themselves (less like "doormats"), and offer strategies for saying "no" without hurting, provoking, or manipulating others (Alberti and Emmons 1988). Assertive behavior contrasts with hostile or belligerent behavior, passive and helpless behavior, and passive–aggressive or indirect manipulation. The exercises included in assertiveness training are nonthreatening, concrete, direct, and enjoyable.

Many intrapersonal prevention concepts, or personal and social skills development concepts, have come and gone, with a trendy "buzz word" accompanying each in the year it was introduced. Many of these concepts overlap, such as life skills training, self-esteem, self-efficacy, resilience training (McIntryre et al. 1990; Norman 1994), and assertiveness training. The danger lies in employing them as gimmicks or slogans that accomplish little. Nevertheless, as Botvin and others have shown, personal and skills training that is carefully based on known cognitive and behavioral change factors, if carefully operationalized, can indeed make a difference (Botvin and Wills 1985; Shiffman and Wills 1987). It is also true that almost any positive lifestyle activity is likely to act as an alternative to participating in a drug-using subculture.

◢ Using Education to Control Drug Use

Education has been used extensively in the past to control the use and abuse of drugs, especially alcohol and tobacco. Drug education actually began in the late 1800s, when most states required that the harmful effects of certain drugs be taught. An example of an early educational attempt to curb or stop drug abuse is the temperance movement in the late nineteenth century. The Women's Christian Temperance Union (WCTU) and the Anti-Saloon League taught that alcohol consumption was harmful and against Christian morality.

Today, school programs, drug education courses, and the mass media are used extensively as mediums for educating the public about the negative consequences of drug abuse. Strategies vary enormously, but can be classified into three general categories:

1. Those that focus on and provide information

2. Those that stress values, beliefs, and attitudes

3. Those that emphasize the consequences of drug use (namely, warnings and scare tactics about drug abuse)

Considering the Audience and Approach

The audience for drug education is composed of both users and nonusers. In analyzing the population of users, categories include the following:

▲ Committed users—those who abuse drugs and have no interest in stopping

▲ Former users

▲ Nonproblem drug users—those who abuse drugs on occasion, mostly for recreation.

▲ Problem users

It is important for individuals involved in drug education to recognize the different types of users so programs can cater to the specific needs of these groups. For committed users, drug education should aim to prevent or delay drug abuse. Former users should be given information that will reinforce their decision to quit abusing drugs. For nonproblem users, drug education programs should examine the abuse of drugs, reinforce the importance of how uncontrolled use leads to abuse, and educate students on how to prevent use from escalating to abuse.

Professionals planning a drug education program have to decide on the type of audience they intend to pursue. A number of questions should be considered: To what type of audience should the drug information be targeted: youths or adults? peers or parents? Should information focus on knowledge, attitudes, or behavior? Should drug education emphasize and recommend abstinence or responsible use?

In most cases, it is appropriate for drug education to focus on knowledge, attitudes, and behavior. The three are clearly related. For instance, if the goal is to increase knowledge, should we assume that attitudes and behavior will change accordingly, or should knowledge about the harmful effects of drugs be kept separate from attitudes and behavior? In other words, if you learn that smoking marijuana is a health hazard, equal to or more destructive than smoking cigarettes, does this knowledge change the satisfaction you derive from smoking marijuana with friends? Some would say yes. Unfortunately, many would say no. In fact, knowledge about the harmful effects of certain types of drugs has very little effect on the personal attitudes and habits of most people. Proof of this statement is cigarette smokers, the number who are aware of the health risks involved with smoking but continue to smoke, day after day and year after year.

Drug education programs have to direct their attention to a small range of behavioral objectives. They will not be effective if they address too many issues.

Finally, drug educators must decide if they will stress total abstinence or responsible use. Abstinence is radically different from responsible use. A program cannot advocate both. Information and "scare tactics" alone have no effect on drug use. Educative models have been modified lately to achieve the following goals:

▲ Convey the message that society is inconsistent concerning drug use. For example, certain drugs that cause serious harm to a large percentage of the population are legal, while other drugs that have less impact are illegal.

▲ Convey that the reasons for drug use are complex and that drug users vary.

▲ Demonstrate to youth that the young and old alike are affected by role models, in that attitudes regarding drug use are often patterned from family members who are role models.

▲ That other influential role models in music, art, drama, business, and education who use

and abuse drugs can affect attitudes toward drug use. (See Chapter 16.)

Curriculum-Based Drug Education Objectives

In an effort to educate students and make them aware of the dangers in using drugs, school-based drug education programs and objectives have been implemented in most U.S. school curriculums. Specific educational goals have been established for elementary, junior high, and senior high and college levels:

Elementary Level

Drugs versus poisons

Effects of alcohol, tobacco, and marijuana on the body

Differences between candy and drugs

Drug overdoses

Dangers of experimentation

Saying no to peers using drugs

Reasons for taking drugs: curing illness, pleasure, escape, parental use, and ceremony

Junior High Level

How peer pressure works

Saying no to peer pressure

How drugs affect the body, physiologically and psychologically

Seeking help when needed

Attitudes toward drug use

Having fun without drugs

Harmful effects of tobacco, alcohol, and marijuana on the body

How advertisers push drugs

Consequences of breaking drug laws

Differences between wine, beer, and distilled spirits

Family drug use

Identifying family drinking problems and identifying family members who may have drug addiction problems

Images of violence and drug use in rock and rap music

Teenage drug abuse and associated problems

"Just say no" programs

Senior High and College Level

Responsible use of medications

How drugs affect the body and the mind

Legal versus illegal drugs

Drinking and driving

Drug effects on the fetus

Recreational drug use

Ways of coping with problems

Detecting problem drug users

Drug education, prevention, and treatment

Positive and negative role models

Criminal sanctions for various types of drug use

"Binge" drinking

Driving

Date rape

Addiction to drugs and alcoholism

"Just say no" programs

Making Drug Education Programs More Effective

The following suggestions have also been made to improve the outcomes of drug education programs:

Practice deliberate planning. Begin by matching imagined needs with real needs. Make a thorough assessment of drug information needed and problems associated with drug use. Program content should be based on this careful assessment.

Review the previous history. Don't assume that people who have been exposed to previous educational campaigns have forgotten all of what they learned. Start by considering the amount and the kind of information to which people have already been exposed. If they have experience with drug education, what was successful in previous campaigns?

Establish links between the messages conveyed and learned and other aspects of students' life experiences. Involve students, teachers, administrators, and even school janitors in the drug education program. Be aware that drug use comes from many sources and that students are involved in many relationships. The drug education program must involve parents and guardians as well as the wider community.

Effectively promote programs. The information to be conveyed must reach important voters and decision makers in the community. The information must be disseminated effectively to a wide audience.

Allocate resources properly. Be mindful that, unless drug use and abuse has become a community-wide burning issue, people will tend to be interested in the drug campaign initially but can quickly lose interest if the drug education program is to take place in schools. For example, make certain that the amounts of curriculum time and staffing are adequate and can be sustained throughout the program's duration.

Evaluate constantly. Is the program effective for the target audience? Are the goals conveyed and understood by the target population? What are the positive and negative outcomes of the strategy employed? Interview staff members of the program as well as the members of the target audience. Are they satisfied? What suggestions do they have for improving the program? These are very important questions. Their answers will reveal if the drug education program is meeting its goals (U.S. Department of Education, 1992).

Alternatives to Drug Use

It has been suggested that people have an innate need to alter their conscious state. This belief is based on the observation that, as part of their normal play, preschoolers deliberately whirl themselves dizzy and even momentarily choke each other to lose consciousness (see Wilson and Wilson 1975, 26). Some young children progress to discovering and using chemicals (such as sniffing shoe polish or gasoline) to alter consciousness and learn to be very secretive about this behavior.

FIGHTING THE DRUG WAR

In 1995, a disturbing study published by a group of researchers at the University of Michigan—and backed by the U.S. Department of Health and Human Services (HHS) and the National Institute on Drug Abuse (NIDA)—showed that the use of illicit drugs by young people had been rising steadily since 1992. The results of this study were all the more confounding because drug use overall had been declining for the same period. *And* the increase was happening despite several seemingly successful efforts to combat drug abuse with high-powered prevention programs.

Since the 1980s, the most funds in drug prevention have been spent in three areas: criminal justice, major ad campaigns, and the D.A.R.E. education program. Compulsory preventive programs have been favored by law enforcement professionals for hard-core addicts, especially in poor urban neighborhoods. According to William N. Brownsberger, Assistant State Attorney General in the Massachusetts Narcotics and Special Investigations Division, addicts who are forced against their will to enter and remain in therapy can overcome their addiction. Roughly 90% of all addicts are arrested at least once every year, giving the criminal justice system plenty of opportunities to help them kick their habits.

One highly visible persuasive effort to end drug abuse has been the publicity and advertising campaign created by the Partnership for a Drug-Free America. The nation's advertising industry developed the Partnership and funded it by collaborating with advertisers and a variety of health and educational agencies. The goal was to promote images designed to make drug use look "uncool"—especially to younger people. In addition to the creative services donated by advertising agencies, media organizations donated more than $2 billion worth of public service and advertising space to the Partnership between the late 1980s and 1990s.

In the early 1990s, the Partnership commissioned surveys to measure the effect of its media campaign on students in the Los Angeles and New York City school systems. On both coasts, increased exposure to the Partnership's messages appeared to dramatically change students' attitudes toward drugs. At the same time, however, the number of students who admitted using drugs actually increased.

Another high-visibility persuasive effort has been the nationwide D.A.R.E. (Drug Abuse Resistance Education) program that was launched in Los Angeles in 1983. Using role-playing techniques and resistance training, uniformed police officers become social workers, talking with students in their classrooms, educating them about the dangers of drugs, and giving them the tools to resist temptation or peer pressure. They generally teach 17 classroom sessions.

Although D.A.R.E. is the most popular drug education program ever developed for children, increasing numbers of critics claim that its effects, if any, are short-lasting. Most D.A.R.E. training begins in the fifth grade. At this age, students accept most of what they hear. By middle school, however, the impact of D.A.R.E. begins to erode. By high school, many students resist participation in the program. According to a researcher from the Research Triangle Institute in Durham, North Carolina, which conducted a $300,000 study on the impact of D.A.R.E., "Unless there's some sort of booster session that reinforces the original curriculum, the effects of most drug use prevention programs decay rather than increase over time."

In light of diminishing returns from various drug prevention programs, in late 1996 the Clinton administration proposed a compulsory drug test for teenagers who are applying for their driver's licenses. Like everything else, the proposal has had both supporters and critics. While it may be part of the answer, the search for prevention programs that have measurable, long-lasting effects is far from over. ∎

Sources: W. N. Brownsberger. "Just Say 'Criminal Justice.'" *Boston Globe* (October 20, 1996).
P. Gordon. "Can Madison Avenue Really Save America by Making Illegal Drugs Totally Uncool?" *Buzz Magazine* (August 1996).
P. Gordon. "The Truth About D.A.R.E." *Buzz Magazine* (July 1996).

They learn to be circumspect or come to feel guilty and repress the desire to alter consciousness when adults catch them in these activities.

If this desire to alter the state of consciousness is inherent in human beings, then the use of psychoactive drugs, legally or illegally, in adulthood is natural. Drug abuse is thus a logical continuation of a developmental sequence that goes back to early childhood (Carroll 1977; Weil 1972).

Other researchers question why, even if there is an innate desire to alter consciousness, only some but not all people progress to abusing chemical substances. It appears that people who do not abuse psychoactive drugs have found positive alternatives to altering consciousness. They feel no need to take chemical substances for this purpose. Involvement in such activities as Boy Scouts and Girl Scouts, youth sports teams, music groups, the YMCA and YWCA, drug-free video game centers, drug-free dances, environmental and historical preservation projects, and social and service projects are viable alternatives to drug use. The rationale for these programs is that youth will find these activities engaging enough to forgo alcohol and drug use (Forman and Linney 1988, 555–6).

This strategy is known as the **alternatives approach.** Workers in the drug abuse field tend to agree on its effectiveness. They note that young ex-abusers of common illicit drugs are more likely to stop when they gain satisfaction from exploring positive alternatives rather than from a fear of

alternatives approach

one approach emphasizing the exploration of positive alternatives to drug abuse, based on replacing the pleasurable feelings gained from drug abuse with involvement in social and educational activities

consequent harm. The alternatives approach assumes the following (Cohen 1971):

1. People abuse drugs voluntarily to fill a need or basic drive.

2. Most people abuse drugs for negative reasons. They may be dealing with negative feelings or situations, such as relieving boredom, anxiety, depression, tension, or other unpleasant emotional and psychological states. They may be rebelling against authority, trying to escape feelings of loneliness or inadequacy, or trying to be accepted by peers. Peer pressure is extremely important as an inducing force.

3. Some people who abuse drugs believe the experience is positive. They may feel enhancement of sensual experiences or listening to music, achieve altered states of consciousness, or simply experience a sense of adventure. Some people may want to explore their own consciousness and reasons for the attraction to drug use.

Whether the reasons for drug use are positive or negative, the effects sought can be achieved through alternative, nondrug means. Such means are preferable to drug use and more constructive because the person is not relying on a psychoactive substance for satisfaction; rather, he or she is finding satisfaction based on personal achievements. Ideally, this approach should lead to a lifetime of self-satisfaction.

Table 17.2 lists various types of experiences, the motives for such experiences, the probable drugs of abuse with which they are associated, and alternatives to these drugs. As shown in the table, any constructive activity can be considered an alternative to drug abuse. For example, a young person who needs an outlet for increased physical energy might respond better to dance and movement training or a project in preventive medicine than to work on ecological projects. In a large alternatives program established in Idaho, the following activities were planned during one month: arts and crafts, karate, reforestation, backpacking, a Humane Society dog show, horseback riding, artwork for posters for various programs, astrology, camping, and volunteering in a local hospital.

Meditation Some of the most intriguing research about the brain is being done on the state of the mind during **meditation.** In certain countries, like India, people have long histories of being able to achieve certain goals through meditation. The word *yoga* is derived from the

meditation

a state of consciousness in which there is a constant level of awareness focusing on one object; for example, yoga and zen Buddhism

Table 17.2   **Experiences, Motives, and Possible Alternatives for a Drug Abuser**

Experience	Corresponding Motives	Drugs Abused	Possible Alternatives
Physical	Desire for physical well-being: physical relaxation, relief from sickness, desire for more energy	Alcohol, sedative-hypnotics, stimulants, marijuana	Athletics, dance, exercise, hiking, diet, carpentry, outdoor work, swimming, hatha yoga
Sensory	Desire to magnify sensorium: sound, touch, taste, need for sensual/sexual stimulation	Hallucinogens, marijuana, alcohol	Sensory awareness training, sky diving, experiencing sensory beauty of nature, scuba diving
Emotional	Relief from psychological pain: attempt to resolve personal problems, relief from bad mood, escape from anxiety, desire for emotional insight, liberation of feeling and emotional relaxation	Narcotics, alcohol, barbiturates, sedative-hypnotics	Competent individual counseling, well-run group therapy, instruction in psychology of personal development
Interpersonal	Desire to gain peer acceptance, break through interpersonal barriers, "communicate"; defiance of authority figures	Any, especially alcohol, marijuana	Expertly managed sensitivity and encounter groups, well-run group therapy, instruction in social customs, confidence training, emphasis on assisting others, e.g.: YMCA or YWCA volunteers.
Social	Desire to promote social change, find identifiable subculture, tune out intolerable environmental conditions, e.g. poverty	Marijuana, psychedelics	Social service community action in positive social change; helping the poor, aged, infirm, or young; tutoring handicapped; ecology action; YMCA or YWCA Big Brother/Sister programs
Political	Desire to promote political change (out of desperation with the social-political order) and to identify with antiestablishment subgroup	Marijuana, psychedelics	Political service, lobbying for nonpartisan projects, e.g.: Common Cause; field work with politicians and public officials
Intellectual	Desire to escape boredom, out of intellectual curiosity, to solve cognitive problems, gain new understanding in the world of ideas, research one's own awareness	Stimulants, sometimes psychedelics	Intellectual excitement through reading, debate, and discussion; creative games and puzzles; self-hypnosis; training in concentration
Creative-aesthetic	Desire to improve creative performance, enhance enjoyment of art already produced, e.g.:, music; enjoy imaginative mental productions	Marijuana, stimulants, psychedelics	Nongraded instruction in producing and/or appreciating art, music, drama, and creative hobbies
Philosophical	Desire to discover meaningful values, find meaning in life, help establish personal identity, organize a belief structure	Psychedelics, marijuana, stimulants	Discussions, seminars, courses on ethics, the nature of reality, relevant philosophical literature; explorations of value systems
Spiritual-mystical	Desire to transcend orthodox religion, develop spiritual insights, reach higher levels of consciousness, augment yogic practices, take a spiritual shortcut	Psychedelics, marijuana	Exposure to nonchemical methods of spiritual development; study of world religions, mysticism, meditation, yogic techniques

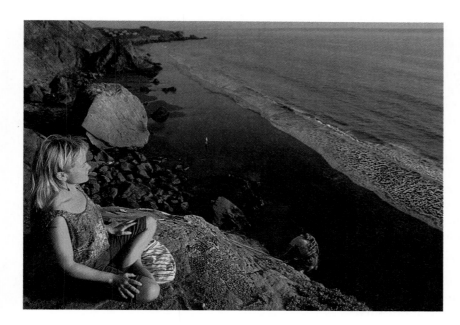

Yoga is one meditation technique that offers a drug-free means of stress-reduction and relaxation.

Sanskrit word for *union,* or *yoking,* meaning "the process of discipline by which a person attains union with the Absolute." In a sense, it refers to the use of the mind to control itself and the body.

Meditation involves brain wave activity centered on ponderous, contemplative, and reflective thought. An individual who meditates is able to decrease oxygen consumption within a matter of minutes as much as 20%, a level usually reached only after four to five hours of sleep in the nonmeditator. However, meditation is physiologically different from sleep, based on the EEG pattern and rate of decline of oxygen consumption. Along with the decreased metabolic rate and changes in EEG, there is also a marked decrease in blood lactate. Lactate is produced by metabolism of skeletal muscle, and the decrease is probably due to the reduced activity of the sympathetic nervous system during meditation. Heart rate and respiration are also slowed.

The Natural Mind Approach Some people who take drugs eventually look for other methods of maintaining the valuable parts of the drug experience. These people may learn to value the meditation "high" and abandon drugs. Long-term drug users sometimes credit their drug experiences with having given them a taste of their potential, even though continued use has diminished the novelty of drug use. Once these individuals become established in careers, they claim to have grown out of chemically induced altered states of consciousness. As Andrew Weil (1972) put it, "One does not see any long-time meditators give up meditation to become acid heads."

Although chemical "highs" are effective means of altering the state of consciousness, they interfere with the most worthwhile states of altered consciousness because they reinforce the illusion that highs come from external, material agents rather than from within your own nervous system.

Some people have difficulty using meditation as an alternative to drugs because, in order to be effective, meditation takes practice and concentration; the effects of drugs are immediate. Nevertheless, it is within everyone's potential to meditate.

◢ Assessing the Success of Prevention Efforts

Measuring the extent of drug use and abuse is important in planning prevention programs to ascertain the distribution of drug abuse behaviors among demographic and social categories. It is also important to target prevention efforts toward groups most at risk, so that we can design programs that respond to their particular needs. We then need to measure the results of these efforts by measuring use patterns before and after the population has taken part in the prevention program. This assessment is known as "pre- and post-testing." While assessment and measurement are valuable enterprises, they have certain limitations (Moscowitz 1989):

1. *Distortion of data due to sampling error.* Survey techniques may omit the following individuals: those unmotivated to respond to our surveys, those who wish to conceal severe abuse, or those who are unavailable (such as those absent due to drug use or dropouts).

2. *Distortion of data due to denial of drug use.*

3. *Difficulty in deciding whether to attribute observed changes to our own efforts or to broad cultural changes.* For example, if our surveys indicate that marijuana use has fallen by 5% at Central High School, does that reflect the effect of our prevention program? Or is it merely due to boredom with marijuana by those who adopted its use two years ago, when we started the prevention program, in response to an overall rise in marijuana use? Or has the "pothead" cohort either dropped out or graduated, leaving behind a new generation of non–drug-oriented students?

4. *Numbers merely measure behavior that is rooted in beliefs, ideas, and attitudes of social and cultural groups.* In Chapter 14 on marijuana, for example, we emphasized the role of student social and cultural groups, and the ritualistic use of marijuana by one type of group. It is important to see drug use from the perspective of users; its importance and meaning to them cannot be garnered from number-crunching alone.

One of the largest studies done in prevention research, although paradoxically one of the least well known, is the Core Instrument. More than 1 million students have taken this survey, which was developed by the U.S. Department of Education-funded Core Institute at the Student Health Program at Southern Illinois University, Carbondale, Illinois. Out of this work have come two monographs that provide a comprehensive profile of alcohol and other drug use at colleges and universities, as well as its consequences in terms of health, criminal justice involvement, and drunk or drugged driving (Presley et al. 1992, 1995).

Sometimes hard measurements bring unwelcome news. As noted earlier, one of the most widespread prevention programs in the nation is Project D.A.R.E. (Drug Abuse Resistance Education), which operates in over 200 communities nationally. Recent evaluations of this program show that, on a short-term basis, D.A.R.E. improved students' views of themselves and increased their sense of personal responsibility. However, the program has not yielded a measurable, significant change in drug use (Drug Strategies 1996, 12). Moreover, Clayton et al. (1991) showed an inconsistency between students' self-reported attitudes about use and actual use behaviors.

Do these studies put prevention efforts in a bad light, or even the components of the strategy put forward by D.A.R.E.? Not necessarily. In fact, many readers have probably picked up on a variable that might throw what seems to be a good mix of prevention plans off track—the fact that D.A.R.E. is offered by police officers. While the officers are well intentioned and their efforts are commendable, they are hardly a mechanism for transmitting new norms that would find converts among students, except perhaps those already successfully socialized (Gopelrud 1991).

Both the NIDA and several individual researchers have evaluated the multitude of drug abuse prevention programs in the United States. The general conclusions of these studies are as follows:

▲ Very few programs have demonstrated clear success or have been adequate in evaluating themselves.

▲ The relationships among information about drugs, attitudes toward use, and actual uses of drugs are unclear in these programs.

Some factors that are key to developing successful programs include the following:

▲ *Coordinating prevention at different levels.* Successful programs involve families, schools, and communities. In most cases, these efforts are not coordinated.

▲ *Integrating ongoing activities of schools, families, and community organizations.* Superficial introduction of drug prevention strategies has limited effects. For instance, door-to-door distribution of literature to households, in-class presentations of the harmful effects of drugs, and posting banners and slogans warning of the consequences of drug abuse in communities are not successful methods. Instead, programs that are integrated into neighborhood clubs, organizations, and church activities are more likely to have a long-term impact on preventing drug use. A more comprehensive, community-wide effort appears to be the most effective. A clear example is the Great American Smokeout launched yearly against tobacco use.

▲ *Including personal autobiographical and social experience accounts of former drug abusers when distributing drug information.* Recipients of drug prevention information should be given real-life accounts of use, abuse, despair, and successful drug rehabilitation. Just getting drug information alone has little impact, either initially or over the long term.

◢ Drug Prevention Programs in Higher Education

Today's average college student spends more money on booze than on books . . . too many young people think that drinking to get drunk, drinking to get blasted, drinking until they pass out—is cool. They have been led to believe that it is an acceptable rite of passage, a necessary path for them to follow . . . [yet] alcohol consumption is one of the leading causes of death among young adults . . . college students get drunk more often than do their counterparts who do not attend college . . . alcohol is a factor in 21% of all college dropouts . . . college students will spend about $4.2 billion yearly for alcoholic beverages—which is more than is spent operating campus libraries, and on college scholarships and fellowships combined throughout the United States . . . among those currently in college, between 240,000 and 360,000

eventually will lose their lives due to drinking . . . the same number of students will probably die eventually from alcohol-related causes as the number of students that will get advanced degrees, masters, and doctorates combined. . . .

Surgeon General Antonia Novello, Press Conference Statement, March 1991

The college campus has long served as a training ground for chemical abuse. Fraternity drunkenness, for example, was decried as early as 1840 (Horowitz 1987, 61). The late Edward Bloustein, Chancellor of Rutgers University, being interviewed on television after an alcohol-poisoning episode at a fraternity pledge party, described fraternities as "organized conspiracies dedicated to the consumption of alcohol."

Chemical abuse on campus is linked to the vast majority of vandalism, fights, accidents, sexually transmitted disease, unplanned pregnancy, racial bias incidents, and date rape and at least one-third of academic attrition (OSAP 1991; Koss et al. 1987). Although campus prevention programs and research date back several decades, such efforts remained isolated and sporadic until the late 1970s.

During 1976–1986, the following developments took place:

▲ The founding of BACCHUS (Boost Alcohol Consciousness Concerning the Health of University Students), a national student organization with over 400 affiliate groups.

▲ The founding of the Interassociation Task Force on Alcohol and Other Drug Issues by 10 professional associations, which sponsored National Collegiate Alcohol Awareness Week and National Collegiate Drug Awareness Week, now combined into a National Collegiate Health and Wellness Week and celebrated in March.

The year 1987 was a watershed time, during which a huge explosion of campus drug prevention programs began. It was spawned by a $14 billion annual budget line for college drug prevention placed in the Drug-Free Schools and Communities Act of 1986 (now titled the Safe and Free Schools and Communities Act). The funding was parceled out by the Department of Education,

Fund for the Improvement of Post-Secondary Education (FIPSE). FIPSE Drug Prevention Programs awarded about 100 grants per year from 1987 until 1996 via a grant competition for colleges to mount "institution-wide" programs. The guiding philosophy included the following points:

▲ A small, isolated program was seen as making little difference, but a comprehensive and institution-wide program reaching into several areas of the institution could send many consistent antiuse messages that would eventually reach "critical mass" and change the campus environment.

▲ There should be well-known, top-down administrative support for prevention programming.

▲ There should be well-written and carefully implemented policies about chemical use on campus.

The hundreds of new programs, whose administrators met together and interacted in annual grantee conferences, generated the sense of a national prevention movement in higher education. The Network of Colleges and Universities Dedicated to Prevention of Alcohol and Other Drug Abuse was founded, incorporating 900 institutions. The Network is supported by a new Higher Education Center for Alcohol and Other Drug prevention funded by the U.S. Department of Education, which provides a range of materials and newsletters (Ryan et al. 1995).

In 1989, FIPSE initiated a grant program for regional campus prevention consortia. By joining a consortium, colleges and universities could pool scarce resources, create support networks, and train new workers. In 1994, over 100 regional consortia were listed on a database maintained on the Higher Education Center Web site. In 1997, more than one half of all 3300 institutions of higher education were affiliates of the Network, belonged to a regional consortium, or had started other programs under the aegis of FIPSE.

Out of this decade-long experience, several exemplary approaches emerged. These strategies might be the predominant focus of a program, or one of a number of complementary components of a comprehensive effort:

Peer-based efforts. Student peers can be utilized in a number of ways—as educators, mentors,

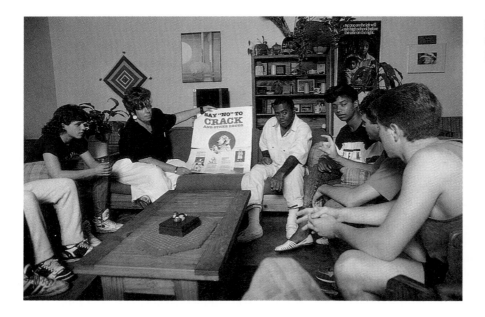

Education and group counseling can effectively prevent drug abuse.

counselors, or facilitators of prevention and outreach work. Such an approach multiplies manpower tremendously, reaches the rank-and-file student, is not perceived as an outside or authoritarian intrusion, speaks the language of students, and works to change the predominant cultural tone on campus. Peers can conduct classroom presentations, man informational tables or drop-in centers, edit and publish prevention newsletters, and establish links to community groups. It is important to carefully train and supervise peer facilitators. Many peer programs are residence hall-based, taking advantage of the training of residence hall assistants and peer facilitators (BACCHUS-GAMMA 1994).

Curriculum infusion. Infusion of a skill or topic across the curriculum has been used in conjunction with classes on writing skills, gender issues, and other areas. This effort can be undertaken at individual institutions or as a consortium project. The advantage of curriculum infusion is that it involves faculty members, achieves open discussion of drug issues in the classroom as part of the normal educational process, and stimulates critical thinking about drug issues.

Improvisational theater groups. Improvisational theater groups that tackle health and wellness issues have been lively, stimulating, and provocative, often breaking through peer and institutional denial, and bringing issues home to students with a dramatic emotional impact. Improvisational topics have included date rape, sexually transmitted disease, children of alcoholics on campus, and denial of chemical dependency.

Strategies to change misperceptions of use. Social psychologists Alan Berkowitz and Wesley Perkins, of Hobart and William Smith Colleges, have done influential research illustrating that students often have incorrect estimates (exaggerated misperceptions) of drug use by their peers (Perkins 1991; Perkins and Berkowitz 1986). Thus, they misperceive the peer norms governing drug use, which may lead them to "follow imaginary peers." This idea is a modification of the traditional understanding that "peers influence peers." It follows logically that activities demonstrating the accurate use pattern to students and correcting misperceptions will indirectly affect overall use patterns. These efforts have included simply publicizing the results of alcohol and drug use surveys, or awarding prizes for coming up with correct estimates.

Alternative events. Alternative events, such as "mocktail" parties, alcohol-free discos, and indoor rockclimbing, especially as alternatives to pre-sporting events and holiday parties, help avoid some events that are traditionally associated with chemical abuse.

Programs that change marketing of alcohol on and near campuses. Institutions of higher education are a major focus of alcohol marketing. Many campus events are sponsored by alcoholic beverage producers, and these companies also buy considerable newspaper advertising. *U—The National College Newspaper,* for example, had a three-year advertising contract with Anheuser-Busch (Magnum and Taylor 1990). This publicity helps send many pro-use messages. Prevention programs have recruited business and advertising majors to work on curtailing such marketing projects.

Finally, it is better to imbed prevention messages within an overall wellness perspective. Students are concerned about health and wellness issues, not programs that appear preachy, moralizing, nagging—perhaps reminding them of life at home!

 REVIEW QUESTIONS

1. What stages would you go through to design a prevention program at a high school where many students don't use drugs?

2. What is the point of teaching assertiveness skills to high school students?

3. Should we teach "responsible use of drugs" to adolescents? Justify your opinion.

EXERCISES FOR THE WEB

Exercise 1: D.A.R.E.

Drug Abuse Resistance Education (D.A.R.E.) is a validated, copyrighted, comprehensive drug and violence prevention education program implemented in kindergarten through 12th grade. D.A.R.E. represents a collaborative effort between school and law enforcement personnel. The D.A.R.E. curriculum is designed to equip elementary, middle, and high school students with the appropriate skills to resist substance abuse, violence, and gangs. More than 22,000 community-oriented law enforcement officers from 7,000 communities throughout the country have taught the core curriculum to more than 25 million elementary school students.

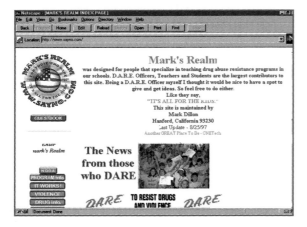

Exercise 2: Youth in Charge

A position paper presented by the Wisconsin Clearinghouse for Prevention Resources, "Putting Youth in Charge" discusses the importance of dealing with youth in prevention programs.

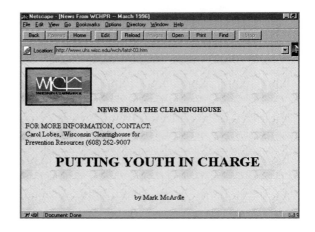

---

4. Is D.A.R.E. effective? Is it a good idea to have police conduct prevention work? Why or why not?

5. How can students help in preventing drug abuse at their schools?

6. Does what students think about what their peers do affect what they do?

7. List some potential topics to include in a drug education program for a junior high school, in addition to those listed in the text.

8. Do you think that teaching meditation techniques has any place in a prevention program? What is the basis for your answer?

9. What are three exemplary programs for higher education drug prevention?

10. What factors make it difficult to measure the success of prevention efforts?

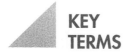

KEY TERMS

primary prevention
secondary prevention
tertiary prevention
alternatives approach
meditation

SUMMARY

1 Concerned parents and teachers face a bewildering array of prevention theories, practices, fads, and activities when designing a prevention program. Prevention specialists at state drug agencies or local councils on alcoholism and drug dependence should be enlisted to cut through this maze.

2 Primary prevention activities are risk-reduction strategies for people who are not yet using drugs.

3 Secondary prevention includes interventions and techniques designed for the early abuser.

4 Tertiary prevention is intervention with advanced abusers and chemically dependent treatment. It is synonymous with treatment.

5 Prevention can occur at the intrapersonal or individual level, the small group level, or the broader systems level.

6 Some well-known approaches to prevention include drug education, alternatives to use such as drug-free events and meditation, personal and social skills development such as assertiveness training, and strengthening of community and family systems.

7 It is difficult to measure the effects of prevention efforts after separating out the validity of the approach, the method and staff used in presentation, and broad cultural drug use patterns.

8 Drug prevention programs in higher education were rare before 1987, but now exist at more than half of the nation's colleges and universities. Comprehensive, institution-wide programs are needed to change campus norms. Particularly effective are peer-based programs, curriculum infu-

sion, improvisational theater, strategies to change misperception of peer norms, and regional consortia of prevention programs.

REFERENCES

Alberti, R. E., and M. L. Emmons. *Your Perfect Right.* Impact Publishers, 1988.

BACCHUS and GAMMA. *Community College Guide to Peer Education.* Denver, CO: The BACCHUS and GAMMA Peer Education Network, 1994.

Botvin, G. J., and T. A. Wills. "Personal and Social Skills Training: Cognitive-Behavioral Approaches to Substance Abuse Prevention." In *Prevention Research: Deterring Drug Abuse Among Children and Adolescents.* NIDA Research Monograph 64. Rockville, MD: NIDA (U.S. HHS, PHS, ADAMHA), 1985.

Clayton, R. R., R. Cattarello, L. E. Cay, and K. P. Walden. "Persuasive Communication and Drug Prevention: An Evaluation of the DARE Program." In *Persuasive Communication and Drug Abuse Prevention,* edited by L. Donohew, H. Sypepher, and W. Bukowski. Hillsdale, NJ: Erlbaum, 1991.

Carroll, E. "Notes on the Epidemiology of Inhalants." In *Review of Inhalants,* edited by C. W. Sharp and M. L. Brehm. NIDA Research Monograph no. 15. Washington, DC: National Institute on Drug Abuse, 1977.

Cohen, A. Y. "The Journey Beyond Trips: Alternatives to Drugs," *Journal of Psychedelic Drugs* 3, no. 2 (Spring 1971): 7–14.

Forman, S. G., and J. A. Linney. "School-Based Prevention of Adolescent Substance Abuse: Programs, Implementation and Future Direction." *School Psychology Review* 17, no. 4 (1988): 550–58.

Gopelrud E. N. ed. *Preventing Adolescent Drug Use: From Theory to Practice.* OSAP Monograph #8, DHHS Publication no. (ADM) 91-1725. Rockville, MD: Office of Substance Abuse Prevention, 1991.

Holstein, M. E., W. E. Cohen, and P. Steinbroner. *A Matter of Balance: Personal Strategies for Alcohol and Other Drugs.* Ashland, OR: CNS Productions, 1995.

Horowitz, H. L. *Campus Life.* New York: Knopf, 1987.

Koss, M. P., C. A. Gidycz, and R. Wisniewski. "The Scope of Rape: Incidence and Prevalence of Sexual Aggression and Victimization in a National Sample of Higher Education Students." *Journal of Consulting and Clinical Psychology* 34 (1987): 186–96.

Magnum, A., and P. Taylor. "Peddling Booze on Campus: How to Spot It, How to Fight It." *Eta Sigma Gamman* 22 (1990): 1.

McIntyre, K., D. White, and R. Yoast. *Resilience among High-Risk Youth.* Madison, WI: University of Wisconsin, 1990.

Moscowitz, J. "The Primary Prevention of Alcohol Problems: A Critical Review of the Research Literature." *Journal of Studies on Alcohol* 50 (1989): 54–88.

Norman, E. "Personal Factors Related to Substance Misuse: Risk Abatement and/or Resiliency Enhancement." In *Substance Abuse in Adolescence,* edited by T. P. Gulotta, G. R. Adamds, and R. Montemayor. Thousand Oaks, CA: Sage Publications, 1994.

Office for Substance Abuse Prevention (OSAP). *Alcohol Practices, Policies, and Potentials of American Colleges and Universities.* OSAP, ADAMHA, U.S. HHS, 1991.

Perkins, H. W. "Confronting Misperceptions of Peer Use Norms Among College Students: An Alternative Approach for Alcohol and Other Drug Education Programs." In *The Higher Education Leaders/Peers Network Peer Prevention Program Resource Manual.* Texas Christian University, U.S. Department of Education (FIPSE), Washington, DC 1991, 18–32.

Perkins H. W., and A. D. Berkowitz. "Perceiving the Community Norms of Alcohol Use Among Students: Some Research Implications for Campus Alcohol Education Programming." *International Journal of the Addictions* 21, nos. 9 and 10 (1986): 861–976.

Presley, C. A., P. W. Meilman, and R. Lyerla. *Alcohol and Drugs on American College Campuses: A Report to College Presidents.* Carbondale, IL: The Core Institute, Southern Illinois University at Carbondale, 1992.

Presley, C. A., P. W. Meilman, and R. Lyerla. *Alcohol and Drugs on American College Campuses,* II. Carbondale, IL: The Core Institute, Southern Illinois University at Carbondale, 1995.

Ryan, B. E., T. Colthurst, and L. Segars. *College Alcohol Risk Assessment Guide.* San Diego: UCSD Extension, University of California at San Diego, 1995.

Shiffman, S., and T. A. Wills, eds. *Coping and Substance Abuse.* New York: Academic Press, 1987.

Weil, A. *The Natural Mind.* Boston, MA: Houghton Mifflin, 1972.

Wilson, M., and S. Wilson, eds. *Drugs in American Life,* Vol. 1. New York: Wilson, 1975.

Appendices

Appendix A
Federal Agencies with Drug Abuse Missions

Drug Enforcement Administration (DEA)

Because of the unique problems of drug abuse in 1930, Congress authorized the establishment of the Bureau of Narcotics in the Treasury Department to administer the relevant laws. This agency remained in the Treasury Department until 1968, when it became part of a new group in the Justice Department, the Bureau of Narcotics and Dangerous Drugs. Harry Anslinger served as head of the bureau for over 30 years, from its creation until his retirement 1962. Anslinger was an agent during Prohibition, and later, as head of the bureau, he played an important role in getting marijuana outlawed by the federal government. In 1973, the Bureau of Narcotics and Dangerous Drugs became the Drug Enforcement Administration (DEA). Today, the DEA has the responsibility of infiltrating and breaking up illegal drug traffic in the United States, as well as controlling the use of Scheduled substances.

Special Action Office for Drug Abuse Prevention (SAODAP)

In 1971, President Richard Nixon set up a temporary agency, SAODAP, to initiate short-term and long-term planning of programs and to coordinate antidrug abuse programs with the states so that proper funding procedures and policies were followed. This office was located in the White House and was intended to advise the president. One major reason for establishing this organization was the initial report of a high heroin addiction rate in returning Vietnam veterans. The program was supposed to fight the increase in addiction in the United States. SAODAP was abolished, as planned, with most of its education, research, treatment, and rehabilitation functions going to a new agency, the National Institute on Drug Abuse (NIDA). An expert on the staff of advisors to the president, the domestic policy staff, assumed the duties of advising the president on drug-related matters and drug abuse programs. The advisor was to keep track of budgets for drug programs and coordinate policy with law enforcement groups. Under the administration of Ronald Reagan, further changes were proposed. A pattern of federal policy was established; that is, control and management of drug programs in the United States change with each new "crisis."

Alcohol, Drug Abuse, and Mental Health Administration (ADAMHA)

In 1973, a new agency was formed after the Department of Health, Education, and Welfare Secretary Casper Weinberger stripped the alcohol and drug abuse sections from the National Institute of Mental Health (NIMH). This action formed the National Institute of Alcohol Abuse and Alcoholism (NIAAA) and the NIDA (see previous section). NIAAA, NIDA, and NIMH were under the agency ADAMHA (Alcohol, Drug Abuse and Mental Health Administration). This shuffling and redesign was part of federal attempts to bring the post-Vietnam War heroin crisis under control and to address the perennial problems of alcoholism and dependence on other drugs. The mission of NIAAA and NIDA was and still is to coordinate both clinical and basic research involved directed at drugs of abuse. Today, these institutes support 80% to 90% of all drug dependence research conducted in the United States. During fiscal year 1996, these institutes controlled budgets of $490 (NIDA) and $212 (NIAAA) million.

In October 1992, ADAMHA was reorganized, and both NIDA and NIAAA officially became Institutes of the National Institutes of Health (NIH) as mandated by the ADAMHA Reorganization Act of 1992 (Greenhouse 1992).

The Substance Abuse and Mental Health Services Administration (SAMHSA)

With passage of the ADAMHA Reorganization Act of 1992, the services programs of NIDA, NIAAA, and NIMH were incorporated into the newly created SAMHSA. This agency was given the lead responsibility for prevention and treatment of addictive and mental health problems and disorders. Its overall mission is to reduce the incidence and prevalence of substance abuse and mental disorders by ensuring the best therapeutic use of scientific knowledge and improving access to high-quality, effective programs (*SAMHSA Bulletin* 1992).

State Regulations

There have always been questions regarding the relative responsibilities of state versus federal laws and their respective regulatory agencies. In general, the U.S. form of government has allowed local control to take precedence over national control. Because of this historic attitude, states were the first to pass laws to regulate the abuse or misuse of drugs. Federal laws developed later, after the federal government gained greater jurisdiction over the well-being and lives of the citizens and it became apparent that, due to interstate trafficking, national drug abuse problems could not be effectively dealt with on a state-by-state basis. Some early state laws banned the use of smoking opium, regulated the scale of various psychoactive drug substances, and in a few instances, set up treatment programs. However, these early legislative actions made no effort to *prevent* drug abuse. Drug abuse was controlled to a great extent by social pressure rather than by law. It was considered morally wrong to be an alcoholic or an addict to opium or some other drug.

The drug laws varied considerably from state to state in 1932, so the National Conference of Commissioners on Uniform State Laws set up the Uniform Narcotic Drug Act (UNDA), which was later adopted by nearly all states. The UNDA provided for the control of possession, use, and distribution of opiates and cocaine. In 1942, marijuana was included under this act because it was classified as a narcotic.

In 1967, the Food and Drug Administration proposed the Model Drug Abuse Control Act and urged the states to adopt it on a uniform basis. This law extended controls over depressant, stimulant, and hallucinogenic drugs, similar to the 1965 federal law. Many states set up laws based on this model.

The federal Controlled Substances Act of 1970 stimulated the National Conference of Commissioners to propose a new Uniform Controlled Substances Act (UCSA). The UCSA permits enactment of a single state law regulating the illicit possession, use, manufacture, and dispensing of controlled psychoactive substances. At this time, most states have enacted the UCSA or modifications of it.

Today, state law enforcement of drug statutes does not always reflect federal regulations, although for the most part, the two statutory levels are harmonious. For example, marijuana has tentatively been approved for medicinal use in California and Arizona but is considered a Schedule I substance by federal regulatory agencies (as of this writing).

Appendix B
Regulating the Development of New Drugs

The amended Federal Food, Drug, and Cosmetic Act in force today requires that all new drugs be registered with and approved by the Food and Drug Administration (FDA). The FDA is mandated by congress to (1) ensure the rights and safety of human subjects during clinical testing of experimental drugs; (2) evaluate the safety and efficacy of new treatments based on test results and information from the sponsors (often health-related companies); and (3) compare potential benefits and risks to determine if a new drug should be approved and marketed. Because of FDA regulations, all pharmaceutical companies must follow a series of steps when seeking permission to market a new drug. (See Figure B.1)

Regulatory Steps for New Prescription Drugs

Step 1: Preclinical Research and Development
A chemical must be synthesized and identified as having potential value in the treatment of a particular condition or disease. The company interested in marketing the chemical as a drug must run a series of tests on at least three animal species. Careful records must be kept of side effects, absorption, distribution, metabolism, excretion, and the dosages of the drug necessary to produce the various effects. Carcinogenic, mutagenic, and teratogenic variables are tested. The dose-response curve must be determined along with potency, and then

Figure B.1

Steps Required by the FDA for Reviewing a New Drug

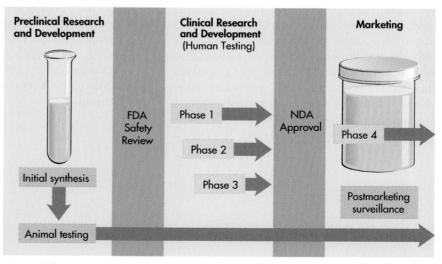

the risk and benefit of the substance must be calculated (see Chapters 5 and 6). If the company still believes there is a market for the substance, it will forward the data to the FDA to obtain an investigational new drug (IND) number for further tests.

Step 2: Clinical Research and Development

Animal tests provide some information, but ultimately tests must be done on the species for which the potential drug is intended—that is, humans. These tests usually follow three phases. Phase 1 is called the *initial clinical stage.* Small numbers of volunteers (usually 20 to 100), both healthy people and patients, are recruited to establish drug safety and dose range for effective treatment and to examine side effects. Formerly, much of this research was done on prison inmates, but because of bad publicity and the possibility of coercion, fewer prisoners are used today. Medical students, paid college student volunteers, and volunteers being treated at free clinics are more often used after obtaining "informed consent." The data are collected, analyzed, and sent to the FDA for approval before beginning the next phase of human subject testing.

Phase 2 testing is called the *clinical pharmacological evaluation stage.* The effects of the drug are tested to eliminate investigator bias and to determine side effects and the effectiveness of the treatment. Because the safety of the new drug has not been thoroughly established, a few patients (100–300 volunteers) with the medical problem the drug is intended to treat are used for these studies. Statistical evaluation of this information is carried out before proceeding with phase 3 testing.

Phase 3 is the *extended clinical evaluation.* By this time, the pharmaceutical company has a good idea of both drug effectiveness and dangers. The drug can be offered safely to a wider group of participating clinics and physicians, who cooperate in administration of the potential drug—when medically appropriate—to thousands of volunteer patients who have given informed consent.

This stage makes the drug available on a wide experimental basis. Sometimes, by this point, there has been publicity about the new drug, and people with the particular disease for which the drug was developed may actively seek out physicians licensed to experiment with it.

During Phase 3 testing, safety checks are made and any side effects are noted that might show up as more people are exposed to the drug. After the testing program is over, careful analysis is made of the effectiveness, side effects, and recommended dosage. If there are sufficient data to demonstrate that the drug is safe and effective, the company will submit a new drug application (NDA) as a formal request that the FDA consider approving the drug for marketing. The application usually comprises many thousands of pages of data and analysis, and the FDA must sift through it and decide whether the risks of using the drug justify its potential benefits. The FDA usually calls for additional tests before the drug is determined safe and effective and granting permission to market it.

Step 3: Permission to Market At this point, the FDA can allow the drug to be marketed under its patented name. It may cost $200 million to $500 million and take up to 12 years to develop a new drug in the United States. The situation is similar elsewhere, although in some European countries, the clinical evaluations are less stringent and require less time. Once the drug is marketed, it continues to be closely scrutinized for adverse effects. This postmarketing surveillance is often referred to as Phase 4 and is important, because in some cases negative effects may not show up for a long time. For example, it was determined in 1970 that diethylstilbestrol (DES), when given to pregnant women to prevent miscarriage, causes an increased risk of a rare type of vaginal cancer in their daughters when these children entered their teens and young adult years. The FDA subsequently removed from the market the form of DES that had been used to treat pregnant women. As described earlier, the thalidomide tragedy resulted in passage of the law that gave the FDA this authority.

Exceptions: Special Drug-Marketing Laws

There is continual concern that the process used by the FDA to evaluate prospective drugs is laborious and excessively lengthy. Recently, an amendment was passed to accelerate the evaluation of urgently needed drugs. The so-called fast-track rule has been applied to testing of certain drugs used for the treatment of rare cancers, AZT (zidovudine) for the treatment of AIDS (the review process only required two years), and other similar drugs. As a result, they have reached the market after a much reduced testing program.

A second amendment, the Orphan Drug Law, allows drug companies to receive tax advantages if they develop drugs that are not very profitable because they are only useful in treating small numbers of patients, such as those who suffer from rare diseases. A rare disease is defined as one that affects less than 200,000 people in the United States or one for which the cost of developing a drug is not likely to be recovered by marketing it.

The federal government and the FDA are continually refining the system for evaluating new drugs in order to assure that new effective therapeutic substances can be made available for clinical use as soon as it is safely possible. Some of these modifications reflect the fact that patients with life-threatening diseases, such as AIDS, are willing to accept greater drug risks in order gain faster access to potentially useful medications. Attempts to accelerate the drug review are illustrated by the *Prescription Drug User Fee Act* of 1992. Under this law, fees are paid by the FDA-regulated pharmaceutical companies to support additional FDA reviewers so as to decrease the average review time for drugs that will treat life-threatening and serious diseases from an average of two years to approximately one year.

The Regulation of Nonprescription Drugs

The Durham-Humphrey Amendment to the Food, Drug, and Cosmetic Act made a distinction between prescription and nonprescription (OTC) drugs and required the FDA to regulate OTC marketing. In 1972, the FDA initiated a program to evaluate the effectiveness and safety of the nonprescription drugs on the market and to ensure that they included appropriate labeling (for more details, see Chapter 15). Each so-called active ingredient in the OTC medications was reviewed by a panel of drug experts, including physicians, pharmacologists, and pharmacists. Based on the recommendations of these panels, the ingredients were placed in one of the following three categories:

I. Generally recognized as safe and effective for the claimed therapeutic indication

II. Not generally recognized as safe and effective or unacceptable indications

III. Insufficient data available to permit final classification

By 1981, the panels had made initial determinations on over 700 ingredients in more than 300,000 OTC drug products and submitted more than 60 reports to the FDA.

In the second phase of the OTC drug review, the FDA evaluated the panels' findings and submitted a tentative adoption of the panels' recommendations (after revision, if necessary), following public comment and scrutiny. After a period of time and careful consideration of new information, the agency issued a final ruling and classification of the ingredients under consideration.

The Effects of the OTC Review on Today's Medications   The review process for OTC ingredients has had a significant impact on the public's attitude about OTC products and their use (both good and bad) in self-medication. It was apparent from the review process that many OTC drug ingredients did not satisfy the requirements for safety and effectiveness. In fact, in 1990 alone, the FDA banned 223 uses of nonprescription drug ingredients, ruling that the ingredients were ineffective against problems ranging from acne to swimmer's ear. Consequently, it is almost certain that, in the future, there will be fewer active ingredients in OTC medicines, but these drugs will be safer and more effective than ever before.

In addition, with heightened public awareness, greater demand has been brought to bear on the FDA to make better drugs available to the public for self-medication. In response to these pressures, the FDA has adopted a switching policy, which allows it to review prescription drugs and evaluate their suitability as OTC products. The following criteria must be satisfied if a drug is to be switched:

1. The drug must have been marketed by prescription for at least three years.

2. Use of the drug must have been relatively high during the time it was available as a prescription drug.

3. Adverse drug reactions must not be alarming, and the frequency of side effects must not have increased during the time the drug was available to the public.

In general, this switching policy has been well received by the public. In fact, 65% of the switched ingredients have ranked first or second in their drug categories within the first five years of being switched. The medical community and the FDA are generally positive about OTC switches as well. There are some concerns, however, that more effective drug products will lead to increased abuse or misuse of OTC products.

William E. Gilbertson, director of the FDA's division of OTC drug evaluation, feels that the agency needs to proceed cautiously with switches and place greater emphasis on adequate labeling and education to assure that consumers have sufficient information to use OTC products safely and effectively. "Most assuredly, making more drugs available will put an added burden on consumers in terms of benefit/risk decisions. In that regard, the ways we disseminate OTC information will be important" (Siegelman 1990).

The Regulation of Drug Advertising

Much of the public's knowledge and impressions about drugs, especially those available OTC, come from advertisements. It is difficult to ascertain the amount of money currently spent by the pharmaceutical industry to promote its products. Because of the intense competition between OTC drugs, it is likely that up to 15% to 20% of the dollar sales for these products is spent on advertising to the general public and that the advertising budget equals a sum of approximately $10 billion annually. For prescription drugs, it is likely that the costs of advertising, promoting, and marketing exceed $10 billion annually.

There is no doubt that these promotional efforts by pharmaceutical manufacturers have a tremendous impact on the drug-purchasing habits of the general public and health professionals. Not surprisingly, drug use based on misleading or false advertising claims, rather than facts, can result in unsatisfactory drug therapy and can be extremely dangerous. Regulations governing the advertising of nonprescription drugs are set and enforced by the Federal Trade Commission. These rules are less stringent than those for prescription medicines.

Prescription Advertising   The economics of prescription drugs is unique because a second party, the health professional, dictates what the consumer, the patient, will purchase. Currently, many pharmaceutical companies advertise medications directly to the public. Direct consumer advertising of prescription drugs has experts concerned that patients will put pressure on physicians to prescribe inappropriately. For example, in 1992 more than $100 million was spent by pharmaceutical companies for public advertising (TV, newspapers, magazines, and so on) of nicotine patches for people trying to quit smoking. Some medical experts argue that, as a consequence, many consumers perceive the patches as a quick cure for their tobacco dependence and ignore the fact that they work only as part of a serious behavior modification program. Critics claim this lack of consumer understanding led to incorrect use of the patches and has resulted in fatal heart attacks.

The vast majority of prescription drug promotion is directed at the health professional and controlled by the FDA. The approaches employed by manufacturers to encourage health professionals to prescribe their products include advertising in prestigious medical journals, direct mail advertising, and some radio and television advertising. All printed and audio materials distributed by drug salespeople are controlled by advertising regulations from the FDA. Perhaps the most effective sales approach is having drug representatives personally visit health professionals; this tactic is harder to regulate.

Unfortunately, many health professionals rely on drug company salespeople for the so-called latest scientific information concerning drugs and their effects. Although these representatives of the drug industry can provide an important informational service, it is essential that health professionals remember that these people make a living by selling their products, and often their information is biased accordingly.

Many people in and out of the medical community have questioned the ethics of drug advertising and marketing in the United States and are concerned about the negative impact that deceptive promotion has on target populations. One of the biggest problems in dealing with misleading or false advertising is defining such deception. Probably the best guideline for such a definition is summarized in the Wheeler-Lea Amendment to the Federal Trade Commission Act:

> The term *false advertisement* means an advertisement, other than labeling, which is misleading in a material respect; and in determining whether any advertisement is misleading, there shall be taken into account not only representations … but the extent to which the advertisement fails to reveal facts.

Tough questions are being asked as to how much control should be exerted over the pharmaceutical industry to protect the public without excessively infringing on the rights of these companies to promote their goods. The solutions to these problems will not be simple; however, efforts to keep drug advertisements accurate, in good taste, and informative are worthwhile and will be necessary if the public is expected to make rational decisions about drug use.

Federal Regulation and Quality Assurance

No matter what policy is adopted by the FDA and other drug-regulating agencies, there will always be those who criticize their efforts and complain that they do not do enough or that they do too much. The FDA has been blamed for being excessively careful and requiring too much testing before new drugs are approved for marketing; on the other hand, when new drugs are released and cause serious side effects, the FDA is condemned for being sloppy in its control of drug marketing.

What is the proper balance, and what do we, as consumers, have the right to expect from government? These are questions each of us should ask, and we have a right to share our answers with government representatives.

On the other hand, regardless of our individual feelings, it is important to understand that the current (and likely future) federal regulations do not assure drug safety or effectiveness for everyone. Too many individual variables alter the way each of us responds to drugs, making such universal assurances impossible. Federal agencies can only deal with general policies and make general decisions. For example, what if the FDA determines that a given drug is reasonably safe in 95% of the population and effective in 70%? Are these acceptable figures, or should a drug be safe in 99% and effective in 90% before it is suitable for general marketing? What of the 5% or 1% of the population who will be adversely affected by this drug? What rights do they have to be protected?

There are no simple answers to these questions. Federal policies are compromises that assume that the clinician who prescribes the drug and/or the patient who buys and consumes it will be able to identify when use of that drug is inappropriate or threatening. Unfortunately, sometimes drug prescribing and drug consuming are done carelessly and unnecessary side effects occur or the drug does not work. The questions surface again: Are federal drug agencies doing all they can to protect the public? Should the laws be changed?

It is always difficult to predict the future, especially when it depends on fickle politicians and erratic public opinion. Nevertheless, with the dramatic increase in new and better drugs becoming available to the public, it is not likely that federal or state agencies will diminish their role in regulating drug use. Now more than ever, the public demands safer and more effective drugs. This public attitude will likely translate into even greater involvement by regulatory agencies in issues of drug development, assessment, and marketing.

Another reason for increased regulation in the future is that many of the larger pharmaceutical companies have become incredibly wealthy. Several of the most profitable companies have become subsidiaries of powerful corporations that are driven more by profit margins than philanthropic interests. In such an environment, governmental agencies are essential to assure that the rights of the public are protected. Only a fool would desire a return to the early days of federal policies based on "buyer beware" principles.

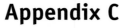

Appendix C
Some National Organizations in the Addictions

Federal Research Entities

National Institute on Drug Abuse

National Institute on Alcohol and Alcoholism

Federal Funding and Coordinating Entities

Center for Substance Abuse Treatment

Center for Substance Abuse Prevention (of the Substance Abuse, Mental Health Services Administration, HHS)

National Clearinghouse for Alcohol and Drug Information (NCADI, the source of all governmental literature and information on alcohol and drug subjects)

Private Advocacy, Informational, and Professional Organizations

National Council on Alcoholism and Drug Dependency (a national association of the local councils on alcoholism and drug dependency in thousands of counties, municipalities, providing referral, information, and prevention services)

National Assoication of Drug Abuse and Alcoholism Counselors (NAADAC)*

International Certification Reciprocity Consortium (ICRC)*(a consortium of state boards certifying addictions counselors)

International Coalition of Addiction Studies Educators

(addiction studies and counselor training programs in higher education)\

National Association of State Alcohol and Drug Abuse Directors

Therapeutic Communities

* NAADAC and ICRC certify alcohol, drug, and addictions counselors.

Appendix D
Drugs of Use and Abuse

The table that follows on pages provides detailed information about the drugs listed. Note that the heading *CSA Schedules* refers to categorization under the Controlled Substances Act (CSA). The roman numeral(s) to the right of each drug name specifies each as a Schedule I, II, III, IV, or V drug. See Chapter 3, for more information on scheduling.

Drugs	CSA Schedules	Medical Uses	Trade or Other Names	Slang Names
Narcotics				
Opium	II III V	Analgesic, antidiarrheal	Dover's Powder, Paregoric, Parepectolin	Opium
Morphine	II III	Analgesic, antitussive	Morphine, MS-Contin, Roxanol, Roxanol-SR	M, Morpho, Morph, Tab, White, Stuff, Miss, Emma, Monkey
Codeine	II III V	Analgesic, antitussive	Tylenol w/Codeine, Empirin w/Codeine, Robitussin A-C, Fiorinal w/Codeine	School Boy
Heroin	I	None	Diacetylmorphine	Horse, Smack, H, Stuff, Junk
Hydromorphone	II	Analgesic	Dilaudid	Little D, Lords
Meperidine (Pethidine)	II	Analgesic	Demerol, Mepergan	Isonipecaine, Dolantol
Methadone	II	Analgesic	Dolophine, Methadone, Methadose	Dollies, Dolls, Amidone
Other Narcotics	I II III IV V	Analgesic, antidiarrheal, antitussive	Numorphan, Percodan, Percocet, Tylox, Tussionex, Fentanyl, Darvon, Lomotil, Talwin*	T. and Blue's, Designer Drugs (Fentanyl Derivatives), China White
Depressants				
Chloral Hydrate	IV	Hypnotic	Noctec	—
Barbiturates	II III IV	Anesthetic, anti-convulsant, sedative, hypnotic, veterinary euthanasia agent	Amytal, Butisol, Fiorinal, Lotusate, Nembutal, Seconal, Tuinal, Phenobarbital	Yellows, Yellow Jackets, Barbs, Reds, Redbirds, Tooies, Phennies
Benzodiazepines	IV	Antianxiety, anticonvulsant, sedative, hypnotic	Ativan, Dalmane, Diazepam, Paxipam, Librium, Xanax, Serax, Valium, Tranxene, Verstran, Versed, Halcion, Restoril	Downers, Goof Balls, Sleeping Pills, Candy
Methaqualone	I	Sedative, hypnotic	Quaalude	Lude, Quay, Quad, Mandrex
Glutethimide	III	Sedative, hypnotic	Doriden	—
Other Depressants	III IV	Antianxiety, sedative, hypnotic	Equanil, Miltown, Noludar, Placidyl, Valmid	Tranquilizers, Muscle Relaxants, Sleeping Pills

* Not designated as a narcotic under C.S.A. (Controlled Substances Act).

Source: Adapted from Drug Enforcement Administration, U.S. Dept. of Justice, Drugs of Abuse. 1989 Edition. Washington, DC: Government Printing office, 1989: and "Let's All Work to Fight Drug Abuse." Dallas, TX: L.A.W. Publications, 1991.

Dependence Physical/ Psychological	Tolerance	Duration (hours)	Administration Methods	Possible Effects	Effects of Overdose	Withdrawal Syndrome
High/High	Yes	3–6	Oral, smoked	Euphoria, drowsiness, respiratory depression, constricted pupils, nausea	Slow and shallow breathing, clammy skin, convulsions, coma, possible death	Watery eyes, runny nose, yawning, loss of appetite, irritability, tremors, panic, cramps, nausea, chills and sweating
High/High	Yes	3–6	Oral, smoked, injected			
Mod./Mod.	Yes	3–6	Oral, injected			
High/High	Yes	3–6	Injected, sniffed smoked			
High/High	Yes	3–6	Oral, injected			
High/High	Yes	3–6	Oral, injected			
High/High–Low	Yes	12–24	Oral, injected			
High–Low/ High–Low	Yes	Variable	Oral, injected			
Mod./Mod.	Yes	5–8	Oral	Slurred speech, disorientation, drunken behavior without odor of alcohol	Shallow respiration, clammy skin, dilated pupils, weak and rapid pulse, coma, possible death	Anxiety, insomnia, tremors, delirium, convulsions, possible death
High–Mod./ High–Mod.	Yes	1–16	Oral			
Low/Low	Yes	4–8	Oral			
High/High	Yes	4–8	Oral			
High/Mod.	Yes	4–8	Oral			
Mod./Mod.	Yes	4–8	Oral			

Table continues on p. 502

Table continued from p. 501

Drugs	CSA Schedules	Medical Uses	Trade or Other Names	Slang Names
Stimulants				
Cocaine†	II	Local anesthetic		Bump, Toot, C, Coke, Flake, Snow, Candy, Crack
Amphetamines	II	Attention deficit disorders, narcolepsy, weight control	Biphetamine, Desoxyn, Dexedrine	Pep Pills, Bennies, Uppers, Truck Drivers, Dexies, Black Beauties, Speed
Phenmetrazine	II	Weight control	Preludin	Uppers, Peaches, Hearts
Methylphenidate	II	Attention deficit disorders, narcolepsy	Ritalin	Speed, Meth, Crystal, Crank, Go Fast
Other Stimulants	III IV	Weight control	Apidex, Cylert, Didrex, Ionamin, Melfiat, Plegine, Sanorex, Tenuate, Tepanil, Prelu-2	—
Hallucinogens				
LSD	I	None		Acid, Microdot, Cubes
Mescaline and Peyote	I	None		Mesc Buttons, Cactus
Amphetamine Variants	I	None	2, 5-DMA, PMA, STP, MDA, MDMA, TMA, DOM, DOB	Ecstasy, Designer Drugs
Phencyclidine	II	None	PCP	PCP, Angle Dust, Hog, Peace Pill
Phencyclidine Analogues	I	None	PCE, PCPY, TCP	—
Other Hallucinogens	I	None	Bufotenine, Ibogaine, DMT, Det, Psilocybin, Psilocyn	Sacred Mushrooms, Magic Mushrooms, Mushrooms
Cannabis				
Marijuana	I	None		Pot, Grass, Reefer, Roach, Maui Wowie, Joint, Weed, Loco Weed, Mary Jane
Tetrahydrocannabinol	I II	Cancer chemotherapy antinauseant	THC, Marinol	THC
Hashish	I	None		Hash
Hashish Oil	I	None		Hash Oil
Inhalants		None	Gasoline, Airplane Glue, Veg. Spray, Hairspray, Deodorants, Spray Paint, Liquid Paper, Paint Thinner, Rubber Cement	Sniffing, Glue Sniffing Snorting

† Designated as a narcotic under C.S.A.

Dependence Physical/ Psychological	Tolerance	Duration (hours)	Administration Methods	Possible Effects	Effects of Overdose	Withdrawal Syndrome
Possible/High	Yes	1–2	Sniffed, smoked, injected	Increased alertness, excitation, euphoria, increased pulse rate and blood pressure, insomnia, loss of appetite	Agitation, increase in body temperature, hallucinations, convulsions, possible death	Apathy, long periods of sleep, irritability, depression, disorientation
Possible/High	Yes	2–4	Oral, injected			
Possible/High	Yes	2–4	Oral, injected			
Possible/Mod.	Yes	2–4	Oral, injected			
Possible/High	Yes	2–4	Oral, injected			
None/Unknown	Yes	8–12	Oral	Illusions and hallucinations, poor perception of time and distance	Longer, more intense "trip" episodes, psychosis, possible death	Withdrawal syndrome not reported
None/Unknown	Yes	8–12	Oral			
Unknown/Unknown	Yes	Variable	Oral, injected			
Unknown/High	Yes	Days	Smoked, oral, injected			
Unknown/High	Yes	Days	Smoked, oral, injected,			
None/Unknown	Possible	Variable	Smoked, oral, injected, sniffed			
Unknown/Mod.	Yes	2–4	Smoked, oral	Euphoria, relaxed inhibitions, increased appetite, disoriented behavior	Fatigue, paranoia, possible psychosis	Insomnia, hyperactivity and decreased appetite occasionally reported
Unknown/Mod.	Yes	2–4	Smoked, oral			
Unknown/Mod.	Yes	2–4	Smoked, oral			
Unknown/Mod.	Yes	2–4	Smoked, oral			
None/Unknown	Yes	30 min.	Sniffed	Euphoria, headaches, nausea, fainting, stupor, rapid heartbeat	Damage to lungs, liver, kidneys, bone marrow, suffocation, choking, anemia, possible stroke, sudden death	Insomnia, increased appetite, depression, irritability, headache

Index